Encyclopedia of Epidemiology

Encyclopedia of
Epidemiology

2

Editor
Sarah Boslaugh
Washington University, St. Louis, School of Medicine
BJC HealthCare, St. Louis

Associate Editor
Louise-Anne McNutt
University at Albany, State University of New York

A SAGE Reference Publication

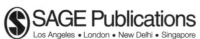

SAGE Publications
Los Angeles • London • New Delhi • Singapore

For information:

SAGE Publications, Inc.
2455 Teller Road
Thousand Oaks, California 91320
E-mail: order@sagepub.com

SAGE Publications Ltd.
1 Oliver's Yard
55 City Road
London EC1Y 1SP
United Kingdom

SAGE Publications India Pvt. Ltd.
B 1/I 1 Mohan Cooperative Industrial Area
Mathura Road, New Delhi 110 044
India

SAGE Publications Asia-Pacific Pte. Ltd.
33 Pekin Street #02–01
Far East Square
Singapore 048763

Printed in the United States of America

Library of Congress Cataloging-in-Publication Data

Encyclopedia of epidemiology/[edited by] Sarah Boslaugh.
    p. ; cm.
Includes bibliographical references and index.
ISBN 978-1-4129-2816-8 (cloth : alk. paper)
   1. Epidemiology—Encyclopedias. I. Boslaugh, Sarah.
[DNLM: 1. Epidemiology—Encyclopedias—English. WA 13 E556 2008]

RA652.E533 2008
614.403—dc22   2007031747

This book is printed on acid-free paper.

07 08 09 10 11 10 9 8 7 6 5 4 3 2 1

Publisher:	Rolf A. Janke
Acquisitions Editor:	Lisa Cuevas Shaw
Developmental Editor:	Diana E. Axelsen
Reference Systems Manager:	Leticia Gutierrez
Production Editor:	Melanie Birdsall
Copy Editor:	QuADS Prepress (P) Ltd.
Typesetter:	C&M Digitals (P) Ltd.
Proofreaders:	Cheryl Rivard and Dennis W. Webb
Indexer:	Kathy Paparchontis
Cover Designer:	Candice Harman
Marketing Manager:	Amberlyn Erzinger

Contents

List of Entries

Reader's Guide

The Reader's Guide provides an overview to all the entries in the *Encyclopedia* as well as a convenient way to locate related entries within an area of interest. Articles are arranged under headings, which represent broad categories of subjects. For instance, the heading Branches of Epidemiology lists the titles for the 20 main entries on fields of study and practice within epidemiology included in this *Encyclopedia*, from Applied Epidemiology to Veterinary Epidemiology. Similarly, under the heading Epidemiologic Data are listed the main entries on that topic, including types of data (e.g., Administrative Data), specific sources of data (e.g., the Behavioral Risk Factor Surveillance System), and issues related to data management (e.g., Biomedical Informatics). The guide is also useful for finding articles related to a particular topic. For instance, if you are interested in Genetic Epidemiology, you will find that topic under the heading Genetics, which also includes articles on topics such as Epigenetics, the Human Genome Project, and Linkage Analysis. Some topics appear under more than one heading (e.g., Genetic Epidemiology appears under both Branches of Epidemiology and Genetics), reflecting the interrelationships among the broad categories represented by the headings.

Behavioral and Social Science

Acculturation
Bioterrorism
Community-Based Participatory Research
Community Health
Community Trial
Cultural Sensitivity
Demography
Determinants of Health Model
Ecological Fallacy
Epidemiology in Developing Countries
EuroQoL EQ-5D Questionnaire
Functional Status
Genocide
Geographical and Social Influences on Health
Health, Definitions of
Health Behavior
Health Belief Model
Health Communication
Health Communication in Developing Countries
Health Disparities
Health Literacy

Life Course Approach
Locus of Control
Medical Anthropology
Network Analysis
Participatory Action Research
Poverty and Health
Quality of Life, Quantification of
Quality of Well-Being Scale (QWB)
Race and Ethnicity, Measurement Issues With
Race Bridging
Rural Health Issues
Self-Efficacy
SF-36® Health Survey
Social Capital and Health
Social-Cognitive Theory
Social Epidemiology
Social Hierarchy and Health
Social Marketing
Socioeconomic Classification
Spirituality and Health
Targeting and Tailoring
Theory of Planned Behavior
Transtheoretical Model

Urban Health Issues
Urban Sprawl

Branches of Epidemiology

Applied Epidemiology
Chronic Disease Epidemiology
Clinical Epidemiology
Descriptive and Analytic Epidemiology
Disability Epidemiology
Disaster Epidemiology
Eco-Epidemiology
Environmental and Occupational Epidemiology
Field Epidemiology
Genetic Epidemiology
Injury Epidemiology
Maternal and Child Health Epidemiology
Molecular Epidemiology
Neuroepidemiology
Nutritional Epidemiology
Pharmacoepidemiology
Psychiatric Epidemiology
Reproductive Epidemiology
Social Epidemiology
Veterinary Epidemiology

Diseases and Conditions

Alzheimer's Disease
Anxiety Disorders
Arthritis
Asthma
Autism
Avian Flu
Bipolar Disorder
Bloodborne Diseases
Cancer
Cardiovascular Disease
Diabetes
Foodborne Diseases
Gulf War Syndrome
Hepatitis
HIV/AIDS
Hypertension
Influenza
Insect-Borne Disease
Malaria

Measles
Oral Health
Osteoporosis
Parasitic Diseases
Plague
Polio
Post-Traumatic Stress Disorder
Schizophrenia
Severe Acute Respiratory Syndrome (SARS)
Sexually Transmitted Diseases
Sick Building Syndrome
Sleep Disorders
Smallpox
Suicide
Toxic Shock Syndrome
Tuberculosis
Vector-Borne Disease
Vehicle-Related Injuries
Vitamin Deficiency Diseases
Waterborne Diseases
Yellow Fever
Zoonotic Disease

Epidemiological Concepts

Attack Rate
Attributable Fractions
Biomarkers
Birth Cohort Analysis
Birth Defects
Case-Cohort Studies
Case Definition
Case-Fatality Rate
Case Reports and Case Series
Cohort Effects
Community Trial
Competencies in Applied Epidemiology for
    Public Health Agencies
Cumulative Incidence
Direct Standardization
Disease Eradication
Effectiveness
Effect Modification and Interaction
Efficacy
Emerging Infections
Epidemic
Etiology of Disease

Epidemiologic Data

Ethics

Genetics

History and Biography

Budd, William
Doll, Richard
Ehrlich, Paul
Epidemiology, History of
Eugenics
Farr, William
Frost, Wade Hampton
Genocide
Goldberger, Joseph
Graunt, John
Hamilton, Alice
Hill, Austin Bradford
Jenner, Edward
Keys, Ancel
Koch, Robert
Lind, James
Lister, Joseph
Nightingale, Florence
Pasteur, Louis
Public Health, History of
Reed, Walter
Ricketts, Howard
Rush, Benjamin
Snow, John
Tukey, John
Tuskegee Study

Infrastructure of Epidemiology and Public Health

American College of Epidemiology
American Public Health Association
Association of Schools of Public Health
Centers for Disease Control and Prevention
Council of State and Territorial Epidemiologists
European Public Health Alliance
European Union Public Health Programs
Food and Drug Administration
Governmental Role in Public Health
Healthy People 2010
Institutional Review Board
Journals, Epidemiological
Journals, Public Health
National Center for Health Statistics

National Institutes of Health
Pan American Health Organization
Peer Review Process
Publication Bias
Public Health Agency of Canada
Society for Epidemiologic Research
Surgeon General, U.S.
United Nations Children's Fund
U.S. Public Health Service
World Health Organization

Medical Care and Research

Allergen
Apgar Score
Barker Hypothesis
Birth Defects
Body Mass Index (BMI)
Carcinogen
Case Reports and Case Series
Clinical Epidemiology
Clinical Trials
Community Health
Community Trial
Comorbidity
Complementary and Alternative Medicine
Effectiveness
Efficacy
Emerging Infections
Escherichia coli
Etiology of Disease
Evidence-Based Medicine
Gestational Age
Intent-to-Treat Analysis
International Classification of Diseases
International Classification of Functioning, Disability, and Health
Latency and Incubation Periods
Life Course Approach
Malnutrition, Measurement of
Medical Anthropology
Organ Donation
Pain
Placebo Effect
Preclinical Phase of Disease
Preterm Birth

K

KAPLAN-MEIER METHOD

The Kaplan-Meier (or product limit) estimator $\hat{S}(t)$ is a nonparametric (or distribution free) estimator of a survival distribution $S(t)$. It was derived by Kaplan and Meier in 1958 as a direct generalization of the sample survivor function in presence of censored data.

In clinical applications, the Kaplan-Meier method is very often used to estimate the probability of dying from specific causes or the probability of occurrence or recurrence of a disease. In general, the Kaplan-Meier method can be used to estimate the probability of occurrence of any event.

The Kaplan-Meier method is generally used to summarize the survival experience of groups of individuals in terms of the empirical survivor function.

Typically, not all individuals under study fail during the observation period. Some individuals may leave the study early while still alive, and some other individuals may finish the study alive. These individuals are called censored.

The Kaplan-Meier estimator does not require any assumptions about the functional form of the distribution of failures and accounts for censored observations. For small data set, the Kaplan-Meier curve can be easily calculated by hand. Most statistical software contains routines for the calculation of the Kaplan-Meier estimator.

Consider a sample of N individuals who are followed up in time prospectively. During the observation period, suppose that K of these individuals die. We also assume that $N - K$ individuals are censored.

Let $t_1 \leq t_2 \leq \cdots \leq t_K$ be the ordered failure times for the K individuals who die during the observation period.

To construct the Kaplan-Meier estimator of the survival distribution, we start by dividing the observation period into small intervals $I_1 = [t_0, t_1)$, $I_2 = [t_1, t_2), \ldots, I_j = [t_{j-1}, t_j), \ldots, I_K = [t_{K-1}, t_K)$, each one corresponding to the survival time of the noncensored individuals. For each interval $I_j (j = 1, \ldots, K)$,

$d_j =$ the number of individuals who die in the interval I_j;

$c_j =$ the number of individuals censored in the interval I_j;

$r_j =$ the number of individuals who are alive and at risk at the beginning of the interval; and

$h_j =$ the hazard of failure, or the conditional probability of an individual surviving through I_j, given that he was alive at the beginning of I_j; this quantity can be well approximated by $\hat{h}_j = d_j / r_j$, the ratio of number of failures over the number of individuals at risk during the interval I_j.

The observed proportion of failures d_{1j} / r_{1j} represent an estimate of the hazard of failure (or instantaneous failure rate) $h(t)$.

At the beginning of the observation period, t_0, all individuals are alive, so that, $d_0 = 0$ and $r_0 = N$. At each step, we calculate $r_j = r_{j-1} - d_{j-1} - c_{j-1}$ to update the number of individuals at risk.

The Kaplan-Meier estimate of the survival distribution $S(t)$ is obtained by the product of all the $1 - \hat{h}_j$:

$$\hat{S}(t) = \prod_{t_j < t} (1 - \hat{h}_j).$$

The Kaplan-Meier estimate $\hat{S}(t)$ is a left continuous, not increasing, step function that is discontinuous at the observed failure times t_j. The intervals I_j may vary in length and depend on the observed data. Observations that are censored at t_j are assumed to occur after t_j. Censored observations contribute to the risk set till the time they are last seen alive. If a failure and a censoring time are tied (i.e., occur at the same point in time), we assume that the failure occurs just before the censoring.

An estimate of the variance of the Kaplan-Meier curve is given by the Greenwood's formula:

$$\hat{V}ar[\ln \hat{S}(t)] = \sum_{j:t_j < t} \frac{d_j}{r_j(r_j - d_j)}$$

(here ln indicates the natural logarithm) from which it is derived that

$$\hat{V}ar[\hat{S}(t)] = [\hat{S}(t)]^2 \sum_{j:t_j < t} \frac{d_j}{r_j(r_j - d_j)}.$$

To calculate an approximate $100(1 - \alpha)\%$ confidence interval for $\hat{S}(t)$, we first calculate a confidence interval for $\ln \hat{S}(t)$ and then we exponentiate to obtain the upper and lower bound of the confidence interval for $\hat{S}(t)$. Note that at extreme values of t such a confidence interval may include unreasonable limits outside the range [0,1].

Example

Consider the following survival times corresponding to the time to death, in days, of 15 patients with advanced squamous cell lung cancer:

$$72, 411, 228, 126, 118, 10, 82, 110,$$
$$314, 100^c, 42, 8, 144, 25^c, 11.$$

The superscript c indicates that the observation is censored. Thus, two patients left the study alive at 25 and 100 days, respectively. All other patients died during the observation period. To construct a Kaplan-Meier estimate of the probability of dying from lung cancer, we follow the steps described above.

Table 1   Lung Cancer Data

t_j	r_j	d_j	c_j	$(1 - \hat{h}_j)$	$\hat{S}(t)$
0	15	0	0	1	1
8	15	1	0	0.9333	0.933
10	14	1	0	0.9286	0.866
11	13	1	0	0.9230	0.800
25 *	12	0	1	1	0.800
42	11	1	0	0.9091	0.7273
72	10	1	0	0.9000	0.6545
82	9	1	0	0.8888	0.5818
100 *	8	0	1	1	0.5818
110	7	1	0	0.8571	0.4987
118	6	1	0	0.8333	0.4156
126	5	1	0	0.8000	0.3325
144	4	1	0	0.7500	0.2494
228	3	1	0	0.6666	0.1662
314	2	1	0	0.5000	0.083
411	1	1	0	0.0000	0.00

Source: Adapted from Kalbfleish and Prentice (2002, Appendix A, p. 378).

Note: Asterisk (*) represents censored observations.

Table 1 summarizes the steps necessary to calculate the Kaplan-Meier estimate of the time to death for these individuals.

The median survival time is calculated from a Kaplan-Meier curve as the time at which the probability of dying is 50%. In the lung cancer data example, the median survival time is 100 days.

To obtain a 95% confidence interval for $\hat{S}(72)$, we first compute a confidence interval for $\ln \hat{S}(72)$

$$\ln S(72) \pm 1.96 \sqrt{\sum_j \frac{d_j}{r_j(r_j - d_j)}}$$
$$= [-0.4761 - 0.0299],$$

and then we exponentiate the lower and the upper bound of this interval to obtain a 95% confidence interval for $\hat{S}(72)$: $[0.6212 - 1.00]$.

—*Emilia Bagiella*

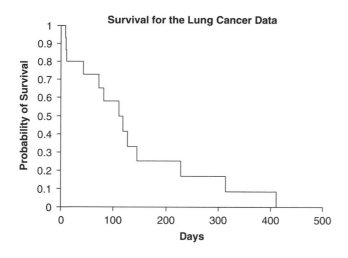

Figure 1   Kaplan-Meier Method Estimates

Source: Adapted from Kalbfleish and Prentice (2002).

See also Censored Data; Hazard Rate; Survival Analysis

Further Readings

Kalbfleish, D. J., & Prentice, R. L. (2002). *The statistical analysis of failure time data* (2nd ed.). Hoboken, NJ: Wiley.

Kaplan, E. L., & Meier, P. (1958). Nonparametric estimation from incomplete observations. *Journal of American Statistical Association, 53,* 457–481.

Prentice, R. L. (1973). Exponential survivals with censoring and explanatory variables. *Biometrika, 60,* 279–288.

KAPPA

The kappa statistic is a measure of agreement, corrected for chance, for a categorical variable. For example, if two radiologists each assess the results for the same set of patients, the kappa is one way to measure how well their conclusions agree. The kappa may be used if the rating system used to grade each patient is binary or categorical. With either a large number of ordinal categories (such as a scale from 0 to 20) or a continuous rating scale, Pearson's correlation coefficient would provide a better assessment of agreement than the kappa.

The formula for the kappa is $\kappa = (p_o - p_e)/(1 - p_e)$, where p_o is the proportion of observed agreement (the sum of the observed values of the cells on the diagonal over the total number of observations), and p_e is the proportion of agreement expected by chance (the sum of the expected values of the same cells on the diagonal over the total number of observations). Notice that the denominator shows the difference between perfect agreement and the amount of agreement expected by chance, representing the best possible improvement of the raters over chance alone. This is contrasted with the numerator, the difference between the observed proportion of agreement and that expected by chance. As a result, the kappa statistic may be interpreted as the proportion of agreement beyond that which is expected just by chance, and kappa values range from less than 0 (less agreement than expected by chance) to 1 (perfect agreement). Kappa values between 0 and 0.4 represent marginal reproducibility or agreement, values between 0.4 and 0.75 show good agreement, and values more than 0.75 indicate excellent agreement.

As the number of possible categories for each rating increases, the associated kappa values tend to decrease. Fortunately, if the categories are ordinal (such as a score from 1 to 10), this can be combated by use of the weighted kappa. In the weighted kappa, the most weight is given to observations with identical ratings, then less weight is given to ratings one unit apart, still less weight is given to observations two units apart, and so on. The user defines how much weight is allotted to each possibility (identical ratings, one unit apart, two units apart, and so on) as well as defining how far apart ratings can be and still contribute toward the weighted agreement.

In the ordinary kappa statistic, only perfect agreement between Raters A and B would count toward

Table 1   Comparison of the Unweighted and Weighted Kappa Statistics

		Rater A			
		I	II	III	IV
Rater B	I	5	(5)	2	2
	II	3	4	4	0
	III	2	2	6	3
	IV	1	0	2	5

agreement. In the weighted kappa statistic, the most weight is given to perfect agreement (dark gray) with less weight given to cells with near perfect agreement (light gray). Specifically, the five observations that Rater A coded as "II" and Rater B coded as "I" would count as disagreement for the ordinary kappa statistic but count as partial agreement in the weighted kappa statistic.

The usual versions of the kappa and weighted kappa statistics allow only two raters to assess each observation. The multirater kappa is an alternative when more than two raters assess each observation. The weighted kappa and the multirater kappa may be interpreted in the same way as the generic kappa statistic.

—Felicity Boyd Enders

See also Interrater Reliability; Pearson Correlation Coefficient

Further Readings

Banerjee, M. (1999). Beyond kappa: A review of interrater agreement measures. *Canadian Journal of Statistics, 27*(1), 3–23.

KEYS, ANCEL
(1904–2004)

Ancel Keys was an American scientist who did pioneering work on the relationship between diet and health, particularly on the relationship between dietary fat and heart disease. Keys and his wife Margaret were the first American promoters of the Mediterranean diet, coauthoring *Eat Well and Stay Well*, an immensely popular cookbook. The discovery of a link between diet and heart disease landed Keys on the cover of *Time* magazine in 1961 and garnered him the nickname "Mr. Cholesterol."

Keys was born in Colorado Springs in 1904, an only child. His family moved to San Francisco just before the devastating April 1906 earthquake, then across San Francisco Bay to Berkeley. While in elementary school, he was identified as one of the 1,528 "gifted" children studied by Stanford psychologist Lewis Terman.

Keys attended the University of California, Berkeley, where he received a B.A. in economics and political science, an M.S. in biology, and a Ph.D. in oceanography and biology. He earned a second Ph.D. in physiology at Cambridge. In 1936, Keys became a professor of physiology at the University of Minnesota. In 1939, Keys founded the Laboratory of Physiological Hygiene. A new quantitative human biology, physiological hygiene combined physiology, nutrition, epidemiology, and prevention research.

In 1944, the U.S. government commissioned Keys to study human performance during nutritional deficiency states and to design lightweight but nutritionally adequate rations for paratroopers. Keys proposed an ambitious project to study the physiology of starvation, selecting 36 conscientious objectors, all volunteers. Keys and his colleagues brought the subjects to a baseline weight, gradually cut their daily diets from 3,500 calories to a semistarvation diet of 1,600 calories, and followed up with a rehabilitation diet. Keys then recorded the physiological changes associated with progressive food deprivation. Out of this research, Keys developed the emergency K-ration, used extensively by the U.S. military.

Immediately following World War II, Keys was perplexed by a set of seemingly counterintuitive observations: U.S. businessmen, presumably among the best-fed persons in the world, had high rates of heart disease, while in postwar Europe, cardiovascular disease rates had decreased sharply in the wake of reduced food supplies. In 1947, Keys helped establish cardiovascular epidemiology by launching the Twin Cities Study, a study of Minnesota businessmen, a few months before the better-known Framingham Heart Study began. Keys identified the relationship between dietary fat, blood cholesterol, and heart disease.

More ambitious was the Seven Countries Study, launched in 1958, which followed a sample of men in 16 distinct populations from seven nations throughout North America, Europe, and Asia. An extensive effort to characterize diet in detail via the collection and biochemical analysis of food samples distinguished the Seven Countries Study from the Framingham Study. Keys and his colleagues established that the risk of chronic disease differed greatly between populations and individuals and that these differences correlated with culturally determined lifestyle and dietary habits.

Keys retired in 1972 and maintained an active lifestyle until his death at age 100.

—Todd M. Olszewski

See also Cardiovascular Disease; Cholesterol; Chronic Disease Epidemiology; Framingham Heart Study; Nutritional Epidemiology

Further Readings

Keys, A., Aravanis, C., Blackburn, H., Buzina, R., Djordjević, B. S., Dontas, A. S., et al. (1980). *Seven countries: A multivariate analysis of death and coronary heart disease.* Cambridge, MA: Harvard University Press.

Keys, A., Brozek, J., Henschel, K., Mickelsen, O., Taylor, H. L., Simonson, E., et al. (1950). *The biology of human starvation.* Minneapolis: University of Minnesota Press.

KOCH, ROBERT
(1843–1910)

Robert Koch is considered one of the founders of modern bacteriology and a key contributor to the etiology of diseases, along with Louis Pasteur. He isolated several disease-causing bacteria, including those for anthrax (1877), tuberculosis (1882), and cholera (1883), and developed Koch's postulates criteria for ascertaining the microbial causes of a specific disease.

Robert Koch was born in Clausthal, Germany, in 1843, one of 13 children. He received a medical degree from the University of Göttingen in 1866. Following this, Koch served as a physician in several German towns, was a field surgeon during the 1870 to 1872 Franco-Prussian war, and then became a medical officer in Wollstein, Germany. It was during this latter part of his career that Koch did most of his research, in a laboratory he developed in Wollstein.

Koch's first major scientific breakthrough occurred when he isolated anthrax bacillus and proved that it caused disease. He did this by injecting healthy mice with spores of *Bacillus anthracis* that had been obtained from the spleens of animals infected with anthrax. Mice injected with these spores later developed anthrax, while mice injected with spores from healthy animals did not. This was the first time that a specific microorganism was causally related to a specific disease.

Following this discovery, Koch developed a set of criteria to prove that a disease is caused by a specific microorganism. These four criteria are commonly referred to as Koch's postulates. Koch argues that for a microorganism to cause a specific disease, each of the four of Koch's postulates had to be fulfilled. While these criteria are not literally believed today, their development contributed significantly to the establishment of the germ theory of disease.

In 1882, Koch isolated the tuberculosis bacillus and then inoculated uninfected animals with it. This induced tuberculosis in the animals and thus established the etiologic role of the bacterium in the causation of disease. He later did further work on tuberculosis by investigating the possible protective effect of injecting a person with dead tuberculin bacilli and then subsequently injecting them with live tuberculosis bacilli and suggesting that he may have discovered a cure for the disease. Although it was not successful as a cure, findings from this work have been important in the development of the tuberculin test currently used today to detect tuberculosis infection in individuals.

Finally, Koch traveled to Egypt and India where he identified the cholera bacillus and determined that its mode of transmission was waterborne. Following this discovery, he did some work investigating vector-borne diseases such as malaria.

Koch not only did work isolating bacteria but also developed many microbiology techniques. These included methods of staining bacteria and investigation using the microscope. Furthermore, Koch introduced the solid culture medium for the cultivation of bacteria. In this way, Koch was an important contributor to the methodology of bacteriology.

Koch received the Nobel Prize in Physiology or Medicine in 1905 for his discoveries in tuberculosis. Koch was married twice during his lifetime and had one child, a daughter. He died in 1910 in Baden-Baden, Germany.

—*Kate Bassil*

See also Koch's Postulates; Pasteur, Louis

Further Readings

Brock, T. D. (1998). *Robert Koch: A life in medicine and bacteriology.* Washington, DC: American Society for Microbiology Press.

Web Sites

Nobel Foundation: http://nobelprize.org/nobel_prizes/medicine/laureates/1905/koch-bio.html.

KOCH'S POSTULATES

Koch's postulates, also known as Henle-Koch postulates, were published by Robert Koch in various forms between 1878 and 1884 to set forth a method of demonstrating that a bacillus causes a particular disease. These postulates follow the process that Koch went through in demonstrating that anthrax and tuberculosis bacilli cause disease. Koch's postulates state that, to establish that an organism causes disease,

- the organism must be present in all cases of the disease;
- the organism must be grown in pure culture outside a diseased animal;
- when inoculated with the organism, healthy test animals must develop the same symptoms as were present in the original cases; and
- the organism must be present in the experimentally infected animals.

Koch believed that satisfying these postulates provided definitive proof that the organism was a necessary and sufficient cause of disease. If fulfilled, these postulates provide powerful evidence that an agent causes disease; however, all these conditions need not be fulfilled to establish causation. Koch noted in his investigations that healthy animals sometimes would not develop disease after being inoculated with the pathogen, leaving the third postulate unfulfilled. Such asymptomatic infections occur in many diseases with well-established causes, such as cholera and influenza. The second postulate, that the organism must be grown in a pure culture outside the diseased animal, cannot be fulfilled for viruses since they are intracellular parasites.

Even when not fulfilled in the strictest sense, Koch's postulates still provide guidelines for establishing disease causation. In modern practice, the first and third postulates are more accurately stated as follows:

- The agent must be significantly more common in individuals with the disease than those without.
- Individuals exposed to the agent must be significantly more likely to develop the disease than those who are not.

There is some debate about the extent to which Koch was influenced by the work of Jacob Henle. Those who feel that Koch was heavily influenced by Henle's work on disease causation refer to the postulates as the Henle-Koch postulates or even as the Henle postulates. While the extent to which Koch was influenced by previous investigators is open to some debate, it is clear that the postulates were significant in Koch's groundbreaking work showing the role of the anthrax and tuberculosis bacilli in the causation of disease. The postulates therefore generally bear only his name.

Modern epidemiological research often focuses on diseases, such as diabetes and cancer, that are not necessarily caused by microorganisms. For these diseases other methods for establishing causation, such as Hill's Considerations for Causal Inference, are used instead of Koch's postulates. An expansion of Koch's postulates was proposed by Alfred S. Evans, who attempted to unify criteria of causation used in the investigation of chronic and acute diseases.

—*Justin Lessler*

See also Causation and Causal Inference; Etiology of Disease; Hill's Considerations for Causal Inference; Koch, Robert

Further Readings

Carter, K. C. (1985). Koch's postulates in relation to the work of Jacob Henle and Edwin Klebs. *Medical History, 29,* 353–374.

Evans, A. S. (1976). Causation and disease: The Henle-Koch postulates revisited. *Yale Journal of Biology and Medicine, 49,* 175–195.

KURTOSIS

Kurtosis is a measure of the thickness of the tails of a statistical distribution and the sharpness of its peak. Kurtosis is also called the fourth moment about the mean and is one of the two most common statistics used to describe the shape of a distribution (the other is skewness).

There are three types of kurtosis: mesokurtosis, platykurtosis, and leptokurtosis. Many times, these are referred to as zero, negative, and positive kurtosis, respectively. The positive and negative descriptors refer to whether the peak of the distribution is "sharper" or higher than a normal distribution or if the peak is "flatter" or lower than the normal distribution.

Kurtosis statistics compare the distribution under study with the normal distribution. A distribution that

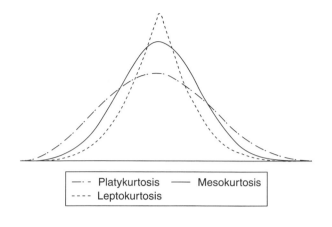

Figure 1   Common Distributions With Type of Kurtosis

Table 1   Illustration of the Three Types of Kurtosis

Distribution	Type of Kurtosis	
Normal	Zero	Mesokurtosis
Student's t	Negative	Platykurtosis (for sample sizes greater than seven)
Uniform	Negative	Platykurtosis
Exponential	Positive	Leptokurtosis
Laplace	Positive	Leptokurtosis
Weibull	Depends on the parameters of the distribution	

resembles the normal distribution in terms of relative peakedness of the distribution is said to be mesokurtic or have zero kurtosis. If a distribution has a higher peak where the width of the peak is thinner and the tails are thinner than the normal distribution, then the distribution is said to be leptokurtic or have positive kurtosis. If a distribution has a lower peak where the width of the peak is wider and the tails are thicker than the normal distribution, then the distribution is said to be platykurtic or have negative kurtosis. A platykurtic distribution may even have a concave peak instead of a rounded peak (see Figure 1).

When analyzing data using an analysis package, a researcher needs to know whether the program uses the kurtosis statistic or the kurtosis *excess* statistic. For the kurtosis statistic, a value of 3 indicates a normal distribution. However, kurtosis excess is a measure of how far the kurtosis statistic is from 3. So a normal distribution has a kurtosis excess of 0. Using the kurtosis excess statistic, the sign of the statistic matches the description of the kurtosis (-1 is negative kurtosis, $+1$ is positive kurtosis).

The most commonly known distributions and their type of kurtosis are given in Table 1.

Many times kurtosis is used to help assess whether a distribution being studied meets the normality assumptions of most common parametric statistical tests. While the normal distribution has a kurtosis of $+3$, it is important to realize that, in practice, the kurtosis statistic for a sample from the population will not be exactly equal to $+3$. How far off can the statistic be and not violate the normality assumption? Provided the statistic is not grossly different from $+3$, then that decision is up to the researcher and his or her opinion of an acceptable difference. For most typically sized (small) samples, the kurtosis statistic is unreliable. To accurately measure the kurtosis of a distribution, sample sizes of several hundred may be needed.

—*Stacie Ezelle Taylor*

See also Inferential and Descriptive Statistics; Skewness

Further Readings

Joanes, D. N., & Gill, C. A. (1998). Comparing measures of sample skewness & kurtosis. *Journal of the Royal Statistical Society: Series D (The Statistician), 47*(1), 183–189 (doi:10.1111/1467-9884.00122).

Reineke, D. M., Baggett, J., & Elfessi, A. (2003). A note on the effect of skewness, kurtosis, and shifting on one-sample *t* and sign tests. *Journal of Statistics Education, 11*(3). Retrieved June 5, 2007, from http://www.amstat.org/publications/jse/v11n3/reineke.html.

L

Latency and Incubation Periods

The starting point of a communicable disease is the exposure of the host to the infectious agent. When communicable diseases are considered as a whole, two different processes have to be distinguished in their evolution over time: infectiveness and disease. Infectiveness consists of two successive periods: the latency period and the period of communicability. The disease process encompasses the incubation period and the clinical signs and symptoms. Whereas the knowledge of infectiveness is of paramount importance for microbiological, pharmacological, and public health purposes, the main interest in the disease process hinges on the clinical care of the patient.

The incubation period is the time that elapses between the initial exposure of the host to the infectious agent and the first appearance of the clinical manifestations (signs or symptoms) associated with the disease. In a vector, it is the time between entrance of an infectious agent into the vector and the time when that vector can transmit the infection (a period known as the extrinsic incubation period).

The duration of the incubation period is determined by the time needed by the infectious agent to grow enough in number in the host to produce symptoms. During the incubation period, the infectious agent can be transferred from one host to another. In many diseases, the communicable period begins before the inception of signs and symptoms, as, for example, in viral hepatitis and some exanthematic infections (those characterized by skin eruptions), such as measles, rubella, scarlet fever, and chickenpox.

The incubation period is known for most diseases. It varies among diseases, and for each particular disease, although in a much lesser degree, depending on the infective dose of the agent, namely, the mean number of microorganisms needed to cause infection. (The infectiveness of an infectious agent is usually expressed as the infectious dose 50 [ID_{50}], and it is defined as the infectious dose needed to produce infection in 50% of the susceptible hosts.) Some examples of incubation periods are as follows: influenza (from 1 to 3 days), diarrhoea caused by *Escherichia coli* (from 3 to 8 days, with a median of 3 to 4 days), measles (from 7 to 18 days, with a median of 10 days), hepatitis A (from 15 to 50 days, depending on the infective dose, with an average of 28 to 30 days), and leprosy (from 9 months to 20 years, with a probable average of 4 years for tuberculoid leprosy and 8 years for lepromatous leprosy).

—*Carlos Campillo*

See also Host; Vector-Borne Disease

Further Readings

Anderson, R. M., & May, R. M. (1992). *Infectious diseases of humans: Dynamics and control.* Oxford, UK: Oxford University Press.

Benenson, A. S. (Ed.). (1995). *Control of communicable diseases manual* (16th ed.). Washington, DC: American Public Health Association.

Thomas, J. C., & Weber, D. J. (2001). *Epidemiologic methods for the study of infectious diseases.* New York: Oxford University Press.

LATENT CLASS MODELS

Many quantities of interest in sociology, psychology, public health, and medicine are unobservable but well-conceived characteristics such as attitudes, temperament, psychological diagnoses, and health behaviors. Such constructs can be measured indirectly by using multiple items as indicators of the unobservable characteristics. The latent class (LC) model can classify individuals into population subgroups based on these unobservable characteristics, by using their responses to questionnaire items that are related to those characteristics. Suppose, for example, we are interested in the construct of nicotine dependence and want to classify respondents into groups corresponding to different types of nicotine dependence we believe are indicated by a number of behaviors relating to cigarette use. We can collect data on several items pertaining to cigarette use and then apply an LC model to this data to identify two or more nicotine dependence types to which smokers might belong. We can use this LC model to classify not only the subjects in our study but also subjects in other studies. The LC model has been widely applied in behavioral and biomedical applications, particularly in the area of substance use prevention and treatment. In physical or psychiatric research, the LC model has been a popular strategy for development and evaluation of diagnostic criteria. The LC model can also be a useful way to address many problems of categorical data analysis in population-based epidemiologic studies.

The Mathematical Model

The LC model explains the relationship among manifest items by positing the assumption that the population comprises different classes related to the construct of interest. In other words, the population is assumed to consist of mutually exclusive and exhaustive groups, called latent classes, and the distribution of the items varies across classes. The LC model comprises two types of parameters: the relative size of each class and the probability of a particular response to each item within a class. To specify an LC model, let $\mathbf{Y} = (Y_1, \ldots, Y_M))$ be M discrete items measuring latent classes, where variable Y_m takes possible values from 1 to r_m. Let $C = 1, 2, \ldots, L$ be the variable of LC membership, and let $I(y = k)$ denote the indicator function that takes the value 1 if $y = k$ and 0 otherwise.

If the class membership were observed, the joint probability that an individual belongs to Class 1 and provides responses $\mathbf{y} = (y_1, \ldots, y_M)$ would be

$$P(Y = y, C = l) = \gamma_l \prod_{m=1}^{M} \prod_{k=1}^{r_m} \rho_{mk|l}^{I(y_m = k)},$$

where

$\gamma_l = P(C = 1)$ represents the probability of belonging to Latent Class 1 and

$\rho_{mk|1} = P(Y_m = k | C = 1)$ represents the probability of response k to the mth item given a class membership in 1.

Therefore, the marginal probability of a particular response pattern $\mathbf{y} = (y_1, \ldots, y_M)$ without regard for the unseen class membership is

$$P(Y = y) = \sum_{l=1}^{L} \gamma_l \prod_{m=1}^{M} \prod_{k=1}^{r_m} \rho_{mk|l}^{I(y_m = k)}.$$

Here, we have assumed *local independence*—that is, the items are assumed to be unrelated within each class. This assumption is the crucial feature of the LC model that allows us to draw inferences about the unseen class variable.

Model Identifiability

Model identification is imperative in estimating parameters of an LC model. The parameters of an LC model are said to be *locally identifiable* if the likelihood function is uniquely determined by the parameters within some neighborhood of a particular value of parameters. A necessary (but not sufficient) condition to make the LC model locally identifiable is that the number of possible response patterns of manifest items must be greater than the number of free parameters in the LC model. Even if this necessary condition is satisfied, it is impossible to say a priori whether or not this model is indeed identifiable. A necessary and sufficient condition for local identifiability is that the first derivative matrix of the log-likelihood function with respect to the parameters evaluated at a particular value must have full column rank. When an LC model is not identifiable, the simplest way to achieve identification is to reduce the number of parameters to be estimated by fixing or constraining parameters.

Estimation

The most common approach to estimate unknown parameters in an LC model is maximum likelihood (ML) estimation using the EM (E-step [expectation] and M-step [maximization]) algorithm. EM is an iterative procedure in which each iteration consists of two steps, the E-step and M-step. Iterating these two steps produces a sequence of parameter estimates that converges reliably to a local or global maximum of the likelihood function. However, researchers should apply several sets of starting values to ensure that the ML estimates represent the best solution (i.e., global maximum). On convergence, standard errors for the estimated parameters are obtained by inverting the Hessian matrix (i.e., the negative second derivative matrix of the log-likelihood function).

As an alternative to ML, one can apply the Bayesian method via a Markov chain Monte Carlo (MCMC) method to estimate unknown parameters in LC models. The most popular MCMC method for the LC model is closely related to EM; it is an iterative procedure whereby each iteration consists of two steps, the I-step (imputation) and the P-step (posterior). Repeating this two-step procedure creates a sequence of iterates converging to the stationary posterior distribution of the LC model parameters. MCMC may produce greater flexibility in model fit assessment and various hypothesis tests without appealing to large-sample approximations.

Model Selection

It is important that a model be assessed adequately at the outset of an analysis. Numerous statistical methods are being adopted to evaluate model fit. However, different methods often suggest different solutions, yielding ambiguity in model selection. The choice of the number of latent classes can be driven, to summarize the distinctive features of the data in as parsimonious a fashion as possible, by a balanced judgment that takes into account the substantive knowledge and objective measures available for assessing model fit.

The log-likelihood-ratio statistics, including the likelihood-ratio test (LRT), are used to assess the absolute model fit of an LC model by comparing the predicted response pattern frequencies with the observed frequencies appearing in the data. For large samples with a relatively small number of response patterns, LRT may be a valid statistic to assess the absolute model fit with the asymptotic chi-square approximation. However, the difference in LRT for testing the relative fit of an L-class model against an $(L+1)$-class alternative does not have limiting chi-square distribution. Therefore, LRT cannot be used to assess the relative model fit of two competing models with different numbers of latent classes. If we do not give up the concept of overall LRT, several solutions to the problems in the asymptotic assumption are available. For example, the adjusted LRT and the parametric bootstrap are popular methods because they are easy to access via software packages such as Mplus and Latent GOLD.

There are numerous other model selection criteria widely used to compare models with different numbers of classes. For example, goodness-of-fit measures based on information theory (e.g., Akaike information criterion, consistent Akaike information criterion, and Bayesian information criterion) can be used to compare LC models with different number of classes. One drawback to this approach is that these methods assess relative model fit only; this says nothing as to whether the best model in a set of competing models actually fits well.

Within a Bayesian framework, there is a tool using the posterior probability check distributions (PPCD) that can be used to assess model fit. The PPCD for the LRT that does not rely on any known distribution can be constructed in the following way: (a) simulate the random draw of parameters from their Bayesian posterior distribution under the current LC model, (b) draw a hypothetical new data set from the same model using the simulated parameters, (c) fit the current model and the competing model to the simulated data set, and (d) compute the LRT difference based on output from (c). Repeating (a) to (d) many times produces a sample of LRT from the PPCD. The area to the right of the observed LRT can be regarded as a Bayesian p value.

—*Hwan Chung*

See also Bayesian Approach to Statistics; Likelihood Ratio; Regression

Further Readings

Goodman, L. A. (1974). Exploratory latent structure analysis using both identifiable and unidentifiable models. *Biometrika, 61,* 215–231.

Lanza, S. T., Collins, L. M., Schafer, J. L., & Flaherty, B. P. (2005). Using data augmentation to obtain standard errors and conduct hypothesis tests in latent class and latent transition analysis. *Psychological Methods, 10*, 84–100.

Lanza, S. T., Flaherty, B. P., & Collins, L. M. (2003). Latent class and latent transition analysis. In J. A. Schinka & W. F. Velicer (Eds.), *Handbook of psychology* (pp. 663–685). Hoboken, NJ: Wiley.

Rubin, D. B., & Stern, H. S. (1994). Testing in latent class models using a posterior predictive check distribution. In A. von Eye & C. C. Clogg (Eds.), *Latent variable analysis: Applications for developmental research* (pp. 420–438). Oxford, UK: Oxford University Press.

LATINO HEALTH ISSUES

As a diverse group, comprising people who differ in national origin, generation, level of acculturation, socioeconomic class, region of residence, and gender, it is not surprising that there is considerable variation in the overall health of the Latino population of the United States. (*Latino* is an umbrella term that covers people of diverse points of origin in Latin American countries.) This diversity among Latinos notwithstanding, reviews of the health status of Latinos relative to the dominant non-Latino white population affirm the importance of health disparities as a prevailing feature of the national health pattern. The average life span of Latinos in the country is 20 years shorter than for non-Latino whites. In terms of specific health differences, Latinos are disproportionately likely to die of violence (homicide being the second leading cause of death for Latinos 15 to 24 years of age), develop late-onset diabetes (11% compared with 5% in the general population), develop cervical cancer (with an incidence rate of 17 per 100,000 for Latinas compared with just under 9 per 100,000 for non-Latinas), suffer from asthma (hospitalization rates for Latino youth in some states are five times higher than for whites), and become infected with HIV/AIDS (although Latinos account for approximately 14% of the population of the United States and Puerto Rico, they comprise 18% of AIDS cases diagnoses since the beginning of the epidemic). Among some Latino subgroups, especially Puerto Ricans and Mexican Americans, there are comparatively high rates of illicit drug, and Mexican Americans have comparatively high rates of heavy drinking compared with non-Latino whites.

Latinas are more likely to report teen pregnancy and have the highest teen birth rate of all ethnic populations in the United States. Of equal significance as these various health disparities, Latinos are the least likely population in the United States to have health insurance and one of the most likely to encounter linguistic and cultural barriers in accessing effective and appropriate health care. For example, research has shown that monolingual Spanish-speaking Latino patients are significantly less likely than non-Hispanic whites to have had a physician visit or an influenza vaccination during the year, while rates for English-speaking Latinos are similar to those of non-Hispanic whites. Despite these challenges, in terms of a number of critical health indicators (e.g., various cancers, cardiovascular and pulmonary disease), Latinos tend to exhibit lower rates of disease and ill health than the dominant population.

Sociodemographic Factors in Latino Health

Latinos now constitute the largest ethnic minority population in the country—5 years earlier than the U.S. Census Bureau had projected they would do so. This population continues to grow at an unprecedented rate of 5.7% each year nationally. It is now estimated that there are 37 million Latinos in the United States, up almost 12% since the completion of the 2000 census. Latinos now comprise almost 13% of the total U.S. population or roughly one of every eight people in the country. As a result, the overall health of the Latino population and the specific health needs of Latinos have a significant impact on health in the country generally.

Generally, Latinos are a comparatively young population, which is a key factor in their exhibiting lower rates of morbidity and mortality relative to diseases commonly associated with aging (e.g., heart disease, cancer). The median age of Latinos in the United States is 25 years, and nearly 40% of Latinos are less than 20 years of age. Moreover, the proportion of Latino children in the total number of children in the United States has increased at a faster pace than that of any other ethnic group, growing from 9% of the child population in 1980 to 19% by 2004. If current trends continue, one in four people living in the United States by 2050 will be Latino, affirming the importance of the health of this population relative to overall health in the United States.

In assessing the health status of the Latino population, it must be stressed that public health researchers generally acknowledge that mortality rates among Latinos tend to be underestimated for several reasons, including misreporting of ethnicity on death certificates and other health-related documents used as health indicators and the return migration of Latinos with life-threatening illnesses to their country of origin. Similarly, morbidity rates for Latinos often are underestimated because of a failure to collect full ethnicity data in many studies or in surveillance monitoring, use of methodologies such as telephone interviewing that do not effectively reach the lowest income populations (because of geographic mobility, inability to pay telephone bills on time, doubling up of families in residential settings, homelessness, etc.), failure of survey research to reach segments of the Latino population, language barriers, and lack of access to health care despite significant health problems. Moreover, because of diversity within the overall Latino population, national statistics on Latinos provide only a rough image of the sociodemographic characteristics and health profiles of Latinos in any particular state. Country of origin (for individuals born outside the United States, or of ancestors for those born in the United States), in particular, differentiates health patterns among Latino subgroups. For example, the frequency of female-headed households among Puerto Ricans is double that of Cubans, the percentage of Latinos of Mexican origin who live in a nonmetropolitan area is more than double that of Puerto Ricans, the rate of asthma among Puerto Ricans is more than double that of Mexicans or Cubans, and the frequency of AIDS-related mortality among Puerto Ricans is more than three times the rate among Mexican Americans.

While Latino health in the United States broadly reflects the overall health profile of the U.S. population, the health disparities found among Latinos reflect broad social disparities relative to the dominant non-Latino white population. Most notably in this regard is the issue of poverty. Poverty has been found to be closely tied with health status, and it is generally considered a risk factor for poor health and disease, especially among children. Moreover, children who grow up in poverty are more likely to do poorly in school, become teen parents, and be unemployed as adults. The poverty rate among Latino is three times the rate of non-Latino whites (approximately 26% vs. 8%). Additionally, the median income for Latino households is about $15,000 a year below that of non-Latino white households. Among Latino subgroups, rates of poverty are highest among Puerto Ricans and lowest among Cubans; nonetheless, even among Cubans, the rate of poverty is about twice as high as among non-Latino whites.

Rates of unemployment among Latinos are almost double that of non-Latino whites. Moreover, while there is a growing Latino middle class, the majority of employed Latinos are disproportionately concentrated in low-salaried jobs with limited room for economic advancement, and, of equal importance, Latinos often hold jobs that do not provide health insurance. Several economic indicators show that there has been a drop in occupational status of Latinos and a growing gap in the respective occupational status of Latinos and non-Latino whites. Data from the 2000 census indicate that about one quarter (27%) of Latino children under the age of 18 years live in poverty, compared with only 9% of non-Latino white children. Poverty rates among Latinos, however, vary significantly by ethnic subgroup. While 16% of Cuban children live in poverty, the rate for Puerto Rican children is 44%. Although rates of poverty are especially high among immigrant Latinos, even among third- and fourth-generation children of Mexican origin, rates of poverty are 2.5 times those of non-Latino white children.

Poverty and related structural violence, such as discrimination and racism, affect health in a number of direct and indirect ways, including unhealthy diets, increased exposure to physical and emotional stressors in the environment (e.g., street violence), heightened exposure to environmental toxins (e.g., lead paint, rodent infestation) and street violence, comparatively high rates of immune system impairments, and limitations on access to preventive care and treatment for existing conditions. For example, Latinos are four times as likely as non-Latino whites to suffer from tuberculosis. Rates of tuberculosis tend to reflect living conditions and residential crowding. Because of poverty, many Latino families live in substandard, poorly ventilated housing, with a higher number of people per square foot of living space than non-Latino whites. These are the conditions under which a communicable disease such as tuberculosis is most likely to spread.

While, as noted, health disparities have been found to be strongly influenced by poverty, they are especially common among poor people who live in areas with a high percentage of poor people in the local population. Thus, poor people in cities with smaller impoverished populations are at lower risk of dying than those in cities with large impoverished populations. Comparisons of findings from the 1990 and 2000 census counts indicate that the size of the Latino population in big cities is increasing, especially in large metropolitan areas such as New York and Los Angeles that already have large concentrations of Latinos. Thus, the number of Latinos who live in neighborhoods in which a majority of residents were Latino grew faster (76%) than in neighborhoods in which Latinos constitute a minority of residents (51%) between 1990 and 2000. In many urban areas with Latino populations, Latinos are disproportionately found in more densely populated inner city zones with comparatively high rates of poverty, a place where disease syndemics involving multiple interacting diseases of diverse kinds are most common.

Moreover, studies of differences in location among the poor show that the sociophysical environment in which people live—that is, their experience of their surrounding community, including issues of danger, stress, comfort, and appeal—is a critical determinant of their health. Feelings of hopelessness and powerlessness in a community have been found to be good predictors of health risk and health status. These are precisely the kinds of sentiments that have been recorded in a number of studies of Latino youth.

This array of factors underlies the disproportionate health burden of Latinos and directly contributes to the specific health problems, discussed below, that are especially common in this population.

Diabetes

The fifth leading cause of death in the United States, diabetes, a disease without a cure, is particularly common among Latinos. Mexican Americans over the age of 20 years, for example, are 1.7 times more likely to develop diabetes than non-Latino whites. Among residents of Puerto Rico, this rate is even somewhat higher. Comparing Latino subgroups, approximately 26% of Puerto Ricans, 24% of Mexican Americans, and 16% of Cubans between the ages of 45 and 74 have diabetes. Diabetes produces several debilitating conditions in different parts of the body, including diabetic retinopathy or damage to the small blood vessels of the retina of the eye and renal disease and kidney failure. Among Mexican Americans with

diabetes, the prevalence of retinopathy is between 32% and 40% while they are 4.5 to 6.6 times more likely to develop end-state renal failure than non-Latino whites.

Asthma

More than 17 million people in the United States suffer from asthma, of whom about a third are below 18 years of age. Asthma has been identified as one of the most common chronic illnesses of childhood in the United States. Recent national surveys report an overall lifetime asthma prevalence of 12.2% for children (below 18 years of age), although there are dramatic differences across ethnic groups and subgroups. Among Latinos, Puerto Ricans have the highest lifetime asthma rate (19.6%), more than three times that for Mexican Americans (6.1%) and almost double the rate of non-Latino whites (11.1%). While alarming, reported rates of asthma among Puerto Ricans probably underestimate the prevalence of this disease in this population because many symptomatic children go undiagnosed for long periods of time. It is estimated that the actual rate of childhood asthma among Puerto Ricans may reach 30%. Research shows that children with asthma are more likely to miss school than children without asthma from the same neighborhoods. An accumulating body of research indicates that low-income Latino families that have young children with asthma lack the necessary information, training in asthma management, and medical resources needed for good asthma control. The problem, however, is not simply one of the health care system failing to adequately prepare Latino parents in asthma management. Research suggests that Latino children are given fewer beta2-agonists (a standard component of asthma management), and Latino children received fewer inhaled steroids from their physicians than non-Latino white children. Even among Latino children in private care, a significant association was found between Latino ethnicity and low inhaled steroid use.

Cancer

Cancer is the second leading cause of death in the United States, with just less than half a million new cancer diagnoses each year. Notably, about half of all new cases of cancer are diagnosed among people 65 years of age and above, a group that while growing among Latinos is still comparatively smaller than in the general populations. Nationally, cancers that are most common among Latinos are of the cervix, esophagus, gallbladder, and stomach, with noticeable rises in female breast and lung cancer rates. Even though breast cancer incidence rates are lower among Latinas than non-Latino white women, Latinas are more likely to die from the disease. Divergent patterns between cancer incidence and mortality rates among Latinas appear to be primarily due to differences in rates of cancer screening (e.g., mammography). Latinas are less likely to obtain cancer screening than whites, which results in later-stage cancer diagnoses and less curable diagnoses, producing lower survival rates from breast cancer among Latinas. A similar pattern exists with cervical cancer. In addition to barriers to health care access, several cultural factors, including the belief that cancer is not curable, may contribute to comparatively low cancer screening rates among Latinos.

Cardiovascular and Pulmonary Health Issues

The number one cause of death in the United States, regardless of ethnicity, is cardiovascular disease, including coronary heart disease, hypertension, and stroke. These diseases, especially coronary heart disease and stroke, kill almost as many people in the United States as all other diseases combined, and they are among the leading causes of disability in the country. A national focus on lowering the rates of such diseases has contributed to a recent decline in rates of heart disease and stroke in the overall population of the country. Nationally, about one fourth of deaths among Latinos stem from cardiovascular conditions, and the rate is expected to rise in coming years as the Latino population ages. Latinas, in particular, are overrepresented among heart disease cases in the country.

Acquired Immune Deficiency Syndrome (AIDS)

Approximately 20% of people in the United States living with HIV infection are Latino, and it is expected that the overall number of new AIDS cases among Latinos will surpass that of non-Latino whites, raising critical questions about the adequacy and appropriateness of AIDS prevention and care

available to Latinos. This concern is sharpened by recognition that while improved prevention and treatment methods contributed to a general decline in AIDS cases for all ages, genders, and ethnicities during the 1990s, the decline was not distributed evenly, resulting in a widening gap between Latinos and non-Latino whites. While the decline nationally in new AIDS cases among non-Latino whites between the years 1993 and 2001 was 73% compared with previous years, among Latinos it was only 56%. Similarly, the number of deaths attributed to AIDS during this period fell by 80% among non-Latino whites but only by 63% among Latinos. The estimated AIDS prevalence (i.e., accumulated cases) among non-Latino whites during this period rose by 68%, in contrast, among Latinos prevalence jumped by 130%, further affirming significant AIDS disparities between Latinos and the majority population.

—*Merrill Singer*

See also Cultural Sensitivity; Health Communication; Health Disparities

Further Readings

Aguirre-Molina, M., Molina, C., & Zambrana, R. (2001). *Health issues in the Latino community.* New York: Jossey-Bass.

Asencio, M. (2002). *Sex and sexuality among New York's Puerto Rican youth.* Boulder, CO: Lynne Rienner.

Diaz, R. (1998). *Latino gay men and HIV: Culture, sexuality and risk behavior.* New York: Routledge.

LaVeist, T. (Ed.). (2002). *Race, ethnicity, and health: A public health reader.* New York: Jossey-Bass.

LaVeist, T. (2005). *Minority populations and health: An introduction to health disparities in the U.S.* New York: Jossey-Bass.

Perez, D. (2006). *Understanding Latino health policy and barriers to care.* New York: ProQuest.

Smedley, B., Stith, A., & Nelson, A. (Eds.). (2002). *Unequal treatment: Confronting racial and ethnic disparities in health.* Washington, DC: National Academies Press.

LEAD

Lead and its compounds have been used in countless ways for thousands of years, despite the equally long history of knowledge about the dangers of lead. Exposure to lead-containing goods and the environmental contamination from their manufacture and use produces considerable mortality and morbidity among workers, children, and the general public. Lead's toxicity appears to have no threshold for harm: Blood-lead levels (BLLs) $< 10 \mu$g/dl (well below those associated with clinical symptoms of lead poisoning) are associated with neurological deficits in children, while slightly elevated BLLs are implicated in increased rates of hypertension and kidney disease in adults. At higher BLLs, clinical signs of lead poisoning appear, including chronic or acute gastrointestinal symptoms and neurological conditions ranging from palsies to paralysis and encephalopathy.

Sources of Exposure to Lead

There are three primary avenues of exposure to lead: (1) environmental sources that are more or less shared by all persons in a given population; (2) occupational exposures from manufacturing or handling lead and lead products; and (3) pediatric exposures, due to the special environmental, behavioral, and metabolic features of early childhood.

Until a few decades ago, people living in industrialized nations routinely faced lead levels higher than those in industrial settings where lead was used, as a result of exposure via air pollution, water supply systems, adulterated foods, medicines, and other sources. Assays of historical lead pollution show a steady increase in bioavailable lead in the general environment from early-modern times, accelerating dramatically in the middle of the 20th century with increased consumption of leaded gasoline. In addition to such airborne sources, lead made its way into foods via insecticide residues and pigments and into drinking water via solid-lead or lead-soldered water supply pipes. Lead-tainted alcohol is implicated in widespread chronic illness from the 18th century through the early 20th century, and alcohol distilled illegally in lead-soldered automotive radiators (e.g., "moonshine") continues to produce occasional outbreaks of saturnism.

At the beginning of the 20th century, the health burden of these universal exposures remained largely hidden beneath the crushing mortality and morbidity from lead in the workplace. From 1910 to 1930, federal mortality statistics reported more than a hundred lead-poisoning deaths annually. But these reports drastically underreported lead-poisoning cases; Leake, a New York physician, complained in 1927 that "there are many plants. . . from which no lead cases are reported, except those failing to 'get by' the coroner" (Leake, 1927). In the Progressive Era (ca. 1890–1913), the fatal conditions in America's lead factories prompted a number of government-sponsored investigations, such as those conducted by Alice Hamilton. The resulting social and political pressure, together with a constricting labor market and the adoption of workers' compensation laws, prompted manufacturers to adopt basic improvements in ventilation and processes. Workers' compensation laws also transformed factory culture, as an empowered force of industrial hygienists sought to control the physical and fiscal costs of occupational sickness. Together, these factors dramatically lowered American workers' exposure to bioavailable lead.

It took considerably longer to fully assess and respond to the ubiquitous dangers lead posed children. Young children in urban and suburban environments were exposed to most of the "universal" sources adults faced, prompting one astute pediatrician, Ruddock, in 1924 to alert his peers that "the child lives in a lead world."

Young children's normal hand-to-mouth activities increase their exposure to any lead dust in their environment (whether from painted surfaces or from air pollution), and teething and oral exploratory activities can lead to the direct ingestion of lead paint. In addition to these behaviors, children's stature and their age-specific metabolic characteristics amplify both the level of exposure and the rate of lead absorption. Despite this, childhood lead poisoning was nearly invisible prior to the 1930s. Federal mortality statistics from 1910 to 1930 typically reported fewer than five pediatric lead-poisoning deaths annually.

Several factors combined to produce this statistical silence. First was the association of lead poisoning with occupational exposure and the dominance of occupational exposure in defining where lead poisoning was to be found and what symptoms and causative factors physicians looked for. Because the typical nursery looked nothing like the typical paint factory, medical professionals assumed that lead poisoning would not occur in the nursery. Second was the dominance of acute infectious diseases as the main health hazard of the young: Several hundred children dying from the toxicants in their environment barely registered compared with the numbers killed annually by contagious diseases. The statistical picture was also confused by a third factor: Lead poisoning's wide symptomatology easily allowed misdiagnosis by doctors who attributed the gastrointestinal and neurological symptoms seriously lead-poisoned children presented to infectious causes. Gradually, a more accurate picture of childhood lead poisoning developed, though this realization was slowed considerably by the fourth factor: As medical interest in pediatric lead poisoning rose, the disease quickly came to be perceived as one of poverty, and of race—just one more tragic problem of the ghetto—and treated with similar complacency; as one researcher, Conway, put it in 1940, "like the poor, lead poisoning is always with us."

Historical Changes in Lead Exposure

Given what we now know about the effects of lead absorption, and with due consideration for the work yet to be done, the dramatic reduction since the 1960s in the amount of bioavailable lead in the environment, and the corresponding drop in average BLLs, must be considered one of the 20th century's greatest public health achievements. Lead production and reliance on lead products have not waned; in fact, annual global production of lead rarely drops far below 3 million metric tons since it peaked in 1977, at 3.5 million. In the United States, the amount of lead consumed (i.e., in the economic sense) remains at near record highs, between 1.3 and 1.7 metric tons annually, with approximately 80% going to storage batteries. But lead consumption (in the metabolic sense) has fallen dramatically, due primarily to the elimination of lead-laced consumer goods, such as ethylized gasoline, lead-based paints, and the widespread use of lead solder in canned foods and plumbing. The impact of leaded gasoline's phase out on average BLL was practically instantaneous, while the impact of shifting from lead-based house paints (well underway in the 1940s as other pigments became economically attractive) has been incremental, with the gradual removal or encapsulation of lead-painted surfaces.

Tracing the body burden of lead in populations is impossible for years prior to the standardization and wide availability of accurate BLL analysis (now routinely done with atomic absorption spectroscopy) and sufficiently robust screening programs, beginning roughly in the 1970s. But case-finding programs in American cities in the 1950s and 1960s suggest that *average* BLLs for urban Americans were >20 μg/dl of whole blood. The distribution of risk was skewed heavily toward the urban poor: for example, a 1956

Baltimore study found that of 333 babies attending well-baby clinics, more than 40% had BLLs >50 μg/dl and 21 of these "asymptomatic" children carried a lead burden in excess of 80 μg/dl. Beginning with the Second National Health and Nutritional Examination Survey (NHANES II), conducted from 1976 to 1980, a much clearer picture of average lead burdens emerged; and together with the subsequent NHANES III and "Continuous NHANES," the series provide dramatic evidence of the progress in reducing average BLLs since the 1970s. Geometric mean BLLs in late 1970s ranged from 10 to 15.8 μg/dl, and the mean for children aged between 1 and 5 years was 15 μg/dl. By 1991, the average BLL had declined to 3.6 μg/dl; by 1999, it stood at 1.9 μg/dl. The prevalence of BLLs > 10 μg/dl fell dramatically as well. Where NHANES II found that 88% of children aged 1 to 5 years had elevated BLLs, by the end of the century that number had fallen from 98% to 1.6%. Racial and ethnic disparities remain, however. NHANES data from 1999 to 2002 show that the percentage of black children aged 1 to 5 years with elevated BLLs (3.1%) was nearly twice (1.6%) that for all children aged 1 to 5 years.

It is only as average BLLs decline that the health effects of lower exposure levels can be determined. The impact of this fact is clear in the federal government's gradual lowering of the "threshold" for harm in pediatric cases. In 1970, the Surgeon General defined BLLs > 70 μg/dl as "undue lead absorption"; a year later the Centers for Disease Control and Prevention (CDC) established 40 μg/dl as the level above which children should be treated for lead. In 1975, this number was reduced to 30; it was lowered to 25 μg/dl 10 years later and to 15 μg/dl in 1990. Since 1991, the CDC has defined 10 μg/dl as "elevated." The agency insists that this is not a "definitive toxicologic threshold," but a useful level for assessing and managing risks. For example, the Department of Health and Human Services "Healthy People 2010" program intends to eliminate all BLLs > 10 μg/dl among children aged 1 to 5 years by 2010. The adequacy of even that goal is challenged by recent studies suggesting that lead's impact on IQ scores increases more sharply between 0 and 10 μg/dl than it does above that "threshold."

—*Christian Warren*

See also Environmental and Occupational Epidemiology; Hamilton, Alice; National Health and Nutrition Examination Survey; Pollution; Urban Health Issues

Further Readings

Bellinger, D. C., & Bellinger, A. M. (2006). Childhood lead poisoning: The torturous path from science to policy. *Journal of Clinical Investigation, 116*, 853–857.

Centers for Disease Control and Prevention. (2005). *Preventing lead poisoning in young children.* Atlanta, GA: Author.

Conway, N. (1940). Lead poisoning: From unusual causes. *Industrial Medicine, 9*, 471–477.

Leake, J. P. (1927). Lead hazards. *Journal of the American Medical Association, 89*, 1113.

Ruddock, J. C. (1924). Lead poisoning in children with special reference to pica. *Journal of the American Medical Association, 82*, 1682.

Warren, C. (2000). *Brush with death: A social history of lead poisoning.* Baltimore: Johns Hopkins University Press.

Life Course Approach

A life course approach to epidemiology is the study of the long-term effects on health and disease risk of biological, behavioral, social, and psychological exposures that occur during gestation, childhood, adolescence, and adulthood. The approach recognizes that exposures and disease pathways may operate independently, cumulatively, and interactively throughout an individual's life course, across generations, and on population-level disease trends. It acknowledges that exposures that occur during certain critical or sensitive developmental periods may have particular long-term health effects. Within chronic disease epidemiology, the life course approach has both challenged and expanded the prevailing adult lifestyle model of chronic disease risk. While many conceptual and methodological challenges remain, this renewed perspective within epidemiology has catalyzed a reconceptualizing of pathways of disease etiology and contributed to an increasingly multilevel and integrative understanding of the social, psychological, and biological determinants of health.

Historical Background

The idea of childhood origins of risk for adult diseases was present in epidemiology and public health thinking during the first half of the 20th century. This paralleled the development of a life course approach in disciplines, such as developmental psychology, demography, sociology, anthropology, human development,

and the biological sciences. After World War II, however, the adult risk factor model of disease, with its focus on clinical and biochemical markers in adults, became the dominant model within chronic disease epidemiology. The identification of the major adult lifestyle risk factors for coronary heart disease (CHD) solidified the success of this approach.

Nonetheless, since the late 1970s and 1980s, a growing body of evidence has documented the potential effects of poor growth, undernutrition, and infectious disease in early life and on the risk of adult cardiovascular and respiratory disease. The most influential of the research from this period originated from David Barker and colleagues in the United Kingdom, who used historical cohort studies to investigate the long-term effects of in utero biological programming associated with maternal and fetal undernutrition. The subsequent proliferation in the 1990s of research on the fetal origins of CHD, which often focused on the proxy of birth weight, met with initial resistance from proponents of the primacy of well-established adult risk factors. Life course epidemiology emerged partly as a synthesis of the two approaches, demonstrating that early life factors may act cumulatively or interactively with adult exposures to influence health and disease in later life.

Conceptual Models

Several conceptual models have emerged within the life course approach to health. One of these, the critical period model, focuses on the importance of the timing of exposure. It holds that biological programming occurring during critical periods of growth and development in utero and in early infancy has irreversible effects on fetal structure, physiology, and metabolism. This model is the basis of the fetal origins of adult disease hypothesis, elaborated by Barker and colleagues and now known as the developmental origins of health and disease (DOHaD), to reflect an expanded developmental time frame.

Research in DOHaD has suggested that the highest risk of CHD, central distribution of body fat, insulin resistance, type 2 diabetes, and the metabolic syndrome may be associated with a phenotype of lower birth weight coupled with a higher body mass index in childhood or adulthood. Many of these studies have explored the potential risk associated with accelerated postnatal catch-up growth. Researchers hypothesized that predictive adaptive responses by the fetus and infant lead to irreversible changes that may, when coupled with environments in childhood and adult life that differ from the one anticipated during early life, increase the risk of adult disease. Populations in the developing world undergoing urbanization and the nutritional transition to Western lifestyles may thus be particularly susceptible to this developmental mismatch risk pattern. Studies have also explored gene-environment interactions, including potential epigenetic modification of fetal genes by the in utero environment.

Another life course model is the accumulation of risk model, which posits that risk may amass gradually over the life course, although the effects may be greater during certain developmental periods. This concept of accumulation of disease risk suggests that as the number and/or duration of insults increase, there is increasing damage to biological systems. Accumulation of risk may occur among independent factors. If the factors are correlated, they may be related through risk clustering or via chains of risk with additive effects or trigger effects, in which only the final link of the chain produces the outcome. The life course perspective has contributed increasingly to the study of social determinants of health and health inequalities, since risk often clusters together in socially patterned ways. For instance, children of low socioeconomic position may also experience low birth weights, poor diets, passive smoke exposure, poor housing conditions, and exposure to violence. Risk accumulation is also reflected in the weathering hypothesis, which describes early health deterioration due to repeated experience with socioeconomic adversity and political marginalization, and a related concept of allostatic load, or the physiological burden imposed by stress.

Research and Policy Implications

Interdisciplinary life course research draws from such disparate fields as clinical medicine, social epidemiology, the social sciences, human development, and the biological sciences. The complex methodological challenges include difficulties inherent in using large prospective birth cohorts with repeated measures and analytical issues associated with modeling latency periods, hierarchical data, latent (unobserved) variables, dynamic disease trajectories, and multiple time-dependent interactions. Multilevel models, path analysis, and Markov models are just a few of the

analytical tools being used to model social and biological pathways and temporal and geographical patterns of disease distribution. As the body of evidence in life course research continues to grow, policymakers may be increasingly challenged to prioritize social and behavioral interventions in pregnancy and early childhood and to address macrolevel determinants of adult health and disease.

—Helen L. Kwon and Luisa N. Borrell

See also Aging, Epidemiology of; Barker Hypothesis; Cardiovascular Disease; Chronic Disease Epidemiology; Geographical and Social Influences on Health; Multilevel Modeling; Social Epidemiology

Further Readings

Barker, D. J. P. (1998). *Mothers, babies, and disease in later life* (2nd ed.). New York: Churchill Livingstone.

Ben-Shlomo, Y., & Kuh, D. (2002). A life course approach to chronic disease epidemiology: Conceptual models, empirical challenges, and interdisciplinary perspectives. *International Journal of Epidemiology, 31,* 285–293.

Kuh, D. L., & Ben-Shlomo, Y. (2004). *A life course approach to chronic disease epidemiology* (2nd ed.). Oxford, UK: Oxford University Press.

Kuh, D. L., & Hardy, R. (2002). *A life course approach to women's health.* Oxford, UK: Oxford University Press.

LIFE EXPECTANCY

Life expectancy is an estimate of the average number of additional years a person of a given age can expect to live. The most common measure of life expectancy is life expectancy at birth. Life expectancy is a hypothetical measure. It assumes that the age-specific death rates for the year in question will apply throughout the lifetime of those born in that year. The process, in effect, projects the age-specific mortality rates for a given period over the entire lifetime of the population born (or alive) during that time. The measure differs considerably by sex, age, race, and geographic location. Therefore, life expectancy is commonly given for specific categories, rather than for the population in general. For example, the life expectancy for white females in the United States who were born in 2003 is 80.5 years; that is, white female infants born in the United States in the year 2003 would be expected to live, on average, 80.5 years.

Life expectancy reflects local conditions. In less developed countries, life expectancy at birth is relatively low compared with more developed countries. In poor countries, life expectancy at birth is often lower than life expectancy at 1 year of age, because of a high infant mortality rate (commonly due to infectious disease or lack of access to a clean water supply).

Life expectancy is calculated by constructing a life table. The data required to construct a life table are the age-specific death rates for the population in question, which requires enumeration data for the number of people, and the number of deaths at each age for that population. By applying the age-specific death rates that were observed during the period, the average life expectancy for each of the age groups within this population is calculated. Life expectancy at any given age is the average number of additional years a person of that age would live if the age-specific mortality rates for that year continued to apply. For example, U.S. males who were 50 years old in 2003 had an average additional life expectancy of 28.5 years.

The potential accuracy of the estimated life expectancy depends on the completeness of the

Table 1   Expectation of Life by Age, Race, and Sex: United States, 2003

Age	All Races			White			Black		
	Total	*Male*	*Female*	*Total*	*Male*	*Female*	*Total*	*Male*	*Female*
0	77.4	74.7	80.0	77.9	75.3	80.4	72.6	68.9	75.9
1	77.0	74.3	79.5	77.4	74.8	79.8	72.6	69.0	75.9
5	73.1	70.4	75.6	73.4	70.9	76.9	68.7	65.2	72.0
10	68.1	65.5	70.6	68.5	65.9	71.0	63.8	60.2	67.1
15	63.2	60.5	65.7	63.5	61.0	66.0	58.9	55.3	62.1
20	58.4	55.8	60.8	58.7	56.2	61.1	54.1	50.6	57.2
25	53.6	51.2	56.0	54.0	51.6	56.3	49.5	46.2	52.4
30	48.9	46.5	51.1	49.2	46.9	51.4	44.9	41.7	47.7
35	44.1	41.8	46.3	44.5	42.2	46.6	40.3	37.3	43.0
40	39.5	37.2	41.5	39.8	37.6	41.8	35.8	32.9	38.4
45	34.9	32.8	36.9	35.2	33.1	37.1	31.5	28.6	34.0
50	30.5	28.5	32.3	30.7	28.7	32.5	27.4	24.7	29.8
55	26.2	24.3	27.9	26.4	24.5	28.0	23.7	21.1	25.7
60	22.2	20.4	23.7	22.3	20.5	23.7	20.1	17.8	21.9
65	18.4	16.8	19.7	18.4	16.8	19.7	16.8	14.8	18.3
70	14.8	13.4	15.9	14.9	13.4	15.9	13.8	12.0	15.0
75	11.7	10.5	12.5	11.6	10.4	12.5	11.1	9.6	12.1
80	8.9	7.9	9.5	8.8	7.9	9.4	8.8	7.6	9.5
85	6.6	5.9	7.0	6.5	5.8	6.9	6.9	6.0	7.3
90	4.8	4.3	5.0	4.7	4.2	4.9	5.3	4.6	5.6
95	3.5	3.1	3.5	3.4	3.0	3.4	4.1	3.5	4.2
100	2.5	2.2	2.5	2.4	2.1	2.4	3.1	2.7	3.1

Source: Arias (2006, p. 3).

census and mortality data available for the population in question. The completeness of this data varies from country to country. In the United States, official complete life tables based on registered deaths have been prepared since 1900, in connection with the decennial census. Beginning in 1945, annual abridged U.S. life tables have been published based on the annual death registration and estimates of the population. Complete life tables show life expectancy for every year of age, and abridged tables show life expectancy for 5- or 10-year age groups, rather than for single years. The U.S. National Center for Health Statistics is the agency that currently publishes national life tables, as well as state and regional life tables. The United Nations publishes national life tables for many countries in its Demographic Yearbook.

The "healthy life expectancy" or "disability-free life expectancy" is the average number of years a person is expected to live in good health, or without disability, given current age-specific mortality rates and disease and disability prevalence rates. Calculation of these figures requires reliable health statistics, as well as mortality and census data.

—*Judith Marie Bezy*

See also Life Tables; Mortality Rates; National Center for Health Statistics

Further Readings

Arias, E. (2006, April). United States life tables, 2003. *National Vital Statistics Reports, 54*(14), 1–40.

Siegel, J. S., & Swanson, D. A. (Eds.). (2004). *The methods and materials of demography* (2nd ed.). San Diego, CA: Elsevier Academic Press.

LIFE TABLES

A life table describes, in terms of various life table functions, the probability distribution of duration time in a tabular form. Duration time is the time interval from an initial time point to the occurrence of a point event such as death or incidence of disease. A point event is a transition from one state to another. For example, death is a transition from the alive state (a transient state) to the dead state (an absorbing state). If the initial time point is taken as birth and the point

event as death, then the time interval from birth to death is called the *life length* or *age-at-death*, and the life table that describes the distribution of the age-at-death is also called a mortality table (particularly by actuaries). In the case of period life tables, the life length random variable X is further decomposed into two random variables, *current age A* and *future lifetime Y*, and the distributions of all three random variables X, A, and Y are described in a period life table.

Construction of life tables has a long history, dating back to the 1662 Bills of Mortality by John Graunt and the famous 1693 mortality table constructed by Halley for the city of Breslau in what is now Poland. Construction of these two life tables, particularly Halley's table, can be regarded as marking the beginning of modern statistics and public health sciences. Modern life table methods are no longer limited to the study of human mortality and to their use in the calculation of life insurance premiums and annuities. They have been used to study the time to the first marriage and the duration of the marriage (as in the construction of nuptiality tables), the duration of intrauterine device use and birth control effectiveness (birth control life tables), labor force participation (working life tables), renewal of animal and plant populations (life cycles life tables), and so on. Epidemiologists are particularly interested in constructing life tables to measure the probabilities of disease incidence, remission, relapse, and death from competing causes as well as to study the expected duration of stay in healthy and morbid states. Morbidity and mortality life table functions can also be combined to measure the burden of diseases and injuries. These epidemiological uses involve many types of life tables, and constructing them requires considerable technical skills. As can be seen in the following descriptions, life table methods are more sophisticated than most other epidemiological methods.

Types of Life Tables

Life table analysis in each situation requires a new definition of the duration time through appropriate choices of the initial time point and the point event to define a life table type. Many types of life tables can be constructed: If the duration time is a *sojourn*—the length of time a stochastic process remains in a state after entering it, then the associated life table is called an *attrition life table*. If the observed sojourn is the sojourn in a single transient state until transiting to a single absorbing state, then the associated life table is called an *ordinary life table*. If more than one absorbing state is present, then the observed sojourn is the minimum of the individual sojourns until transiting to each respective absorbing state, and the resulting attrition life tables may include *multiple-decrement life table, net life table, cause-deleted life table*, and *cause-reduced life table*. Construction of these life tables requires consideration of competing risks, as death from one cause automatically prevents an individual from dying from another cause. If the duration time is the *total lifetime*—sum of different sojourns, then the associated life table is known as the *multistate* or *increment-decrement life table*. Whether it is an attrition life table or a multistate life table, two types of life tables can be constructed for use in each case. A *cohort* (or *generation*) *life table* is constructed from data on the initial birth cohort size and vital events as they occur in time in a real birth cohort and reflects the probability distribution of the life length and vital event in question in that cohort. In epidemiology and biostatistics, *modified cohort life tables* have also been constructed for follow-up studies of patient cohorts. *Period* (or *current*) *life table*, on the other hand, is constructed from cross-sectional data, namely, the schedule of vital rates observed during a short calendar time period (usually 1 or 3 years known as the *base period*), and reflects the probability distribution of the life length and vital event in question in a hypothetical cohort in the *stationary population*.

Depending on how finely the age axis is partitioned into intervals, each type of life table defined above can be constructed as an abridged, a complete, or a continuous life table. In an abridged life table, the first two age intervals are of lengths 1 and 4 years, respectively, with the remaining age intervals all having length 5 years. In a complete life table, all age intervals are 1 year long. In a continuous life table, age is treated as a continuous variable and the life table functions can be computed for any age (i.e., any nonnegative real number within the life span). Finally, each type of life table can be constructed for each stratum obtained from cross-classification by calendar time period, geographic region, sex, race, socioeconomic class, occupation, and so on. Table 1 is an abridged period life table for the male population in Canada, constructed from the age-specific

population, birth and death data observed in the base period 1990 to 1992.

Period Life Table and Stationary Population

Almost all published life tables are period life tables. Besides providing the basis for probability theory, stochastic processes, mathematical statistics, and population models, period life tables, rather than cohort life tables, are the more common applications for two reasons. (1) Data for constructing period life tables are more readily available, as they are routinely collected by governments, which is not the case with data for constructing cohort life tables. (2) Period life tables can be constructed to provide comparisons of mortality conditions at any past time point up to the present, while cohort life tables cannot be so constructed, as extinction of an entire birth cohort requires the whole life span and so the most recent cohort life table that can be constructed would have to be started a 100 or more years ago. A period life table depicts the distribution of the life length in a hypothetical cohort in the stationary population uniquely determined by the current mortality schedule of the observed population.

A stationary population is a special case of the stable population. It is a population that is closed against migration and characterized by (1) a constant annual number of births and (2) a constant mortality schedule over calendar time. Consequently, the annual number of births always equals the annual number of deaths and so the size of the population is stationary. In a stationary population, a death at any age at a given calendar time is instantly replaced by a birth at that calendar time. Moreover, the age distribution is fixed over calendar time so that the chance of surviving any given age interval is also constant over time. It, therefore, follows that the sequence of instantaneous age-specific death rates (i.e., the *force of mortality*) for any calendar year (period analysis) is identical to the sequence of instantaneous age-specific death rates for any cohort (cohort analysis), and so in a stationary population, a period life table is identical to a cohort life table. That is to say, one can regard a period life table as a hypothetical cohort life table constructed on a stationary population. The age distribution of such stationary population is uniquely determined by the

Table 1   Abridged Life Table for Canadian Males, 1990 to 1992

(1)	(2)	(3)	(4)	(5)	(6)	(7)	(8)	(9)	(10)
Start of the ith Age Interval $[x_i, x_{i+1})$	Conditional Probability of Dying in Interval	First-Order Survival Function	Death Density Function at Age	Hazard Function at Age x_i	Second-Order Survival Function at Age x_i	Stationary Population Segment	Individual Life Expectancy at Age x_i	Third-Order Survival Function at Age x_i	Population Life Expectancy at Age x_i
x_i	q_i	$l(x_i)$	$f(x_i)$	$h(x_i)$	$T(x_i)$	L_i	$e(x_i)$	$Y(x_i)$	$\varepsilon(x_i)$
0	.00758	100,000	.03947	.03947	7,433,284	99,357	74.33	289875994	39.90
1	.00157	99,242	.00094	.00095	7,333,927	395,991	73.90	282491142	38.52
5	.00103	98,946	.00016	.00016	6,937,936	494,480	70.12	253945670	36.60
10	.00131	98,845	.00017	.00017	6,443,456	493,979	65.19	220489298	34.22
15	.00462	98,715	.00056	.00057	5,949,477	492,552	60.27	189504426	31.85
20	.00581	98,259	.00112	.00114	5,456,925	489,872	55.54	160986563	29.50
25	.00580	97,688	.00114	.00116	4,967,053	487,029	50.85	134925085	27.16
30	.00648	97,121	.00117	.00120	4,480,024	484,079	46.13	111305673	24.84
35	.00794	96,492	.00138	.00143	3,995,945	480,611	41.41	90114252	22.55
40	.01052	95,726	.00170	.00177	3,515,334	476,276	36.72	71334841	20.29
45	.01684	94,719	.00248	.00262	3,039,058	469,921	32.08	54948149	18.08
50	.02751	93,124	.00399	.00428	2,569,137	459,739	27.59	40928175	15.93
55	.04632	90,562	.00650	.00718	2,109,398	443,164	23.29	29234364	13.86
60	.07629	86,367	.01054	.01220	1,666,234	416,510	19.29	19801232	11.88
65	.11915	79,778	.01604	.02011	1,249,724	376,338	15.67	12522223	10.02
70	.17784	70,273	.02186	.03110	873,386	321,515	12.43	7231441	8.28
75	.27287	57,775	.02855	.04942	551,871	250,498	9.55	3691536	6.69
80	.39491	42,010	.03351	.07977	301,373	168,162	7.17	1588560	5.27
85	.54434	25,420	.03153	.12404	133,211	90,716	5.24	533752	4.01
90+	1	11,583	.02293	.19797	42,495	42,495	3.67	120504	2.84

Source: Based on the method developed by the author described in Hsieh 1991a and 1991b.

mortality schedule used to construct the period life table. Thus, different mortality schedules would determine different stationary age distribution and hence different period life tables.

In interpreting the life table functions, the fact that the life table population is a stationary population should always be borne in mind. Thus, the life expectancy function computed from mortality rates observed in the year 1921, say, will underestimate the mean life length of the generation born that year because of the reduction in the force of mortality since then. In general, with the trend toward lower mortality, the expectation of life at birth computed from a period life table would understate the average length of life of a newly born generation. To determine the actual life expectancy for a generation, it is necessary to construct many period life tables at consecutive time periods and to concatenate them to form a generation life table. The direct application of period life tables is for comparative studies. Period life tables provide valid comparisons of mortality among different populations because the life table death rates, or equivalently the life expectancies, arise from the stationary population rather than from the actual observed population and hence are independent of the age distribution of the observed populations and so are devoid of any confounding by differential age distributions among the different observed populations.

Description of Period Life Table Functions

A period life table consists of many columns with age being the first column followed by several life table functions (see Table 1). Each life table function is a function of age and describes the distribution of the life length in a different way—in terms of density function, conditional distribution function, survival function, generalized survival function, and conditional expectation. The purpose of the tabular display is to provide simultaneously several life table function values at each of many different ages. A cohort life table has two life table columns less than a period life table, with the last two columns $Y(x_i)$ and $\varepsilon(x_i)$ excluded.

In Table 1, the first column, age, is the independent variable, which ranges from 0 to 90+, or 100+, or 110+, depending on the type of life table to be constructed. The age axis is partitioned into

age intervals $[x_i, x_{i+1})$ with interval length $\Delta x_i \equiv x_{i+1} - x_i = 1$ for all integral values x_i for a complete life table and $\Delta x_i = 5$ except for the first two age intervals in which $\Delta x_i = 1$ for the first age interval and $\Delta x_i = 4$ for the second interval, for $x_i = 0$, 1, 5 (5) 90 for an abridged life table. The remaining columns are the life table functions. The ordinary life table may include up to nine or more main life table functions (nine or more for period life table and seven or more for cohort life table). The unconditional life table functions in Columns 3, 4, 6, and 7 have two interpretations: The first depicts the probability distribution of the life length in a hypothetical cohort, and the second describes the stationary population structure. The remaining conditional life table functions have only one interpretation with Columns 2, 5, and 8 having the first (hypothetical cohort) interpretation and Columns 9 and 10 having the second (stationary population) interpretation.

Column 2, conditional probability of death, $q_i = \Pr\{X < x_{i+1} | x \ge x_i\} = 1 - l(x_{i+1})/l(x_i)$, which is the conditional probability of dying before age x_{i+1} given survival to age x_i (hypothetical cohort interpretation).

Column 3, survivorship function, $l(x_i) = 10^5 \Pr\{X > x_i\}$, which is the expected number surviving to age x_i out of the initial cohort of 100,000 live births (hypothetical cohort interpretation). This implies that $l(x_i)$ is proportional to the survival function $S(x_i) = \Pr\{X > x_i\}$ of the life length X or the expected number alive at age x_i per year in a stationary population supported by 100,000 annual live births (stationary population interpretation), which implies that $l(x_i)$ is proportional to the density function of the current age A and of the future lifetime Y.

Column 4, death density function,

$$f(x_i) = \lim_{\Delta x_i \downarrow 0} \frac{\Pr\{x_i \le X < x_i + \Delta x_i\}}{\Delta x_i},$$

which is the probability per unit time of dying in the age interval $[x_i, x_i + \Delta x_i)$ $(M-1)$ as Δx_i tends to 0, for a member of the initial cohort of live births (hypothetical cohort interpretation) or the expected proportion of deaths per year in the age interval $[x_i, x_i + \Delta x_i)$ $(M-1)$ as Δx_i tends to 0, among the live births during any fixed calendar time period in a stationary population (stationary population interpretation).

This function describes the left-skewed distribution of the life length X, implying that the mean (74.34 years, obtained from Column 8 below) is less than the median (77.4 years, obtained from Column 3 above), which in turn is less than the mode (81.2 years, obtained from Column 4). Note that this curve has two peaks, one at the start of life and the other at age 81.2 years and that the area under the whole curve is one.

Column 5, hazard function (force of mortality),

$$h(x_i) = \lim_{\Delta x_i \downarrow 0} \frac{\Pr\{X < x_i + \Delta x_i | X \geq x_i\}}{\Delta x_i},$$

which is the probability per unit time of dying in the age interval $[x_i, x_i + \Delta x_i)$ as Δx_i tends to 0, for a member of the cohort surviving to age x_i (hypothetical cohort interpretation). Note that $h(0) = f(0)$ and $h(x) = f(x)/S(x) > f(x)$ for all $x > 0$, so that $S(x) = \exp(-\int_0^x h(u)du)$. Notice also the almost exponential growth of the hazard function after age 30 years.

Column 6, second-order survivorship function, $T(x_i) = \int_{x_i}^{\omega} l(u)du$, which is the expected number of person-years lived beyond age x_i by the $l(x_i)$ survivors of the initial cohort of 100,000 live births (hypothetical cohort interpretation), which implies that $T(x_i)$ is proportional to the second-order survival function $S^{(2)}(x_i) \equiv \int_{x_i}^{\infty} S(u)du$ of the life length X or the expected population size beyond age x_i in a stationary population supported by 100,000 annual live births (stationary population interpretation), which implies that $T(x_i)$ is proportional to the survival function of the current age A and of the future lifetime Y. The second interpretation of this function can be used to estimate the annual number of births from the observed population size.

Column 7, stationary population segment, $L_i = \int_{x_i}^{x_{i+1}} l(u)du$, which is the expected number of person-years lived in the age interval $[x_i, x_i + \Delta x_i)$ by the $l(x_i)$ survivors of the 100,000 initial birth cohort (hypothetical cohort interpretation) or the expected population size in the age interval $[x_i, x_i + \Delta x_i)$ in a stationary population supported by 100,000 annual live births (stationary population interpretation). The second interpretation of this function can be used to make population projection. This column can also be used in combination with Column 3 to form age-specific life table death rates $m_i \equiv [l(x_i) - l(x_{i+1})]/L_i$ for precise age-adjusted mortality comparisons and other uses.

Column 8, individual life expectancy function, $e(x_i) \equiv E\{X - x_i | X > x_i\} = T(x_i)/l(x_i)$, which is the expected remaining life length conditional on

survival to age x (hypothetical cohort interpretation). This function may be used to compare summary mortality levels of different populations.

Column 9, third-order survivorship function, $Y(x_i) = \int_{x_i}^{\omega} T(u)du$, which is the expected future person-years lived by the $T(x)$ people aged x and above in the stationary population supported by 100,000 annual live births (stationary population interpretation).

Column 10, population life expectancy function, $\varepsilon(x_i) \equiv E[Y|A \geq x_i] = Y(x_i)/T(x_i)$, which is the expected remaining lifetime for the $T(x_i)$ people aged x_i and above in the stationary population supported by 100,000 annual live births (stationary population interpretation). This function is a statistically more robust estimator of summary mortality than Column 8, $e(x_i)$.

In addition to these main life table functions, higher-order survival functions and the variances of their empirical life table functions can also be calculated, which are needed for statistical inference (see Application section below).

Construction of Period Life Tables

To construct a life table means to calculate the life table functions from the observed age-specific exposure and decrement data. Large population cohort life tables can be directly constructed from the cohort data by using simple arithmetic operations, division, multiplication, addition, and subtraction, to calculate the life table functions. However, for human populations, construction of a complete cohort life table would require more than 100 years of follow-up data that are rather difficult to obtain. To construct a period (current) life table is a totally different matter, as it requires conversion of the cross-sectional observed data on age-specific deaths and populations or their combinations, death rates, observed in a short base period of 1 to 3 years into the hypothetical cohort (stationary population) life table functions in terms of conditional probabilities and expectations. Construction of period (current) life tables requires a great deal of mathematical skill, because conversion from observed age-specific death rates M_i into conditional probability of death q_i requires accurate approximations and so are the evaluation of death density function $f(x)$, hazard function $h(x)$, and person-year functions $T(x)$ and $Y(x)$ that are all derived from the q_i function. Different life table methods render different solutions to these approximation problems and so produce slightly different life table function values. The life table shown in Table 1 is constructed using Hsieh's method of 1991 that has been tested to be more accurate than other existing methods. For detailed methods of life table construction and derivation of the standard errors of empirical life table functions, see references listed in Further Readings, particularly those of Chiang, Hsieh, and Keyfitz.

Applications of Life Table Functions

The superiority of the life table method over other epidemiological methods, such as direct and indirect standardization, is that comparisons using standardization methods depend on the choice of the standard population to adjust the age-specific rates and such adjustment can lead to opposing conclusions due to arbitrariness of the choice of the standard population. On the other hand, all period (current) life tables are defined by the stationary population model whose age-sex distribution has a fixed bell shape and so the comparison using period life tables is independent of the age distribution of the observed populations. Thus, the life table method provides a standardized comparison free of age confounding with definitive conclusion. Life table functions have many applications, several of which have been described in the previous sections. Here, we shall concentrate on their applications in epidemiology and public health.

Ordinary cohort and period (current) life tables may be used to compare the intensity of the point event of interest between two strata (such as two geographic regions) by using two-sample Z-test on any of the corresponding life table functions from each stratum. This is because all empirical life table functions are asymptotically Gaussian. For example, to compare mortality for a given age interval $[x, x + \Delta x]$ between two strata, we may use the function $\Delta x q_x$. To compare mortality for ages beyond x, we may use the function $e(x)$; and to compare mortality for ages before x, we may use the function $l(x)$; to compare mortality for all ages, we may use the value $e(0)$. The same four life table functions from the net life table may be used to compare mortality from a given cause between the two strata, adjusting for the competing risks.

To evaluate the impact of a given cause on longevity of a given population, we can compare a cause-deleted life table with the ordinary life table in terms of the differences of three ordinary life table functions and the corresponding functions with cause k eliminated: $\Delta x q_x - \Delta x q_x^{\bullet k}, [l^{\bullet k}(x) - l(x)]/1(0)$, and $e^{\bullet k}(x) - e(x)$, which represent potential reduction in age-specific mortality rate, gain in survival probability, and gain in life expectancy, respectively, if cause k were eliminated as a risk of death. We may also compare the percentage change by computing $[\Delta x q_x - \Delta x q^{\bullet k} x]/\Delta x q_x, [l^{\bullet k}(x) - l(x)]/l(x)$, and $[e^{\bullet k}(x) - e(x)]/e(x)$.

As the survivorship function increases toward its natural rectangular limit, ordinary cohort and period (current) life tables become less useful as health measures. But they can be used to compute disability-free life expectancy (DFLE) by combining the life table function $l(x)$ (mortality) with the age-specific disability prevalence estimated from cross-sectional survey data (morbidity), as done in Sullivan's method. Disability-adjusted life expectancy (DALE) can also be calculated by weighting different levels of disabilities. Alternatively, DFLE may be obtained by constructing a multistate life table with three states: healthy, disabled, and dead. DFLE may be calculated as the area between the survival curve against the disable state and the survival curve against the dead state to the right divided by the height of the survival curve against the dead state.

Ordinary cohort and period (current) life tables may be used to compute years of life lost (YLL) by summing the products of observed number of death at each age and the age weighted, discounted life expectancy at that age for the loss of life through death. We can also compute years lived with disability (YLD) to account for loss of quality of life through disability by summing the products of observed number of disability incidences at each age, the severity score of the disability, and the duration of disability, the last being obtainable by constructing a multistate life table with two transient states: healthy, disability (illness) and one absorbing state (death), and by subtracting the area under the survival curve for death from the area under the survival curve for disability (or illness). Addition of YLL to YLD yields DALY, disability-adjusted life years that have been used to measure and compare the burden of disease.

Counts of survivors and deaths in an ordinary life table may be treated as point processes and used to compute quantities of use in epidemiology and demography, such as conditional probabilities of death and expected life lengths, in any regions of the Lexis diagram given surviving a certain region of the Lexis diagram. For multiple decrement and multistate life tables, the point process methods can be used to compute conditional probabilities of stay in each state and expected duration of stay in any transient state given surviving a certain region of the Lexis diagram.

The survivorship function $l(x)$, the second-order survivorship function $T(x)$, and the third-order survivorship function $Y(x)$ in the ordinary and net life tables can be used to compute the Lorenz curve $1 - [T(x) + xl(x)]/T(0)$, scaled total-time-on-test $1 - T(x)/T(0)$, Gini index $2\int_0^1\{x - 1 + [T(x) + xl(x)]dx\}/T(0)$ and variances of their empirical estimates for comparative statistical analysis of morbidity and mortality in public health using Central Limit Theorem for Brownian bridge and Brownian motion processes.

—John J. Hsieh

See also Birth Cohort Analysis; Direct Standardization; Global Burden of Disease Project; Graunt, John; Hazard Rate; Life Expectancy; Mortality Rates

Further Readings

Bowers, N., Gerber, H., Hickman, J., Jones, D., & Nesbitt, C. (1986). *Actuarial mathematics.* Itasca, IL: Society of Actuaries.

Chiang, C. L. (1968). *Introduction to stochastic processes in biostatistics.* New York: Wiley.

Chiang, C. L. (1984). *The life table and its applications.* Malabar, FL: Robert E. Krieger.

Colvez, A., & Blanchet, M. (1983). Potential gains in the life expectancy free of disability: A tool for health planning. *International Journal of Epidemiology, 12,* 224–229.

Ebert, T. A. (1999). *Plant and animal populations: Methods in demography.* New York: Academic Press.

Hsieh, J. J. (1985). Construction of expanded infant life tables: A method based on a new mortality law. *Mathematical Biosciences, 76,* 221–242.

Hsieh, J. J. (1989). A probabilistic approach to the construction of competing-risk life tables. *Biometrical Journal, 31,* 339–357.

Hsieh, J. J. (1991a). A general theory of life table construction and a precise abridged life table method. *Biometrical Journal, 33,* 143–162.

Hsieh, J. J. (1991b). Construction of expanded continuous life tables: A generalization of abridged and completed life tables. *Mathematical Biosciences, 103,* 287–302.

Keyfitz, N., & Caswell, H. (2005). *Applied mathematical demography.* New York: Springer.

Preston, S. H., Heuveline, P., & Guillot, M. (2001). *Demography: Measuring and modelling population process.* Oxford, UK: Blackwell.

Preston, S. H., Keyfitz, N., & Schoen, R. (1972). *Causes of death: Life tables for national populations.* New York: Seminar Press.

Rogers, A. (1995). *Multiregional demography: Principles, methods and extensions.* Chichester: Wiley.

Salomon, J. A., & Murray, C. (2002). The epidemiologic transition revisited: Compositional models for causes of death by age and sex. *Population and Development Review, 28,* 205–228.

Schoen, R. (1988). *Modeling multigroup populations.* New York: Plenum Press.

Sullivan, D. F. (1971). A single index of mortality and morbidity. *Health Services and Mental Health Administration Health Reports, 86,* 347–354.

LIKELIHOOD RATIO

The likelihood ratio is used to compare different data models, perform hypothesis tests, and construct confidence intervals. The likelihood of a model is a measure of how well the model fits the observed data. Model likelihood is most often used when fitting a parametric model (e.g., a normal distribution) to data to find the parameters that best describe the data. The general formula for the likelihood function is

$$L(\theta|D) = P(\mathbf{D}|\theta),$$

where

θ is the model parameterization,

$\mathbf{D}$ is the observed data,

$L(\theta|D)$ is the likelihood of the model parameterization given the observed data $\mathbf{D}$, and

$P(\mathbf{D}|\theta)$ is the probability density function of the data given the model parameterization θ.

The basis for this formulation of the likelihood function is best understood by using Bayes's theorem to calculate the probability of the model given the observed data:

$$P(\theta|\mathbf{D}) = \frac{P(\mathbf{D}|\theta)P(\theta)}{P(\mathbf{D})}.$$

If we assume that all models are equally likely and note that the probability of the observed data is fixed, this formula is proportional to the likelihood formula given above. That is, for any two model parameterizations if the likelihood of one parameterization is greater than that of the other, then the probability of that parameterization is also greater by the above formula.

When comparing two models, we use their likelihood ratio. The formula for the likelihood ratio is

$$\lambda(\mathbf{D}) = \frac{L(\theta_0 | \mathbf{D})}{L(\theta_1 | \mathbf{D})}.$$

In hypothesis testing, the top model parameterization (θ_0) represents the null hypothesis and the bottom parameterization (θ_1) represents the alternative hypothesis. We will reject the null hypothesis in favor of the alternative hypothesis if $\lambda(\mathbf{D}) < c$, where c is some preselected critical value. Confidence intervals, sometimes referred to as supported intervals when using this approach, can be calculated in a similar manner. In this approach, the value of θ that maximizes the likelihood (the maximum likelihood estimate) is used to determine the denominator (θ_1) and alternative parameterizations are used in the numerator (θ_0). The supported region consists of those values of (θ_0) where $\lambda(\mathbf{D}) < c$, where c is some critical value. Some statisticians and epidemiologists argue that these approaches are superior to traditional approaches because they incorporate the probability of the observed data given the alternative models into the calculation, not only the probability under the null hypothesis.

Another common use of the likelihood ratio occurs when performing a likelihood ratio test. A likelihood ratio test is used when comparing a model with fewer parameters with a more complex one (i.e., one with more parameters). In general, the more complex model will fit the observed data better. To determine if this increase in goodness of fit is enough to justify the increase in model complexity, we first calculate the likelihood ratio test statistic:

$$LR = -2\frac{\ln L_0}{\ln L_1},$$

where

L_0 is the likelihood of the simpler model using the maximum likelihood parameter estimate and

L_1 is the likelihood of the more complex model using the maximum likelihood parameter estimate.

This statistic is then used as the test statistic in a chi-squared test with n degrees of freedom, where n is the number of additional parameters in the more complex model. If the chi-squared test is greater than the $1 - \alpha$ region of a chi-squared distribution, the more complex model is accepted as valid; otherwise the simpler model is used.

—Justin Lessler

See also Bayes's Theorem; Chi-Square Test; Degrees of Freedom; Likelihood Ratio

Further Readings

Goodman, S. N. (1993). P-values, hypothesis tests, and likelihood: Implications for epidemiology of a neglected historical debate. *American Journal of Epidemiology, 137*, 485–495.

Hills, M. (1996). *Statistical models in epidemiology.* Oxford, UK: Oxford University Press.

LIKERT SCALE

Likert scales are rating scales used in questionnaires that measure people's attitudes, opinions, or perceptions. Subjects choose from a range of possible responses to a specific question or statement, such as "strongly agree," "agree," "neutral," "disagree," "strongly disagree." Often, the categories of response are coded numerically, in which case the numerical values must be defined for that specific study, such as $1 = strongly\ agree$, $2 = agree$, and so on. Likert scales are named for Rennis Likert, who devised them in 1932.

Likert scales are widely used in social and educational research. Epidemiologists may employ Likert scales in surveying topics such as attitudes toward health or toward specific behaviors that affect health (e.g., smoking); opinions about the relative importance, efficacy, or practicality of different treatment options; and public perceptions about health care, the role of health professionals, or risk factors for specific diseases. When using Likert scales, the researcher must consider issues such as categories of response (values in the scale), size of the scale, direction of the scale, the ordinal nature of Likert-derived data, and appropriate statistical analysis of such data.

Categories of Response

Generally, a Likert scale presents the respondent with a statement and asks the respondent to rate the extent to which he or she agrees with it. Variations include presenting the subject with a question rather than a statement. The categories of response should be mutually exclusive and should cover the full range of opinion. Some researchers include a "don't know" option, to distinguish between respondents who do not feel sufficiently informed to give an opinion and those who are "neutral" on the topic.

Size of Likert Scales

The size of Likert scales may vary. Traditionally, researchers have employed a 5-point scale (e.g., strongly agree, agree, neutral, disagree, strongly disagree). A larger scale (e.g., seven categories) could offer more choice to respondents, but it has been suggested that people tend not to select the extreme categories in large rating scales, perhaps not wanting to appear extreme in their view. Moreover, it may not be easy for subjects to discriminate between categories that are only subtly different. On the other hand, rating scales with just three categories (e.g., poor, satisfactory, good) may not afford sufficient discrimination. A current trend is to use an even number of categories, to force respondents to come down broadly "for" or "against" a statement. Thus, 4-point or 6-point Likert scales are increasingly common.

Directionality of Likert Scales

A feature of Likert scales is their directionality: The categories of response may be increasingly positive or increasingly negative. While interpretation of a category may vary among respondents (e.g., one person's "agree" is another's "strongly agree"), all respondents should nevertheless understand that "strongly agree" is a more positive opinion than "agree." One important consideration in the design of questionnaires is the use of reverse scoring on some items. Imagine a questionnaire with positive statements about the benefits of public health education programs (e.g., "TV campaigns are a good way to persuade people to stop smoking in the presence of children"). A subject who strongly agreed with all such statements would be presumed to have a very positive view about the benefits of this method of health education. However, perhaps the subject was not participating wholeheartedly and simply checked the same response category for each item. To ensure that respondents are reading and evaluating statements carefully, it is good practice to include a few negative statements (e.g., "Money spent on public health education programs would be better spent on research into new therapies"). If a respondent answers positively to positive statements and negatively to negative statements, the researcher may have increased confidence in the data. Thus, it is good practice to employ reverse scoring of some items.

Ordinal Measures and the Use of Descriptive and Inferential Statistics

Likert scales fall within the ordinal level of measurement: The categories of response have directionality, but the intervals between them cannot be presumed equal. Thus, for a scale where $1 = strongly\ agree$, $2 = agree$, $3 = neutral$, $4 = disagree$, and $5 = strongly\ disagree$, we can say 4 is more negative than 3, 2, or 1 (directionality); but we cannot infer that a response of 4 is twice as negative as a response of 2.

Deciding which descriptive and inferential statistics may legitimately be used to describe and analyze the data obtained from a Likert scale is a controversial issue. Treating Likert-derived data as ordinal, one should employ the median or mode as the measure of central tendency. In addition, one may state the frequency/percentage frequency of responses in each category. The appropriate inferential statistics for ordinal data are those employing nonparametric tests, such as chi-square, Spearman's rho, or the Mann-Whitney U test.

However, many researchers treat Likert-derived data as if it were at the interval level (where numbers on the scale not only have directionality but also are an equal distance apart). They use the mean and standard deviation to describe their data and analyze it with "powerful" parametric tests, such as ANOVA or Pearson's product-moment correlation, arguing this is legitimate provided one states the assumption that the data are interval level. Calculating the mean, standard deviation, and parametric statistics requires arithmetic manipulation of data (e.g., addition, multiplication).

Since numerical values in Likert scales represent verbal statements, one might question whether it makes sense to perform such manipulations. Moreover, Likert-derived data may fail to meet other assumptions for parametric tests (e.g., a normal distribution). Thus, careful consideration must also be given to the appropriate descriptive and inferential statistics, and the researcher must be explicit about any assumptions made.

—Susan Jamieson

See also Chi-Square Test; Measures of Central Tendency; Nonparametric Statistics; Normal Distribution; Questionnaire Design

Further Readings

Burns, R. B. (2000). Attitude surveys. In R. B. Burns (Ed.), *Introduction to research methods* (4th ed., pp. 555–565). London, UK: Sage.

Clegg, F. (1998). *Simple statistics.* Cambridge, UK: Cambridge University Press.

Cohen, L., Manion, L., & Morrison, K. (2000). *Research methods in education* (5th ed.). London, UK: Routledge Falmer.

Jamieson, S. (2004). Likert scales: How to (ab)use them. *Medical Education, 38,* 1217–1218.

LIND, JAMES
(1716–1794)

James Lind, the founder of British naval hygiene, was a Scottish physician who discovered the cause of scurvy, a dietary deficiency due to lack of vitamin C. His legacy as one of the first modern clinical investigators reflected his desire to improve the health of soldiers and sailors.

Lind was born in Edinburgh, Scotland, the son of Margaret Smelum and James Lind, a merchant. In 1731, Lind registered as an apprentice to George Langlands, an Edinburgh physician. Lind began his naval career in 1739 as a surgeon's mate and was promoted to surgeon in 1747.

While serving on the *H.M.S. Salisbury* in 1747, Lind carried out experiments on scurvy. He selected 12 men from the ship, all suffering from symptoms of scurvy and divided them into six pairs. He then gave each group different supplements to their basic diet. Two men were given an unspecified elixir three times a day; two were treated with seawater; two were fed with a combination of garlic, mustard, and horseradish; two were given spoonfuls of vinegar; two received a quart of cider a day; and the last two were given two oranges and one lemon every day. Lind recorded no improvement with the first four diets, slight improvement in the men given cider, and significant improvement in those fed citrus fruit.

In 1748, Lind left the navy and obtained his M.D. from the University of Edinburgh later that year. In 1750, Lind became fellow of the Royal College of Physicians of Edinburgh and later served as treasurer from December 1756 to 1758. He published *A Treatise of the Scurvy* in 1753. Although the *Treatise* garnered little acclaim at the time, it attracted the attention of Lord Anson, then first Lord of the Admiralty, and to whom it was dedicated. Lord Anson was influential in securing Lind's appointment to the Royal Naval Hospital at Haslar in 1758. During the 1760s, Lind published several treatises on preventive and tropical medicine, proposing a simple method of supplying ships with fresh water distillation and providing advice on the prevention of tropical fevers. When Lind retired from the Naval Hospital in 1783, his son John succeeded him as chief physician.

Lind was never elected a fellow of the Royal Society, nor were his dietary recommendations immediately realized. Forty years passed before an official Admiralty Order on the supply of lemon juice to ships was issued in 1795, a year after his death. When this order was implemented, scurvy disappeared from the Fleets and Naval hospitals.

—Todd M. Olszewski

See also Nutritional Epidemiology; Vitamin Deficiency Diseases

Further Readings

Carpenter, K. J. (1986). *The history of scurvy and vitamin C.* Cambridge, UK: Cambridge University Press.

Lind, J. (1753). *A treatise of the scurvy.* Edinburgh, UK: Millar.

Lind, J. (1757). *An essay on the most effectual means of preserving the health of seamen in the Royal Navy.* London: D. Wilson.

Lind, J. (1768). *An essay on diseases incidental to Europeans in hot climates, with the method of preventing their fatal consequences.* London: T. Becket & P. A. de Hondt.

LINEAR REGRESSION

See REGRESSION

LINKAGE ANALYSIS

Linkage analysis is used to pinpoint the location of disease genes within the genome. Given genetic data from a family with a strong history of a disease, it is possible to trace the inheritance of the disease through the family, and thereby localize the genetic region (or locus) responsible for disease in that family. In practice, linkage analysis combines the biological rules of inheritance with statistical inference to identify a linked locus.

Linkage analysis is based on research conducted by Gregor Mendel in the 1860s. Mendel's second law of inheritance states that genetic loci are inherited independently of one another. This independent assortment occurs because genes are located on individual chromosomes, which are redistributed randomly every time an egg or sperm cell is produced. This is why siblings have similar, but not identical, traits; each sibling arose from a unique assortment of parental chromosomes. When two loci are located on separate chromosomes, they will be inherited independently, meaning that the loci will be distributed to the same offspring about 50% of the time. However, loci on the same chromosome are inherited together more frequently. Because portions of each chromosome are rearranged during meiosis, two loci that are near each other are inherited together more frequently than loci distant from each other on the same chromosome. Thus, it is possible to determine the relative position of loci by examining inheritance patterns in a family.

Linkage analysis traces inheritance patterns, and therefore must use genetic and phenotypic data collected from groups of related individuals, some of which have the trait of interest. In most linkage studies, genetic data are collected by genotyping family members for several hundred genetic markers distributed at known locations throughout the genome. Commonly used markers are microsatellite markers and single nucleotide polymorphisms. Researchers then use statistical software to determine which markers are likely to be near the trait locus, based on marker inheritance patterns in affected and unaffected family members.

Linkage analysis requires making several assumptions. First, it is assumed that the trait of interest is genetic. This is usually established by performing a familial aggregation analysis, which can determine if relatives of an affected individual are more likely to have a trait than individuals in the general population. However, familial aggregation of a trait can also be caused by nongenetic factors, including shared environmental exposures and shared behaviors. Second, linkage analysis assumes that the trait follows Mendelian rules of inheritance and that the mode of inheritance is known. This assumption can be tested via segregation analysis that uses statistical tests to identify the most likely mode of inheritance for a trait.

Several phenomena can complicate linkage analyses. Genetic heterogeneity, a situation in which several distinct genes cause the same phenotype via different pathways, can make it nearly impossible to establish linkage. Epistasis, a state in which two or more genes interact to cause a phenotype, will also obscure linkage. While linkage analysis can provide clues about the location of a gene associated with a phenotype, it does not identify a causal allele or mutation. Linkage analyses in several families may identify the same locus linked to the same disease, but each family's disease may be caused by a unique genetic variant. For this reason, linkage analyses are often followed by a genetic association study, which can identify causal alleles in the candidate gene identified by linkage analysis.

In 1990, Hall and colleagues published results of a linkage analysis that linked a region on Chromosome 17 to early-onset familial breast cancer. This analysis used data from 329 individuals within 23 families with a history of early-onset breast cancer. This gene was later identified as a tumor suppressor and named BRCA1. Today, many women from high-risk families choose to be tested for BRCA1 mutations to predict their personal risk for early-onset breast and ovarian cancer.

—*Megan Dann Fesinmeyer*

See also Association, Genetic; Family Studies in Genetics; Genetic Epidemiology; Genetic Markers

Further Readings

Altmuller, J., Palmer, L. J., Fischer, G., Scherb, H., & Wjst, M. (2001). Genomewide scans of complex human diseases: True linkage is hard to find. *American Journal of Human Genetics, 69*(5), 936–950.

Elston, R. C. (1998). Methods of linkage analysis and the assumptions underlying them. *American Journal of Human Genetics, 63*(4), 931–934.

Hall, J. M., Lee, M. K., Newman, B., Morrow, J. E., Anderson, L. A., Huey, B., et al. (1990). Linkage of early-onset familial breast cancer to Chromosome 17q21. *Science, 250*(4988), 1684–1689.

Khoury, M. J, Beaty, T. H., & Cohen, B. H. (1993). *Fundamentals of genetic epidemiology.* New York: Oxford University Press.

LISTER, JOSEPH

(1827–1912)

Joseph Lister was a British surgeon best remembered today for pioneering antiseptic techniques to reduce infection rates, and thus morbidity and mortality, following surgical procedures. Lister was born to a Quaker family in Upton, Essex, England; his father was the physicist Joseph Jackson Lister, who invented the achromatic microscope. Joseph Lister studied medicine at University College, London, and graduated in 1852. He served as a resident in University Hospital, London, and was then appointed as an assistant surgeon at the Edinburgh Royal Infirmary in 1856, where he worked under James Syme. In 1859, Lister was appointed to the Regius Professorship of Surgery at Glasgow University, and in 1861, he became surgeon of the Glasgow Royal Infirmary.

When Lister began his career, the mortality rate for surgery was nearly 50%, and a common complication of surgery was infection. It was commonly believed that wound infections or sepsis were caused by oxidation that could be prevented by not allowing exposure to the air. However, following an idea of Louis Pasteur's, Lister believed that wound infection was caused by microorganisms and if the organisms could be prevented from entering the wound site, the infection could be prevented.

Lister began using carbolic acid (previously demonstrated to kill parasites in sewage) as an antiseptic solution in the wards he supervised at the Glasgow Royal Infirmary; it was used to clean and dress wounds and to disinfect surgical instruments, the air in the operating theatre was sprayed with a mist of carbolic acid, and surgeons were required to wash their hands with a carbolic acid solution before operating. There were some complications, primarily skin irritation, from the carbolic acid, but infection rates plummeted with the adoption of these practices. Lister reported, at a British Medical Association meeting in 1867, that the wards he supervised at the Glasgow Royal Infirmary had remained free of sepsis for 9 months. Despite these obvious successes, Lister's ideas were slow to gain support in England, where many surgeons resented having to perform extra procedures they felt were unnecessary, and who rejected the implication that they might be a cause of infection. His ideas were adopted more readily in Germany, and antiseptic procedures saved many lives during the Franco-Prussian War (1870–1871). Lister's theory that wound infections were caused by microorganisms was further reinforced by the demonstration in 1878 by the German physician Robert Koch that heat sterilization of surgical instruments and dressings dramatically reduced infection rates.

Lister became Chair of Surgery in King's College, London, in 1877, and was knighted by Queen Victoria in 1883. He converted many skeptics to the merits of antiseptic surgery following a successful operation to repair a fractured patella (kneecap), an operation considered inordinately risky at the time. He was also one of the first British surgeons to operate on a brain tumor and developed improved techniques for mastectomy and for the repair of the patella.

—*Sarah Boslaugh*

See also Observational Studies; Public Health, History of

Further Readings

Fisher, R. B. (1977). *Joseph Lister, 1827–1912.* London: Macdonald & James.

Goldman, M. (1987). *Lister Ward.* Bristol, UK: Adam Hilger.

Lister, J. (2004). *On the antiseptic principle of the practice of surgery.* (Originally published 1867). Retrieved October 20, 2006, from http://etext.library.adelaide.edu.au/l/lister/joseph/antiseptic/index.html.

LOCUS OF CONTROL

The construct *locus of control,* also referred to as perceived control, is one of the most studied and cited dispositional constructs in psychology and the social behavioral sciences, and it plays an important role in public health research and health behavior interventions. Locus of control may be either internal or external. Rotter (1990) explains this distinction in terms of the degree to which people assume that the results of their behavior depend on their own actions or personal characteristics rather than on chance, luck, or the influence of powerful others. The popularity of the locus of control construct in health research is demonstrated by the existence of almost 2,500 publications in the *PsycInfo* database for the years 1967 to 2006, which are indexed by the combination of keywords *locus of control* and *health.*

Understanding Locus of Control

The locus of control construct is rooted in social learning theory, and the foundation for this work comes out of research on human and animals. For example, Herbert Lefcourt notes that when rats were able to exercise control over an aversive stimulus, they exhibited less fear of that stimulus than if they could not exercise such control. Similar results have been found in human studies. For example, when participants believed that their behavior could reduce electric shock duration, they gave lower ratings of the painfulness and aftereffects of shocks, compared with when they thought they did not have control. Anecdotal clinical observations support the importance of the perceived control construct in behavior change; for instance, Lefcourt noted that some clients learned from psychological therapy and other new experiences and subsequently changed their behavior, but other clients did not change their behavior as a result of these experiences. Often, the latter would attribute their lack of change to the belief that it was really other people, not themselves, who controlled relevant outcomes for them. In social learning theory terms, the construct of perceived control is a generalized expectancy of external or internal control of reinforcement, for either positive or negative events. It is an abstraction derived from many expectancy-behavior-outcome cycles in which people viewed the causes of their success or failure as being under internal or external control. A person's actions are a function of the situation, expectations, and values. More specifically, the probability that behavior B by person P will occur in situation S, given reinforcement R, is a function of P's expectation that reinforcement R will occur after P's behavior B in situation S, and of the value V to P of the reinforcement R in situation S.

For example, while in college, Pat has tried to lose weight through diet and exercise many times in the past, and he has always been unsuccessful. Therefore, he has developed a low generalized expectancy of success resulting from his memory of and reflection on years of specific expectancy-behavior-outcome sequences. Based on past experience, Pat has a fairly stable estimate of the probability that certain behaviors will lead to the goal of losing weight. In addition, Pat has developed some beliefs as to why his weight loss efforts have been unsuccessful for so long. Perceived locus of control, then, is Pat's abstraction of why weight loss has been unsuccessful all those times— a generalized expectancy of internal (e.g., "I have no willpower when it comes to food") or external (e.g., "My busy class and work schedules prevent me from losing weight"). The above example used Pat's failure as an illustration, but Pat's success could also be used as an example. It is important to note that both successes and failures may be related to either internal or external loci of control. So even with successful weight loss efforts, Pat may have external perceived control ("My family's support, my doctor's instructions, and a gym on campus will make it very easy for me to lose weight"). Therefore, perceived locus of control focuses on how the individual perceives self in relationship to things that happen to him or her and the meaning that the self makes of those experiences.

In many ways, this is very similar to constructs in attribution theory found in social psychology, which has also been applied to interventions to change health behaviors. Attribution theory provides a framework to explain the process that people use information to make inferences about the causes of behaviors or events. For example, we might ask ourselves why Matt can't stop smoking. Our reasons or attributions may be, similar to locus of control theory, internal (Matt does not have much willpower) or external (All Matt's friends smoke, so it is hard for him to quit with them around). There are other dimensions of attributions as well (e.g., temporary vs. permanent aspects).

Measuring Locus of Control

Lefcourt strongly suggests that researchers and practitioners tailor or target the locus of control measure to their populations and their specific domains of interest rather than depending on the more global measures that are quite probably irrelevant to the people and behavior of interest. This recommendation is very similar to findings from the attitude-behavior consistency literature that suggests that if we want to predict a particular behavior (e.g., jogging behavior) from attitudes, then we should assess specific attitudes toward that specific behavior (attitudes toward jogging) instead of more global attitudes (e.g., attitudes toward health).

The first measures of perceived control were created as part of dissertations in the 1950s at Ohio State University by Phares and James. Phares used a Likert-type scale and found that participants with more external attitudes behaved in a fashion similar to participants who received "chance" instructions for a task. James used a longer scale, referred to as the James-Phares Scale, based on what seemed to be the most useful items from Phares's scale. James also found modest correlations between his measure of locus of control and his participants' responses to failure and success. The items from these scales provided the basis for the well-known and often used Rotter Internal-External Control Scale developed by Rotter. The Rotter scale used forced-choice items (e.g., participants had to choose the internal response or the external response) and included items from many different domains (e.g., war, personal respect, school grades and examination performance, leadership, being liked and respected, personality, getting a good job), as well as filler items. It became clear that expectancies of internal-external control were assessable with paper-and-pencil measures, although Lefcourt, who developed such a measure, warns against strict interpretation of locus of control as a trait or typology based on scales.

Consistent with the early writings of Rotter and Lefcourt, many social science researchers have attempted to develop and tailor perceived control scales to their populations and domains of interest, including many for health-related domains. Interestingly, many of the measures are multidimensional. Factor analyses often suggest several dimensions that are not highly intercorrelated. There seems to be an increasing acceptance that locus of control is a multidimensional construct and that internal and external are not just opposite ends of a single bipolar dimension. These results suggest that perceived control is more complex than early researchers thought, since scholars have found that respondents may score high on both internal and external dimensions (e.g., highly religious or spiritual persons may believe that weight loss will be due both to God and their own exercise and dieting efforts), high on one and low on the other, or even low on both internal and external dimensions (perhaps indicating that the domain is not relevant to that individual). Furthermore, there is also some recognition that there may be multiple internal and multiple external dimensions. Even early scholars realized, for example, that luck, chance, God, and powerful others may reflect different dimensions of external perceived control. For example, someone with a high external score in the domain of weight loss may attribute his or her successes or failures mostly to God, and less to luck, chance, and powerful others (e.g., their physician), while those with high internal scores on weight loss may attribute their successes or failures to ability, motivation, or effort. These findings suggest that other dimensions must be considered along with perceived control. For example, stability over time may be an important part of perceived control, with ability reflecting internal perceived control and fixed stability, and effort reflecting internal control and variable stability (e.g., Pat may put more effort into losing weight in January, right after overeating during the holidays, than in September when classes are starting). Similarly, external control and fixed stability might characterize task difficulty, and external control and variable stability may characterize luck. Some of the scales developed to measure locus of control include the Crandall, Katkovsky, and Crandall Intellectual Achievement Responsibility Questionnaire, which assesses children's beliefs about their control and responsibility for failure and success in intellectual achievement; the Nowicki-Strickland Internal-External Control Scale for Children, which assesses generalized expectancies among children, with items from a variety of domains, such as catching a cold, getting good grades, being punished, being good at sports, choosing friends; the Lefcourt, von Bayer, Ware, and Cox Multidimensional-Multiattributional Causality Scale, which assesses perceived control in areas of affiliation and achievement for older/university students; the Miller, Lefcourt, and Ware Marital Locus of Control Scale, which assesses perceived control of marital satisfaction; and the Campis, Lyman, and Prentice-Dunn Parenting Locus of Control Scale, which assesses perceived control beliefs regarding parents' perspective of child rearing successes and failures.

Measuring Health-Related Perceived Control

Health-related control scales are increasing in popularity. Among the scales that measure control in health-related areas are the Wallston, Wallston, and

DeVellis Multidimensional Health Locus of Control Scale, which assesses control beliefs relevant to health; the Hill and Bale Mental Health Locus of Control Scale, which assesses perceived control of therapeutic changes by patient/internal or therapist/external; the Keyson and Janda Drinking Locus of Control Scale, which assesses control expectancies for drinking-related behaviors; the Saltzer Weight Locus of Control Scale, which assesses internal and external control beliefs regarding determinants of weight; and the Catania, McDermott, and Wood Dyadic Sexual Regulation Scale, which assesses control beliefs relevant to sexual activity. Recently, Holt and colleagues have developed and revised their Spiritual Health Locus of Control Scale, which assesses African Americans' perceived control beliefs regarding health, including several dimensions regarding the influence of God, as well as internal control beliefs.

Lefcourt has suggested that higher perceived control is associated with better access to opportunities, so that those who are able to more readily reach valued outcomes that allow a person to feel satisfaction are more likely to hold internal control expectancies (i.e., an internal locus of control). He suggests that, compared with whites in the United States, members of ethnic minority groups who do not have such access are more likely to hold external control and fatalistic beliefs. However, Banks, Ward, McQuater, and DeBritto (1991) have warned against making such a sweeping generalization about ethnic groups, in particular African Americans. They have reviewed some of the research and noted some of the methodological and theoretical weaknesses of the original construct and method. Some researchers have also suggested that the domains studied are usually those in which individuals have at least some control; rarely, if ever, are domains studied in which the individual has no actual control. These domains may be ones in which it is not beneficial to have internal perceived control. Not inconsistently with these ideas, both Lefcourt and Rotter have suggested that perceived control should have a curvilinear relationship with measures of psychological adjustment.

Another measurement issue is one of construct validity. Researchers sometimes confuse constructs in developing measures of perceived locus of control, self-efficacy, perceived behavioral control, and comparable variables. For example, Albert Bandura, who was instrumental in the development of social learning theory, has argued strongly that the construct of perceived locus of control is very different from self-efficacy, even though both originate from social learning theory. However, it is not clear that all measures of perceived control (or efficacy, for that matter) reflect these theoretical differences. More care is needed in developing and validating locus of control scales.

Lefcourt recommends that researchers place more emphasis on a neglected aspect of perceived control: the value or importance of the domain and the reinforcement. According to social learning theory, the value of the reinforcement, not just the expectancy, is an important part of the process, yet few researchers assess this variable or incorporate it into their interpretation of their results. Some researchers have suggested that locus of control best predicts performance in areas that are highly valued, and both Lefcourt and Rotter emphasize the importance of embedding perceived control into the larger social learning theory when designing research and interpreting research findings.

Interventions: Changing Perceived Control

Lefcourt suggests that perceived locus of control can be changed, at least as assessed by current scales, and at least for short periods of time. He notes that there is less evidence for long-term change of perceived control. In fact, change in locus of control may be an important goal of physicians, physical therapists, and other health and mental health professionals. Lefcourt suggests that people can change their attributions if they have experiences that change the perception of contingencies between their behavior and the perceived outcomes. However, another approach is not to attempt to change someone's locus of control but to develop health education materials and other interventions that are tailored to the individual's current locus of control and thus are perceived as more relevant by the participants. Such efforts should take into account the fact that perceived control may change if the individual is more likely to use the health information. (For example, if a woman with an external locus of control regarding her health is induced by health education materials tailored to obtain a mammogram, this may influence her to change to a more internal locus of control, at least for that particular health behavior.) Research that has tested the possibility of changing an individual's locus of control in this manner has been performed, but with somewhat related construct of self-efficacy. Like many dispositional variables and behaviors, accomplishing long-term change in locus of control will probably require more than a one-time intervention and will need to include follow-up sessions aimed at maintaining the change over time and preventing relapse.

Locus of Control and Health Behaviors

Catherine Sanderson suggests that locus of control and other personality/dispositional variables may influence health behaviors but that this influence may depend on other mediating variables. For example, locus of control may influence the perceptions of a stressor, the coping strategies used, how well the individual gathers social support, and the amount of physiological reaction the individual has to the situation. These variables, in turn, then influence the health behavior of interest. The study of possible mediators is providing new information in answering the how and why questions regarding the role of perceived control in related health behavior.

—*Eddie M. Clark*

See also Health Behavior; Health Communication; Self-Efficacy

Further Readings

Bandura, A. (1997). *Self-efficacy: The exercise of control.* New York: W. H. Freeman.

Banks, W. C., Ward, W. E., McQuater, G. V., & DeBritto, A. M. (1991). Are blacks external: On the status of locus of control in Black populations. In R. L. Jones (Ed.), *Black psychology* (3rd ed., pp. 181–192). Berkeley, CA: Cobb & Henry.

Holt, C. L., Clark, E. M., & Klem, P. R. (2007). Expansion and validation of the spiritual locus of control scale: Factor analysis and predictive validity. *Journal of Health Psychology, 12*(4), 597–612.

Holt, C. L., Clark, E. M., Kreuter, M. W., & Rubio, D. M. (2003). Spiritual health locus of control and breast cancer beliefs among urban African American women. *Health Psychology, 22,* 294–299.

Lefcourt, H. M. (Ed.). (1981). *Research with the locus of control construct: Vol. 1. Assessment methods.* New York: Academic Press.

Lefcourt, H. M. (1982). *Locus of control: Current trends in theory and research* (2nd ed.). Hillsdale, NJ: Erlbaum.

Lefcourt, H. M. (1991). Locus of control. In J. P. Robinson, P. R. Shaver, & L. S. Wrightsman (Eds.), *Measures of personality and social psychological attitudes* (pp. 413–499). San Diego, CA: Academic Press.

Lefcourt, H. H., von Bayer, C. L., Ware, E. E., & Cox, D. V. (1979). The multidimensional-multiattributional causality scale: The development of a goal specific locus of control. *Canadian Journal of Behavioural Science, 11,* 286–304.

Rotter, J. B. (1966). Generalized expectancies for internal versus external control of reinforcement. *Psychological Monographs, 80*(1, Whole No. 609).

Rotter, J. B. (1990). Internal versus external control of reinforcement: A case history of a variable. *American Psychologist, 45,* 489–493.

Saltzer, E. B. (1982). The weight locus of control (WLOC) scale: A specific measure for obesity research. *Journal of Personality Assessment, 46,* 620–628.

Sanderson, C. A. (2004). *Health psychology.* Hoboken, NJ: Wiley.

Wallston, K. A., Wallston, B. S., & DeVellis, R. (1978). Development of the multidimensional health locus of control scales. *Health Education Monographs, 6,* 161–170.

LOG-BINOMIAL REGRESSION

See REGRESSION

LOGISTIC REGRESSION

Logistic regression is a statistical technique for analyzing the relationship of an outcome or dependent variable to one or more predictors or independent variables when the dependent variable is (1) *dichotomous*, having only two categories, for example, the presence or absence of symptoms, or the use or non-use of tobacco; (2) *unordered polytomous*, a nominal scale variable with three or more categories, for example, type of contraception (none, pill, condom, intrauterine device) used in response to services provided by a family planning clinic; or (3) *ordered polytomous*, an ordinal scale variable with three or more categories, for example, whether a patient's condition deteriorates, remains the same, or improves in response to a cancer treatment. Here, the basic logistic regression model for dichotomous outcomes is examined, noting its extension to polytomous outcomes and its conceptual roots in both log-linear analysis and the general linear model. Next, consideration is given to methods for assessing the goodness of fit and predictive utility of the overall model, and calculation and interpretation of logistic regression coefficients and associated inferential statistics to evaluate the importance of individual predictors in the model. Throughout, the discussion assumes an interest in prediction, regardless of whether causality is implied; hence the language of "outcomes" and "predictors" is preferred to the language of "dependent" and "independent" variables.

The equation for the logistic regression model with a dichotomous outcome is $\text{logit}(Y) = \alpha + \beta_1 X_1 + \beta_2 X_2 + \cdots + \beta_K X_K$, where Y is the dichotomous outcome; $\text{logit}(Y)$ is the natural logarithm of the odds of Y, a transformation of Y to be discussed in more detail momentarily; and there are $k = 1, 2, \ldots K$ predictors X_k with associated coefficients β_k, plus a constant or intercept, α, which represents the value of $\text{logit}(Y)$ when all the X_k are equal to 0. If the two categories of the outcome are coded 1 and 0, respectively, and P_1 is the probability of being in the category coded as 1, and P_0 is the probability of being in the category coded as 0, then the odds of being in Category 1 is $P_1/P_0 = P_1/(1 - P_1)$ (since the probability of being in one category is one minus the probability of being in the other category). Logit(Y) is the *natural logarithm of the odds*, $\ln[P_1/(1 - P_1)]$, where ln represents the natural logarithm transformation.

Polytomous Logistic Regression Models

When the outcome is polytomous, logistic regression can be implemented by splitting the outcome into a set of dichotomous variables. This is done by means of contrasts that identify a reference category (or set of categories) with which to compare each of the other categories (or sets of categories). For a nominal outcome, the most commonly used model is called the *baseline category logit model*. In this model, the outcome is divided into a set of dummy variables, each representing one of the categories of the outcome, with one of the categories designated as the reference category, in the same way that dummy coding is used for nominal predictors in linear regression. If there are M categories in the outcome, then $\text{logit}(Y_m) = \ln(P_m/P_0) = \alpha_m + \beta_1 m X_1 + \beta_2 m X_2 + \cdots + \beta_K m X_K$, where P_0 is the probability of being in the reference category and P_m is the probability of being in Category $m = 1, 2, \ldots, M - 1$, given that the case is either in Category m or in the reference category. A total of $(M - 1)$ equations or logit functions is thus estimated, each with its own

intercept α_m and logistic regression coefficients $\beta_{k,m}$, representing the relationship of the predictors to $\text{logit}(Y_m)$.

For ordinal outcomes, the situation is more complex, and there are several different contrasts that may be used. In the *adjacent category logit* model, for example, each category is contrasted only with the single category preceding it. In the *cumulative logit* model, for the first logit function, the first category is contrasted with all the categories following it; then, for the second logit function, the first *two* categories are contrasted with all the categories following them, and so forth; until for the last $(M - 1)$ logit function, all the categories preceding the last are contrasted with the last category. Other contrasts are also possible. The cumulative logit model is the model most commonly used in logistic regression analysis for an ordinal outcome, and has the advantage over other contrasts that splitting or combining categories (representing more precise or cruder ordinal measurement) should not affect estimates for categories other than the categories that are actually split or combined, a property not characteristic of other ordinal contrasts. It is commonly assumed in ordinal logistic regression that only the intercepts (or *thresholds*, which are similar to intercepts) differ across the logit functions. The ordinal logistic regression equation can be written (here in the format using intercepts instead of thresholds) as $\text{logit}(Y_m) = \alpha_m + \beta_1 X_1 + \beta_2 X_2 + \cdots + \beta_K X_K$, where $\alpha_m = \alpha_1, \alpha_2, \ldots, \alpha_{M-1}$ are the intercepts associated with the $(M - 1)$ logit functions, but $\beta_1, \beta_2, \ldots, \beta_K$ are assumed to be identical for the $(M - 1)$ logit functions, an assumption that can be tested and, if necessary, modified.

Logistic Regression, Log-linear Analysis, and the General Linear Model

Logistic regression can be derived from two different sources, the general linear model for linear regression and the logit model in log-linear analysis. Linear regression is used to analyze the relationship of an outcome to one or more predictors when the outcome is a continuous interval or ratio scale variable. Linear regression is extensively used in the analysis of outcomes with a *natural metric*, such as kilograms, dollars, or numbers of people, where the unit of measurement is such that it makes sense to talk about larger or smaller differences between cases (the difference between the populations of France and Germany is smaller than the difference between the populations of France and China), and (usually) it also makes sense to talk about one value being some number of times larger than another ($10,000 is twice as much as $5,000), comparisons that are not applicable to the categorical outcome variables for which logistic regression is used. The equation for linear regression is $Y = \alpha + \beta_1 X_1 + \beta_2 X_2 + \cdots + \beta_K X_K$, and the only difference from the logistic regression equation is that the outcome in linear regression is Y instead of logit(Y). The coefficients β_k and intercept α in linear regression are most commonly estimated using ordinary least squares (OLS) estimation, although other methods of estimation are possible.

For OLS estimation and for statistical inferences about the coefficients, certain assumptions are required, and if the outcome is a dichotomy (or a polytomous variable represented as a set of dichotomies) instead of a continuous interval/ratio variable, several of these assumptions are violated. For a dichotomous outcome, the predicted values may lie outside the range of possible values (suggesting probabilities >1 or <0), especially when there are continuous interval or ratio scale predictors in the model; and inferential statistics are typically incorrect because of *heteroscedasticity* (unequal residual variances for different values of the predictors) and nonnormal distribution of the residuals. It is also assumed that the relationship between the outcome and the predictors is linear; however, in the *general linear model*, it is often possible to linearize a nonlinear relationship by using an appropriate nonlinear transformation. For example, in research on income (measured in dollars), it is commonplace to use the natural logarithm of income as an outcome, because the relationship of income to its predictors tends to be nonlinear (specifically, logarithmic). In this context, the logit transformation is just one of many possible linearizing transformations.

An alternative to the use of linear regression to analyze dichotomous and polytomous categorical outcomes is logit analysis, a special case of log-linear analysis. In log-linear analysis, it is assumed that the variables are categorical, and can be represented by a *contingency table* with as many dimensions as there are variables, with each case located in one cell of the table, corresponding to the combination of values it has on all the variables. In log-linear analysis, no distinction is made between outcomes and predictors, but in logit analysis, one variable is designated as the outcome and the other variables are treated as predictors, and each unique combination of values of the predictors represents a covariate pattern. Logit model equations are typically presented in a format different from that used in linear regression and logistic regression, and log-linear and logit models are commonly estimated using *iterative maximum likelihood (ML) estimation*, in which one begins with a set of initial values for the coefficients in the model, examines the differences between observed and predicted values produced by the model (or some similar criterion), and uses an algorithm to adjust the estimates to improve the model. This process of estimation and adjustment of estimates is repeated in a series of steps (*iterations*) that end when, to some predetermined degree of precision, there is no change in the fit of the model, the coefficients in the model, or some similar criterion.

Logistic regression can be seen either as a special case of the general linear model involving the logit transformation of the outcome or as an extension of the logit model to incorporate continuous as well as categorical predictors. The basic form of the logistic regression equation is the same as for the linear regression equation, but the outcome, logit(Y), has the same form as the outcome in logit analysis. The use of the logit transformation ensures that predicted values cannot exceed observed values (for an individual case, the logit of Y is either positive or negative infinity, $+\infty$ or $-\infty$), but it also makes it impossible to estimate the coefficients in the logistic regression equation using OLS. Estimation for logistic regression, as for logit analysis, requires an iterative technique, most often ML, but other possibilities include iteratively reweighted least squares, with roots in the general linear model, or some form of quasi-likelihood or partial likelihood estimation, which may be employed when data are clustered or nonindependent. Common instances of nonindependent data include multilevel analysis, complex sampling designs (e.g., multistage cluster sampling), and designs involving repeated measurement of the same subjects or cases, as in longitudinal research. Conditional logistic regression is a technique for analyzing related samples, for example, in matched case-control studies, in which, with some minor adjustments, the model can be estimated using ML.

Assumptions of Logistic Regression

Logistic regression assumes that the functional form of the equation is correct, and hence the predictors X_k are linearly and additively related to logit(Y), but variables can be transformed to adjust for nonadditivity and nonlinearity (e.g., nonlinearly transformed predictors or interaction terms). It also assumes that each case is independent of all the other cases in the sample, or when cases are not independent, adjustments can be made in either the estimation procedure or the calculation of standard errors (or both) to adjust for the nonindependence. Like linear regression, logistic regression assumes that the variables are measured without error, that all relevant predictors are included in the analysis (otherwise the logistic regression coefficients may be biased), and that no irrelevant predictors are included in the analysis (otherwise standard errors of the logistic regression coefficients may be inflated). Also, as in linear regression, no predictor may be perfectly collinear with one or more of the other predictors in the model. Perfect collinearity means that a predictor is completely determined by or predictable from one or more other predictors, and when perfect collinearity exists, there exist an infinite number of solutions that maximize the likelihood in ML estimation, or minimize errors of prediction more generally. Logistic regression also assumes that the errors in prediction have a binomial distribution, but when the number of cases is large, the binomial distribution approximates the normal distribution. Various diagnostic statistics have been developed and are readily available in existing software to detect violations of assumptions and other problems (e.g., outliers and influential cases) in logistic regression.

Goodness of Fit and Accuracy of Prediction

In logistic regression using ML (currently the most commonly used method of estimation), in place of the sum of squares statistics used in linear regression, there are log-likelihood statistics, calculated based on observed and predicted probabilities of being in the respective categories of the outcome variable. When multiplied by -2, the difference between two log-likelihood statistics has an approximate chi-square distribution for sufficiently large samples involving independent observations. One can construct -2 log-likelihood statistics (here and elsewhere designated as

D) for (1) a model with no predictors, D_0, and (2) the tested model, the model for which the coefficients are actually estimated, D_M. D_M, sometimes called the *deviance statistic*, has been used as a goodness-of-fit statistic, but has somewhat fallen out of favor because of concerns with alternative possible definitions for the saturated model (depending on whether individual cases or covariate patterns are treated as the units of analysis), and the concern that, for data in which there are few cases per covariate pattern, D_M does not really have a chi-square distribution. The Hosmer-Lemeshow goodness-of-fit index is constructed by grouping the data, typically into deciles, based on predicted values of the outcome, a technique applicable even with few cases per covariate pattern. There appears to be a trend away from concern with goodness of fit, however, to focus instead on the model chi-square statistic, $G_M = D_0 - D_M$, which compares the tested model with the model with no predictors. G_M generally does follow a chi-square distribution in large samples, and is analogous to the multivariate F statistic in linear regression and analysis of variance. G_M provides a test of the statistical significance of the overall model in predicting the outcome. An alternative to G_M for models not estimated using ML is the multivariate Wald statistic.

There is a substantial literature on coefficients of determination for logistic regression in which the goal is to find a measure analogous to R^2 in linear regression. When the concern is with how close the predicted probabilities of category membership are to observed category membership (quantitative prediction), two promising options are the likelihood ratio R^2 statistic, $R_L^2 = G_M/D_0$ applicable specifically when ML estimation is used, and the OLS R^2 statistic itself, calculated by squaring the correlation between observed values (coded 0 and 1) and the predicted probabilities of being in Category 1. Advantages of R_L^2 are that it is based on the quantity actually being maximized in ML estimation, it appears to be uncorrelated with the *base rate* (the percentage of cases in Category 1), and it can be calculated for polytomous as well as dichotomous outcomes. Other R^2 analogues have been proposed, but they have various problems that include correlation with the base rate (to the extent that the base rate itself appears to determine the calculated accuracy of prediction), having no reasonable value for perfect prediction or for perfectly incorrect prediction, or being limited to dichotomous outcomes.

Alternatively, instead of being concerned with predicted probabilities, one may be concerned with how accurately cases are qualitatively classified into the categories of the outcome by the predictors (qualitative prediction). For this purpose, there is a family of indices of predictive efficiency, designated lambda-p, tau-p, and phi-p, that are specifically applicable to qualitative prediction, classification, and selection tables (regardless of whether they were generated by logistic regression or some other technique), as opposed to contingency tables more generally. Finally, none of the aforementioned indices of predictive efficiency (or R^2 analogues) takes into account the ordering in an ordered polytomous outcome, for which one would naturally consider ordinal measures of association. Kendall's tau-b is an ordinal measure of association which, when squared (τ_b^2), has a proportional reduction in error interpretation and seems most promising for use with ordinal outcomes in logistic regression. Tests of statistical significance can be computed for all these coefficients of determination.

Unstandardized and Standardized Logistic Regression Coefficients

Interpretation of unstandardized logistic regression coefficients (b_k, the estimated value of β_k) is straightforward and parallel to the interpretation of unstandardized coefficients in linear regression: a one-unit increase in X_k is associated with a b_k increase in logit(Y) (not in Y itself). If we raise the base of the natural logarithm, e = 2.718 . . . , to the power b_k, we obtain the odds ratio, here designated ω_k, which is sometimes presented in place of or in addition to b_k, and can be interpreted as indicating that a one-unit increase in X_k multiplies the odds of being in Category 1 by ω_k. Both b_k and ω_k convey exactly the same information, just in a different form. There are several possible tests of statistical significance for unstandardized logistic regression coefficients. The univariate Wald statistic can be calculated either as the ratio of the logistic regression coefficient to its standard error, $b_k/SE, (b_k)$, which has an approximate normal distribution, or $[b_k/SE(b_k)]^2$, which has an approximate chi-square distribution. The Wald statistic, however, tends to be inflated for large b_k, tending to fail to reject the null hypothesis when the null hypothesis is false (Type II error), but it may still be the best available option

when ML is not used to estimate the model. Alternatives include the Score statistic and the likelihood ratio statistic (the latter being the difference in D_M with and without X_k in the equation). When ML estimation is used, the likelihood ratio statistic, which has a chi-square distribution and applies to both b_k and ω_k, is generally the preferred test of statistical significance for b_k and ω_k.

Unless all predictors are measured in exactly the same units, neither b_k nor ω_k clearly indicates whether one variable has a stronger impact on the outcome than another. Likewise, the statistical significance of b_k or ω_k tells us only how sure we are that a relationship exists, not how strong the relationship is. In linear regression, to compare the *substantive significance* (strength of relationship, which does not necessarily correspond to statistical significance) of predictors measured in different units, we often rely on standardized regression coefficients. In logistic regression, there are several alternatives for obtaining something like a standardized coefficient. A relatively quick and easy option is simply to standardize the predictors (standardizing the outcome does not matter, since it is the probability of being in a particular category of Y, not the actual value of Y, that is predicted in logistic regression). A slightly more complicated approach is to calculate $b_k^* = (b_k)(s_x)(R)/s_{logit(Y)}$, where b_k^* is the fully standardized logistic regression coefficient, b_k is the unstandardized logistic regression coefficient, s_x is the standard deviation of the predictor X_k, R is the correlation between the observed value of Y and the predicted probability of being in Category 1 of Y, $s_{logit(Y)}$ is the standard deviation of the predicted values of logit(Y), and the quantity $s_{logit(Y)}/R$ represents the estimated standard deviation in the observed values of logit(Y) (which must be estimated, since the observed values are positive or negative infinity for any single case). The advantage of this fully standardized logistic regression coefficient is that it behaves more like the standardized coefficient in linear regression, including showing promise for use in path analysis with logistic regression, a technique under development as this is being written.

Logistic Regression and Its Alternatives

Alternatives to logistic regression include probit analysis, discriminant analysis, and models practically identical to the logistic regression model but with different distributional assumptions (e.g., complementary log-log or extreme value instead of logit). Logistic regression, however, has increasingly become the method most often used in empirical research. Its broad applicability to different types of categorical outcomes and the ease with which it can be implemented in statistical software algorithms, plus its apparent consistency with realistic assumptions about real-world empirical data, have led to the widespread use of logistic regression in the biomedical, behavioral, and social sciences.

—Scott Menard

See also Chi-Square Test; Collinearity; Discriminant Analysis; Likelihood Ratio; Regression

Further Readings

Fienberg, S. E. (1980). The analysis of cross-classified categorical data (2nd ed.). Cambridge: MIT Press.

Hosmer, D. W., & Lemeshow, S. (2000). Applied logistic regression (2nd ed.). New York: Wiley.

McCullagh, P., & Nelder, J. A. (1989). Generalized linear models (2nd ed.). London: Chapman & Hall.

Menard, S. (2000). Coefficients of determination for multiple logistic regression analysis. The American Statistician, 54, 17–24.

Menard, S. (2002). Applied logistic regression analysis (2nd ed.). Thousand Oaks, CA: Sage.

Menard, S. (2004). Six approaches to calculating standardized logistic regression coefficients. The American Statistician, 58, 218–223.

Pregibon, D. (1981). Logistic regression diagnostics. Annals of Statistics, 9, 705–724.

Raudenbush, S. W., & Bryk, A. S. (2002). Hierarchical linear models: Applications and data analysis methods (2nd ed.). Thousand Oaks, CA: Sage.

Simonoff, J. S. (1998). Logistic regression, categorical predictors, and goodness of fit: It depends on who you ask. The American Statistician, 52, 10–14.

LOG-RANK TEST

The log-rank test is a statistical method to compare two survival distributions—that is, to determine whether two samples may have arisen from two identical survivor functions. The log-rank test is easy to compute and has a simple heuristic justification and is therefore often advocated for use to nonstatisticians. The log-rank test can also be thought as a censored data rank test.

Suppose we obtain two samples from two populations and we are interested in the null hypothesis

$$H_0 : S_1 = S_2$$

that the survival distribution from Sample 1 is identical to the survival distribution in Sample 2.

The idea behind the log-rank test is to compare the observed number of deaths at each failure time with the expected number of deaths under the null hypothesis (i.e., assuming that the null hypothesis is true).

To do this, we consider the ordered failure times for the combined samples $t_1 \leq t_2 \leq \cdots t_j \cdots \leq t_k$. We then divide the observation period into small intervals ($I_1 = [t_0, t_1)$ $(M - 1)$ $I_2 = [t_1, t_2), \ldots, I_j = [t_j - 1, t_j), \ldots, I_K = [t_K - 1, t_K))$, each one corresponding to the survival time of the noncensored individuals. For each interval I_j $(j = 1, K)$,

d_j is the number of individuals who die at t_j and

r_j is the number of individuals who are alive and at risk just before t_j.

For each table, the quantities d_{1j}/r_{1j} and d_{2j}/r_{2j} are hazard estimates.

To perform the log-rank test, we construct a 2×2 table at each of the failure times t_j.

	Dead	Alive	Total
Sample 1	d_{1j}	$r_{1j} - d_{1j}$	r_{1j}
Sample 2	d_{2j}	$r_{2j} - d_{2j}$	r_{1j}
Total	d_j	$r_j - d_j$	r_j

From this table, define

$O_j = d_{1j}$,

$E_j = \frac{d_{1j}r_{1j}}{r_j}$, and

$V_j = \text{Var}(E_j) = \frac{d_j(r_j - d_j)r_{1j}r_{2j}}{r_j^2(r_j - 1)}$,

and calculate

$O_\bullet = \sum_j O_j$ = Total number of deaths in Sample 1,

$E_\bullet = \sum_j E_j$ = Total number of expected deaths in Sample 1 under the null hypothesis of no difference between the two survival distributions, and

$V_\bullet = \sum_j V_j$ = Variance term for the failures in Sample 1.

The log-rank test is given by

$$T_{L-R} = \frac{(O_\bullet - E_\bullet)^2}{V_\bullet}.$$

This test statistic follows a chi-square distribution with 1 degree of freedom under the null hypothesis (although the tables are not really independent, the distributional result still holds).

Large values of the test statistic indicate that the observed distribution of deaths in Sample 1 diverges from the expected number of deaths if the two survival distributions were identical. Although different censoring patterns do not invalidate the log-rank test, the test can be sensitive to extreme observations in the right tail of the distribution.

The log-rank test is particularly recommended when the ratio of hazard functions in the population being compared is approximately constant. For small data set, the log-rank test can be easily calculated by hand. Most statistical software contains routines for the calculation of the log-rank test.

—Emilia Bagiella

See also Hypothesis Testing; Kaplan-Meier Method; Survival Analysis

Further Readings

Mantel, N. (1966). Evaluation of survival data and two new rank order statistics arising in its consideration. *Cancer Chemotherapy Reports, 50,* 163–170.

Savage, I. R. (1956). Contribution to the theory of rank order statistics: The two sample case. *Annals of Mathematical Statistics, 27,* 590–615.

LONGITUDINAL RESEARCH DESIGN

In epidemiology, a longitudinal study refers to the collection of data from the same unit (e.g., the same person) at two or more different points in time. The great advantage of longitudinal studies is that each subject serves as his or her own control in the study of change across time. This reduces between-subject variability and requires a smaller number of subjects compared with independent subject designs, and it allows the researcher to eliminate a number of competing explanations for effects observed—most important, the cohort effect. The main disadvantages of longitudinal designs are that they are expensive and time-consuming relative to cross-sectional designs, and that they are subject to difficulties with retention, that is, subjects may drop out of the study. In addition, special statistical techniques are needed to account for the fact that repeated measurements taken on the same person or unit will be more similar than the same number of measurements taken on different people.

Designing a longitudinal study is a complex task that involves a number of decisions. The primary decision is whether the data should be recorded prospectively (from the starting point of the study into the future) or retrospectively (collecting data on events that have already occurred). The investigator must also determine how to select a sample of subjects that will represent the target population and how large a sample is needed to have adequate power. Finally, the investigator must choose the variables that will represent the phenomenon under investigation and the frequency at which these variables should be measured.

Methods for the analysis of data in longitudinal studies depend primarily on whether time is considered as a covariate or as an outcome. When the time is viewed as a covariate, regression techniques that account for within-subject association in the data can be used to study the change across time. For time-to-event data, survival analysis that takes into account the potential censoring of data, that is, the unavailability of end points, is required. This entry is concerned with studies in which time is considered to be a covariate. Survival analysis and related methods, which consider time-to-event as the outcome, are treated in a separate entry.

Types of Longitudinal Studies

Longitudinal studies allow the separation of the cohort effect (e.g., the effect of being born in 1956 vs. being born in 1966) from the time effect (e.g., the change in risk behavior for someone at age 20 vs. age 30). They are more difficult and time-consuming to perform than cross-sectional studies, but they allow the investigator to make more convincing conclusions about cause and effect. In addition, longitudinal designs generally need fewer subjects than cross-sectional designs, and the fact that the same subjects are studied repeatedly reduces the variability due to subjects and increases the study's power.

There are several variations of longitudinal studies, but the most common ones are prospective, retrospective, and nested case-control designs. In a prospective study, the investigator plans a study ahead of time, deciding what data to gather, and then records pertinent information on the exposures, outcomes, and potential confounders. The main advantage of this design is that the researcher can collect data that are needed to answer a particular research question, as opposed to simply gleaning whatever existing data are available from other sources. In a retrospective study, the events that are being studied occurred in the past, and the researcher is studying data gleaned from existing sources, such as hospital records. This type of study is feasible only if adequate data about the risk factors, potential confounders, and main outcomes are available on a cohort that has been assembled for other reasons. The main advantage of a retrospective design is that it is possible to gather data in a relatively short period, and these designs are particularly useful in studying rare diseases.

The third type of longitudinal study is the nested case-control design. As the name suggests, nested case-control designs have a case-control study nested within a prospective or retrospective study. They are most useful for predictor variables that are costly to collect, such as the analysis of human specimens. One good example of a nested case-control study is the Baltimore Longitudinal Study on Aging, an ongoing study that started in 1958. The primary objective of this prospective study is to study the process of normal human aging. Participants in the study are volunteers who return approximately every 2 years for 3 days of biomedical and psychological examinations. As reported by Geert Verbeke and Geert Molenberghs, this study is a unique resource for rapidly evaluating longitudinal hypotheses because of the availability of data from repeated examinations and a bank of frozen blood samples from the same participants above 35 years of follow-up. For example, to study the natural history of prostate cancer, subjects with the disease (cases) are matched with their peers who are disease free (controls) and compared according to their previously recorded prostate-specific antigen profiles across time. The disadvantage of this type of study is that development of prostate cancer may have been influenced by many covariates that were not recorded in the study and that, therefore, cannot be examined as risk factors;

the advantage is that the research begins with existing cases of prostate cancer rather than beginning with a large number of healthy subjects and observing them over many years to see which will become ill.

Observation Time Points, Duration, Sample Size, and Power of the Study

The type of design the investigator chooses for the study and the nature of the outcome have a major impact on the observation time points (time points at which data will be collected) and the time lag between these time points, sample size, and power of the study. All power calculations involve considerations of effect size, effect variability, and sample size; however, in a longitudinal design, two other factors are involved—the number of time points at which data will be collected and the time lag between these time points. Typically, these observation time points as well as the time lags between them are preselected by the researcher based on the etiology of the phenomenon under investigation. Generally, one of the factors is computed, usually through simulations, assuming that the remaining factors are prespecified by the investigator. As an example, to compute the sample size necessary for a given statistical power, the investigator has to specify the smallest worthwhile effect size representing the smallest effect that would make a difference to the interpretation of the research question, the number of observation time points, and the time lags between these points and the variance. The smallest worthwhile effect size and the variance are typically estimated from a pilot study, or previously conducted studies with similar objectives. Alternatively, the sample size, variance, effect size, number of design time points, and time lags can be fixed for acceptable power to be calculated.

Statistical Analysis in Longitudinal Studies

When the time variable is viewed as a covariate, regression models known as growth curve models are typically used to summarize longitudinal profiles of the dependent variable under investigation. These models include the popular linear mixed models, generalized linear mixed models, and generalized estimating equation (GEE) models.

Modeling Continuous Outcomes

Linear mixed-effects models are a useful tool to analyze normal continuous repeated measurements recorded on the same subject. They are likelihood-based models for which the conditional expectations (given random effects) are made of two components, a fixed-effects term and a random-effects term. The fixed-effects term represents the average effects of time-dependent covariates, such as the time itself and the effects of time-independent covariates, that is, those whose values may not change during the course of the study, such as baseline covariates. The random effects represent a deviation of a subject's profile from the average profile, and they account for the within-subject correlation across time. These random effects adjust for the heterogeneity of subjects, which can be viewed as unmeasured predispositions or characteristics. These models have an appealing feature in that the fixed-effects parameters have both a subject-specific interpretation and a population-averaged one. Specifically, the effects of time-dependent covariates are interpreted using the conditional expectations given random effects, whereas that of time-independent covariates are conducted using the marginal mean (unconditional of random effects). Before the advent of linear mixed models, longitudinal data were analyzed using techniques, such as repeated measures analysis of variance (ANOVA). This approach has a number of disadvantages and has generally been superseded by linear mixed modeling, which is now available in commonly used statistical packages. For example, repeated measures ANOVA models require a balanced design in that measurements should be recorded at the same time points for all subjects, a condition not required by linear mixed models.

Modeling Discrete and Categorical Outcomes

Although there are a variety of standard likelihood-based models available to analyze data when the outcome is approximately normal, models for discrete outcomes (such as binary outcomes) generally require a different methodology. Kung-Yee Liang and Scott Zeger have proposed the so-called generalized estimating equations model, which is an extension of generalized linear model to correlated data. The basic idea of this family of models is to specify a function that links the linear predictor to the mean response and use the so-called sandwich estimator to adjust the standard errors for association in the data. As a result, the within-subjects association is not modeled explicitly, but treated as a nuisance parameter. GEE regression parameter estimates have a population-averaged interpretation analogous to those obtained from a cross-sectional data analysis. A well-known alternative to this class of models is the generalized linear mixed models, which explicitly model the association in the data using random effects. These models are also likelihood based and are typically formulated as hierarchical models. At the first stage, the conditional distribution of the data given random effects is specified, usually assumed to be a member of the exponential family. At the second stage, a prior distribution is imposed on the random effects. One of the drawbacks of these models is that the fixed-effects parameters, with the exception of few link functions, have a subject-specific interpretation in that they give the magnitude of change occurring within an individual profile. To assess changes between subjects, the investigator is then required to integrate out the random effects from the quantities of interest. There exist other likelihood methods for analyzing discrete data for which parameters have a population-averaged interpretation. One good example is the multivariate Probit model for binary and ordered data that uses the Pearson's correlation coefficient to capture the association between time point responses. Another alternative is the multivariate Plackett distribution that uses odds ratios for association. One drawback of these marginal models is that they require the time points to be the same for all subjects.

Missing Data

The problem of missing data is common to all studies in epidemiological research. In the context of longitudinal studies, missing data take the form of dropouts, intermittent missing data, or both. A dropout occurs when a subject begins the study but fails to complete it, and intermittent missingness refers to the situation where a subject misses at least one visit but ultimately completes the study. When the missing data process is not properly investigated by the investigator, inferences may be misleading. Any attempt to accommodate missing data in the modeling process depends primarily on the missing data process—that is, the underlying mechanism by which the data are missing. Little and Rubin (1987) have developed a terminology that is helpful in categorizing and understanding different types of missing data. Data are classified as missing completely at random (MCAR), missing at random (MAR), and missing not at random (MNAR), depending on whether the fact of missingness is related to (1) none of the outcomes, (2) the observed outcomes only, or (3) both observed and unobserved outcomes, respectively. Under an MCAR mechanism, subjects with complete data may be considered a random sample of all subjects, and a simple remedy to the missing data problems is to delete all subjects with incomplete records. Although the analysis of the resulting complete data set is reasonably straightforward to perform using standard commercial software, this approach may result in substantial loss of subjects, particularly in studies with a large amount of incomplete data. In addition, the MCAR assumption seldom applies to dropouts in longitudinal studies: More typically, those who drop out differ from those who do not drop out with respect to the outcome under investigation. Under an MAR mechanism, imputation techniques that are available with many standard software packages can be used to fill in the missing holes. These techniques range from simple to multiple imputation methods. Such methods, particularly simple imputation, must be used with care because they can introduce new types of bias into the data.

From a modeling standpoint, likelihood-based models produce valid inferences under the MAR mechanism. GEE-based models only produce valid inferences under an MCAR process, but when properly weighted, these models have been shown to be also valid under an MAR mechanism. When the MNAR mechanism applies, that is, when the missingness mechanism depends on the unobserved outcomes, both likelihood and GEE-based models are known to produce biased inferences. The missing data process then needs to be modeled explicitly. Several authors have proposed a family of models that incorporates both the information from the response process and the missing data process into a unified estimating function. This has provoked a large debate about the identifiability of such models, which is possible only on the basis of strong and untestable assumptions. One then has to impose restrictions to recover identifiability. Such restrictions are typically carried out by considering a minimal set of parameters, conditional on which the others are estimable. This, therefore, produces a range of models that form the basis of sensitivity analysis, the only meaningful analysis when the missing data process is likely to be informative.

Software Packages

Longitudinal data analysis has been greatly facilitated by the development of routines for longitudinal analysis within standard statistical packages. SAS, STATA, and SPSS are the most common statistical analysis packages used to analyze data from longitudinal studies. SAS has great data management capabilities and is suitable for standard statistical problems, but may be difficult to master for the practicing epidemiologist. STATA is becoming increasingly popular among epidemiologists because of its interactive nature. Most important, STATA has many procedures tailored to sophisticated biomedical analysis. SPSS is easier to learn and very popular among socioepidemiologists. These statistical software packages come with manuals that explain the syntax of the routines as well as the underlying theories behind the statistical techniques. Despite these advances, it should be noted that there are some complex data that may not be analyzed using standard statistical software with appropriate methods. The investigator is then required to generate his or her own computer codes using matrix-oriented programming languages to answer a specific research question. This then necessitates a good collaboration between the epidemiologist and the statistician or the computer programmer.

—*David Todem*

See also Cohort Effects; Missing Data Methods; Study Design; Survival Analysis

Further Readings

Diggle, P. D., & Kenward, M. G. (1994). Informative dropout in longitudinal data analysis (with discussion). *Applied Statistics, 43*, 49–93.

Hulley, S. B., & Cummings, S. R. (1988). *Designing clinical research.* Baltimore: Williams & Wilkin.

Liang, K.-Y., & Scott, L. Z. (1986). Longitudinal data analysis using generalized linear models. *Biometrika, 73*, 13–22.

Little, R. J. A., & Rubin, D. B. (1987). *Statistical analysis with missing data.* New York: Wiley.

Molenberghs, G., & Verbeke, G. (2005). *Models for discrete longitudinal data.* New York: Springer.

Plackett, R. L. (1965). A class of bivariate distributions. *Journal of the American Statistical Association, 60*, 516–522.

Singer, J. B., & Willett, J. B. (2003). *Applied longitudinal data analysis.* New York: Oxford University Press.

Verbeke, G., & Molenberghs, G. (2000). *Linear mixed models for longitudinal data.* New York: Springer-Verlag.

LOVE CANAL

In the late 1970s, Love Canal—first a toxic waste site, then a neighborhood in southeastern Niagara Falls, New York—ignited national concerns on hazardous waste disposal and its possible health effects. Following closure of the waste facility in 1953, the land surrounding Love Canal was developed into a blue-collar neighborhood. From the time of its development, residents complained of contamination and health problems. In 1978, high groundwater levels surfaced toxic waste, leading President Jimmy Carter to declare the first man-made federal emergency. Two years later, the crisis at Love Canal provided the impetus for the creation of the Comprehensive Environmental Response, Compensation, and Liability Act, or Superfund.

Background

By the end of the 19th century, Niagara Falls, New York, was a heavily industrialized city. To provide hydroelectricity for local industries, in 1894, Love began construction of a canal connecting the Niagara River and Lake Ontario. A few years later following the discovery of alternating current, financial support for Love's canal bottomed out and construction ceased. Then, in 1942, Hooker Chemicals and Plastics Corporation purchased the incomplete canal and its surrounding land for use as a toxic waste dump. A decade later, the canal filled to capacity with almost 22 tons of mixed chemical waste, the site was closed and covered with dirt. During its 10 years as a toxic waste dump, hundreds of chemicals, including halogenated organics, pesticides, chlorobenzenes, and dioxin, were disposed of at Love Canal. In 1953, Hooker Chemicals sold the property to the Niagara Falls Board of Education for $1. Within the year, a school (the 99th Street School) and residences were built around the former landfill.

From the late 1950s through the early 1970s, Love Canal residents complained of chemical odors, surfacing chemicals, and minor explosions and fires. But it was not until 1976 and 1977 that high groundwater levels due to heavy rains revealed widespread contamination. According to firsthand reports, corroding waste-disposal drums surfaced, vegetation began dying off, and pools of noxious chemicals formed in yards and basements. Testing for toxic chemicals in soil, air, and water by health agencies, prompted by unremitting reporting by the *Niagara Falls Gazette*, confirmed the presence of contamination.

Government Response

In 1978, the New York State Department of Health Commissioner, Robert Whalen, responded to the crisis by declaring a health emergency. Immediately, the 99th Street School was closed, and pregnant women and children below 2 years of age residing closest to the site were evacuated. Over the next 2 years, President Jimmy Carter declared the site a federal state of emergency twice, and about 950 families were relocated from within a 10-mile radius of the site. The use of federal disaster assistance at Love Canal marks the first time federal emergency funds were granted for a nonnatural disaster. In 1980, the Carter Administration passed the Comprehensive Environmental Response, Compensation, and Liability Act, or Superfund, largely in response to the Love Canal crisis.

Health Consequences

Early epidemiological studies of the potential health effects experienced by Love Canal residents have had inconclusive or conflicting results. These studies were limited by a number of factors, including the lack of precise exposure data, small sample size and selection bias, recall bias, and lack of control for confounders. A 2006 study by the New York State Department of Health investigated mortality, cancer incidence, and reproductive outcomes of Love Canal residents. Although this study had limitations similar to those of the earlier research, it suggested increased rates of congenital malformations and proportions of female births. The study also revealed an increased number of adverse reproductive outcomes for women exposed as a child or whose mothers resided in Love Canal during pregnancy.

—*Michelle Kirian*

See also Birth Defects; Environmental and Occupational Epidemiology; Pollution

Further Readings

Beck, E. (1979). *History: The Love Canal tragedy. The United States environmental protection agency.* Retrieved December 11, 2006, from http://www.epa.gov/history/topics/lovecanal/01.htm.

Center for Environmental Health, New York State Department of Health. (2006). *Love Canal follow-up health study-project report to ATSDR (Public Comment Draft).* Love Canal: Author. Retrieved December 12, 2006, from http://www.health.state.ny.us/nysdoh/lcanal/docs/report_public_comment_draft.pdf.

Ecumenical Task Force of the Niagara Frontier. (1998). *Love Canal collection.* Buffalo: University Archives, University Libraries, State University of New York at Buffalo. Retrieved December 13, 2006, from http://ublib.buffalo.edu/libraries/projects/lovecanal/.

M

MALARIA

Malaria is a parasitic disease that causes between 1 million and 3 million deaths each year, mainly African children. Three billion persons—close to 50% of the world's population—live in 107 countries and territories in which malaria is endemic. Most mortality is due to *Plasmodium falciparum*, a protozoan parasite transmitted by the Anopheles mosquito, which is responsible for more than 515 million cases of disease annually: In addition, almost 5 billion febrile episodes resembling malaria, but which cannot be definitively identified as such, occur in endemic areas annually. The medical, epidemiologic, and economic burdens due to malaria have greatly impeded development in endemic countries, particularly in Africa.

Cause of Malaria and Natural Cycle

The four species of the genus *Plasmodium* that cause malarial infections in humans are *P. falciparum*, *P. vivax*, *P. ovale*, and *P. malariae*. Human infection begins when the malaria vector, a female anopheline mosquito, inoculates infectious plasmodial sporozoites from its salivary gland into humans during a bloodmeal. The sporozoites mature in the liver and are released into the bloodstream as merozoites. These invade red blood cells, causing malaria fevers. Some forms of the parasites (gametocytes) are ingested by anopheline mosquitoes during feeding and develop into sporozoites, restarting the cycle.

Manifestations

The complex interrelationships of the malaria parasite, the female Anopheles mosquito vector, and the human target, along with environmental factors and control measures, determine the expression of disease manifestations and epidemiology.

The first symptoms of malaria are nonspecific: Patients are unwell and have headache, fatigue, abdominal discomfort, and muscle aches followed by fever—all similar to a minor viral illness. Later, fever spikes, chills, and rigors occur. Anemia, hypoglycemia, cerebral manifestations, and low birthweight newborns result frequently from malaria as do neurocognitive sequelae after severe illness. Those who have been exposed to malaria develop partial immunity, but not protection from infection, such that they have parasitemia but not illness: This condition is called premunition and is the reason that adults living in malarious areas have much less illness, despite being bitten by infected mosquitoes. In addition, many persons may have comorbidity—malaria parasitemia or illness at the same time that they have other diseases, complicating the diagnosis.

Case Fatality Rates and Sequelae

Correctly and promptly treated, uncomplicated falciparum malaria has a mortality rate of approximately 0.1%. Once vital organ dysfunction occurs or the proportion of erythrocytes infected increases to more than 3%, mortality rises steeply. Coma is a characteristic and ominous feature of falciparum malaria and,

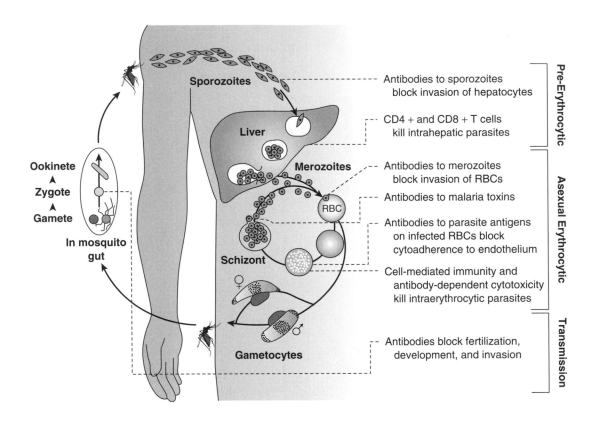

Figure 1   Natural Cycle of Malaria

Source: White and Breman (2005). Copyright © 2006 by The McGraw-Hill Companies, Inc. Reproduced with permission of The McGraw-Hill Companies.

despite treatment, is associated with death rates of some 20% among adults and 15% among children. Convulsions, usually generalized and often repeated, occur in up to 50% of children with cerebral malaria (CM). Whereas less than 3% of adults suffer neurological sequelae, roughly 10% to 15% of children surviving CM—especially those with hypoglycemia, severe malarial anemia (SMA), repeated seizures, and deep coma—have some residual neurological deficit when they regain consciousness. Protein-calorie undernutrition and micronutrient deficiencies, particularly zinc and vitamin A, contribute substantially to the malaria burden.

Where, When, and Why Malaria Occurs

P. falciparum predominates in Haiti, Papua New Guinea, and sub-Saharan Africa. *P. vivax* is more common in Central America and the Indian subcontinent and causes more than 80 million clinical episodes of illness yearly. The prevalence of these two species is approximately equal in the Indian subcontinent, eastern Asia, Oceania, and South America. *P. malariae* is found in most endemic areas, especially throughout sub-Saharan Africa, but is much less common than the other species. *P. ovale* is unusual outside Africa, and where it is found accounts for less than 1% of isolates.

While more than 40 anophelines can transmit malaria, the most effective are those such as *Anopheles gambiae*, which are long-lived, occur in high densities in tropical climates (particularly sub-Saharan Africa), breed readily, and bite humans in preference to other animals. Females require blood for nourishing their eggs; therefore, they bite animals. The entomological inoculation rate (EIR)—that is, the number of sporozoite-positive mosquito bites per person per year—is the most useful measure of malarial transmission and varies from less than 1 in some parts of Latin America and Southeast Asia to more than 300 in parts of tropical Africa. Also important is the basic reproduction rate (Ro), the number of infected persons

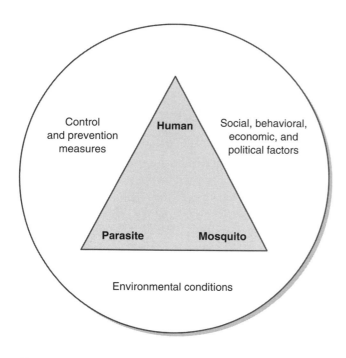

Figure 2   Malaria Ecology and Burden: Intrinsic and Extrinsic Factors

deriving from a single infected person. Ro for malaria may range from 1 to > 1,000.

Geographic and climate-driven (mainly rainfall) models of suitability for malaria transmission characterize the diversity of malaria transmission. The African continent illustrates four distinct areas of transmission that also exist in Latin America and Asia:

- Class 1, no transmission (northern and parts of southern Africa)
- Class 2, marginal risk (mainly in some areas of southern Africa and in high-altitude [> 1,500 m] settings)
- Class 3, seasonal transmission with epidemic potential (along the Sahara fringe and in highlands)
- Class 4, stable and unstable malarious areas (most areas south of the Sahara to southern Africa and below an altitude of around 1,500 m)

The epidemiology of malaria may vary considerably within relatively small geographic areas. In tropical Africa or coastal Papua New Guinea, with *P. falciparum* transmission, more than one human bite per infected mosquito can occur per day and people are infected repeatedly throughout their lives. In such areas, morbidity and mortality during early childhood are considerable. For survivors, some immunity against disease develops in these areas, and by adulthood, most malarial infections are asymptomatic. This situation, with frequent, intense, year-round transmission and high EIRs is termed *stable malaria*. In areas where transmission is low, erratic, or focal, full protective immunity is not acquired and symptomatic disease may occur at all ages. This situation is termed *unstable malaria*. An epidemic or complex emergency can develop when changes in environmental, economic, or social conditions occur, such as heavy rains following drought or migrations of refugees or workers from a nonmalarious to an endemic region. A breakdown in malaria control and prevention services intensifies epidemic conditions. Epidemics occur most often in areas with unstable malaria, such as Ethiopia, northern India, Madagascar, Sri Lanka, and southern Africa. Many other African countries situated in the Sahelian and sub-Saharan areas are susceptible to epidemics. Public health specialists have only recently begun to appreciate the considerable contribution of urban malaria, with up to 28% of the burden in Africa occurring in rapidly growing urban centers.

Burden

In 2001, the World Health Organization (WHO) ranked malaria as the eighth highest contributor to the global disease burden, as reflected in disability-adjusted life years (DALYs), and the second highest in Africa after HIV/AIDS. Malaria is the biggest killer of African children below the age of 5 years (more than 1 million deaths per year), followed by pneumonia and diarrhea. Alarmingly, the burden of malaria in children in Africa has been growing since 1990, whereas overall childhood mortality is dropping.

The DALYs attributable to malaria were estimated largely from the effects of *P. falciparum* infection as a direct cause of death and the much smaller contributions of short-duration, self-limiting, or treated mild febrile events, including malaria-specific mild anemia and neurological disability following CM. The estimate assumes that each illness event or death can be attributed only to a single cause that can be measured reliably. Table 1 shows deaths and DALYs from deaths attributable to malaria and to all causes by WHO region. It does not include the considerable toll caused by the burden of malaria-related moderate and severe anemia, low birthweight, and comorbid events. Sub-Saharan African children below 4 years represent

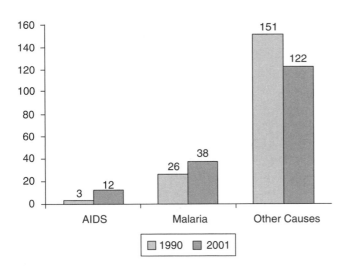

Figure 3   Under-5 Deaths per 1,000 Births

Source: Jamison (2006).

82% of all malaria-related deaths and DALYs. Malaria accounts for 2.0% of global deaths and 2.9% of global DALYs. In the African region of WHO, 9.0% of deaths and 10.1% of DALYs are attributable to malaria.

While the malaria incidence globally is 236 episodes per 1,000 persons per year in all endemic areas, it ranges from about 400 to 2,000 (median 830) episodes per 1,000 persons per year in areas with intense, stable transmission; these areas represent 38% of all falciparum endemic areas.

The vast majority of deaths and illness in developing countries occur outside the formal health service, and in Africa, most government civil registration systems are incomplete. Newer demographic and disease-tracking systems are being used globally and should help rectify the woefully inadequate vital statistics available for malaria and other diseases. The current woeful health system coverage and registration of health events is analogous to "the ears of a hippopotamus".

Health personnel usually attribute causes of death during demographic surveillance system surveys through a verbal autopsy interview with relatives of the deceased about the symptoms and signs associated with the terminal illness. Both the specificity and the sensitivity of verbal autopsy vary considerably depending on the background spectrum of other common diseases, such as acute respiratory infection, gastroenteritis, and meningitis, which share common clinical features with malaria.

In most of the countries where malaria is endemic, laboratory confirmation occurs infrequently. Clinical impressions and treatments are based on febrile illness, which may occur 5 to 10 times a year in young children and may have causes other than malaria. In malarious Africa, some 30% to 60% of outpatients with fever may have parasitemia. Monthly surveillance of households will detect a quarter of the medical events that are detected through weekly surveillance, and weekly contacts with cohorts identify approximately 75% of events detected through daily surveillance. Given the predominance of fevers, malaria case management in Africa and other endemic areas usually centers on presumptive diagnosis.

Estimates of the frequency of fever among children suggest one episode every 40 days. If we assume that the perceived frequency of fever in Africa is similar across all transmission areas (and possibly all ages), African countries would witness approximately 4.9 billion febrile events each year. Estimates indicate that in areas of stable malaria risk, a minimum of 2.7 billion exposures to antimalarial treatment will occur each year for parasitemic persons, or 4.93 per person per year. While these diagnostic, patient management, and drug delivery assumptions are debatable, they indicate the magnitude of the challenges that malaria presents.

Studies of neurological sequelae after severe malaria indicated that 3% to 28% of survivors suffered from such sequelae, including prolonged coma and seizures. CM is associated with hemiparesis, quadriparesis, hearing and visual impairments, speech and language difficulties, behavioral problems, epilepsy, and other problems. The incidence of neurocognitive sequelae following severe malaria is only a fraction of the true residual burden, and the impact of milder illness is unknown.

Indirect and Comorbid Risks

The DALY model of malaria does not sufficiently take it into account as an indirect cause of broader morbid risks. Some consider anemia to be caused indirectly unless linked to acute, high-density parasitemia. Similarly, low birthweight may also be indirectly attributable to malaria, and a child's later undernutrition and growth retardation linked to malaria infection enhances the severity of other concomitant

Table 1 Deaths and DALYs From Deaths Attributable to All Causes and to Malaria by WHO Region, 2000

Region	Population Thousands	Deaths, 2000 — All Causes		Deaths, 2000 — Malaria		Malaria Deaths as a Percentage of All Deaths	DALYs From Deaths, 2000 — All Causes		DALYs From Deaths, 2000 — Malaria		Malaria DALYs as a Percentage of All DALYs
		Thousands	Percentage	Thousands	Percentage		Thousands	Percentage	Thousands	Percentage	
World	6,122,211	56,554	100.0	1,124	100.0	2.00	1,467,257	100.0	42,279	100.0	2.90
Africa	655,476	10,681	18.9	963	85.7	9.00	357,884	24.4	36,012	85.2	10.10
Americas	837,967	5,911	10.5	1	<0.1	0.02	145,217	9.9	108	0.2	0.07
Eastern Mediterranean	493,091	4,156	7.3	55	4.9	1.30	136,221	9.3	2,050	4.8	1.50
Europe	874,178	9,703	17.2	<1	<0.1	<0.010	151,223	10.3	20	0.04	0.01
Southeast Asia	1,559,810	14,467	25.6	95	8.5	0.70	418,844	28.5	3,680	8.7	0.90
Western Pacific	1,701,689	11,636	20.6	10	0.9	0.09	257,868	17.6	409	1.0	0.20

Source: Breman, Mills, and Snow (2006).

Note: Percentages may not add up to 100 because of rounding.

627

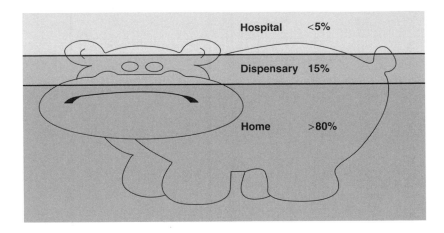

Figure 4   The Ears of the Hippopotamus: Where Malaria Patients Are Managed ... and Die

Source: Breman, Egan, and Keusch (2001, p. 6). Reprinted with permission.

or comorbid infectious diseases through immune suppression. Thus, malaria infection contributes to broad causes of mortality beyond the direct fatal consequences of infection and is probably underestimated.

In Africa, pregnant women experience few malaria-specific fever episodes but have an increased risk of anemia and placental sequestration of the parasite. Maternal clinical manifestations are more apparent in areas with less intense transmission, particularly in Asia. Estimates indicate that in sub-Saharan Africa, malaria-associated anemia is responsible for 3.7% of maternal mortality, or approximately 5,300 maternal deaths annually. Prematurity and intrauterine growth retardation resulting in low birthweight associated with maternal malaria account for 3% to 8% of infant mortality in Africa. Assuming an infant mortality rate of 105 per 1,000 live births in 2000, 71,000 to 190,000 infant deaths were attributable to malaria in pregnancy. Other studies indicate that malaria-associated low birthweight accounted for 62,000 to 363,000 infant deaths.

Anemia among African children is caused by a combination of nutritional deficiencies and iron loss through helminth infection, red cell destruction, decreased red cell production as a result of infectious diseases, and genetically determined hemoglobinopathies. Chronic or repeated infections, often associated with parasite resistance to drugs, are more likely to involve bone marrow suppression.

It is estimated that 190,000 to 974,000 deaths per year in sub-Saharan Africa are attributable to SMA. Children residing in areas where the prevalence of *P. falciparum* was more than 25% had a 75% prevalence of anemia. By modeling the relationship between anemia and parasite prevalence, it was found that mild anemia rose 6% for every 10% increase in the prevalence of infection. Reducing the incidence of new infections through insecticide-treated nets (ITNs) or the prevalence of blood-stage infections through chemoprophylaxis or intermittent preventive treatment (IPT) for children halved the risk of anemia.

Iron, zinc, and protein-calorie deficits are responsible for a considerable amount of malaria-related mortality and morbidity and indicate that 57.3% of deaths of underweight children below 5 years are attributable to nutritional deficiencies. One striking feature of the global distribution of anthropometric markers of undernutrition is its congruence with the distribution of endemic malaria.

Early during the HIV epidemic, it was demonstrated that malaria-associated anemia treated with unscreened blood transfusions contributed to HIV transmission. At the same time, two longitudinal cohort studies in Kenya and Uganda and one hospital-based case-control study in Uganda demonstrated that HIV infection approximately doubles the risk of malaria parasitemia and clinical malaria in nonpregnant adults and that increased HIV immunosuppression is associated with higher-density parasitemias. In pregnant women, the presence of HIV increases the rate and intensity of parasitemia and frequency of anemia.

Malaria accounts for 13% to 15% of medical reasons for absenteeism from school, but little information is available on the performance of parasitized schoolchildren. A randomized placebo control study of chloroquine prophylaxis in Sri Lankan schoolchildren demonstrated an improvement in mathematics and language scores by those who received chloroquine but found no difference in absenteeism. As noted earlier, malaria may result in low birthweight, and low birthweight can lead to a range of persistent impaired outcomes, predominantly behavioral difficulties, cerebral palsy, mental retardation, blindness, and deafness. The recently launched studies of intermittent preventive treatments during infancy (IPTi) should provide a more precise means of examining the benefits of IPTi and consequences on learning and performance of infection early in life.

Interventions and Their Effectiveness

Malaria will be conquered only by full coverage, access to, and use of antimalarial services by priority groups; prompt and effective patient management (rapid, accurate diagnosis, treatment, counseling and education, referral); judicious use of insecticides to kill and repel the mosquito vector, including the use of ITNs; and control of epidemics. All interventions must be applied in a cost-effective manner. Eliminating malaria from most endemic areas remains a huge, but surmountable challenge because of the widespread *Anopheles* breeding sites, the large number of infected people, the use of ineffective antimalarial drugs, and the inadequacies of resources, infrastructure, and control programs. WHO Global Malaria Programme and the Roll Back Malaria Partnership, which began in 1998, aim to halve the burden of malaria by 2010; they have developed strategies and targets for 2005 (Table 2).

While ambitious, the initiative is making substantial progress by means of effective and efficient deployment of currently available interventions. Indeed, Brazil, Eritrea, India, Vietnam, and other countries are reporting recent successes in reducing the malaria burden. Despite the enormous investment in developing a malaria vaccine administered by means of a simple schedule and recent promising results in the laboratory and in field trials in Africa, no effective, long-lasting vaccine is likely to be available for general use in the

Table 2   Targets Established at the Abuja Malaria Summit, April 2000

The goal of Roll Back Malaria (RBM) is to halve the burden of malaria by 2010. The following targets for specific intervention strategies were established at the Abuja Malaria Summit, April 2000.

RBM Strategy	*Abuja Target (by 2005)*
• Prompt access to effective treatment • Insecticide-treated nets (ITNs) • Prevention and control of malaria in pregnant women • Malaria epidemic and emergency response	• 60% of those suffering with malaria should have access to and be able to use correct, affordable, and appropriate treatment within 24 hr of the onset of symptoms • 60% of those at risk for malaria, particularly children below 5 years of age and pregnant women, will benefit from a suitable combination of personal and community protective measures, such as ITN • 60% of pregnant women at risk of malaria will be covered with suitable combinations of personal and community protective measures, such as ITN • 60% of pregnant women at risk of malaria will have access to intermittent preventive treatment[a] • 60% of epidemics are detected within 2 wk of onset • 60% of epidemics are responded to within 2 wk of detection

Source: Breman, Mills, and Snow (2006).

a. The original Abuja declaration included the recommendation for chemoprophylaxis as well, but present WHO and RBM policy strongly recommends intermittent preventive treatment, and not chemoprophylaxis, for prevention of malaria during pregnancy.

near future. Yet the search for new and improved interventions continues, and discovery of better drugs, vaccines, diagnostics, and vector control inventions will someday lead to the conquest of this disease.

—Joel Breman

See also Epidemiology in Developing Countries; Insect-Borne Disease; Parasitic Diseases

Further Readings

Breman, J. G., Alilio, M. S., & Mills, A. (2004). Conquering the intolerable burden of malaria: What's new, what's needed: A summary. *American Journal of Tropical Medicine and Hygiene, 71*(Suppl. 2), 1–15.

Breman, J. G., Egan, A., & Keusch, G. (2001). The ears of the hippopotamus: Manifestations, determinants, and estimates of the malaria burden. *American Journal of Tropical Medicine and Hygiene, 64*(Suppl. 1/2), 1–11.

Breman, J. G., Mills, A., & Snow, R. (2006). Conquering malaria. In D. T. Jamison, J. G. Breman, A. R. Measham, G. Alleyne, M. Claeson, D. B. Evans, et al. (Eds.), *Disease control priorities in developing countries* (2nd ed., pp. 413–431). New York: Oxford University Press.

Craig, M. H., Snow, R. W., & le Sueur, D. (1999). A climate-based distribution model of malaria transmission in sub-Saharan Africa. *Parasitology Today, 15*, 105–111.

Greenberg, A. E., Ntumbanzondo, M., Ntula, N., Mawa, L., Howell, J., & Davachi, F. (1989). Hospital-based surveillance of malaria-related paediatric morbidity and mortality in Kinshasa, Zaire. *Bulletin of the World Health Organization, 67*(2), 189–196.

Holding, P. A., & Kitsao-Wekulo, P. K. (2004). Describing the burden of malaria on child development: What should we be measuring and how should we be measuring it? *American Journal of Tropical Medicine and Hygiene, 71*(Suppl. 2), 71–79.

Jamison, D. T. (2006). Investing in health. In D. T. Jamison, J. G. Breman, A. R. Measham, G. Alleyne, M. Claeson, D. B. Evans, et al. (Eds.), *Disease control priorities in developing countries* (2nd ed., pp. 3–34). New York: Oxford University Press.

Mendis, K., Sina, B. J., Marchesini, P., & Carter, R. (2001). The neglected burden of *Plasmodium vivax* malaria. *American Journal of Tropical Medicine and Hygiene, 64*(Suppl. 1), 97–105.

Mung'Ala-Odera, V., Snow, R. W., & Newton, C. R. J. C. (2004). The burden of the neurocognitive impairment associated with falciparum malaria in sub-Saharan Africa. *American Journal of Tropical Medicine and Hygiene, 71*(Suppl. 2), 64–70.

Snow, R. W., Guerra, C. A., Noor, A. M., Myint, H. Y., & Hay, S. I. (2005). The global distribution of clinical episodes of *Plasmodium falciparum* malaria. *Nature, 434*, 214–217.

Steketee, R. W., Wirima, J. J., Hightower, A. W., Slutsker, L., Heymann, D. L., & Breman, J. G. (1996). The effect of malaria and malaria prevention in pregnancy on offspring birthweight, prematurity, and intrauterine growth retardation in rural Malawi. *American Journal of Tropical Medicine and Hygiene, 55*(Suppl.) 33–41.

White, N. J., & Breman, J. G. (2005). Malaria and babesiosis: Diseases caused by red blood cell parasites. In D. Kasper, E. Braunwald, A. S. Fauci, S. L. Hauser, D. L. Longo, & J. L. Jameson (Eds.), *Harrison's principles of internal medicine* (16th ed., pp. 1218–1233). New York: McGraw-Hill.

World Health Organization. (2005). *The World Malaria Report 2005: Roll Back Malaria.* Geneva, Switzerland: Author.

Worrall, E., Rietveld, A., & Delacollette, C. (2004). The burden of malaria epidemics and cost-effectiveness of interventions in epidemic situations in Africa. *American Journal of Tropical Medicine and Hygiene, 71*(Suppl. 2), 136–140.

MALNUTRITION, MEASUREMENT OF

Malnutrition is a serious global issue, affecting more than 2 billion people worldwide. The problem has two principal constituents—protein-energy malnutrition and deficiencies in micronutrients—and affects women and young children in particular. Malnutrition is the most important risk factor for illness and death in developing countries. Of the many factors that may cause malnutrition, most are related to poor intake of food or to severe or frequent infection, especially in underprivileged populations. Because malnutrition and social factors are closely linked, the nutritional status of a population is a good indicator of the quality of life in a community.

Assessment of Nutritional Status

Nutritional status can be measured at the individual or population level. Population-based assessments are typically performed to measure the extent of malnutrition in a community, identify high-risk groups, and estimate the number of people requiring interventions such as supplementary and therapeutic feeding. Estimates of the burden of malnutrition are important at the national and local levels to define strategies for improving the health of the population.

Methods to assess malnutrition include anthropometry, biochemical indicators (e.g., decrease in serum albumin concentration), and clinical signs of malnutrition (e.g., edema, changes in the hair and skin, visible thinness). Anthropometry is the preferred method to assess malnutrition in both individual people and surveyed populations because body measurements are sensitive over the full spectrum of malnutrition, while biochemical and clinical indicators are useful only when malnutrition is advanced. The purpose of the assessment should guide the choice of measurement methods.

Common anthropometric indicators of malnutrition in childhood include combinations of body measurements (e.g., either length or height combined with weight) according to age and sex. Anthropometric measurements of children below the age of 5 years are used to draw conclusions about the nutritional well-being of the population in which they live, because children are more vulnerable to adverse environments and respond more rapidly than adults to dietary changes.

To interpret anthropometric data and determine an individual child's level of malnutrition, the child's height and weight are compared with reference curves of height-for-age, weight-for-age, and weight-for-height. The internationally accepted references were developed by the Centers for Disease Control and Prevention (CDC) using data collected from a population of healthy children in the United States. More recently, the World Health Organization (WHO) released international standards for child growth that were based on a pooled sample from six countries. Anthropometric data can be plotted using software available from the CDC (www.cdc.gov/epiinfo) or WHO (www.who.int/childgrowth/software). The internationally recommended indicators used to characterize the different types of malnutrition in childhood include the following:

- Low height-for-age: Assess stunting or shortness
- Low weight-for-height: Assess wasting or thinness
- Low weight-for-age: Assess underweight

Stunting reflects a failure to reach one's linear growth potential (maximum height) because of chronic malnutrition due to either inadequate intake of food or recurrent illness; wasting, in contrast, indicates recent loss of weight, usually as a consequence of famine or severe disease. Underweight reflects both wasting and stunting, and thus in many cases, it reflects a synthesis of undesirable body proportions and reduced linear growth. The choice of anthropometric indicator depends on the purpose of the assessment. For example, in emergency situations, weight-for-height is the index most often used, because wasting has the greatest potential for causing mortality or widespread morbidity. Other anthropometric indices, such as mid-upper-arm circumference and triceps skinfold thickness, are sometimes used but are less reliable.

Three different classification systems can be used to distinguish "normal" from "not normal" growth in childhood: z scores, percentiles, and percentage of median. Although percentiles are typically used in the United States, WHO recommends the use of the z score (a z score of 1 represents 1 standard deviation from the reference median). Malnutrition is defined as a z score of less than -2 for weight-for-height, height-for-age, or weight-for-age. A cutoff point of a z score of -3 is used to identify severely malnourished children. Abnormal findings in an individual child may reflect normal variation in growth (e.g., low height-for-age because both parents are short).

A simple clinical examination can help detect certain causes of malnutrition. For example, examining a sample of children for pretibial or pedal edema (swelling of the foot/ankle) can determine community rates of kwashiorkor (malnutrition with edema). Children with edema should always be classified as having severe acute malnutrition regardless of their weight-for-height or weight-for-age z scores. To detect malnutrition in adults, particularly nonpregnant women of childbearing age, it is recommended that underweight be used as a proxy for malnutrition. The body mass index (BMI) can be used to measure the prevalence of underweight. BMI is determined by dividing the weight in kilograms by the square of the height in meters. Levels of malnutrition can be classified as follows using the BMI:

- Mild: 17 to < 18.5
- Moderate: 16 to < 17
- Severe: < 16

Conducting a Population-Based Assessment of Nutritional Status

In most population-based assessments of nutritional status, the children are between the ages of 6 and 59 months. Children in this age group are highly vulnerable to increased morbidity and mortality during a nutrition crisis and will often be the first to exhibit signs of malnutrition.

Before any data are collected, it is important to define what an appropriate population-based sample would be and determine a sample size that gives results of sufficient precision and power. Criteria for obtaining data of good quality include using the right equipment to collect the data and employing standard measuring techniques. Children should be weighed in their underwear without shoes, and the scale should read to the nearest 0.1 kg. For height, children below the age of 2 years should lie on a suitable board to have their length measured; children above 2 years should stand up to have their height determined. Accurate measurements of weight, height, and age are required for the identification of malnutrition to be made. To maintain a high level of data quality, field-workers should be trained to collect data in a standardized format and should be supervised.

Once a comparison has been made for every child in the sample between his or her nutritional status and the reference population, the prevalence of malnutrition in the population can be calculated. For example, if the intention is to calculate the prevalence of wasting, one can count all the children in the sample with a weight-for-height z score less than -2 and divide the final count by the total number of children in the sample. A prevalence of wasting $>10\%$ is cause for concern and indicates a need for rapid intervention. A prevalence of stunting $>30\%$ and a prevalence of underweight $>20\%$ are also indicators of severe malnutrition in a community.

Data from a nutritional assessment should be presented in a standard format. Items to report include the general characteristics of the population, the design of the survey used to collect the data, methods of measurement, summary statistics, and the prevalence of malnutrition (stunting, wasting, and underweight) at z scores of less than -2 and less than -3. As needed, prevalence might be presented by age group or sex. The ability to produce meaningful estimates by subgroup will depend on having sufficiently large samples for these classifications.

—*Parminder S. Suchdev*

See also Body Mass Index (BMI); Centers for Disease Control and Prevention; Nutritional Epidemiology; Sampling Techniques; Vitamin Deficiency Diseases; World Health Organization

Further Readings

Blossner, M., & de Onis, M. (2005). *Malnutrition: Quantifying the health impact at national and local levels.* Geneva, Switzerland: World Health Organization.
Kleinmann, R. (Ed.). (2004). *Pediatric nutrition handbook* (5th ed.). Elk Grove Village, IL: American Academy of Pediatrics.
Muller, O., & Krawinkel, M. (2005). Malnutrition and health in developing countries. *Canadian Medical Association Journal, 173,* 279–286.
World Food Programme. (2005). *A manual: Measuring and interpreting malnutrition and mortality.* Rome: Author.

Web Sites

Centers for Disease Control and Prevention: http://www.cdc.gov.
World Health Organization: http://www.who.int.

MANAGED CARE

Many Americans hold strong opinions about managed care. Audiences in movie houses across the nation famously broke into cheers when actress Helen Hunt's character cursed it in the 1997 movie *As Good as It Gets.* Managed care is an important element of the health care delivery system in the United States today, and familiarity with it is a prerequisite to understanding the contemporary health care context. However, managed care is not neatly defined. Instead, it is an umbrella term covering a historically changing collection of administrative practices, organizational forms, and business strategies intended to make provision of health care more efficient.

Defining efficiency in this context has posed challenges. Some efficiencies focus on information, including electronic medical records, and profiling provider quality to facilitate informed choice by consumers; however, advocates of managed care like to stress that providing better medical care can itself save money. Examples include preventive care and monitoring of chronic conditions, both of which can avert more expensive care. More problematic are instances when there are real or perceived conflicts between reducing costs and providing good care. These conflicts usually focus on restrictions of various kinds, since for every procedure denied, there is a provider or a patient unhappy to be told no.

Managed Care Practices

It is useful to describe common practices that may be bundled together in various organizational forms. *Gatekeeping* is a role assigned to primary care physicians that aims to limit use of high cost specialty services by requiring patients to get referrals from their primary care physician, who provides it only when judged warranted. *Utilization review* is an administrative practice that aims to limit use of unwarranted treatments by hiring third parties to evaluate them. *Capitation* is a payment practice in which the physician receives a set payment based on the number of patients under care, and in turn assumes the financial risk of providing for those patients' care, a strategy that aims to make physicians cost conscious. This strategy aims to reverse an incentive system that rewards physicians for multiple procedures, some of which might be unnecessary or inefficient. Instead, the healthier a patient remains, the greater the savings for the physician. In theory, the physician could retain the entire payment for the patient who needs no care, although in fact some of the capitation payment may be used to pay for insurance that physicians in capitated plans generally hold to limit their liability for patients with very high medical expenses. *Case management* is a practice in which a role is assigned to someone—typically a nonphysician, managed care employee—whose job it is to limit losses due to fragmentation of care and inadequate services.

Background and Development

Despite experiments outside the United States, the managed care story is overwhelmingly an American one, reflecting the distinctive challenges posed by U.S. employer-based insurance, extensive development and use of high cost technologies, and the relative absence of direct government influence on costs. Early elements of managed care can be found in the 20th century in prepaid group plans, such as the one established for workers in Kaiser Industries in 1945, or the Health Insurance Plan of New York, initially created for city workers in New York City in the 1940s.

The term *health maintenance organization* (HMO), coined in 1970 by physician Paul Ellwood, refers to an organized system of care that, in return for a fixed premium, provides (or contracts for) health care for members. HMOs can be classified as a *staff model* (that hires physicians who treat members, and often

also owns hospitals, labs, and other services), a *group model* (that contracts with a physician group that is responsible for paying physicians and contracting with hospitals), or a *network model* (that contracts with multiple physician groups for services).

A second phase in the development of managed care can be dated from the HMO Act of 1973, which was a federal legislation passed as part of a new health policy initiative of the Nixon administration. The bill aimed to expand the proportion of the population with HMO coverage, removed legal barriers to HMO development, tried to seed new HMOs by providing federal dollars to ease the initial financing burden, and spurred entry into existing insurance markets by requiring employers with 25 or more employees to accompany traditional plans with an opportunity to participate in an HMO that met certain federal guidelines. The legislation spurred institutional development, but the overall growth of HMOs fell short of what was anticipated. Only when cost control gained new urgency in the 1980s did managed care gain momentum. Importantly, when rapid growth in managed care organizations (MCOs) was demanded by employers, it was supplied less often by HMOs that directly provided care than by for-profit, largely administrative structures with lower start-up costs. Independent practice associations (IPAs), for example, were formed by individual medical practices that contracted as an organization with an HMO for a per capita fee rate paid for patients.

Context of Growth

The flagging U.S. economy of the late 1980s strengthened the appeal of HMOs to purchasers of managed care. Real per capita health care costs had been increasing for years, but the rate of increase accelerated in the 1980s. Employers had to pay an even greater proportion of labor costs to provide health insurance for their employees, making it harder to compete with foreign counterparts unburdened by employer-based insurance. Health economist Uwe Reinhardt has credited the impact of job insecurity with providing employers with the leverage needed to move employees into health coverage that limited access and benefits to reduce costs. Put simply, Reinhardt believes that employees decided that accepting restricted insurance looked better than being unemployed.

The federal government was a major payer for health care through entitlement-based programs, such as Medicaid and Medicare (both created in 1965), and so also felt pressure from rising health care costs. Bill Clinton was elected president in 1992 with a vague mandate to reform health care, and his administration saw control of health care costs as a key to restoring economic vitality and combined this economic argument with a political case for equity. Clinton created the Task Force on National Health Care Reform, with the mandate to develop a plan to provide universal health care to all Americans. The Clinton logic appealed to some large employers, but once the Clinton plan was defeated in 1994, employers had little reason to hope for cost relief by government intervention. Many shifted their strategies and began contracting with for-profit MCOs.

Doctors' private practices had long functioned like small businesses, providing care to patients who chose their services. But so long as third parties paid the bills, neither doctor nor patient had strong financial incentives to pay attention to costs. Profit-conscious MCOs are intended to introduce price sensitivity by giving physicians and patients an incentive to shop for the best price for medical care and to negotiate tough deals with providers. Many MCOs initially focused on increasing market share, sometimes sacrificing some short-term profits, to gain negotiating leverage and achieve economies of scale. As more and more insured patients moved into restricted plans, MCOs were able to stimulate price competition among hospitals and providers. Physicians often found themselves in the position of subcontractors, vulnerable to being excluded from health plan panels, that is, not having their services covered by health plans, if their practices did not conform to various plan expectations regarding price and practice style.

Power and Backlash

The tools of managed care proved successful in containing costs for a certain time period. Cost increases were constrained through the mid-1990s, and many benefited from low premiums. But most commentators agree that, sometime in the late 1990s, a widespread backlash against managed care occurred. Public distrust grew. Critics pushed for regulation. Hospitals and providers organized to increase negotiating power. Several explanations have been suggested for this shift in mood. Sheer visibility probably played some role because, although mistakes and inequities have always existed, managed care gave

patients someone to blame. Certainly, value conflicts played some role. The shift to managed care ran headlong into the value Americans place on consumer choice of provider and their distaste for limits that connote rationing. In fact, any health care system requires resource allocation choices because it is not possible to provide unlimited health care with limited resources, but the MCOs made these choices explicit. Even if these dissatisfactions had long been present, the upturn in the economy and lower unemployment put employees in a stronger position to gain a hearing for their unhappiness. Once the rise in real per capita health care spending again turned upward after 1997, purchasers could no longer feel confident that economic benefits were being provided in return for the extensive administrative-control-granted MCOs.

MCOs responded with products that allow more choices, but require the patient to pay more for certain services, for instance, to see a physician outside the plan. Examples include reliance on preferred provider organizations (PPOs), point of service (POS) plans, and most recently, a variety of "tiered" plans. In a PPO, physicians contract to offer services to plan participants for a favorable rate. Patients are encouraged to use them by lower co-payments and deductibles, but they can go elsewhere. Facing a similar set of incentives, the patient in a POS plan can go to an individual plan physician for the prepaid fee or opt to go to an outside physician for a higher co-payment. However, these concessions to consumer desire for choice may have loosened the MCO grip on costs. Some see evidence of a modest return to stricter controls, such as utilization review. Also, some firms are building "tiered networks," created by classifying hospitals and providers based on their cost of care, then using cost-sharing incentives to encourage patients to rely on lower-cost sources.

The long-term significance of managed care for U.S. health care is far from clear. The most straightforward narrative stresses its slow development, followed by its rapid rise, the backlash against it, and its subsequent downfall. Yet an alternative version might stress, not the downfall of managed care, but its protean adaptability and the survival of its component mechanisms, as these have been shuffled, reshuffled, and reassembled. Ultimately, any persuasive assessment should acknowledge, first, that it helped end an era of unprecedented professional and patient autonomy, largely financed by third-party payers with remarkably limited attention to costs; second, that the expansion of market strategies to increase competition was accompanied by widespread consolidation in the health care sector; and, third, that despite the constraints it introduced, there is little reason to believe that it can on its own provide a satisfactory solution to rising costs.

—*James Walkup*

See also Formulary, Drug; Governmental Role in Public Health; Health Care Delivery; Health Care Services Utilization

Further Readings

Mechanic, D. (2004). The rise and fall of managed care. *Journal of Health and Social Behavior*, 45(Suppl. 1), 76–86.

Reinhardt, U. (2001). *On the meaning of a rational health system: The American Health System—past, current, future*. Retrieved December 1, 2006, from http://conferences.mc.duke.edu/privatesector/dpsc2001/da.htm.

Schlesinger, M. (2002). On values and democratic policy making: The deceptively fragile consensus around market-oriented medical care. *Journal of Health Politics, Policy, and Law*, 27, 889–925.

MATCHING

Matching is the process of selecting a comparison group so that it is equivalent in terms of certain characteristics (e.g., age or gender) to the group to which it will be compared. Matching is most often used for selection of controls in case-control studies; however, it may be applied in cohort studies as well. This entry describes benefits and drawbacks of matching, as well as the analysis methods applied to matched data. Unless otherwise stated, the discussion refers to matching in case-control studies.

Matching can be performed in different ways. In *individual matching*, one or several controls are selected for each case so that they are equivalent to the case for their values of the variables being matched on. For example, if a case was a female non-smoker, one or more female nonsmokers would be selected as controls. To match on a continuous variable, such as age, controls can be matched to cases within defined categories (age 20 to 29, 30 to 39, etc.) or within a given increment of the case's value (e.g., ±3 years). The latter strategy is termed *caliper* matching.

Frequency matching involves selecting controls so that their distribution matches that of the cases for the variables of interest. Using the example above, where matching was on sex and smoking status, if 30% of cases were female nonsmokers, then 30% of controls would also be selected with these characteristics. Frequency matching will tend to require that all cases are identified before control selection to determine the required proportions, whereas individual matching is more conducive to concurrent identification of cases and controls.

Advantages of Matching

There are benefits to matching in addition to the intuitive appeal of comparing groups that appear similar to one another. Matching can facilitate the selection of a referent group without requiring identification of the entire base population. For example, it may be fairly easy to select as a matched control the "next" patient at a hospital or clinic where cases are identified. On the other hand, it may be much more difficult to enumerate and then enroll a random sample of all patients from the hospital or all potential patients from the surrounding geographic area. Matching can also be an efficient way to identify controls when controlling for factors such as neighborhood or sibship is of importance. Because there would be very few existing appropriate control subjects (people from the same neighborhood or sibship as cases) in the overall base population, choosing a random sample of this population is unlikely to yield a suitable control group. Finally, matching may result in a gain in precision of the estimate of association. This will be most apparent when the matching variable is a strong confounder.

Disadvantages of Matching

Matching also has disadvantages that should be carefully considered. Matching on many variables may make it difficult to locate matched controls, and information on the matching factors needs to be collected for "extra" controls that will not actually end up matching to cases. These factors may decrease cost efficiency of the study. Also, matching variables cannot be considered as independent risk factors themselves. This is because they have been set by design to be distributed similarly in cases and controls. (It *is* still possible to assess effect modification by the matching variables.) Finally, overmatching may result in reduced statistical precision or a biased estimate of association. Matching on strong correlates of exposure, variables associated with exposure but not disease, or factors that are affected by the outcome or exposure of interest should be avoided.

Analysis of Matched Data

Matched data require special consideration in the analysis. This is because the process of matching induces selection bias, so an unmatched analysis will generally lead to a biased estimate of the odds ratio. For individually matched pairs, a crude odds ratio can be calculated using a 2×2 table, set up as shown in Figure 1.

In this table, pairs, rather than individuals, contribute to the cell counts. The matched pairs odds ratio (OR) is calculated as $OR = b/c$ based on the discordant pairs only. To calculate an odds ratio adjusted for multiple covariates, conditional logistic regression is used. For frequency matched data, the methods used are similar to those for unmatched data, with the matching variables included as covariates in all analyses. For individually matched data, it may be possible to conduct a frequency matched analysis if the pairs or sets can be condensed into strata where all sets have equal values for the matching variables.

Matching in Other Study Types

The concept of matching is implicit in certain specific study designs. A case-crossover study is a special instance of matching in which individuals serve as their own controls, while in a nested case-control study with incidence density sampling, controls are matched to cases according to follow-up time. Matching of unexposed to exposed subjects in cohort studies can also be done, and may increase precision. However, this benefit is not guaranteed and the practice is not very common. Other strategies for matching that fall somewhere in between random and fully matched sampling have been described using terms such as partial, marginal, and flexible matching. The term *countermatching* refers to a strategy of choosing controls in a nested study based on their exposure or a proxy of exposure, rather than a confounder. Instead of making members of matched case-control sets similar to one another, as accomplished by the typical matching strategy, countermatching aims to maximize variability within these sets.

—Keely Cheslack-Postava

See also Control Group; Overmatching; Stratified Methods; Study Design

Further Readings

Kelsey, J. L., Whittemore, A. S., Evans, A. S., & Thompson, W. D. (1996). Case-control studies: II. Further design considerations and statistical analysis. In *Methods in observational epidemiology* (2nd ed., pp. 214–243). New York: Oxford University Press.

Langholz, B., & Clayton, D. (1994). Sampling strategies in nested case-control studies. *Environmental Health Perspectives, 102*(Suppl. 8), 47–51.

Rothman, K. J., & Greenland, S. (1998). Matching. In *Modern epidemiology* (2nd ed., pp. 147–161). Philadelphia: Lippincott Williams & Wilkins.

Szklo, M., & Nieto, F. J. (2000). Basic study designs in analytical epidemiology. In *Epidemiology beyond the basics* (pp. 3–51). Gaithersburg, MD: Aspen.

MATERNAL AND CHILD HEALTH EPIDEMIOLOGY

Maternal and child health epidemiology is concerned with determinants of health in populations of women, infants, children, and families, with a particular focus on women's health during pregnancy and after giving birth and on neonatal and early childhood health. This entry describes frequently used indicators of maternal and child health from different parts of the world. It also discusses problems related to obtaining valid data

Figure 1 Calculation of the Odds Ratio Using Individually Matched Data.

about child and maternal health and puts these issues into a public health perspective.

The Mother-Child Relationship

Mother and child form the most basic partnership in evolution, and the health of the child is to a large extent determined by the health of the mother. In the very early phase of life, they also compete for nutrition. An example of this competition is that the average birthweight is less than the optimal birthweight (the birthweight with the lowest mortality). The mother needs to reserve a certain amount of her supply of nutrition to take care of the child and to be able to reproduce in the future. The fetus needs to grow as large as possible to survive the risks it meets outside the uterus.

The unborn child has a remarkable developmental plasticity. The fetus must adapt to the uterine environment and prepare for extrauterine life. When these adaptations are appropriate to the reality of the child's life outside the womb, they are beneficial; but in other cases, they may be inappropriate, and the health consequences may be serious. For example, insulin resistance may be a fetal response to a temporary insufficient food supply to slow down growth in order to preserve the limited energy available for brain development and to prepare for a life with an expected shortage of food. Insulin resistance may be an advantage in such an environment, since it facilitates storing fat in time periods when food is plentiful. On the other hand, if food becomes unduly plentiful, insulin resistance may predispose an individual to obesity and diabetes because glucose transport to cells is impaired and insulin production may not be able to keep up with demands. Lack of food, stress, infections, and environmental exposures not only affect the health of the pregnant mother but may also have lifelong implications for the unborn child.

Indicators of Maternal and Child Health

A number of specific indicators have been developed to facilitate surveillance and research on maternal and child health issues. Data on the following indicators based on the definitions of the World Health Organization (WHO) are available in many countries. Except for the fertility rate, they deal with causes of mortality.

- *Perinatal Mortality Rate.* The risk of fetal or infant death during late pregnancy (at 22 completed weeks of gestation and more), during childbirth, and up to 7 completed days of life, expressed per 1,000 total births.
- *Neonatal Mortality Rate.* The risk of dying between birth and within the first 28 days of life, expressed per 1,000 live births.
- *Infant Mortality Rate.* The risk of dying between birth and exactly 1 year of life, expressed per 1,000 live births.
- *Child Mortality Rate, Under 5.* The risk of dying before age 5, expressed per 1,000 live births.
- *Maternal Death.* The pregnancy-related death of a woman, either during pregnancy or within 42 days of termination of pregnancy.
- *Maternal Mortality Ratio.* The number of maternal deaths per 100,000 live births.
- *Total Fertility Rate.* Estimated number of live births that a woman will have from her 15th year through her childbearing years.

Child and Maternal Mortality

One of the main contributors to the improvements in life expectancy in the 20th century was the reduction in child mortality; in 2003, the global mortality rate in children under 5 reached a low of 79 per 1,000. However, the most progress has been made in high-income countries. There is an enormous gap in child mortality between the richest and the poorest parts of the world.

During the past 30 to 40 years, many national and international organizations have tried to reduce inequalities in health by improving vaccination coverage and breastfeeding practices, and by reducing malnutrition and deaths from diarrhea. The global mortality rate for children below 5 years of age was halved from 1960 to 1990. The WHO aims at reaching a two-thirds reduction from 1990 to 2015, but progress has been modest in recent years. Communicable diseases such as pneumonia, diarrhea, measles, malaria, and tuberculosis are still the main killers in poor countries, and the HIV/AIDS epidemic in sub-Saharan Africa has even erased the survival and health gains in these countries. About 11 million children below the age of 5 still die annually from preventable causes.

The global neonatal mortality rate in 2000 was estimated at 30 per 1,000, but with large geographical variations. Moreover, better survival has been achieved mainly in children who have survived the first month of life, while neonatal mortality, especially in the

Table 1 Neonatal and Maternal Mortality in Countries Where the Decline in Child Mortality Has Stagnated or Reversed

Decline in Child Mortality (1990–2003)	Number of Countries	Percentage of Live Births (2000–2005)	Under-5 Mortality Rate (1990)	Under-5 Mortality Rate (2003)	Neonatal Mortality Rate (2000)	Maternal Mortality Rate (2000)
On track	30 (OECD)	11%	22	13	7	29
	63 (non-OECD)	23%	78	39	19	216
Slow progress	51	44%	92	72	35	364
In reversal	14	6%	111	139	41	789
Stagnating	29	16%	207	188	47	959

Source: Adapted from the World Health Organization, "The World Health Report 2005. Make every mother and child count."

first critical days of life, has undergone more modest reductions. Almost 30% of all child deaths in 2000 happened in the first week of life and were due mainly to infections, birth asphyxia, and prematurity. To reach the WHO goal for child mortality, comprehensive health care programs during pregnancy, during childbirth, and in the postnatal period are needed. However, these interventions may be more expensive to implement than the interventions needed later in infancy.

In 2000, 529,000 women died as a result of pregnancy or childbirth, which is equivalent to a global maternal mortality ratio of 400 per 100,000. Only 1% of these deaths occurred in high-income countries. Most causes of maternal deaths are preventable complications to pregnancy and childbirth, such as hemorrhage, obstructed labor, sepsis, eclampsia, unsafe abortion, and anemia. In Africa, HIV/AIDS, malaria, and the tradition of genital mutilation contribute to and worsen these complications. Better health care during pregnancy and childbirth not only improves neonatal survival but also reduces maternal mortality and the numbers of stillbirths. At present, it is estimated that 3.3 million babies are stillborn—a number that approaches that of the 4 million infants who die within the first 28 days of life. The provision of skilled perinatal care is crucial to further reduce child and maternal mortality.

Other factors related to maternal mortality are birth spacing, use of contraceptives, and use of safe methods of abortion. It is estimated that 19% of married women in low-income countries have unmet contraceptive needs.

Other Aspects of Child and Maternal Health

In most high-income countries, maternal mortality is now low, but other aspects of maternal health are reasons for concern. The frequency of preterm deliveries (birth before 37 weeks of pregnancy) is often high (more than 10% in some countries) and may be increasing.

Global fertility rates (the total number of children a woman has over her lifetime) fell from six to three after the introduction of contraception in the last part of the 20th century, and in some countries, the rate is now only slightly above one. It is not known whether the increasing use of infertility treatments in high-income countries reflects increasing infertility problems. However, part of the decrease in fertility rates is an artifact related to delayed reproduction. The measure depends on a steady state situation where age-specific fertility rates do not change over calendar time.

The substantial increase in the rate of caesarean sections cannot be explained by purely medical indications or related improvements in neonatal outcome. The rates are as high as 30% to 50% in some countries of South America. Although caesarean section in a well-functioning health care system is considered a safe mode of delivery, the consequences for future pregnancies are still uncertain.

Children are more vulnerable to many environmental stressors because of their rapid growth, and during intrauterine life, the unborn child is not well protected from external exposures that cross the placenta barrier. The fetus may be unable to metabolize some of these toxic compounds, and the brain may have vulnerable time periods where lesions could have long-lasting effects. Western lifestyle factors that may interfere with child and maternal health are in great contrast to some of the problems observed in the poorest parts of the world. The abundance of energy-rich foods combined with a lack of physical activity among both parents and children is related to obesity problems in many parts of the world, with an obesity prevalence of 10% to 25% among women of childbearing age in affluent countries and growing obesity problems in childhood. The total burden of diseases related to childhood obesity is still to be discovered, but it is expected that the occurrence of diabetes and cardiovascular diseases will increase and have an earlier onset, accompanied with reduced life quality and physical impairment.

Congenital malformations may be serious or trivial and are difficult to count because some are invisible or are simply deviations from normal structures. Estimates of the frequency of malformations at birth, therefore, ranges from 1% to 7% among all births, depending on how thoroughly the newborns are examined. Some causes of congenital malformations are known, such as radiation, some infections during pregnancy, or specific types of medicine, but in most situations the causes of a specific malformation are unknown. Whether this frequency is increasing or decreasing is unknown.

Asthma and atopic diseases are frequent (about 20% in some countries). The increasing prevalence and the worldwide variation indicate that environmental factors play an important role in the etiology of these diseases, but the underlying mechanisms are poorly understood.

Behavioral problems such as attention-deficit hyperactivity disorder (ADHD) have a frequency of 3% to 15% in affluent societies, and an increasing trend has been suggested in these countries. It should, however, be considered that the condition and therefore also its frequency are defined by manmade cutoff levels in a continuous distribution of behavioral problems.

Measurement Issues in Maternal and Child Health Epidemiology

Health is a broad concept, and data sources that allow international comparisons and comparisons over time cover only part of this concept while those that are available are often far from perfect. Even data on mortality, especially cause-specific mortality, are difficult

to get from many countries. For instance, although death is well-defined, death rates may be difficult to calculate because accurate information on the total population may not be known in populations with poor demographic statistics. In addition, the validity of data on causes of death depends on the availability of diagnostic facilities for all who die in the population. In some cases, the causes of death rely on a "verbal autopsy," which is a retrospective interview of close relatives done by people with limited clinical training.

Some of the concepts used in maternal and child health epidemiology are also difficult to operationalize, such as "a pregnancy-related death" used to estimate maternal mortality. If a woman dies of eclamptic seizures or during labor, the death is clearly related to the pregnancy, but if she dies from a stroke or commits suicide, either of which may be related to the pregnancy, the death may not be counted as "pregnancy-related."

All mortality or disease rates are expressed as events per unit of time, and in reproduction the counting time starts at either the time of conception or at the time of birth. Deaths that happen during fetal life would normally be seen as a function of time since conception, but this period is only estimated, and the estimates may lack precision because the exact time of conception is unknown. Stillbirths are therefore routinely calculated not as a function of the number of fetuses in the population under study at the time of death but as a proportion of all births because data on births may be available.

The change from fetal time to extrauterine time normally starts at 266 days after conception. When variation from this time exceeds certain limits (< 37 weeks or > 42 weeks) the terms *preterm birth* or *postterm birth* are used, but these terms are purely descriptive and based on the estimate of gestational age. Estimating gestational age is key and unfortunately not easy. Traditionally, the estimates have been based on Naegel's rule, which states that the due date of birth can be calculated by adding 7 days and then subtracting 3 months to the first day of the last menstrual period. This works well only if menstrual periods are regular, which often is not the case. In affluent societies, estimates are now based on measures of growth by using ultrasound techniques. This principle rests on the assumption that growth in the early phase of life follows the same velocity. This assumption is good enough for making clinical predictions but have some limitations when used in epidemiologic studies.

Since the pregnant woman may carry more than one child, there may even be ambiguity in whether preterm births or preterm confinements have been counted. Preterm births would, for example, increase over time in countries that increasingly use infertility treatments leading to more twins.

Congenital anomalies are by definition present at birth but they may not be diagnosed at birth. For example, some malformations may not manifest themselves until much later in life, although their onset occurs during fetal life, usually in the 2nd and 3rd months of pregnancy. Also, many—perhaps most—of these malformations lead to spontaneous abortions. The number of anomalies (the prevalence) present at birth therefore reflects only some of the cases that occur during fetal life. Abortions that are induced as part of prenatal screening will also affect the prevalence of congenital malformations.

Most data on maternal and childhood health come from ad hoc data collections or review of medical records. Data on some conditions that do not always lead to hospitalization, such as obesity, asthma, pregnancy nausea, or even early spontaneous abortions, depend on results generated in specific studies. For example, it is expected that about 30% of all pregnancies end in spontaneous abortions, but only part of these will be known because they happen before the pregnancy is clinically recognized. These abortions will be detected only if it is possible to follow women trying to become pregnant over time and measure sensitive biological markers of a pregnancy in urine or blood.

Other studies would have to rely on asking questions on nausea, asthma symptoms, or behavioral problems during childhood. Most of these measures will come with some measurement errors. Measures of behavioral problems during childhood will be heavily influenced by actual and present problems when filling in the questionnaires. Such studies will also be biased by people who are invited to take part in the study but refuse or drop out during follow-up.

Public Health Implications

Maternal and child health is not only a medical concern. Social and economic factors play major roles (in particular because women and children are often a low priority in poor countries), and, in turn, poor maternal and child health lead to undesirable social consequences. Poverty and inequity, unstable and unjust political systems, and lack of education are important determinants of maternal and child health. These factors contribute to a vicious cycle that may require political actions to be broken. A child who grows up in poverty and with a shortage of food will not reach his or her optimal growth potential and may suffer reduced mental capacity. A girl with only a limited education will be at high risk of getting pregnant at a young age, and she will be less prepared to care for her own and her baby's health.

During pregnancy, she may have a too low weight gain and be more susceptible to infections, which will impair her chances of surviving the challenges of childbirth. Her short stature due to restricted growth during childhood will furthermore place her in higher risk of preterm birth, prolonged or obstructed labor, and giving birth to a low birthweight baby, and both of them may be at high risk of death or severe impairment. Furthermore, limited energy supplies and other hazards during intrauterine life may alter organ functions and the child may be more susceptible to diseases in later life. Unfortunately, most research takes place in countries where the health problems are smallest, and it is not certain that research results generated in one region can be applied in a different region with different resources and risk factors. Information on child and maternal health in low-income countries often stems from rather crude data of poor quality but is sufficient to demonstrate that the world's poorest countries carry the largest burden of diseases. They have serious health problems that impair long-term health, and they have the smallest capacity to cope with these problems.

—Ellen Aagaard Nohr and Jorn Olsen

See also Child and Adolescent Health; Fertility, Measures of; Fetal Death, Measures of; Health, Definitions of; Reproductive Epidemiology

Further Readings

Bellamy, C. (2002). Child health. In R. Detels, J. McEwen, R. Beaglehole, & H. Tanaka (Eds.), *Oxford textbook of public health* (pp. 1603–1622). Oxford, UK: Oxford University Press.

Gluckman, P. D. (2004). Living with the past. Evolution, development, and patterns of disease. *Science, 305,* 1733–1736.

Janssen, I., Katzmarzyk, P. T., Boyce, W. F., Vereecken, C., Mulvihill, C., Roberts, C., et al. (2005). Comparison of overweight and obesity prevalence in school-aged youth from 34 countries and their relationships with physical activity and dietary patterns. *Obesity Reviews, 6,* 123–132.

Krickeberg, K., Kar, A., & Chakraborty, A. K. (2005). Epidemiology in developing countries. In W. Ahrens & I. Pigeot (Eds.), *Handbook of epidemiology* (pp. 545–1590). Berlin: Springer-Verlag.

Olsen, J., & Basso, O. (2005). Reproductive epidemiology. In W. Ahrens & I. Pigeot (Eds.), *Handbook of epidemiology* (pp. 1043–1110). Berlin: Springer-Verlag.

Pearce, N., & Douwes, J. (2006). The global epidemiology of asthma in children. *The International Journal of Tuberculosis and Lung Disease, 10,* 125–132.

Wang, S., An, L., & Cochran, S. D. (2002). Women. In R. Detels, J. McEwen, R. Beaglehole, & H. Tanaka (Eds.), *Oxford textbook of public health* (pp. 1587–1602). Oxford, UK: Oxford University Press.

WHO 2005 Global Survey on Maternal and Perinatal Health Research Group. (2006). Caesarean delivery rates and pregnancy outcomes: The 2005 WHO global survey on maternal and perinatal health in Latin America. *Lancet, 367,* 1819–1829.

World Health Organization. (2003). Diet, nutrition and chronic diseases in context. In *Diet, Nutrition and the Prevention of Chronic Diseases. Report of a Joint WHO/FAO Expert Consultation.* WHO Technical Report Series, No. 916. Geneva, Switzerland: Author. Retrieved July 26, 2006, from http://whqlibdoc.who.int/trs/WHO_TRS_916.pdf.

World Health Organization. (2005). Make every mother and child count. *The World Health Report.* Geneva, Switzerland: Author. Retrieved July 26, 2006, from http://www.who.int/whr/2005/whr2005_en.pdf.

Measles

Measles is a highly contagious viral infection, which prior to the introduction of effective vaccines was a common experience of childhood, sometimes with fatal consequences. Unfortunately, even today not all children receive the vaccine despite its efficacy and availability. In May 2003, the World Health Assembly endorsed resolution WHA56.20 urging Member countries to achieve a goal to reduce global measles deaths by half by end of 2005 compared with the 1999 estimates. Based on results from surveillance data and a natural history model, overall, global measles mortality decreased 48% from an estimated 871,000 deaths in 1999 to an estimated 454,000 deaths in 2004. Many of the recommended World Health Organization (WHO)

measles control strategies now in place had been developed and first used during the early 1990s in the Americas, when the countries of the Caribbean and Latin America adopted a multi-tiered vaccination approach combining routine vaccination and mass vaccination campaigns.

Among the WHO regions, the Region of the Americas has had the most success in controlling measles. Starting in 1999, countries throughout the Region of the Americas embarked on accelerated measles elimination activities, using strategies building on the accomplishments of the polio elimination program. Implementing a measles elimination program was clearly an ambitious task, requiring the collaboration of ministries of health, the private sector, nongovernmental organizations, and multilateral and bilateral international partners. The last occurrence of widespread measles virus transmission in the Americas dates to November 2002. Sporadic cases and outbreaks have continued to occur, although 51% of the 370 measles cases reported in the Americas between January 2003 and April 2006 were positively linked to an importation.

Infectious Agent and Transmission

Measles virus is a member of the genus *Morbillivirus* of the Paramyxoviridae family. The virus appears to be antigenically stable—there is no evidence that the viral antigens have significantly changed over time. The virus is sensitive to ultraviolet light, heat, and drying.

Measles virus is transmitted primarily by respiratory droplets or airborne spray to mucous membranes in the upper respiratory tract or the conjunctiva. Man is the only natural host of measles virus. Although monkeys may become infected, transmission in the wild does not appear to be an important mechanism by which the virus persists in nature.

Measles is highly contagious and is most communicable 1 to 3 days before the onset of fever and cough. Communicability decreases rapidly after rash onset. Secondary attack rates among susceptible household contacts have been reported to be more than 80%. Due to the high transmission efficiency of measles, outbreaks have been reported in populations where only 3% to 7% of the individuals were susceptible.

Prior to the development of effective vaccines, measles occurred worldwide. Presently, in countries that have not embarked on eradication or elimination campaigns or achieved a very high level of sustained measles immunization coverage, the disease still exists. In temperate climates, outbreaks generally occur in late winter and early spring. In tropical climates, transmission appears to increase after the rainy season. In developing countries with low vaccination coverage, epidemics often occur every 2 to 3 years and usually last between 2 and 3 months. Even countries with relatively high vaccination coverage levels may experience outbreaks when the number of susceptible children becomes large enough to sustain widespread transmission.

Epidemiology

Since the introduction of effective measles vaccines, the epidemiology of measles has changed in both developed and developing countries. As vaccine coverage has increased, there has been a marked reduction in measles incidence; and, with decreased measles virus circulation, the average age at which infection occurs has increased. Even in areas where coverage rates are high, outbreaks may still occur. Periods of low incidence may be followed by a pattern of periodic measles outbreaks, with increasing number of years between epidemics. Outbreaks are generally due to the accumulation of susceptibles, including both unvaccinated children and vaccine failures. Approximately 15% of children vaccinated at 9 months and 5% to 10% of those vaccinated at 12 months of age are not protected after vaccination. Outbreaks among older children also occur and usually involve those children who have not been vaccinated and have previously escaped natural measles infection because of the relatively low measles incidence. Since measles vaccine is less than 100% effective, some vaccinated children may also contract measles, especially during periods of intense transmission.

In large urban areas, even where measles vaccine coverage is high, the number of susceptible infants and children may still be sufficient to sustain transmission. Conditions such as high birth rates, overcrowding, and immigration of susceptible children from rural areas can facilitate transmission. Measles remains endemic in such areas, and a large proportion of cases occurs in infants before their first birthday. In endemic areas, only a brief period exists between the waning of maternal antibody and children's exposure to circulating measles virus. The highest age-specific measles case-fatality rates occur in children below 1 year of age.

Clinical Features

The incubation period is approximately 10 days (with a range of 8 to 13 days) from the time of exposure to the onset of fever and about 14 days from exposure to the appearance of the rash. Measles infection presents with a 2- to 3-day prodrome of fever, malaise, cough, and a runny nose. Conjunctivitis and bronchitis are commonly present, and the patient is highly contagious. A harsh, nonproductive cough is present throughout the febrile period, persists for 1 to 2 weeks in uncomplicated cases, and is often the last symptom to disappear. Generalized lymphadenopathy commonly occurs in young children. Older children may complain of photophobia (light sensitivity) and, occasionally, of arthralgias (joint pains). Koplik's spots, slightly raised white dots 2 to 3 mm in diameter on an erythematous base, may be seen shortly before rash onset in 80% of the cases. Initially, there are usually one to five of these lesions, but as rash onset approaches there may be as many as several hundred.

Within 2 to 4 days after the prodromal symptoms begin, a characteristic rash made up of large, blotchy red areas initially appears behind the ears and on the face. At the same time, a high fever develops. The rash peaks in 2 to 3 days and becomes most concentrated on the trunk and upper extremities. The density of the rash can vary. It may be less evident in children with dark skin. The rash typically lasts from 3 to 7 days and may be followed by a fine desquamation (shedding of the outer layers of skin). Some children develop severe exfoliation, especially if they are malnourished.

Complications

Complications from measles include otitis media, pneumonia, diarrhea, blindness, and encephalitis. It is estimated that otitis media plus pneumonia occurs in 10% to 30% of infants and young children with measles. Respiratory infections are the most common cause of significant morbidity and mortality in infants and children with measles. Pneumonia may be due to the measles virus alone or to secondary infection with other viral agents or bacterial organisms. Diarrhea is one of the major factors contributing to the adverse impact of measles on the nutritional status in children in developing countries. Measles infection is more severe among children who are already malnourished.

Neurological complications occur in 1 to 4 of every 1,000 infected children. The most common manifestation is febrile convulsions. Encephalitis or postinfectious encephalopathy occurs in approximately 1 of every 1,000 infected children. Subacute sclerosing panencephalitis (SSPE; an infection of the nervous system) with an incidence of approximately 1 per 100,000 measles cases and may develop several years after a measles infection.

In developed countries, the case-fatality rate for measles tends to be low (between 0.1 and 1.0 per 1,000 cases). In developing countries, the overall case-fatality rate has been estimated at between 3% and 6%; the highest case-fatality rate occurs in infants 6 to 11 months of age, with malnourished infants at greatest risk. These rates may be an underestimate because of incomplete reporting of outcomes of severe measles illnesses. In certain high-risk populations, case-fatality rates have been reported to be as high as 20% or 30% in infants below 1 year of age.

Other than supportive therapies, there is currently no specific treatment for measles infection. Administration of vitamin A to children at the time of measles diagnosis has been shown to decrease both the severity of disease and the case-fatality rate. Accordingly, the WHO has recommended that vitamin A be administered to all children diagnosed with measles infection.

Immunity and Vaccination

Prior to the availability of measles vaccine, measles infection was virtually universal by 10 years of age. Infants are generally protected until 5 to 9 months of age by passively acquired maternal measles antibody. Some infants who are immunized before they are 9 months old may not develop detectable immunity because of interference by maternal measles antibody. Immunity following natural infection is believed to be lifelong, and vaccination with measles vaccine has been shown to be protective for at least 20 years.

Serologic studies have demonstrated that measles vaccines induce seroconversion in about 95% of children 12 months of age and older. Immunity conferred by a single dose vaccination against measles has been shown to persist for at least 20 years and is generally thought to be lifelong for most individuals. Studies indicate that antibody responses to the measles component when given as multiple antigens is equivalent to receiving the measles vaccine separately.

The likelihood of detecting immunoglobulin M (IgM) antibodies decreases with time. Aspirates, throat swabs, or nasopharyngeal swabs are the preferred

sample for viral detection/isolation for measles viruses, but urine samples are an acceptable alternative. Data on viral genotypes are critical for tracking transmission pathways, investigating suspected vaccine-related cases, documenting the elimination of endemic strains, and supporting the hypothesis of importations from other regions.

Vaccine Schedule

Routine immunization schedules usually recommend that the first dose of measles vaccine be administered to children aged ≥ 12 months. However, if measles is present in a community, consideration may be given to lowering the age of measles vaccination to 6 months (with an additional dose at 12 months of age.) All children should have a second opportunity to receive a measles-containing vaccine. This may be provided either as a second dose in the routine immunization schedule or through periodic mass vaccination campaigns.

Vaccine Safety

The measles vaccines are generally extremely safe. Adverse events range from pain and swelling at the injection site to rare systemic reactions such as anaphylaxis. They tend to occur among people who have never been vaccinated and are very rare after revaccination. There are only two major contraindications to measles vaccination; those who have experienced an anaphylactic or severe hypersensitivity reaction to a previous dose of measles vaccine or to neomycin. In addition, pregnant women or those who have severe immunosuppressive diseases should not be vaccinated.

Vaccination Strategies

Vaccination of each successive birth cohort with a single dose of measles vaccine delivered through routine health services was a strategy originally used in many countries to control measles. Nevertheless, while vaccine coverage increased, measles outbreaks continued to occur. Since measles vaccine is less than 100% effective and coverage is rarely universal via routine health services, an accumulation of nonimmune children results over time. With each successive birth cohort, the number of children susceptible to measles increases (including both children who were never vaccinated and those who are vaccine failures). This buildup of susceptible children over time in a population is the most serious obstacle to measles elimination.

To improve measles control, a number of countries have adopted a vaccination schedule that recommends two doses of a measles vaccine. The first dose is usually given at or after 12 months of age; the second dose is often given when children start school. For those countries with sufficient resources, a well-developed health services delivery system, and school attendance by the majority of children, this schedule reduces the number of susceptible children and ultimately interrupts measles transmission. However, the routine addition of a second dose is not an appropriate strategy for measles elimination in those countries where large segments of the population do not have access to routine health services and/or where many children do not attend school. Unfortunately, children who never received the first routine dose of measles vaccine are also those who are unlikely to receive the scheduled second routine dose.

To rectify this shortcoming, the Pan American Health Organization (PAHO) developed a three-tiered vaccination strategy. Its implementation allowed significant interruption of transmission of the measles virus in the Region of the Americas. The three main components of the PAHO vaccination strategy are as follows:

• First, measles virus circulation in a community is rapidly interrupted by conducting a one-time-only "catch-up" measles vaccination campaign over a wide age cohort of infants, children, and adolescents.

• Second, to maintain the interruption of measles virus circulation, routine immunization programs (or "keep-up" vaccination) must provide measles vaccine to at least 95% of each new birth cohort of infants before the age of 2 years in every district of the country.

• Finally, to counter the inevitable buildup of children susceptible to measles, periodic "follow-up" vaccination campaigns among preschool-aged children are carried out every 4 years. In addition to these three components, special intensive efforts, known as "mop-up" vaccination, may be required to provide measles vaccine to children living in high-risk areas who missed routine vaccination and also escaped vaccination during the "catch-up" and "follow-up" campaigns.

Surveillance and Global Eradication

A sensitive surveillance system is essential to monitor progress toward and to sustain measles elimination. In the initial stages of measles elimination efforts, the primary purpose of measles surveillance is to detect in a timely manner all areas where the measles virus is circulating, not necessarily to investigate every suspected measles case. However, once endemic transmission has become rare or has been interrupted, the surveillance goal becomes to detect and investigate all suspected measles cases, including those imported, and to implement activities that prevent or limit secondary transmission. This goal requires rapid notification and investigation of all suspected measles patients.

Both the successful smallpox eradication program and the efforts to control polio suggest that achieving measles eradication depends on several factors: the biological characteristics of the organism, vaccine technology, surveillance and laboratory identification, effective delivery of vaccination programs, and international commitment. Clearly, experience in the Americas has shown that these factors favor a measles eradication effort. There is also growing international support for such an initiative both from governmental and donor agencies.

—Marc Strassburg

Note: The author worked as a consultant for the PAHO measles elimination program, and in that capacity assisted in writing a number of earlier versions of the measles elimination field guide. Sections from both previous and current field guides were liberally adapted for this article.

See also Child and Adolescent Health; Disease Eradication; Public Health Surveillance; Vaccination

Further Readings

Clements, J. C., Strassburg, M. A., Cutts, Ft., Milstien, J. B., & Torel, C. (1992). Global control of measles: New strategies for the 1990s. In E. Kurstak (Ed.), *Control of virus diseases* (2nd ed., pp. 179–210). New York: Marcel Dekker.

Clements, J. C., Strassburg, M. A., Cutts, Ft., Milstien, J. B., & Torel, C. (1993). Challenges for global control of measles in the 1990's. In E. Kurstak (Ed.), *Measles and poliomyelitis* (pp. 13–24). Vienna, Austria: Springer-Verlag.

Clements, J. G., Strassburg, M., Cutts, Ft., & Torel, C. (1992). The epidemiology of measles. *World Health Statistics Quarterly, 45*, 285–291.

de Quadros, C., Olive, J. M., Hersh, B., Strassburg, M. A., Henderson, D. A., Brandling-Bennet, D., et al. (1996).

Measles elimination in the Americas: Evolving strategies. *Journal of the American Medical Association, 275,* 224–229.

Drotman, D. P., & Strassburg, M. A. (2001). Sources of data. In J. C. Thomas & D. J. Weber (Eds.), *Epidemiologic methods for the study of infectious diseases* (pp. 119–137). New York: Oxford University Press.

Galindo, M. A., Santin, M., Resik, S., Ribas, M. L. A., Guzman, M., Lago, P. M., et al. (1998). The eradication of measles from Cuba. *Pan American Journal of Public Health, 4*(3), 171–177.

Morgan, O. W. C. (2004). Following in the footsteps of smallpox: Can we achieve the global eradication of measles? [Electronic version]. *BMC International Health and Human Rights, 4*(1), doi: 10.1186/1472-698X-4-1. Retrieved February 28, 2007, from http://www.pubmedcentral.nih.gov/articlerender.fcgi?artid=387835.

Pan American Health Organization. (2005). *Measles elimination: Field guide.* Washington, DC: Author. (Scientific and Technical Publication No. 605). Retrieved February 28, 2007, from http://www.paho.org/english/ad/fch/im/fieldguide_measles.pdf.

Pan American Health Organization. (2006). *Immunization Newsletter, 28*(4) [Electronic version]. Retrieved February 28, 2007, from http://www.paho.org/English/AD/FCH/IM/sne2804.pdf.

Weekly Epidemiological Record. (2006, March 10). *81*(10), 89–96.

Measurement

Scientists from numerous disciplines frequently make sense of the world by using yardsticks that they hope will show how their study participants are performing, what they are thinking, and how they interact with others. Numbers are faithfully recorded, spun through various forms of software, and prepared for publication. All this is fine if the yardsticks themselves are true—all the time, in every single place they are used, regardless of who is doing the actual recording of the numbers, and regardless of the circumstances in which the numbers are obtained. But what if the yardsticks themselves are shaky?

In epidemiologic analyses based strictly on counting, a few units in dispute here or there may seem rather unlikely to significantly change the overall interpretation of the data set. However, even a single reclassification of a case from one cell to another, for instance, can force a confidence interval to bracket 1.0 where it otherwise might not do so, or a statistical test to just miss threshold. Although it might not

appear as an issue when the data are highly differentiable, the need for quality measurement is fundamentally inescapable. Equally important, whole sections of the field of epidemiology have long ago been unbound from the simple exercise of counting, working instead in arenas in which measurements take the form of scores, scales, and other assessments. In such settings, the challenges to designing and conducting strong and reproducible studies are magnified.

The domain of psychometrics gives criteria concerning the quality of a measurement. Although "psychometrics" has been a label narrowly applied to a particular specialized branch of mathematical and statistical thinking within educational research, this entry uses the term in a broader sense. It explores a handful of concepts that are crucial to all measurements and considers recent examples in the epidemiologic literature that show the importance of such considerations.

Reliability

Psychometricians have been preaching for decades that the core considerations of good measurement must not be simply assumed whenever a set of assessments is made. Principal among these considerations is that the measurements be reliable and valid. Reliability is defined as the consistency of measurements made by a specific group of persons using the measurement instrument, working under the same conditions. In the most elementary sense, high reliability means that data will be consistent if the identical study is run again. Even in closely monitored laboratory conditions, however, there are numerous possible contaminants that can interfere with obtaining reliable data. To reduce error and improve reliability, laboratories make constant use of standardizing and correcting baseline values for all their measurement devices. Likewise, measurements made in the field need comparable standardizations: One often-used method for standardization is to be sure that different field workers show high levels of agreement when facing the same situations for data collection. A simple but informative analysis is to evaluate overall agreement between workers using varying tolerances: A tolerance of zero (equivalent to exact agreement) results in a overall percentage between 0 and 100, then (if not 100%) tolerances are widened step by step (i.e, liberalizing the definition of agreement) until 100% agreement is achieved. (Software to accomplish this task is available in the R package.*) The climb toward full agreement as tolerances are made less restrictive is a direct reflection of the reliability of the sources of data.

Three other classical methods to assess reliability are test-retest, multiple forms, and split-half assessments. In test-retest, the specific test instrument is used by the same workers at different times. The correlation coefficients between the scores achieved at the differing times serve as coefficients of reliability. In multiple forms, the testing sequence is systematically varied, given to either the same workers twice or to two or more different groups of workers. Split-half reliability is estimated by analyzing half the results from the test instrument in comparison with the results of the overall analysis. Both Cronbach's alpha and the Kuder-Richardson coefficient called KR-20 provide readily interpretable statistics describing the amount of reliability in the measurements.

A measurement tool that does not yield reliable scores leads to the possibility that every subsequent interpretation will be suspect. If measurements are unreliable, there are few good ways of disentangling how much the variation within those measurements is explainable and how much is due simply to error. Even when excellent research designs and high-level statistical procedures are employed, in general whatever real effects are present will be underestimated.

An example of the importance of understanding test reliability is seen in Schiffman and Schatzkin's (1994) analysis of two earlier studies in molecular epidemiology conducted by their research team. In analyses of the relationship between human papillomavirus (HPV) infection and cervical neoplasia, the issue in brief was whether molecular assays produced consistent results across many clinical specimens collected over a period of months or years. Two different case-control studies had been conducted several years apart to investigate the presence of HPV and cervical intraepithelial neoplasia. While both used the same case definitions, HPV testing underwent significant transformation during the intervening years and the

resulting assays differed. In the first study, comparisons of results between laboratories found poor agreement, but in the second study, data were far less often misclassified. The association between HPV and neoplasia was an order of magnitude greater in the second study. Indeed, the conclusions of the two studies differed dramatically—the first pointed to HPV infection as a risk factor but not the key etiologic agent, while in the second, HPV was found to have a central, causal role. The authors concluded that measurement error can be a common problem in studies that rely on highly technical assays and can lead directly to wrong conclusions.

Validity

The term *validity* refers to a number of different concerns about measurements. Internal validity is an indication of how measurements perform in settings or with cases that are similar to those for which the measurement was first developed. A close synonym for internal validity is reproducibility. External validity is an indication of how the measurements perform in new settings or in cases with characteristics different from the original. A close synonym for external validity is generalizability. Face validity is obtained by having experts vet the measurement in question to assure that the measurement appears to reflect ground truth. Content validity can be ascertained by study of the relationships between different measurement dimensions. Criterion validity can be assessed by benchmarking one measurement against a gold standard; additionally, criterion validity can be separated into the success with which the measurements estimate concurrent events and the success with which they predict future events. Construct validity can be appraised by how well the measurement tool matches the underlying theory or model of what is being measured; additionally, construct validity can be separated into the degree to which the elements within the measurement scales converge on the same result, and the degree to which the measurements succeed in discriminating between cases that diverge from one another by greater or lesser amounts.

An important consideration is that a given measurement tool can have high reliability but poor validity. This is not unlike achieving great success with a bow and arrow, hitting the same target repeatedly, but then discovering that the target is not the one we had been aiming at. On the other hand, a given

---

* R is an international collaborative open-source software product for data manipulation, calculation, and graphical display—available at no charge—that is highly extensible, integrating contributions from numerous statistical professionals by means of packages of code and documentation built to strict criteria. R is a product of the R Foundation for Statistical Computing, Vienna, Austria. Extensive information is available at http://www.r-project.org.

measurement tool cannot have high validity without also being reliable. That is, a broad sweep of arrow volleyed toward the vague area of the target will not lead to a well-focused series of strikes. Many authors on this topic have discussed threats to validity and reliability and the essential need to assure optimal research designs to standardize measurement and reduce error.

An example of a noteworthy analysis of validity is seen in Hukkelhoven et al.'s (2006) detailed comparison of prediction success using competing models of outcome after traumatic brain injury. The authors identified 10 competing prognostic models in the recent literature. Each had been developed from careful study of samples of brain-injured patients assessed by numerous measurement tools, with the final product in every instance being touted as the best combination of indicators of outcome. Hukkelhoven et al. systematically applied each of these models to validation populations composed of 4,238 brain-injured patients from published sources. The success or failure of each model was examined in terms of discrimination and calibration, two terms that are underpinned by strong statistical methods. Discrimination refers to a given model's capacity to distinguish between patients who have different outcomes and can be immediately determined from the receiver operating characteristic (ROC) curve (see R package "ROCR"). Calibration refers to the degree to which a model's estimates match reality by producing unbiased estimates and can be tested by goodness-of-fit statistics.

Hukkelhoven et al. (2006) found that the selected models demonstrated substantial variability in discrimination: The range was from 0.61 to 0.89 (where perfect discrimination would be 1.0 and no discrimination would be 0.50). Additionally, the same models varied in discrimination depending on which validation population was being considered. Calibrations for four of the six competing prognostic models were poor, with the direct implication that predicted mortality was too high compared with actual mortality. For example, one model suggested that one of the validation populations should have a mortality of 60% when in fact the observed mortality was merely 35%. Calibration curves were often nonlinear, signifying that some of the models might be relatively more correct for some cases but not for others. Reasons for the diminished success of prognostic models undergoing the process of external validation can include small original sample sizes that limit statistical power and precision, insufficient numbers of predictors, and differences in study populations and therapeutic approaches.

Item Response Theory

An elemental point of reference in psychometrics has long been that a given individual can be assigned a score that truly (or, perhaps, adequately) represents that person's condition, capacity, or characteristic. Entire generations of psychometric analysts were imbued with rules for their work that stemmed from enumerating pupil skills in settings involving educational or psychological testing. Classical test theory, however, has become increasingly supplanted by other techniques because the underlying assumptions were found to be either unrealistic or too restrictive for broader applications. A spectrum of analytic tools is now available for performing detailed psychometric statistics across many different professional domains. Item response theory (IRT) is one of the leading sources of these new rules for measurement.

IRT is a collection of statistical methods and models that rely on the probabilistic relationship between a person's response to test items and that person's position on an underlying construct on which the test is attempting to focus. Within IRT, two key assumptions are made. First is that whatever model is used is adequate to explain how changes in the level of the characteristic being measured related to changes in the probabilities of responding to items. Second is that the terms included in the model fully explain the interrelationships between the persons being tested and the items used for testing. From these two assumptions, it follows that there might be a proliferation of models. Indeed there are at least a hundred separate IRT models, all of which are mathematical expressions of how unidimensional or multidimensional data should fit together to reflect the underlying construct being measured. They differ primarily in how many mathematical terms are estimated and how many constraints are placed on the estimation process.

Embretson and Reise (2000) point out that IRT draws on analogies to clinical inference, asking how plausible a certain diagnosis might be in the face of selected behaviors and test responses. How likely is that diagnosis to explain the presenting behaviors? What level of the measured characteristic is most likely to explain the person's test responses? In IRT-based analyses, identifying that measurement level is a matter of seeking the highest likelihood for the responses observed. To find the most likely level or score, the likelihood of the person's actual response pattern is evaluated within the mathematical model. The likelihood calculation allows evaluation of any point along a hypothetical line that represents the full range of the condition or behavior.

To explain response patterns in the simplest of terms, imagine a short test constructed out of only five items, which can only either be scored true or false, correct or wrong, present or absent. If the test items are lined up properly in terms that reflect their inherent difficulty—that is, they are tied to the construct being tested in an orderly manner, then only a limited series of response patterns from persons taking this test make sense. One acceptable pattern is that a given person misses every item (and the resulting vectors of scores reads "00000"). That pattern ought to signify that the person is at the bottom of the test construct. Equally acceptable is a vector that reads "11111," signifying a person at the top of the construct. In theory, we can easily make sense of "10000," "11000," "11100," and "11110" as well-ordered score vectors. If the difficulty steps between items are equal—the difference between each item reflects the same difference no matter which side-by-side pair is evaluated—then the individual performances shown by these vectors are themselves readily interpretable.

Matters get more interesting when score vectors are unexpected (such as "10001"—succeeding on both the easiest and most difficulty items but failing on the others) and the underlying interpretability of the person's performance on the test is thrown into some doubt. Probabilistically, such a score vector should be quite rare, if everything else about the test is well constructed. IRT allows explicit methods to sort out just how interpretable a given person's performance is, and where the test items themselves may be poorly functioning. Work on understanding the nature of disorderly response patterns harks back to the delightful phrase "higgledy-piggledy," which was used to label this phenomenon in the earliest attempts to formally describe systematic testing.

Formal evaluation of the score vector for every respondent is made through IRT software analyses that address the simultaneous computation of likelihoods for each response, each person, and each test item. Trait levels are developed by maximizing the likelihood of a person's response pattern in the context of the particular IRT model employed. Most common are models that invoke only a single parameter reflecting item difficulty, or an additional parameter keyed to how each item differs in its discrimination between low-performing and high-performing responses, or yet another parameter reflecting the role of success by guessing or chance. The one-parameter IRT approach is known as the Rasch model, after the Danish professor Georg Rasch who discovered its properties. Rasch models are directly able to estimate reliability and provide detailed information about individual person performance and test score error. Several IRT software products are available, including TESTFACT, BILOG, MULTILOG, RUMM, WINSTEPS, and the R package "ltm."

Structural Equation Modeling

A different approach to understanding the relationship between outcome measures and a set of indicators or constructs is contained in the analytic technique called structural equation modeling (SEM). Like IRT, the probability of a certain indicator being positive for a certain outcome measures is directly assessable in SEM. Unlike IRT, additional analysis can be made of relations among factors and between factors and other variables that may be plausible covariates. One way in which the SEM approach is used is the creation of uni- and bidirectional paths that describe regression relationships and correlations, respectively, among the variable sets.

An SEM approach to understanding how cerebral white matter abnormalities relate to cognitive functioning in elderly persons is shown in a recent study by Deary, Leaper, Murray, Staff, and Whalley (2003). Questions about this association included whether it was independent of mental ability during youth and whether it was related to general and/or specific mental abilities. Ratings were made of periventricular and subcortical and deep white matter abnormalities seen on magnetic resonance images taken of each participant. SEM techniques found that white matter abnormalities accounted for 14% of the variance found in cognitive function in old age.

SEM can be extended to encompass factor analyses, modeling of multiple indicators and multiple causes, and analyses involving complex longitudinal data. A variety of SEM software products are available, including LISREL, EQS, M-PLUS, and AMOS, as well as an R package called "sem."

It is entirely possible that some measurements can be demonstrated to be both reliable and valid yet will never conform to IRT or SEM specifications. Both IRT and SEM also risk having computational complexity grow to be enormous as sample sizes and test batteries are enlarged. However, both have distinctive mathematical underpinnings that can be used to examine features of research that are otherwise exceedingly difficult to analyze.

Robustness

Understanding how data sets fit models, and how model inferences can be affected by both misspecifications in the model and particular points within the data that have high influence, is the goal of robustness analyses. The principal question pursued in such analyses is how outliers are identified and how might such outliers affect the ultimate interpretation of a study. Two different directions have been actively pursued: The first is to use analytic methods that are themselves robust in the sense that underlying assumptions of normal distributions and common variances found in traditional statistics are entirely supplanted by far more powerful techniques. Wilcox (2005) explores the foundation for robust statistical analysis and provides systematic solutions (including R code) for estimating robust measures of location and scale, developing robust confidence intervals, and working with robust solutions to correlation and regression problems. The second direction is the development of tools for sensitivity analyses, which rely on changing various model assumptions and parameters and checking whether relatively large changes have negligible effects on calculated quantities. This approach also allows especially thorny analytic problems, such as the failure of estimates in logistic regression to converge, to be addressed systematically (see R package "accuracy").

Developments over the last several decades in psychometrics and statistics have been extraordinary in terms of the potency with which such improvements can be made. We have not sought to impugn any extant epidemiologic study for failure to address its quality of measurement. But, as the reader surely has sensed, we are making a case for assessing data quality (and analysis quality) on a regular basis. Anytime we allow imprecise measurements to be included in a study, we have reduced the quality of the science itself.

—*David L. McArthur*

See also Quantitative Methods in Epidemiology; Reliability; Validity

Further Readings

Altman, M., Gill, J., & McDonald, M. P. (2003). *Numerical issues in statistical computing for the social scientist.* Hoboken, NJ: Wiley-Interscience.

Andrich, D. (1988). *Rasch models for measurement.* Newbury Park, CA: Sage.

Cook, D. A., & Beckman, T. J. (2006). Current concepts in validity and reliability for psychometric instruments: Theory and application. *American Journal of Medicine, 119*(2), 166.e7–166.e16.

Deary, I. J., Leaper, S. A., Murray, A. D., Staff, R. T., & Whalley, L. J. (2003). Cerebral white matter abnormalities and lifetime cognitive change: A 67-year follow-up of the Scottish Mental Survey of 1932. *Psychology and Aging, 18,* 140–148.

Embretson, S. W., & Reise, S. P. (2000). *Item response theory for psychologists.* Mahwah, NJ: Lawrence Erlbaum.

Hukkelhoven, C. W. P. M, Rampen, A. J. J, Maas, A. I. R., Farace, E., Habbema, J. D. F, Marmarou, A., et al. (2006). Some prognostic models for traumatic brain injury were not valid. *Journal of Clinical Epidemiology, 59,* 132–143.

Kaplan, D. (2000). *Structural equation modeling: Foundations and extensions.* Thousand Oaks, CA: Sage.

Rasch, G. (1960/1980). *Probabilistic models for some intelligence and attainment tests.* Chicago: University of Chicago Press.

Schiffman, M. H., & Schatzkin, A. (1994). Test reliability is critically important to molecular epidemiology: An example from studies of human papillomavirus infection and cervical neoplasia. *Cancer Research, 54*(Suppl.), 1944s–1947s.

Wilcox, R. R. (2005). *Introduction to robust estimation and hypothesis testing* (2nd ed). Amsterdam: Elsevier.

MEASURES OF ASSOCIATION

Measures of association encompass methods designed to identify relationships between two or more variables and statistics used to measure the relationship when it exists. Although the terms *correlation* and *association* are often used interchangeably, correlation in a stricter sense refers to linear correlation and association refers to any relationship between variables, including the relationship between two categorical variables.

Choosing the Correct Method

Choosing the correct method to measure association involves a determination of the data characteristics for each variable. Data may be measured on an interval/ratio scale, an ordinal/rank scale, or a nominal/categorical scale. These three characteristics can be thought of as continuous, integer, and qualitative categories.

Pearson's Correlation Coefficient

A typical example for measuring the association between two variables measured on an interval/ratio scale is the analysis of relationship between a person's height and weight. Each of these two characteristic variables is measured on a continuous scale. The appropriate measure of association for this situation is the Pearson's correlation coefficient.

The Pearson's correlation coefficient, ρ (rho), measures the strength of the linear relationship between the two variables measured on a continuous scale. The coefficient ρ takes on the values of -1 through $+1$. Values of -1 or $+1$ indicate a perfect linear relationship between the two variables, whereas a value of 0 indicates no linear relationship. Correlation coefficients that differ from 0 but are not $+1$ or -1 indicate a linear relationship, although not a perfect linear relationship. Negative values simply indicate the direction of the association: As one variable increases, the other decreases. In practice, ρ (the population correlation coefficient) is estimated by r, the correlation coefficient derived from sample data.

Although the Pearson's correlation coefficient is a measure of the *strength* of an association (specifically the linear relationship), it is not a measure of the *significance* of the association. The significance of the association is a separate analysis of the sample correlation coefficient, r, using a t test to measure the difference between the observed r and the expected r under the null hypothesis.

Spearman Rank-Order Correlation Coefficient

The Spearman rank-order correlation coefficient (Spearman rho) is designed to measure the strength of a monotonic (in a constant direction) association between two variables measured on an ordinal or ranked scale. Examples that indicate the Spearman rho should be used to include data obtained on preferences where the data result from ranking. It is also appropriate for data collected on a scale that is not truly interval in nature,

such as data obtained from Likert-scale administration. Any interval data may be transformed to ranks and analyzed with the Spearman rho, although this results in a loss of information; for instance, this may be done if one variable of interest is measured on an interval scale and the other is measured on an ordinal scale. Like the Pearson's correlation coefficient, the Spearman rho may be tested for its significance. A similar measure of strength of association is the Kendall tau, which may also be applied to measure the strength of a monotonic association between two variables measured on an ordinal or rank scale.

As an example of when Spearman rho would be appropriate, consider the case where there are seven substantial health threats to a community. Health officials wish to determine a hierarchy of threats in order to most efficiently deploy their resources. They ask two credible epidemiologists to rank the seven threats from 1 to 7, where 1 is the most significant threat. The Spearman rho or Kendall tau may be calculated to measure the degree of association between the epidemiologists indicating the collective strength of the action plan. If there is a significant association between the two sets of ranks, health officials will feel more confident in their strategy than if a significant association is not evident.

Chi-Square Test

The chi-square test for association (contingency) is a standard measure for association between two categorical variables. The chi-square test, unlike the Pearson's correlation coefficient or the Spearman rho, is a measure of the significance of the association rather than a measure of the strength of the association.

A simple and generic example follows. If a scientist was studying the relationship between gender and political party, then he could count people from a random sample belonging to the various combinations: female-Democrat, female-Republican, male-Democrat, and male-Republican. He could then perform a chi-square test to determine whether there was a significant disproportionate membership among these groups indicating an association between gender and political party.

Relative Risk and Odds Ratio

Several other measures of association between categorical variables are used in epidemiology, including the relative risk and odds ratio. The relative risk is appropriately applied to categorical data derived from an epidemiologic cohort study. The relative risk measures the strength of an association by considering the incidence of an event in an identifiable group (numerator) and comparing that with the incidence in a baseline group (denominator).

A relative risk of 1 indicates no association; a relative risk other than 1 indicates an association. For example, if 10 of 1,000 people exposed to X developed liver cancer, but only 2 of 1,000 people (who were never exposed to X) developed liver cancer, then we can say the relative risk is $(10/1000)/(2/1000) = 5$. The strength of the association is 5: People exposed to X are five times more likely to develop liver cancer than others. If the relative risk was < 1, perhaps 0.2, then the strength of the association is equally evident but with another explanation: Exposure to X reduces the likelihood of liver cancer fivefold—a protective effect. The categorical variables are exposure to X (yes or no) and the outcome of liver cancer (yes or no). Of course, this calculation of the relative risk does not test whether the relative risk $= 5$ is statistically significant or not. Questions of significance may be answered by calculation of a 95% confidence interval: If the confidence interval does not include 1, the relationship is considered significant.

Similarly, an odds ratio is an appropriate measure of strength of association for categorical data derived from a case-control study. The odds ratio is often interpreted the same way that a relative risk is interpreted when measuring the strength of the association, although this is somewhat controversial when the risk factor being studied is common.

Additional Methods

There are a number of other measures of association for a variety of circumstances. For example, if one variable is measured on an interval/ratio scale and the second variable is dichotomous, then the point-biserial correlation coefficient is appropriate. Other combinations of data types (or transformed data types) may require the use of more specialized methods to measure the association in strength and significance.

Other types of association describe the way data are related but are usually not investigated for their own interest. Serial correlation (also known as autocorrelation), for instance, describes how in a series of events occurring over a period of time, events that occur closely spaced in time tend to be more similar than those more widely spaced. The Durbin-Watson test is a procedure to test the significance of these correlations. If these correlations are evident, then we may conclude that these data violate the assumptions of independence, rendering many modeling procedures invalid. A classical example of this problem occurs when data are collected over time for one particular characteristic. For example, if an epidemiologist wanted to develop a simple linear regression for the number of infections by month, there would undoubtedly be serial correlation: Each month's observation would depend on the prior month's observation. This serial effect (serial correlation) would violate the assumption of independent observations for simple linear regression and accordingly render the parameter estimates for simple linear regression as not credible.

Inferring Causality

Perhaps the greatest danger with all measures of association is the temptation to infer causality. Whenever one variable causes changes in another variable, an association will exist. But whenever an association exists, it does not always follow that causation exists. The ability to infer causation from an association in epidemiology is often weak because many studies are observational and subject to various alternative explanations for their results. Even when randomization has been applied, as in clinical trials, inference of causation is often limited.

—*Mark Gerard Haug*

See also Causation and Causal Inference; Chi-Square Test; Hill's Considerations for Causal Inference; Pearson Correlation Coefficient

Further Readings

Freedman, D. A. (2005). *Statistical models: Theory and practice.* Cambridge, UK: Cambridge University Press.

Kutner, M. H., Nachtsheim, C. J., Neter, J., & Li, W. (2005). *Applied linear statistical models* (5th ed.). New York: McGraw-Hill.

Rawlings, J. O., Pantula, S. G., & Dickey, D. A. (1998). *Applied regression analysis: A research tool* (2nd ed.). New York: Springer.

Sheskin, D. J. (1997). *Handbook of parametric and nonparametric statistical procedures.* Boca Raton, FL: CRC Press.

Tietjen, G. L. (1986). *A topical dictionary of statistics*. Boca Raton, FL: Chapman & Hall.

MEASURES OF CENTRAL TENDENCY

Measures of central tendency provide a single summary number that captures the general location of a set of data points. This measure should be a good representation of the set of data. There are three common measures of central tendency used: the mean, the median, and the mode. Depending on the characteristics of the data, one measure may be more appropriate to use than the others.

The mean and the median are most commonly used to summarize data that can take on many different values (i.e., continuous data); the mode is often used to summarize data that can only take on a finite number of specific values (i.e., categorical data). The construction of each measure is illustrated with the gender and height data in Table 1 collected from 22 subjects.

The Mean

The mean is the most commonly used measure of central tendency. It is often referred to as *x-bar*, $\bar{x}$, and is found by using the formula,

$$\bar{x} = \frac{1}{n} \sum_{i=1}^{n} x_i$$

where

> x_i represents the individual observation from the *i*th subject;

> $\sum$ is the summation sign that indicates that you sum over everything that follows it. The limits below and above the sign indicate where you start, and stop, the summation, respectively. As it is written above, it says you should begin summing with x_1 and stop with x_n; and

> n represents the number of observations in your data set.

For illustrative purposes, consider the data in Table 1. To compute the mean height, we do the following:

1. Sum over all the observations (the x_i values).

2. Divide the quantity in Step 1 by the total number of observations.

Table 1   Heights of 22 Students in an Introductory Statistics Class

Observation	Gender	Height in Inches
x_1	Female	61
x_2	Female	62
x_3	Female	63
x_4	Female	63
x_5	Female	64
x_6	Female	64.5
x_7	Female	65
x_8	Female	65
x_9	Female	65
x_{10}	Female	65
x_{11}	Female	66
x_{12}	Female	66
x_{13}	Female	66
x_{14}	Male	67
x_{15}	Female	67
x_{16}	Male	67
x_{17}	Male	68
x_{18}	Female	68
x_{19}	Male	69
x_{20}	Female	69.5
x_{21}	Male	72
x_{22}	Male	74

For the data set above, the above formula gives

$$\bar{x} = \frac{1}{22} \sum_{i=1}^{22} x_i = \frac{1}{22}(1457) = 66.2 \text{ in.}$$

Additional Notes About the Mean

- The small n represents the sample size when computing the mean for a sample. When computing the mean for a population, a large N is generally used.
- The sample mean represents the population mean better than any other measure of central tendency.

- The mean can be thought of as being like a fulcrum that balances the weight of the data.
- The sum of deviations of each observation from the mean is 0.
- The mean is in the same units of measurement as the observations in your data set.
- The mean is very sensitive to outliers, that is, extreme values. An observation that lies far away from the others will pull the mean toward it. For example, if the last observation in Table 1 were 740 instead of 74, the mean would jump to 96.5 (an increase of more than 30 in.).
- The mean is generally the preferred measure of central tendency for data that are symmetric (evenly distributed about their center), but is not generally recommended to be used to describe data with outliers, or data that are not symmetric.

The Median

The median is used less often than the mean to describe the central tendency of a set of continuous data, but is still a commonly used measure. It is the midpoint of the data, and is often denoted with the letter M. To find the median, the following steps are taken:

1. Sort the observations from smallest to largest (sorting from largest to smallest is also valid).

2. Choose the correct step below depending on the number of observations in the data set:
   a. If you have an odd number of observations, observation number $(n + 1)/2$ is the median.
   b. If you have an even number of observations, the average of observation number $n/2$ and observation number $(n/2) + 1$ is the median.

Consider the data in Table 1. The observations have already been sorted in ascending order according to height. Since there is an even number of observations (22) in the data set, the median is the average of the 11th and 12th observations. Thus,

$$M = \frac{x_{11} + x_{12}}{2} = \frac{132}{2} = 66 \text{ in.}$$

Note that if the 22nd observation (x_{22}) were not in the data set, the median would be the 11th observation ($M = 66$ in.).

Additional Notes About the Median

- The median is often called the 50th percentile since it marks the midpoint of the data. That is, half the observations are less than the median and half the observations are greater than the median.
- The median is in the same units of measurement as the observations in your data set.
- The median is not sensitive to outliers unlike the mean. For example, if the last observation in the table above were 740 instead of 74, the median would still be 66 in.
- The median is the recommended measure of central tendency for data that have outliers or that are not symmetric.

The Mode

The mode is most commonly used for data that are categorical (data that can only take on one of a set of distinct values). It is defined as the most frequently occurring value. In Table 1, the mode of the gender variable is "female" since there are 16 females, but only 6 males. The mode can also be used to summarize continuous data, although this is less common. The height variable in Table 1 has a mode of 65 in. since it occurs more often than any other height. The mode is in the measurement units of the variable it is summarizing.

—*Liam M. O'Brien*

See also Box-and-Whisker Plot; Histogram; Measures of Variability; Percentiles

Further Readings

Rosner, B. (2006). *Fundamentals of biostatistics* (6th ed.). Belmont, CA: Duxbury Press.

MEASURES OF VARIABILITY

Numerical summaries used to describe a set of data generally include a measure of central tendency. While this provides a single estimate that describes where the data are located, it does not describe how spread out the data are about this central point. There are several numerical summaries that describe the variability in a data set. Four of the most common are the variance, the standard deviation, the interquartile range (IQR), and the range. They are illustrated in Table 1 using data collected on height from 22 subjects.

Table 1 Measures of Variability for the Heights of 22 Students in an Introductory Statistics Class

Observation	Height in Inches	Deviation From Mean	Deviation From Mean Squared
x_1	61.0	−5.2	27.04
x_2	62.0	−4.2	17.64
x_3	63.0	−3.2	10.24
x_4	63.0	−3.2	10.24
x_5	64.0	−2.2	4.84
x_6	64.5	−1.7	2.89
x_7	65.0	−1.2	1.44
x_8	65.0	−1.2	1.44
x_9	65.0	−1.2	1.44
x_{10}	65.0	−1.2	1.44
x_{11}	66.0	−0.2	0.04
x_{12}	66.0	−0.2	0.04
x_{13}	66.0	−0.2	0.04
x_{14}	67.0	0.8	0.64
x_{15}	67.0	0.8	0.64
x_{16}	67.0	0.8	0.64
x_{17}	68.0	1.8	3.24
x_{18}	68.0	1.8	3.24
x_{19}	69.0	2.8	7.84
x_{20}	69.5	3.3	10.89
x_{21}	72.0	5.8	33.64
x_{22}	74.0	7.8	60.84

The Variance

The variance is approximately equal to the average squared distance of each observation about the mean and is generally denoted by s^2. This is most easily seen in its formula, which is given by

$$s^2 = \frac{1}{n-1} \sum_{i=1}^{n} (x_i - \bar{x})^2$$

where

x_i represents the individual observation from the ith subject;

the mean of the data is given by $\bar{x}$;

$\sum$ is the summation sign, which indicates that you sum over everything that follows it. The limits below and above the sign indicate where you start, and stop, the summation, respectively. As it is written above, it says you should begin summing with the squared deviation of x_1 from the mean and stop with the squared deviation of x_n from the mean; and

n represents the number of observations in your data set.

For illustrative purposes, consider the data in Table 1 above. To compute the variance of the height measurements, do the following:

1. Calculate the mean height $\bar{x}$.

2. For each observation, calculate the deviation from the mean $x_i - \bar{x}$.

3. Square the deviation of each observation from the mean $(x_i - \bar{x})^2$.

4. Sum over all the squared deviations.

5. Divide this sum by $n - 1$, where n is the sample size.

Table 1 gives the quantities described in Steps 2 and 3 above for each observation. For this set of data the procedure above gives

$$s^2 = \frac{1}{(22-1)} \sum_{i=1}^{22} (x_i - \bar{x})^2$$

$$= \frac{1}{21} \sum_{i=1}^{22} (x_i - 66.2)^2 = \frac{200.38}{21}$$

$$= 9.54 \text{ in.}^2$$

Additional Notes About the Variance

- The small n represents the sample size when computing the mean for a sample. When computing the mean for a population, you divide the sum of the squared deviations from the population mean and divide that sum by the population size N. This is done only if you have data from a census, that is, when you collected data from every member of a population.

- The units of the variance are the *square* of the measurement units of the original data.
- The variance is very sensitive to outliers. It is generally not the recommended measure of variability to use if there are outliers in the data or if the data are not symmetric.

The Standard Deviation

The standard deviation is the most commonly used measure of variability for data that follow a bell-shaped (or normal) distribution. It is generally denoted by s, and is simply the square root of the variance. Formally, it is given by the formula

$$s = \sqrt{\frac{1}{n-1} \sum_{i=1}^{22} (x_i - \bar{x})^2}$$

where the quantities in the formula are defined in the same way as described above for the variance. If we consider the data in Table 1, we can calculate the standard deviation easily using the value that we calculated for the variance:

$$s = \sqrt{s^2} = \sqrt{9.54 \text{ in.}^2} = 3.09 \text{ in.}$$

Additional Notes About the Standard Deviation

- The standard deviation has the same measurement units as the original data.
- The standard deviation is sensitive to outliers just like the variance.
- The standard deviation is not recommended as a measure of variability if there are outliers, or if the data are not symmetric.
- The standard deviation is the recommended measure of variability for data that are symmetric. It is generally used to describe the variability when the mean is used to describe central tendency.
- If the data are bell shaped, then the "empirical rule" states that
- approximately 67% of the data fall within 1 *SD* of the mean,
- approximately 95% of the data fall within 2 *SD* of the mean, and
- approximately 99.7% of the data fall within 3 *SD* of the mean.

The Interquartile Range

The IQR is a measure that describes the range of the middle half of the data. It is found by locating the points in the data set that mark the 25th and 75th percentiles. The IQR is then the 75th percentile minus the 25th percentile. This can be found by performing the following steps:

1. Sort your data from the smallest observation to the largest observation.
2. Divide your data into two equally sized halves. If you have an odd number of observations, remove the midpoint (i.e., the median) and divide the remaining data into halves.
3. The median of the lower half of the data marks the 25th percentile.
4. The median of the upper half of the data marks the 75th percentile.
5. Subtract the 25th percentile from the 75th percentile.

The resulting quantity is the IQR. For the data in Table 1, the lower half of the data consists of observations 1 through 11, and the upper half consists of observations 12 through 22. The IQR is found by

$$\text{25th percentile} = x_6 = 64.5 \text{ in.}$$
$$\text{75th percentile} = x_{17} = 68.0 \text{ in.}$$
$$\text{IQR} = 68.0 - 64.5 = 3.5 \text{ in.}$$

Additional Notes About the IQR

- The IQR has the same measurement units as the original data.
- The IQR is a *single number* that describes the range of the middle half of the data.
- The IQR is not sensitive to outliers or data that are not symmetric.
- It is the preferred measure of variability for data that have outliers or that are not symmetric. It is used when the median is the preferred measure of central tendency.

The Range

The range is the simplest measure of variability to calculate. It is the largest observation minus the smallest observation. For the data in Table 1, the range is given by

$$x_{22} - x_1 = 74 - 61 = 13 \text{ in.}$$

Additional Notes About the Range

- The range is very sensitive to outliers. Due to its extreme sensitivity, it is the least commonly used of the four measures described here.
- The range is in the same measurement units as the original data.

—*Liam M. O'Brien*

See also Box-and-Whisker Plot; Histogram; Measures of Central Tendency; Percentiles

Further Readings

Rosner, B. (2006). *Fundamentals of biostatistics* (6th ed.). Belmont, CA: Duxbury Press.

Mediating Variable

A mediator is a variable that explains, totally or partially, the relationship between a predictor and an outcome. In other words, a mediating variable is a mechanism through which a predictor exerts its effect on an outcome variable. Mediation is important in epidemiology because health events are rarely due to direct causes. For instance, low socioeconomic condition increases the risk of low birthweight (LBW) through a complex mechanism mediated by food supply to the pregnant woman and weight gain during pregnancy. If the predictor is an intervention, identifying mediating variables is essential to understand how some actions produce certain outcomes.

Given any two correlated variables, X and Y, and no outside theoretical information, it is impossible to say whether changes in X cause changes in Y, changes in Y cause changes in X, some third variable, Z, produces changes in both X and Y, or any combination of these alternatives. This is, of course, an oversimplification of the analysis, because in practice the problem is never confined to just three variables.

Confounding, Mediation, and Effect Modification

Most often the influence of one variable on another is affected by the confounding, mediating, or modifying effect of a third one. It is important to clearly distinguish between these three concepts.

Given D (disease) and E (exposure), E may cause D, but it can also be related to D if both are caused by factor F. This case is illustrated in Figure 1, in which poverty has been depicted as a *confounder*. If we had concluded that migration causes disease, when, in fact, they have no true causal relationship, we would say that the relationship between migration and disease is confounded by poverty. People migrate because they are poor, and for the same reason they have higher rates of disease. Migration by itself does not cause disease.

However, not every factor associated with both the exposure and the disease is a confounder. It may also be a *mediating variable*. Mediating variables are associated with both the independent variable and the outcome, but are also part of the causal chain between them. In the diagram depicted in Figure 2, Z is the mediator between X and Y. If path c completely disappears when controlling for Z, then there is complete mediation. If, on the contrary, path c is not zero, then there is only partial mediation. Again, low socioeconomic status (SES) affects maternal nutrition and a deficient maternal nutrition increases the risk of LBW. However, there is a marginal effect of low SES on LBW, which cannot be completely accounted for by maternal nutrition.

The failure to distinguish between a confounder and a mediator is one of the most frequent errors in epidemiology. This distinction cannot be made on statistical grounds. An understanding of the process leading from the exposure to the disease is necessary.

When analyzing the probable causal relationship between an exposure and a disease, controlling for mediators can potentially lead to false conclusions. For instance, babies born to mothers with lower SES tend to have higher mortality rates. Controlling for birthweight reduces or nearly eliminates the differences between strata of SES. However, this does not mean that SES is not important as a causal factor of infant mortality. It just means that all or most of its

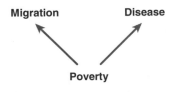

Figure 1   Poverty as a Confounder of the Relationship Between Migration and Disease

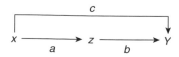

Figure 2 Z as a Mediating Variable Between X and Y

effect is expressed through the causal pathway represented by LBW.

There is yet a third way in which a factor F can influence the exposure-disease relationship. Factor F is said to be a *modifier or moderator* if it modifies the way in which the exposure and the disease are related. If exposure has different effects on disease at different levels of values of a variable, that variable is a modifier.

If a treatment is effective in cancer patients at Stages 1 or 2, and is ineffective in patients at Stages 3 or 4, then the stage of the disease modifies the effect of treatment on disease. In individuals with high cholesterol levels, smoking produces a higher relative risk of heart disease than it does in individuals with low cholesterol levels. Cholesterol is a modifier of the effect of smoking on heart disease. It can also be said that smoking *interacts* with cholesterol in its effects on heart disease.

As with confounding and mediation, the distinction between mediation and effect modification cannot be made on statistical grounds but on theoretical grounds.

Testing for Mediation

Several authors have provided algorithms to test for mediation. The best-known references are listed in the Further Readings. All these algorithms are based on linear regression. They can be summarized in the following steps (refer to Figure 2).

1. Show that the independent variable X is correlated with the outcome Y. To do this, regress Y on X and estimate the slope of the overall effect, which is given by the slope of the regression equation. By doing this, it has been established that there exists an effect that may be mediated.

2. Show that X is correlated with Z. For this, regress Z on X, which is equivalent to using the mediator as if it were an outcome, and estimate and test path a.

3. Show that Z is independently correlated with the outcome variable. To do this, regress Y on X and Z, and estimate and test path b. Observe that the

regression is fitted with both X and Z as predictors. The purpose of this is to control for X in assessing the effect of the mediator on the outcome, and to avoid overlooking the fact that they could be both caused by the initial variable X. In this step, path c is also estimated and tested. If it does not significantly differ from zero, then complete mediation has been established. Otherwise, there is only partial mediation.

In Figure 2 and in the previous three-step algorithm, path c measures the direct effect of X on Y, while the product ab measures the indirect effect. It is important to note, however, that going through these steps and showing that ab is not zero does not conclusively prove that mediation has occurred, but only that it is consistent with the data.

—Jorge Bacallao Gallestey

See also Causal Diagrams; Causation and Causal Inference; Effect Modification and Interaction

Further Readings

Baron, R. M., & Kenny, D. A. (1986). The moderator-mediator distinction in social psychological research: Conceptual, strategic, and statistical considerations. *Journal of Personality and Social Psychology, 51,* 1173–1182.

Hoyle, R. H., & Kenny, D. A. (1999). Statistical power and tests of mediation. In R. H. Hoyle (Ed.). *Statistical strategies for small sample research.* Thousand Oaks, CA: Sage.

Judd, C. M., & Kenny, D. A. (1981). Process analysis: Estimating mediation in treatment evaluations. *Evaluation Review, 5,* 602–619.

MacKinnon, D. P. (1994). Analysis of mediating variables in prevention and intervention research. In A. Cazares & L. A. Beatty (Eds.), *Scientific methods in prevention research* (pp. 127–153). NIDA Research Monograph 139. DHHS Pub. No. 94-3631. Washington, DC: Government Printing Office.

MacKinnon, D. P., & Dwyer, J. H. (1993). Estimating mediated effects in prevention studies. *Evaluation Review, 17,* 144–158.

MacKinnon, D. P., Lockwood, C. M., Hoffman, J. M., West, S. G., & Sheets, V. (2002). A comparison of methods to test mediation and other intervening variable effects. *Psychological Methods, 7,* 83–104.

Shrout, P. E., & Bolger, N. (2002). Mediation in experimental and nonexperimental studies: New procedures and recommendations. *Psychological Methods, 7*(4), 422–445.

MEDICAID

Medicaid, created by Title XIX of the Social Security Act of 1965, is a program that provides health insurance coverage for qualifying low-income individuals and their families. The program is administered through a state-federal partnership, with states having the authority to establish standards for eligibility, coverage of benefits, and payment rates. Over the past two decades, eligibility for Medicaid programs has been expanded to a variety of populations within the United States as a result of amendments to the original statute.

Overview of Benefits

Medicaid is administered by the states and territories of the United States. Each of the state Medicaid programs is financed jointly by the state and the federal government through a system of matching rate expenditures, as well as an allocation of federal funds to certain hospitals that treat a large number of Medicaid patients. Although the funding of the program is partly federal, the states have some control over how their particular program is structured and which health care services are covered by the program. Under the statute of Title XIX, each state has the ability to structure a Medicaid benefits package and payment system that fits their particular population needs.

While states are charged with designing and implementing their particular Medicaid program, all states must cover certain basic services. These core services include inpatient and outpatient care, visits to a physician, laboratory and imaging services, home health services, skilled nursing services, family planning, and general checkup and treatment services for children. Medicaid will also cover services provided in a nursing home or long-term care facility for those persons who have exhausted most of their financial assets. In addition to these services, states have the option to cover other services under Medicaid. These optional services include hospice care, other home and community-based services, dental care, physical and occupational therapy, rehabilitative services, coverage for eyeglasses, and prescription drug coverage. It is at the discretion of the state whether to include these optional services as part of the standard Medicaid benefits package.

Eligibility and Enrollment

Beneficiaries of the program include the categorically needy (families with children or certain groups of adults who meet specific income criteria), the medically needy (those who are blind and/or disabled), certain Medicare beneficiaries, the elderly, and persons who have very high medical bills. In recent years, federal legislation has expanded the traditional eligibility criteria to include additional groups that may receive Medicaid benefits.

Two pieces of legislation, in particular, give states the option of providing coverage to certain young adults; these eligible youth include those who are either in the foster care system or who are able to demonstrate financial independence. The Foster Care Independence Act of 1999 allows the state the ability to cover those individuals below the age of 21 who were in foster care on their 18th birthday. The other piece of legislation, the Benefits and Improvement Act of 2000, enables states to expand their eligibility criteria to include children below the age of 19 who qualify as Medicaid eligible based on information given to a school, homeless shelter, tribal program, or other qualified organization.

Additional federal legislation in the late 1990s and early 2000s expanded coverage to additional groups of disabled persons and women suffering from breast or cervical cancer. The Ticket to Work and Work Incentives Improvement Act of 1999 expands coverage to those disabled individuals who want to work and increase their earning capacity. Prior to this legislation, these individuals had been at risk for losing Medicaid coverage if they earned above a certain percentage of the federal poverty level. This act also establishes a program to allow states the option of providing Medicaid to people who will become blind or disabled as a consequence of their current illness. Additionally, the Breast and Cervical Prevention and Treatment Act of 2000 endows states with the ability to provide Medicaid assistance to women diagnosed with breast or cervical cancer and who are in need of treatment. Women who are eligible for Medicaid under this statute are entitled to all the services provided by the state Medicaid plan.

Each individual state is responsible for establishing the eligibility criteria for its Medicaid program, under the guidance of broad federal guidelines. In general, Medicaid eligibility is limited to the elderly, blind, and disabled, but may also include the parents or caretakers of a child as well as pregnant women and their children. In addition to these qualifications, some beneficiaries must meet certain income criteria, with personal income and other resources below a percentage of the federal poverty level, as specified by the state. There are also state eligibility requirements that apply in certain circumstances, such as state residency and/or U.S. citizenship.

Administration of Medicaid

All the 50 states, Washington D.C., and the territories of Puerto Rico, Guam, American Samoa, the Virgin Islands, and the Northern Mariana Islands administer Medicaid programs. The state agency that administers this program is usually the state Department of Health and Human Services, which follows the guidelines set forth by the federal statute in Title XIX. In close coordination with this agency, the Centers for Medicare and Medicaid Services (CMS) assists in setting broad policy guidelines and monitoring the administration of the program.

While each state has a wide amount of discretion in the design and administration of the Medicaid program, each state must submit an administration plan for approval by CMS in accordance with the federal guidelines. States must specify eligibility criteria, benefits to enrollees, implementation guidelines and payment rates, and other requisite information. If a state wishes to change its current program, amendments must also be submitted to CMS for approval.

—*Ashby Wolfe*

See also Governmental Role in Public Health; Health Disparities; Medicare; Poverty and Health

Further Readings

Centers for Medicare and Medicaid Services. (2004). *CMS congressional guide: Medicare, Medicaid, SCHIP* (OCLC No. 57491652). Baltimore: Department of Health and Human Services, Center for Medicare and Medicaid Services, Office of the Administrator.
Centers for Medicare and Medicaid Services. (2005). *Medicaid-at-a-glance: A Medicaid information source* (Publication No. CMS-11024–05). Baltimore: Department of Health and Human Services. Retrieved July 26, 2007, from http://www.cms.hhs.gov/MedicaidGenInfo/Downloads/MedicaidAtAGlance2005.pdf.
Williams, B., Claypool, H., & Crowley, J. S. (2005, February). *Navigating Medicare and Medicaid: A resource guide for people with disabilities, their families and their advocates.* Washington, DC: Henry J. Kaiser Family Foundation. Retrieved July 26, 2007, from http://www.kff.org/medicare/loader.cfm?url=/commonspot/security/getfile.cfm&PageID=50946.

Web Sites

Department of Health and Human Services, Centers for Medicare and Medicaid Services: http://www.cms.hhs.gov.

MEDICAL ANTHROPOLOGY

Medical anthropology is a subdiscipline within anthropology that addresses sociocultural dimensions of health and illness, as well as the epistemologies and practices associated with diverse systems of healing. This entry examines medical anthropology's contribution to the study of the social production of health and illness. Although medical anthropologists move through the terrain of human health in various ways, this entry concentrates on a select few examples of theoretical and methodological contributions to the anthropological understanding of the political economy of health.

According to medical anthropologist Morgan (1987), the political economy of health is "a macroanalytic, critical, and historical perspective for analyzing disease distribution and health services under a variety of economic systems, with particular emphasis on the effects of stratified social, political, and economic relations within the world economic system" (p. 132). Political-economic medical anthropologists argue that health-threatening conditions are the result of historically based social, political, and economic systems of inequality. This perspective is bolstered by a methodological and conceptual commitment to the delineation of structures of inequality and their reproduction over time. The political-economic medical anthropology (PEMA) research framework thus engages the notion of change as an important part of the context of health.

PEMA research focuses on ideological and material foundations of inequality by examining the lived experiences of class relations and state-sponsored policies and practices. It expands microlevel, culturally based analyses of health and illness in particular communities or societies by illuminating the broader context through which health phenomena are unevenly distributed among social groups. PEMA research thus explores the interaction among macrosocial forces and microlevel circumstances. As a result, PEMA studies emphasize the multifactorial nature of disease causality.

According to Morsy (1996), power is the central analytical construct within the PEMA framework. Power is a relational concept that describes the privileges of one group and concomitant subordination of others. Analyses of power allow researchers such as Ida Susser to make the connections between material and social resource distribution and structures of social inequality. In turn, focusing on the various and interconnecting dimensions of power enables PEMA scholars to understand population health and sickness as socially produced phenomena.

Political Economy in Population Health

On the basis of this political economic framework, PEMA scholarship raises a variety of questions about the social mechanisms of health and illness. Some biocultural anthropologists work to understand how environmental, social, and biological factors interact to produce differential health outcomes and the uneven spread of disease in populations. As Wiley (1992) explains, these researchers discern the effects of inequality on population health by focusing on biological variation and change that is associated with disease, psychophysiologic symptoms, and malnutrition. For example, Dressler (2005) elucidates the connections between hypertension, stress, and structurally mediated culture change for African Americans and Brazilian families. He finds that downward social mobility and the resulting inability to fulfill culturally based consumer norms induce stress-related illnesses such as hypertension and depression within these populations.

Another emerging trend in biocultural research involves the conceptual integration of social and human biological processes to examine health and illness as the direct outcome of political economic inequities. In their edited volume, Goodman and Leatherman (1998) provide a framework for applying political economic perspectives to biocultural studies. The contributions to this volume engage with diverse topics such as malnutrition, infant mortality, epidemic disease, and the impact that illness has on household production and reproduction. Swedlund and Ball (1998), for example, argue that poverty was the root cause of high infant mortality rates in a northeastern United States town in the early 20th century. Early studies that did not take into account the regional political-economic context blamed child death on the mothering skills of poor women rather than nutritional and ecological factors. Like Swedlund and Ball, other contributors working primarily on communities across the Americas illustrate how political-economic processes influence human biology, producing biological variation among groups that is expressed as illness and disease. Subsequently, human biological events affect the social fabric of communities and societies.

Focusing on the social construction of race, Mwaria (2001) argues that due to the history and ongoing patterns of racial/ethnic discrimination in the United States, researchers need to be aware of the potential for epidemiologic data to be misused. For example, Mwaria notes that certain genetic diseases are more common in some populations than others, as a result of historical and environmental factors. Thus, sickle cell disease (SCD) and sickle cell trait (SCT) are found in greater frequency among populations living in Africa, the Mediterranean, Saudi Arabia, and the Americas. However, to understand what this means in practice—in this instance, how SCT affects African Americans in the United States—requires moving from the level of medical ecology to that of critically informed biocultural anthropology. According to Molnar (1998) and Duster (1990), during the 1970s, institutions including the military considered African Americans as a population to be at high risk for developing sickle cell disease. Recruits who tested positive for SCT were considered unsuited for strenuous activities and especially for work conducted at high altitudes, including flying airplanes. The ban on recruits with SCT was ended in 1981, but the practice of testing prospective employees for SCT continues at some corporations. Put another way, Mwaria (2001) argues the importance of considering how medical information is used to understand the impact of genetic diseases that differentially affect specific racial/ethnic groups.

Political Economy in International Health

Medical anthropologists concerned with international health clarify the connections between macrolevel global power relations and population health. More generally, they show that global power relations, structured along the lines of financial and political wealth, culminate in an uneven global distribution of adverse health effects. This body of research includes, but is not limited to, three broad research topics.

First, researchers such as Kim, Millen, Irwin, and Gershman (2000), Michele Rivkin-Fish (2005), and Paul Farmer (2001) participate in discussions concerning the uneven distribution of public health and health care resources among nations. For example, Farmer notes that prevention resources are concentrated in the United States, to address potential disease outbreaks, with considerably less attention given to ongoing epidemics in Haiti and elsewhere in the Global South.

Second, Imrana Qadeer, Nalini Visvanathan, and other medical anthropologists examine what kinds of health programs and issues are given priority within the context of international development programs. In their analysis of reproductive health programs in India, Qadeer and Visvanathan (2004) find that family planning services are designed to be compatible with strategies for national economic growth rather than the health of populations. International financial institutions encourage the Indian state to curb population growth to reduce internal expenditures, thereby freeing resources to service foreign debt.

Third, medical anthropologists draw attention to the ways in which international power structures shape local understandings of illness and disease. Adams (1998) explores how the Chinese-Tibetan conflict and international human rights discourses have affected the ways in which Tibetan dissidents define health and illness. Given these political, historical, and cultural factors, Adams argues, it is important to focus on the collective needs of Tibetans rather than health at the individual level.

The relationship between poverty and poor health is complicated. Accordingly, anthropologists, such as public health practitioners, point to the importance of research on multiple social forces that affect health. The topics discussed above are not discrete categories of analysis, but represent the broader discussions to which medical anthropology can contribute. Analyses often contribute to all three research foci and the interplay among them.

For example, in her book *Life Exposed: Biological Citizens after Chernobyl*, Petryna (2002) examines the making of "biological citizenship," or persons whose health needs and rights as citizens have been redefined as the result of their exposure to the 1986 Chernobyl nuclear disaster. In the context of international public health responses to the disaster, Petryna examines the ways in which scientific precision masked the arbitrariness of diagnosis with radiation illness. Narrowly defined categories of radiation-induced illness proved beneficial to strategies for economic development in post-Socialist Ukraine, insofar as they minimized the political and economic costs of this event. The use of these categories likewise meant that many survivors were not diagnosed with radiation illness and were thus considered ineligible for state-sponsored social support.

Political Economy at the Intersections of Social Life

Intersectionality theory is one of the primary theoretical tools that PEMA researchers use to guide political-economic analyses. This theoretical approach was developed by black feminist scholars as a way to understand the ways that racial/ethnic, class, and gendered inequalities work synergistically, producing outcomes that far exceed any of these constitutive factors. Consequently, intersectionality studies criticize the use of race, class, and gender as discrete variables. Applied to anthropology, intersectionality theorists use the ethnographic case study to understand the relationship between these various dimensions of social identity, and how they are experienced in daily life. The challenge in intersectionality studies is to move out of the abstract realm of social identities to identify specific processes through which health inequalities are produced. The following examples explore intersectionality as it relates to the political economy of health.

In her ethnography of health and healing in Egypt, Morsy (1993) focuses on the historical contexts of sickness and healing for poor women. Morsy explores the connections among the historical trajectories of state economic and social service policies, the unfolding of international development programs in Egypt, and transformations in production and the labor force. These changes are reflected in household gender dynamics that produce unequal chances for health and access to certain forms of healing. The consequence is that women, and poor women in particular, have fewer health care choices than men. As a result, Morsy's analysis brings into focus the interlocking nature of social locations and social inequality, macrolevel political economic relationships, and human health and illness.

Mullings and Wali's (2001) ethnographic research in central Harlem illustrates that African American women's experiences with problematic birth outcomes are shaped by resource inequality, institutionalized racism, and gender discrimination. Stressors such as unemployment, impoverishment, occupational duress, violence, and the lack of affordable (and well-maintained) housing are the results of inadequate urban planning, along with changes in welfare policies implemented at national and local levels during the 1990s. These stressors are compounded by pregnancy, decreasing black women's chances for positive reproductive health outcomes. By examining the context of women's daily lives, Mullings and Wali highlight the multicausal nature of high infant mortality rates among black women.

In their edited volume, Parker, Barbosa, and Aggleton (2000) explore the complex interplay among social, cultural, political, and economic processes that sustain power imbalances at the level of communities and in the daily lives of residents. The contributors to this volume argue that it is insufficient to focus on sexuality or sexual risk taking in isolation; rather, sexual practices should be considered within broader political, cultural, and historical contexts. The chapters in this volume provide diverse examples from Indonesia, Brazil, Argentina, the United States, Costa Rica, Mexico, South Africa, and the Philippines to examine ways in which global relations of power, as well as local cultural tradition, articulate with experiences of sexuality. For example, in an analysis drawn from ethnographic research in developing countries, Mane and Aggleton (2000) examine the ways in which class and prevailing gender relations exacerbate women's vulnerability to sexually transmitted diseases. They find that, although the female condom is a potentially empowering technology, economic and social factors impinge on women's abilities to insist on protected sex. While sex workers generally reported higher use of condoms, especially the female condom, poor women who lacked power in marital relationships were most likely to be forced to have unprotected sex. Analyses such as Mane and Aggleton's reveal the complex interplay between gender and sexuality, the local and the global, power and resistance.

In her study among pregnant drug addicted women, Whiteford (1996) explores the ways in which poor, African American women experience discrimination in the medical and law enforcement systems. She focuses on a Florida statute that mandated drug testing and prison sentences for pregnant women who, on testing

positive, could be charged with fetal endangerment. However, only the public hospitals that primarily served poor and African American women conducted drug testing at prenatal appointments. In contrast, middle- and upper-income women with access to private health care were shielded from this kind of surveillance during their pregnancies. The result of this policy was that low-income African American women were disproportionately subject to incarceration during which time they were denied access to health care. Rather than address important public health concerns, including the need for accessible prenatal care and drug treatment programs tailored to the specific concerns of pregnant women, such laws simply punish women of color for being poor and pregnant.

From Theory to Practice

In addition to theoretical contributions to medical anthropology, PEMA studies making use of the intersectionality approach seek to move beyond the realm of purely academic research. Their aim is to apply study findings to improve the material conditions in which health and illness are produced, and thereby reduce inequities in health. To this end, many PEMA scholars engage with the research process and research participants in a participatory manner.

Specifically, PEMA scholars seek to build collaborative relationships with community activists to understand the inner workings of health organizations and coalitions that are endeavoring to effect a movement for social change. Morgen (2002), for example, conducted ethnographic research in a feminist clinic in the United States to better grasp what it means for women to take control of their health. Studying women's experiences with running the clinic sensitized Morgen to the racialized politics of the women's health movement. In the clinic, women of color struggled for autonomy as well as inclusion within a dominantly white framework of activism and devised new strategies to address issues heretofore neglected by the women's movement.

According to Lock and Kaufert (1998), research that is guided by the perspectives of participants engenders new social scientific definitions and local strategies of resistance, agency, choice, and compliance. For example, Lopez (1998) points out that the reproductive "choices" of Puerto Rican women can only be understood when their perspectives concerning sterilization are placed in historical context. In the early 1900s, the convergence of poverty, colonialism, the eugenics movement, and the commodification of family planning positioned sterilization as an economically and morally effective means of birth control. While the sterilization of Puerto Rican women has its roots in this context of coercion, the contemporary choice to undergo the procedure is often seen by women as a strategy for resisting the increased responsibilities that accompany large families. For Lopez, choice and resistance must be viewed through the perspectives of research participants.

The capacity for research to foster collaborative relationships and garner input from all participants is not serendipitous and must, instead, be built into the framework of the study. Inhorn (2001) argues that health research methodologies are most effective when they combine qualitative, quantitative, and community participatory research strategies. Participant observation, longitudinal case studies, and focus groups provide the means for data verification and enrichment of quantitative analyses. Various forms of community input can then guide ethnographic interpretations, the selection of fieldwork locations, and lines of inquiry. These diverse approaches to data collection, in turn, promote more holistic understanding of health-affecting circumstances and processes. Honing methodological dimensions of the PEMA framework are, for many political-economic medical anthropologists, an essential piece of the research process that warrants interdisciplinary dialogue.

Developing Interdisciplinary Dialogue

From the early work of Janes, Stall, and Gifford (1986) to the more recent efforts by Inhorn (1995) and Trostle (2005), medical anthropologists have explored points of convergence between medical anthropology and epidemiology. These include mutual interest in health as a human right, concerns about the health of populations at large, and attention to social dimensions in the prevention and treatment of disease. Medical anthropologists and epidemiologists alike examine multiple factors involved with the social production of disease. Through its focus on the contextualization of health inequities, medical anthropological research such as that of Carole Browner deepens understandings of the relationships between structures of inequality and individual health behaviors. Interdisciplinary exchange between medical anthropology and epidemiology contributes to the

development of measures of health that link inequality with the physical expression of ill-health and disease. In this interdisciplinary framework, researchers redirect attention from the biomedical understanding of disease as solely or predominantly biological and toward an understanding of the social relations of poor health. This more holistic approach has the potential to create more effective social action to facilitate health and prevent or treat disease.

—Alyson Anthony, Mary Alice Scott,
and Mary K. Anglin

See also African American Health Issues; Community Health; Health Disparities; Immigrant and Refugee Health Issues; Sexual Risk Behavior; Syndemics; Urban Health Issues; Women's Health Issues

Further Readings

General

Morgan, L. M. (1987). Dependency theory in the political economy of health: An anthropological critique. *Medical Anthropology Quarterly, 1*(2), 131–154.

Morsy, S. A. (1996). Political economy in medical anthropology. In T. Johnson & C. F. Sargent (Eds.), *Medical anthropology: Contemporary theory and method* (2nd ed., pp. 21–40). Westport, CT: Praeger.

Susser, I. (1996). The construction of poverty and homelessness in U.S. cities. *Annual Review of Anthropology, 25*, 411–435.

Political Economy in Population Health

Dressler, W. W. (2005). What's cultural about biocultural research? *Ethos, 33*(1), 20–45.

Duster, T. (1990). *Backdoor to eugenics*. New York: Routledge.

Goodman, A. H., & Leatherman, T. L. (Eds.). (1998). *Building a new biocultural synthesis: Political-economic perspectives on human biology*. Ann Arbor: University of Michigan Press.

Kevles, D. J. (1995). *In the name of eugenics*. Cambridge, MA: Harvard University Press.

Molnar, S. (1998). *Human variation: Races, types, and ethnic groups*. Upper Saddle River, NJ: Prentice Hall.

Mwaria, C. (2001). Diversity in the context of health and illness. In I. Susser & T. C. Patterson (Eds.), *Cultural diversity in the United States* (pp. 57–75). Malden, MA: Blackwell.

Swedlund, A. C., & Ball, H. (1998). Nature, nurture, and the determinant of infant mortality: A case study from Massachusetts, 1830–1920. In A. H. Goodman &

T. L. Leatherman (Eds.), *Building a new biocultural synthesis: Political-economic perspectives on human biology* (pp. 191–228). Ann Arbor: University of Michigan Press.

Wiley, A. (1992). Adaptation and the biocultural paradigm in medical anthropology: A critical review. *Medical Anthropology Quarterly, 6*(3), 216–236.

Political Economy in International Health

Adams, V. (1998). Suffering the winds of Lhasa: Politicized bodies, human rights, cultural difference, and humanism in Tibet. *Medical Anthropology Quarterly, 12*(1), 74–102.

Farmer, P. (2001). *Infections and inequalities: The modern plagues.* Berkeley: University of California Press.

Kim, J. Y., Millen, J. V., Irwin, A., & Gershman, J. (Eds.). (2000). *Dying for growth: Global inequality and the health of the poor.* Monroe, ME: Common Courage Press.

Petryna, A. (2002). *Life exposed: Biological citizens after Chernobyl.* Princeton, NJ: Princeton University Press.

Qadeer, I., & Visvanathan, N. (2004). How healthy are health and population policies? The Indian experience. In A. Castro & M. Singer (Eds.), *Unhealthy health policy: A critical anthropological examination* (pp. 145–160). Walnut Creek, CA: Altamira Press.

Rivkin-Fish, M. (2005). *Women's health in post-Soviet Russia: The politics of intervention.* Bloomington: Indiana University Press.

Political Economy at the Intersections of Social Life

Mane, P., & Aggleton, P. (2000). Cross-national perspectives on gender and power. In R. Parker, R. M. Barbosa, & P. Aggleton (Eds.), *Framing the sexual subject: The politics of gender, sexuality, and power* (pp. 104–116). Berkeley: University of California Press.

Morsy, S. A. (1993). *Gender, sickness, and healing in rural Egypt: Ethnography in historical context.* Boulder, CO: Westview Press.

Mullings, L., & Schulz, A. J. (2006). Intersectionality and health: An introduction. In A. J. Schulz & L. Mullings (Eds.), *Gender, race, class, and health: Intersectional approaches* (pp. 3–17). San Francisco: Jossey-Bass.

Mullings, L., & Wali, A. (2001). *Stress and resilience: The social context of reproduction in Central Harlem.* New York: Kluwer Academic.

Parker, R., Barbosa, R. M., & Aggleton, P. (Eds.). (2000). *Framing the sexual subject: The politics of gender, sexuality, and power.* Berkeley: University of California Press.

Whiteford, L. M. (1996). Political economy, gender, and the social production of health and illness. In C. F. Sargent & C. B. Brettell (Eds.), *Gender and health: An international perspective* (pp. 242–259). Upper Saddle River, NJ: Prentice Hall.

From Theory to Practice

Inhorn, M., & Whittle, K. L. (2001). Feminism meets the "new" epidemiologies: Toward an appraisal of antifeminist biases in epidemiological research on women's health. *Social Science & Medicine, 53,* 553–567.

Lock, M., & Kaufert, P. A. (Eds.). (1998). *Pragmatic women and body politics.* New York: Cambridge University Press.

Lopez, I. (1998). An ethnography of the medicalization of Puerto Rican women's reproduction. In M. Lock & P. A. Kaufert (Eds.), *Pragmatic women and body politics* (pp. 240–259). New York: Cambridge University Press.

Morgen, S. (2002). *Into our own hands: The women's health movement in the United States, 1969–1990.* New Brunswick, NJ: Rutgers University Press.

Singer, M. (1995). Beyond the ivory tower: Critical praxis in medical anthropology. *Medical Anthropology Quarterly, 9*(1), 80–106.

Interdisciplinary Dialogue

Browner, C. (1999). Ethnicity, bioethics, and prenatal diagnosis: The Amniocentesis decisions of Mexican-origin women and their partners. *American Journal of Public Health, 89*(11), 1658–1666.

Inhorn, M. (1995). Medical anthropology and epidemiology: Divergences or convergences? *Social Science & Medicine, 40*(3), 285–290.

Janes, C., Stall, R., & Gifford, S. M. (1986). *Anthropology and epidemiology: Interdisciplinary approaches to the study of health and diseases.* Boston: Kluwer Academic.

Trostle, J. A. (2005). *Epidemiology and culture.* New York: Cambridge University Press.

MEDICAL EXPENDITURE PANEL SURVEY

The Medical Expenditure Panel Survey (MEPS), conducted by the Agency for Healthcare Research and Quality (AHRQ), is an ongoing study conducted in the United States that collects data on health care utilization and costs and insurance coverage. It consists of four separate components: the Household Component (HC), the Nursing Home Component (NHC), the Medical Provider Component (MPC), and the Insurance Component.

The MEPS HC is a nationally representative survey of the U.S. civilian, noninstitutionalized population, using a sampling frame drawn from the previous year's National Health Interview Study sampling frame. The HC, which has been conducted continuously since 1966, collects data on all members of a sampled household or family from a single member of the household and uses an overlapping panel design so that data are collected from each participating family or household for 2 years. Topics covered by the HC include family demographics; health conditions; health status; health care utilization, including physician visits, hospital utilization including inpatients care and visits to the Emergency Department and Outpatient Department, dental care, home health care, use of prescription and over-the-counter medications; health care expenditures; health insurance coverage; and household income and assets.

The MPC of the MEPS is a survey conducted with providers and facilities that provided health care to individuals included in the HC; this includes hospitals, physicians, and medical providers working under their supervision; home health care agencies; and long-term care institutions. Data collected by the MPC are used to verify and supplement data collected in the HC about charges, payments, and sources of payment for health services and are used to estimate the expenses of people enrolled in managed care plans; MPC data are not released as a stand-alone file. Collection of MPC data requires that the HC respondents give their consent to have MEPS contact their care providers, so not all providers of care to HC respondents are included, and the MPC sample for this reason is not nationally representative.

The IC, which collects data on employer-based health insurance, has been conducted annually since 1996. IC data were originally collected from two different samples, the *household sample* and the *list sample*. The household sample was originally selected from the insurance providers (unions and insurance companies) and employers of respondents to the previous year's HC: These providers and employers acted as proxy respondents who provided insurance information for the HC respondents. The data collected were then attached to the respondent's HC record. The definition of who was included in the household sample has changed several times, and this survey is no longer conducted: Data were collected in 1996, 1997, 1998, 1999, 2001, and 2002. The list sample collects information from a nationally representative sample of workplaces about the types and costs of health insurance offered through employers, including governments.

The NHC was conducted in 1996 only on a nationally representative sample of nursing homes and residents of nursing homes. Data collected about the facilities include structure (e.g., if it was part of a hospital or retirement center), ownership, staffing, number of beds, number of residents, and type and size of special care units. Data collected from residents include demographics, insurance coverage, health status, and medical conditions.

Most researchers will be interested in analyzing MEPS HC data, which are publicly accessible and available for download from the MEPS data site for the years 1996–2004. Due to confidentiality concerns, data from the NHC, MPC, and IC components are not publicly accessible. Researchers may apply for access to NHC and MPH data at the AHRQ's Center for Financing, Access, and Cost Trends Data Center; researchers cannot access the IC data directly but can produce tables using IC data through the MEPSnet online interface.

—*Sarah Boslaugh*

See also Health Care Delivery; Health Care Services Utilization; Health Economics; Secondary Data

Further Readings

Agency for Health Care Policy and Research. (1997). *Design and methods of the Medical Expenditure Panel Survey Household Component*. Rockville, MD: Author. Retrieved July 26, 2007, from http://www.meps.ahrq.gov/mepsweb/data_files/publications/mr1/mr1.shtml.

Web Sites

Medical Expenditure Panel Survey: http://www.meps.ahrq.gov/mepsweb/index.jsp.

MEDICARE

Medicare, established under Title XVIII as part of the Social Security Act of 1965, is the federal health care financing program that provides health insurance for the elderly, the disabled, and those with end-stage renal disease (ESRD). Generally, Medicare covers care that is reasonable, necessary, and related to a diagnosed illness or injury. Medicare currently has four programs, which provide a variety of services to its enrollees (beneficiaries). These programs include Part A for inpatient services, Part B for outpatient and physician services, Medicare Advantage for those services provided by private health plans, and Part D for those prescription drugs not covered under Parts A or B.

The Medicare program has evolved significantly since its inception, as a result of changes to the original statute. Originally, Medicare included Parts A and B and was available only to those above 65 years of age. The law was amended in 1972 to include those individuals entitled to disability benefits and in 1976 to include those with ESRD. The Medicare law was amended in 1997 as a result of the Balanced Budget Act to establish the Medicare + Choice program (Part C), which provides private health plan choices to beneficiaries. Additionally, as a result of the Medicare Prescription Drug, Improvement and Modernization Act of 2003, the Part D program was added to provide additional prescription drug benefits and to replace the Medicare + Choice program with Medicare Advantage.

Overview of the Medicare Programs

Medicare Part A

Medicare Part A is the portion of this program that pays for hospital, or inpatient, services. Covered services include inpatient hospital care, care at a skilled nursing facility, home health care, and hospice care. To receive these benefits, each person must meet certain eligibility qualifications. Most beneficiaries who receive coverage under Medicare Part A do not pay a premium, because the program is financed through payroll taxes that were deducted while beneficiaries were working. Part A is known as a fee-for-service benefit, whereby coverage is determined based on the services rendered by the health care provider.

Medicare Part B

The Medicare Part B program provides supplementary medical insurance to those electing to receive the benefit. There is a premium associated with this portion of the program, which is paid monthly by the beneficiary. Part B provides coverage for outpatient health services provided in local clinics or home health service organizations, as well as coverage for specific medical devices and equipment. Covered services include physician services, other outpatient care, drugs and biologicals, durable medical equipment, and preventive services (such as annual screenings). Services that are not covered by Part B include routine physicals, foot care, hearing aids or eyeglasses, dental care, and outpatient prescription drugs. Part B is also a fee-for-service program.

Medicare Advantage (Part C)

Formerly known as Medicare Part C or the Medicare + Choice program, Medicare Advantage is the Medicare program that allows beneficiaries to receive covered benefits through a private health plan. Specifically, if a person is enrolled in Medicare Advantage, there is no need to be enrolled in Medicare Parts A, B, or D. Medicare Advantage provides coverage of inpatient and outpatient services, in addition to prescription drug coverage, in one plan, which is administered by a variety of private health plans. Medicare Advantage is not a fee-for-service program.

Medicare Part D

Medicare Part D, the newest program within Medicare, provides coverage for prescription drugs for those who choose to enroll in the program. Benefits include coverage for certain prescription drugs not covered under Parts A or B of the Medicare program. Coverage is provided in two ways: (1) by private plans that offer drug-only coverage or (2) through the Medicare Advantage program, which offers both drug benefits and health insurance coverage. Covered drugs under this program include those drugs available by prescription, as well as vaccines, insulin, and the associated medical supplies required to administer the medication.

Eligibility and Enrollment

Using the Medicare guidelines, the Social Security Administration is responsible for determining those eligible to receive Medicare benefits. Each portion of the Medicare program has particular criteria. In general, those Americans aged 65 or older are entitled to receive hospital insurance under Medicare Part A. In addition to these beneficiaries, those with disability and most patients with ESRD or kidney failure are entitled to receive benefits under Part A. Persons are able to enroll 3 months prior to, and 3 months following, the day on which they become 65.

Medicare Part B is a voluntary program, and those who are able to receive Part A are also eligible to enroll in Part B to receive supplemental insurance for outpatient services. Additional eligible individuals include those permanent residents of the United States who have lived in the United States for 5 years. Part B has a general enrollment period in January through March of each calendar year; beneficiaries are also able to enroll during the 3 months prior to, and 3 months following, their becoming 65. There are additional requirements, and certain penalties, for those eligible individuals who choose not to enroll during the period in which they are initially eligible.

Medicare Advantage (Part C) is available to those beneficiaries who are eligible for Parts A and B but choose instead to enroll in a private health plan. Beneficiaries do have the option of returning to their original Medicare coverage under Parts A and B if they elect to do so.

Medicare Part D is available to those beneficiaries who quality for Parts A and B. The initial enrollment period for this program occurred between November 2005 and May 2006; however, subsequent enrollment will occur annually between November 15 and December 31 of each calendar year. For those eligible beneficiaries who choose not to enroll during these periods, a late fee surcharge, similar to the penalty for Part B late enrollment, is assessed.

Administration of Medicare

Medicare is administered by the Centers for Medicare and Medicaid Services (CMS), a federal administration agency under the supervision of the Department of Health and Human Services. Formerly known as the Health Care Financing Administration (HCFA), today CMS coordinates both Medicare operations at the federal level and assists each state with the administration and operation of Medicaid.

CMS contracts with several agents outside of the federal government to provide payment and insurance services to its beneficiaries. Each of these companies processes claims relating to particular services under the separate parts of the Medicare program. Under Part A of the program, those companies processing claims for inpatient, skilled nursing or home health/hospice services are known as *fiscal intermediaries.* Those companies, which pay claims relating to Medicare Part B and all medical supplier claims, are known as carriers. Also contracting with CMS are organizations known as integrity program contractors, which investigate fraud and abuse claims.

For those beneficiaries seeking information about Medicare, agencies equipped to provide such information include the Social Security Administration, the Department of Health and Human Services, and the Centers for Medicare and Medicaid Services.

—Ashby Wolfe

See also Aging, Epidemiology of; Governmental Role in Public Health; Medicaid

Further Readings

Centers for Medicare and Medicaid Services. (2004). *CMS Congressional Guide: Medicare, Medicaid, SCHIP* (OCLC No. 57491652). Baltimore: Department of Health and Human Services, Center for Medicare and Medicaid Services, Office of the Administrator.

Centers for Medicare and Medicaid Services. (2006). *Medicare and Medicaid Statistical Supplement* (Publication No. 03469). Baltimore: Department of Health and Human Services, Center for Medicare and Medicaid Services, Office of Research, Development and Information.

Web Sites

Department of Health and Human Services, Center for Medicare and Medicaid Services: http://www.cms.hhs.gov. Medicare: http://www.medicare.gov.

MEN'S HEALTH ISSUES

Men in the United States suffer more severe chronic conditions, have higher death rates for most of the leading causes of death, and die nearly 5 1/2 years younger than women. Why are there such gender differences, and why are some men healthy and others are not? The definition of health is complex, as is the answer to these questions. To improve the health of men, health care providers and public health professionals must better understand the determinants of men's health and become advocates for change of the social and economic factors that affect these determinants.

This entry presents an overview of (1) selected epidemiologic aspects of men's health; (2) the reported causes and "actual" causes of death for men; (3) the role of "gender" as a determinant of health; (4) the influence of selected dimensions of the social and economic environment, such as poverty, education, socioeconomic status, racism, and social capital, on health status and outcomes in men; and (5) the role of stress as a mediator between these dimensions and health.

Epidemiology

Health, United States, 2005 (National Center for Health Statistics) provides extensive data on trends and current information on selected determinants and measures of health status relevant to the health of men and differences between men and women. These data raise many questions and suggest areas for further study and interventions related to differences in health outcomes by gender, race, education, and other variables. The information in this report includes the following:

• *Life Expectancy.* In 2002, life expectancy for males (at birth) was 74.5 years, while for females, 79.9 years. Between 1990 and 2002, life expectancy at birth increased more for the Black population than for the White population, thereby narrowing the gap in life expectancy between these two racial groups. In 1990, life expectancy at birth was 7.0 years longer for the white than for the black population. By 2003, the difference had narrowed to 5.2 years. However, for black men, the difference was 6.3 years.

• *Death Rates.* For males and females, age-adjusted death rates for all causes of death are three to four times higher for those with 12 years or less education compared with those of educational attainment of 13 years or more. Males continued to have higher death rates due to diseases of the heart (286.6 vs. 190.3), malignant neoplasms (233.3 vs. 160.9), chronic liver disease and cirrhosis (12.9 vs. 6.3), HIV disease (7.1 vs. 2.4), motor vehicle injuries (21.6 vs. 9.3), suicide (18.0 vs. 4.2), and homicide (9.4 vs. 2.6). In 2002, adolescent boys (15 to 19 years) were five times as likely to die from suicide as adolescent girls, in part reflecting their choice of more lethal methods, such as firearms.

• *Cancer Incidence.* Incidence rates for all cancers combined declined in the 1990s for males. Cancer incidence was higher for black males than for males of other racial and ethnic groups. In 2001, age-adjusted cancer rates for black males exceeded those for white males by 50% for prostate, 49% for lung and bronchus, and 16% for colon and rectum.

• *Tobacco Use.* In 2003, 24% of men were smokers, compared with 19% of women. Cigarette smoking by adults is strongly associated with educational attainment. Adults with less than a high school education were three

times more likely to smoke than were those with at least a bachelor's degree or more from college.

• *Alcohol Use.* Among current drinkers 18 years and older, 40% of men and 20% of women reported drinking five or more alcoholic drinks on at least one day (binge drinking) in the past year. Among males in Grades 11 and 12, 22.4% drove after drinking alcohol, compared with 12.3% of females.

• *Seat Belt Use.* In 2003, 22% of male high school students rarely or never used a seat belt compared with 15% of female high school students.

• *Access to Health Care and Health Insurance.* Working-age males 18 to 64 years were nearly twice as likely as working-age females to have no usual source of health care (22% vs. 12%). Men of all ages, particularly between the ages of 18 and 54, are less likely than women to visit physician offices and hospital outpatient and emergency departments. For all persons below 65 years of age, males are less likely to have health insurance than are females.

"Real" Versus "Actual" Causes of Death

The mortality data presented above represent the reported causes of death on death certificates and indicates the primary pathophysiologic conditions identified at the time of death, as opposed to the root causes of the death. Major external (nongenetic) modifiable factors that contribute to death have been labeled "the actual causes of death." Half of the deaths that occurred among U.S. residents in 1990 were potentially preventable and could be attributed to the following factors: tobacco use (19%), diet/activity patterns (14%), alcohol (5%), microbial agents (4%), toxic agents (3%), firearms (2%), sexual behavior (1%), motor vehicles (1%), and illicit use of drugs (< 1%). A similar analysis of the "actual causes of death" in 2000 showed that tobacco smoking remains the leading cause of mortality but diet and physical inactivity may soon overtake tobacco as the leading cause of death.

Gender

These striking differences in health status and outcomes for men and women result from a complex mix of beliefs, behaviors, biology, and socialization. Many sociocultural factors, including gender, are associated with, and influence, health-related beliefs and behaviors.

There are gender differences in health beliefs. Compared with men, women rely less on "provider control" of health (doctors being in charge), express greater "nutritional consciousness," and believe more that psychological factors play an important part in the etiology of illness. There are gender differences in perceptions of cancer. Women are more frightened than men of cancer. Men are more frightened of heart disease than cancer. The greatest fear of cancer was its perceived incurability and the associated suffering. The greatest fear of heart disease was perceived susceptibility. Men are more likely than women to hold a more negative attitude toward cancer information and more likely to identify a cause of cancer as behavior rather than heredity. The greatest barrier to seeking services in male college students is their socialization to be independent and to conceal vulnerability.

The concept of masculinity may vary among communities and cultures, but the development and maintenance of male identity usually requires taking risks that are hazardous to health—more dangerous jobs, more homicides and car accidents, excess drinking of alcohol, smoking, and substance abuse. Unwillingness to admit weakness may prevent many men from consulting a doctor when an illness arises, from taking health promotion messages seriously, or admitting to and seeking care for mental illness. Factors such as ethnicity, economic status, educational level, sexual orientation, and social context influence the kind of masculinity that men construct and contribute to the differential health risks among men in the United States.

Poverty and Social Status

Poverty and social inequalities may be the most important determinants of poor health worldwide. Poverty is a multidimensional phenomenon that can be defined in both economic and social terms. Poverty leads to a person's exclusion from the mainstream way of life and activities in a society. Socioeconomic differences in health status exist even in industrialized countries where access to modern health care is widespread. There is convincing evidence of an increase in differential mortality rates according to socioeconomic level in the United States. Not surprisingly, mortality rates from most major causes are higher for persons in lower social classes. The Whitehall studies of British civil servants showed that mortality rates are three times greater for the lowest employment grades (porters) than for the highest grades (administrators). Conventional risk factors (smoking, obesity, low levels of physical activity, high blood pressure, and high plasma cholesterol) levels explain only about 25% to 35% of the differences in mortality rates among persons of different incomes. Income disparity, in addition to absolute income level, is a powerful indicator of overall mortality. Male mortality is more unequal than female mortality across socioeconomic groups.

Variables that have been postulated to intervene between income inequality and health status include civic engagement and levels of mutual trust among community members, and dimensions of social capital. One's control of the work environment may be an important connection between social and occupational class and mortality. Some researchers suggest that education is the critical variable.

Social Capital

Studies across the world indicate that social support (marriage, family, group affiliations) affects mortality after controlling for baseline differences in health status. A consistent pattern exists in which high levels of social capital are associated with desirable health outcomes.

Social capital has been shown to be associated with decreasing depression, suicide, colds, heart attacks, strokes, and cancer. It has also been associated with sociological factors such as reduced crime, juvenile delinquency, teen pregnancy, child abuse, drug abuse, and increased graduation rates/test scores.

Multiple studies have demonstrated an association between reported well-being and social connectedness. The protective effects of social connectedness have been shown for family ties, friendship networks, participation in social events, and association with religion and other civic organizations. These protective factors reduce the likelihood of developing colds, heart attacks, strokes, cancer, depression, and many sources of premature death. In fact, the strength of social integration and social support on health is believed to be as great as well-known risk factors such as smoking, obesity, and physical inactivity. How and/or why social connectedness is associated with well-being is uncertain, but researchers believe that the support (emotional and financial) that social networks provide decreases stress and, as such, reduces illness. Social networks increase communication between people, may support healthy norms in the community such as not smoking and physical activity, and social cohesion may promote activism around important issues such as health insurance.

A nationwide study that related social capital and state-level health outcomes using data on trust and group membership in 39 states revealed that levels of social trust and group membership were significantly associated with heart disease, malignant neoplasms, and infant mortality. Increased trust and group membership decreased mortality rates even after controlling for income and poverty levels.

Racism, Discrimination, and Bias

Another important determinant of male health is access to, and the quality of, the health care "system." However, access and quality of care are not equal for all men. Numerous studies have found that racial and ethnic minorities tend to receive a lower quality of health care than nonminorities, even when access-related factors such as patients' insurance status and income are controlled. The sources of these disparities are complex and rooted in historic and contemporary inequities, and involve many participants at many levels. As one of the participants, health care providers may contribute to the racial and ethnic disparities found among men. Three mechanisms may be operative: bias or prejudice against minorities, greater clinical uncertainty when interacting with minority patients, and beliefs or stereotypes held by the provider about the behavior or health of minorities.

External stressors such as racism may contribute directly to the physiological arousal that is a marker of stress-related diseases. In addition, anger in young men has been associated with premature cardiovascular disease.

Stress as a Mediator

Individuals experience objective psychological and environmental conditions—such as discrimination, racism, mistrust, poverty, and diminished social capital—that are conducive to stress. The perception of stress is influenced by social, psychological, biophysical factors, genetics, and behavior. When the brain perceives an experience as stressful, physiological and behavioral responses are initiated, leading to allostasis (homeostasis) and adaptation. Wear and tear across multiple physiological systems becomes a significant contributor to overall health risk. Such wear and tear is hypothesized

to result from repeated exposures to social relationship conflicts. Over time, allostatic load can accumulate, and overexposure to mediators of neural, endocrine, and immune system stress have adverse effects on various organ systems, leading to enduring negative health outcomes—physiological (e.g., hypertension and cardiovascular disease), psychological (e.g., depression), and behavioral (e.g., alcoholism and drug abuse).

—James Plumb, Rickie Brawer,
and Lara Carson Weinstein

See also Cardiovascular Disease; Health Disparities; Social Capital and Health; Stress

Further Readings

Committee on Health and Behavior: Research, Practice, and Policy Board on Neuroscience and Behavioral Health. (2001). *Health and behavior: The interplay of biological, behavioral and societal influences.* Washington, DC: National Academy Press.

Doyal, L. (2001). Sex, gender, and health: The need for a new approach. *British Medical Journal, 323,* 1061–1063.

Kaplan, G. A., Pamuk, E. R., Lynch, J. W., Cohen, R. D., & Balfour, J. L. (1996). Inequality in income and mortality in the United States: Analysis of mortality and potential pathways. *British Medical Journal, 312,* 999–1003.

McCally, M., Haines, A., Fein, O., Addington, W., Lawrence, R. S., & Cassel, C. K. (1998). Poverty and health: Physicians can, and should, make a difference. *Annals of Internal Medicine, 129*(9), 726–733.

Mustard, C. A., & Etches, J. (2003). Gender differences in socioeconomic inequality in mortality. *Journal of Epidemiology and Community Health, 57,* 974–980.

National Center for Health Statistics. (2005). *Health, United States, 2005 with chartbooks on trends in the health of Americans.* Hyattsville, MD: Government Printing Office

Putnam, R. D. (2000). *Bowling alone: The collapse and revival of American community.* New York: Simon & Schuster.

van Ryn, M., & Fu, S. S. (2003). Paved with good intentions: Do Public Health and Human Service Providers contribute to racial/ethnic disparities in health? *American Journal of Public Health, 93*(2), 248–255.

Wender, R. C., & Haines, C. (2006). *Men's health, an issue of primary care: Clinics in office practice.* A title in The Clinics: Internal Medicine series. Philadelphia: Saunders Elsevier.

MERCURY

Mercury, also known as *quicksilver*, has been known since ancient times and is represented in the periodic table by the symbol "Hg," which stands for *hydrargyrus*, or liquid silver, in Latin. It is a silvery transitional metal that is liquid at or near standard room temperature. Mercury has many uses, both in homes and in industry, and it has also been used as a medicine, although it has been acknowledged as being toxic to humans.

Mercury exists predominantly in three forms: elemental, inorganic, and organic. Methylmercury is the most important organic form of mercury in terms of human health effects. It has a high affinity for the brain, particularly the posterior cortex. It is neurotoxic (damaging to the nervous system), toxic to the developing fetus, and genotoxic (damaging to the DNA), and it can cause effects such as numbness and tingling, stumbling gait, weakness and fatigue, vision and hearing loss, spasticity and tremors, and in high enough concentrations, coma. Efforts have been made to decrease mercury exposure through public policy initiatives such as those of the U.S. Environmental Protection Agency.

History

There is evidence to suggest that mercury was known to the ancient Chinese and Hindus and was found in Egyptian tombs dating back to about 1500 BCE. Mercury has found many uses in ancient civilizations, including making of ointments, cosmetics, amalgams with other metals, and in alchemy. It was thought to prolong life, heal fractures, and preserve health. Indeed, it was named after the Roman god Mercury, known for his speed and mobility. It has been used as a diuretic, disinfectant, laxative, as a treatment for syphilis and worm infestation, in thermometers, in sphygmomanometers (blood pressure measuring devices), and as an antidepressant.

In the 18th and 19th centuries, mercury was used in the industrial process of carrotting, a method of treating fur in the process of making felt. Animal skins were rinsed in a solution of mercuric nitrate that helped open the sheaths surrounding each fur fiber and permitted matting (felting) of fibers in subsequent operations for making felt hats. The process, however, produced highly toxic mercury vapors and led to mercury poisoning among hatters. Many experienced tremors, emotional lability, insomnia, dementia, and hallucinations, and these symptoms led to the phase commonly used in medical parlance, "mad as a hatter," which refers to someone poisoned by mercury. It was also

known as Danbury shakes, due to the effects seen in Danbury, Connecticut, a center of hat making. The U.S. Public Health Service banned the use of mercury in the felt industry in December 1941.

Some prominent historical personalities known or believed to be affected by mercury toxicity include Sir Isaac Newton, King Charles II, and Sir Michael Faraday. Their erratic behavior was thought to correspond to their work with mercury. Abraham Lincoln also exhibited erratic behavior that was thought to be due to the mercury in the "blue pill" he took for depression.

Toxicology and Clinical Manifestations

Metallic or elemental mercury volatilizes to odorless mercury vapor at ambient air temperatures, and it can be absorbed via inhalation, with concerns particularly in poorly ventilated spaces. Inhalation of mercury vapors may produce inflammation of the respiratory passages and a pneumonitis-like syndrome and the triad of excitability, tremors, and gingivitis (the mad hatter syndrome). Inorganic mercury salts can be divalent (mercuric salts) or monovalent (mercurous salts). They are generally white powder or crystals, with the exception of cinnabar (mercuric sulfide), which is red. The greatest concentrations of mercury after exposure to the inorganic salts or vapors can be found in the kidney. Mercuric salts are more corrosive and toxic than the mercurous salts. "Pink disease" has been seen in children when teething powders containing mercurous mercury has been used and is characterized by fever; pink rash; swelling of the spleen, lymph nodes, and fingers; constipation or diarrhea; hair loss and irritability. Organic mercury compounds are formed when mercury combines with carbon. As noted above, methylmercury is the most important organic form of mercury in terms of human health effects.

Mercury Exposure

The major sources of mercury exposure today are the natural degassing of the earth's crust, mining, and the consumption of fish containing mercury. In addition to miners, others subject to occupational risks of mercury exposure include technicians, nurses, those doing dental work, and machine operators. Workers involved in industrial production of elemental mercury, cinnabar (ore containing mercury) mixing and processing, and the manufacturing and use of instrumentation containing elemental mercury are at a higher risk. Average urinary mercury among dentists in the United States was well above the general population mean, but it dropped after an educational campaign on mercury hygiene sponsored by the American Dental Association. Mercury exposure to patients filled with dental amalgam is somewhat controversial. Although it has been shown that routine activities such as tooth brushing, chewing gum, and cleaning and polishing of teeth result in high concentrations of mercury in the mouth in patients with amalgam tooth fillings, the average absorbed dose has been shown to be much less than environmentally absorbed mercury. Some other common uses of mercury today are in barometers, cell batteries, calibration instruments, fluorescent and mercury lamps, photography, silver and gold production, thermometers, fungicides, paper manufacturing, and wood preservatives.

On August 11, 2006, the U.S. Environmental Protection Agency (EPA) announced the National Vehicle Mercury Switch Recovery Program to remove mercury-containing light switches from scrap vehicles. During dismantling of discarded cars, a significant amount of mercury is released into the environment during melting of the scrap metal to make new steel and steel products. This can be prevented if mercury-containing switches are removed from scrap vehicles before they are shredded. This program aims at helping cut mercury air emissions by up to 75 tons over the next 15 years.

Some of the more recent mass exposures of mercury include the famous Minamata Bay incident in Japan (1960) and methylmercury-treated grain in Iraq (1960, 1970). The former refers to the contamination of the Minamata Bay in Japan by tons of mercury compounds dumped into it by a nearby company. Thousands of people whose normal diet consisted of fish from the bay developed mercury poisoning. The methylmercury incident in Iraq was one involving import of wheat grain contaminated with methylmercury used as a pesticide.

Diagnosis, Evaluation, Treatment, and Prevention

Acute inhalation exposure to high concentrations of elemental mercury vapors is a medical emergency. Aggressive supportive care is needed. Development of acute pneumonitis should be watched for. Mercury can be chelated with agents such as penicillamine, dimercaprol, or dimercaptosuccinic acid. Measurement of mercury in a 24-hr specimen is used to confirm exposure. Acute ingestion of mercuric chloride, usually with suicidal intent, is another medical emergency. Chelation can help excretion, and hemodialysis may be required in severe cases.

Chronic exposure is best assessed by measuring urine mercury, preferably from 24-hr collected urine. It should be remembered, however, that correlation of urine or blood mercury levels with toxicity is poor. For methylmercury, body burden can be estimated from measurement of mercury in whole blood or hair, although the reliability of these, especially the latter, is often questioned in clinical medicine.

Once the exposure and signs and symptoms are confirmed, the person should be removed from the exposure to avoid further ongoing toxicity. Pregnant women, or women intending to become pregnant in the near future, should limit the intake of food that contains elevated mercury levels, such as swordfish, shark, mackerel, and certain tuna.

—*Abhijay P. Karandikar*

See also Environmental and Occupational Epidemiology; Pollution

Further Readings

Diner, B., & Brenner, B. *Mercury toxicity*. Retrieved September 8, 2006, from http://www.emedicine.com/EMERG/topic813.htm.

Klaassen, C. D., & Watkins, J. B., III. (1999). *Casarett & Doull's toxicology companion handbook* (5th ed.). New York: McGraw-Hill.

Rosenstock, L., Cullen, M. R., Brodkin, C. A., & Redlich, C. A. (2004). *Textbook of clinical occupational and environmental medicine* (2nd ed.). Philadelphia: Elsevier Saunders.

U.S. Environmental Protection Agency. (2007). *Mercury*. Retrieved September 8, 2006, from http://www.epa.gov/mercury.

META-ANALYSIS

In epidemiology, the proliferation of multiple and sometimes contradictory studies can be a challenge for interpretation of health risk and health policy formulation. One approach to synthesizing the results of separate but related studies is meta-analysis—the systematic identification, evaluation, statistical synthesis, and interpretation of separate study results. For example, for many years, conflicting results were reported in observational studies of the effect of diet on breast cancer risk. The lower rate of breast cancer incidence for women in Asian countries suggested a protective effect for soy-based diets; yet migration patterns and changes in diet yielded conflicting results. A synthesis of epidemiologic studies showed a moderately protective effect for soy intake (odds ratio $[OR] = 0.89$, 95% confidence interval $[CI]$ $0.75 - 0.99$), with a stronger effect among premenopausal women ($OR = 0.70$, 95% $CI = 0.58 - 0.85$).

This entry reviews the elements of a well-conducted meta-analysis, summarizes recent research, and discusses two important examples of the use of meta-analysis in epidemiology: *The Guide to Community Preventive Services* and the Human Genome Epidemiology Network.

The technique of using a quantitative synthesis probably was used first by Karl Pearson in 1904 to increase statistical power in determining the efficacy of a vaccine for enteric fever; Gene Glass coined the term *meta-analysis* in 1976 to apply to systematic review and quantitative synthesis. From the social sciences, use of meta-analysis quickly spread to medicine in the 1980s. Later, meta-analysis was used increasingly to combine results from observational studies.

Over time, meta-analysis has become more prominent in epidemiology, extending to important policy decisions and determining the effectiveness of interventions. To address the quality of reporting of meta-analytic reviews, guidelines were developed for reporting randomized controlled trials (RCTs) to facilitate synthesis, meta-analysis of RCTs, and meta-analysis of observational studies.

Elements of a Well-Conducted Meta-Analysis

Stating the Problem and Conducting the Literature Search

A well-conducted meta-analysis should start with an explicit statement of the research problem, which can be framed by population, intervention (or exposure), comparison, or outcome. After specifying the study question, the next step is a systematic search for relevant studies. Computerized databases have aided this step, particularly in meta-analyses of RCTs. However, limiting a search to two or three electronic databases might produce incomplete evidence. A comprehensive search will include multiple databases, the reference lists of recent review articles and meta-analyses, and frequently contact with experts to find unpublished results.

With the proliferation of meta-analyses in the epidemiologic literature and the availability of electronic repositories of research, variably skilled researchers are conducting searches. Recognizing the importance of knowledge and skills in complex bibliographic retrieval and verification of information, the Medical Library Association has developed a policy that health science librarians should contribute to the search process for health and information research.

Collection of Data

Abstraction of data from the search should begin with explicit inclusion and exclusion criteria for studies. Commonly used criteria include period covered in the review, operational definitions of the variables, the quality of a study, and the language of publication. To the extent possible, inclusion or exclusion criteria should be based on valid scientific principles (e.g., treatment changes over time), not the convenience of the researcher.

The procedures for abstracting data should be developed in detail and documented. Blinding the abstractor(s) to the identity of the journal or the results, for example, can reduce bias; however, blinding is difficult to achieve, time-consuming, and might not substantially alter results. If possible, multiple abstractors should assess the data, and the report should include a calculation of interrater reliability.

Assessment of Study Quality

One of the most controversial questions related to meta-analysis is the question of whether to include studies that are of doubtful or poor quality. Critics argue that any meta-analysis that summarizes studies of widely differing quality is likely to be uninformative or flawed. Indeed, studies with methodologic flaws have been demonstrated to overestimate accuracy in studies of a medical test. One study of published cost-effectiveness studies reported that studies funded by industry, studies of higher methodologic quality, and those published in Europe and the United States were more likely to report favorable cost-effectiveness ratios.

Other researchers counter by noting that assessing methodologic quality is often difficult, and researchers often disagree on what constitutes quality. Despite a researcher's best attempts to provide an objective measure of quality, decisions to include or exclude studies introduce bias into the meta-analysis.

Still others note that the quality of a study might not have an effect on the study's outcome. When in doubt, include the study in the meta-analysis and use an independent variable to code the quality of a study; for example, using quality to stratify the estimates. Guidelines have been developed to assess quality of RCTs, but even here, improvement is needed.

Evaluation of the Body of Evidence Collectively

Assessment of Publication Bias

Reporting of publication bias, the tendency to publish findings (or not) based on bias at the investigator or editorial level (e.g., failure to publish results of studies demonstrating negative results), is a major problem for meta-analysis in epidemiology. This bias

can be related to strength or direction of results, author's native language, the sex of the author, or country of publication.

Of the methods developed to address publication bias, perhaps the simplest is the funnel plot, a type of scatter plot with estimate of sample size on one axis and effect size estimate on the other (Figure 1). The utility of the funnel plot to assess publication bias is based on the statistical principle that sampling error decreases as sample size increases. Other statistical tests can help assess deviation from symmetry, but these are controversial because of high Type I error rates. A more robust approach includes a comprehensive search and estimating contribution from the components of publication bias.

Assessment of Heterogeneity

When studies to be combined in a meta-analysis are heterogeneous, the interpretation of any summary effect might be difficult. Tests for heterogeneity most often use a formulation of Hedges Q statistic; however, this method has been reported to have low power when the variance of the effect size differs among studies (which is the case most of the time). This problem can be addressed with meta-regression techniques and graphical approaches. Statistical methods have been developed to assist with determining

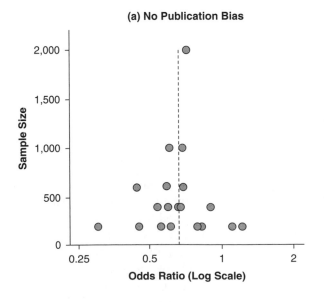
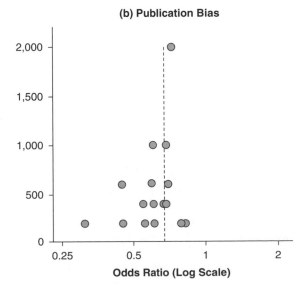

Figure 1   Sample Funnel Plots Illustrating Publication Bias

the source and nature of heterogeneity. Whether the heterogeneity is important, however, requires judgment beyond the statistics.

Consideration of Quantitative Synthesis of Evidence

A quantitative synthesis might not be useful if the number of studies is limited, the studies are of low quality, or important conceptual or empirical heterogeneity exists. If the studies located are appropriate for a quantitative synthesis, fixed-effects or random-effects models can be used in a meta-analysis, depending on the presence or absence of heterogeneity. The fixed-effects model applies to a situation that assumes each study result estimates a common (but unknown) pooled effect. The random-effects model assumes that each study result estimates its own (unknown) effect, which has a population distribution (having a mean value and some measure of variability). Thus, the random-effects model allows for between- and within-study variability. Summary estimates from heterogeneous studies should be interpreted with caution, even when using a random-effects model, bearing in mind that the source of heterogeneity might be as important to identify estimate of risk.

Recently, Bayesian meta-analysis has been used more frequently, allowing both the data and the model itself to be random parameters. Bayesian methods allow the inclusion of relevant information external to the meta-analysis. Although use of Bayesian meta-analysis methods is hindered by software limitations and not easily understood p value, it leads easily to a framework that can consider costs and utilities when making decisions based on epidemiologic studies.

Cumulative meta-analysis is the process of performing a new (or updated) meta-analysis as results become available. For certain public health problems, and indeed for the majority of situations with limited resources, adding additional information for an already established effect is of limited value. Thus, methods to determine when sufficient evidence exists to establish intervention effectiveness are critical.

Emerging Methods

As meta-analysis becomes more widely used, numerous aspects can be handled by emerging methods. For example, meta-analysis is often complicated by lack of information on standard deviation of estimates in reports; the validity of various methods of imputing this information from other sources has been studied. Combining information from different study designs or evidence on multiple parameters is of interest to researchers. Models for this situation are complex but provide opportunities to assess whether data are consistent among studies. Finally, availability of computer packages has aided in the conduct of meta-analysis in epidemiology.

Meta-Analysis in Epidemiologic Practice: Two Examples

The Guide to Community Preventive Services (Community Guide) provides decision makers recommendations regarding population-based interventions to promote health and to prevent disease, injury, disability, and premature death. The Task Force on Community Preventive Services makes its recommendations on the basis of systematic reviews of topics in three general areas: changing risk behaviors; reducing diseases, injuries, and impairments; and addressing environmental and ecosystem challenges. Systematic reviews (and quantitative synthesis where appropriate) are conducted for selected interventions to evaluate the evidence of effectiveness that is then translated into a recommendation or a finding of insufficient evidence. For those interventions where evidence of effectiveness is insufficient, the *Community Guide* provides guidance for further prevention research.

The completion of sequencing of the human genome and advances in genomic technology provide tremendous opportunities for using genetic variation in epidemiology. The Human Genome Epidemiology Network (HuGENet™) is a global collaboration committed to the assessment of the impact of human genome variation on population health and how genetic information can be used to improve health and prevent disease. To address the quality of reporting of genotype prevalence and gene disease association, an interdisciplinary group of epidemiologists has developed guidelines for appraising and reporting such studies. Such guidelines will contribute to the quality of meta-analyses. Furthermore, systematic reviews of genetic studies and publication of results increase the utility of this discipline.

The use of meta-analysis in epidemiology has moved beyond just recognizing the need to stay current with the literature in a field experiencing an explosion of studies. The method has driven recommendations about improved reporting of abstracts and primary studies, identified research gaps, and shifted attention away from statistical significance to consideration of effect size and confidence interval. The term *evidence-based* will continue to have varying interpretations, but the role of meta-analysis in epidemiology is pushing the science of public health further.

—*Stephen B. Thacker and Donna F. Stroup*

See also Bayesian Approach to Statistics; Evidence-Based Medicine; Publication Bias

Further Readings

Cochrane Collaboration. (2006). *The Cochrane Collaboration: The reliable source of evidence in health care*. Oxford, UK: Author. Retrieved April 20, 2006, from http://www.cochrane.org/index.htm.

Dickersin, K. (2002). Systematic reviews in epidemiology: Why are we so far behind? *International Journal of Epidemiology, 31,* 6–12.

Egger, M., Stern, J. A. C., & Smith, G. D. (1998). Meta-analysis software [Electronic version]. *British Medical Journal, 316.* Retrieved April 20, 2006, from http://bmj.bmjjournals.com/archive/7126/7126ed9.htm.

Glass, G. V. (1976). Primary, secondary, and meta-analysis of research. *The Educational Researcher, 10,* 3–8.

Glasziou, P., Irwig, L., Bain, C., & Coldtiz, G. (2001). *Systematic reviews in health care: A practical guide.* New York: Cambridge University Press.

Greenhalgh, T., & Peacock, R. (2005). Effectiveness and efficacy of search methods in systematic reviews of complex evidence: Audit of primary sources. *British Medical Journal, 331,* 1064–1065.

Hedges, L. V., & Olkin, I. (1985). *Statistical methods for meta-analysis.* New York: Academic Press.

Jadad, A. R., Moher, D., & Klassen, T. P. (1998). Guides for reading and interpreting systematic reviews. II. How did the authors find the studies and assess their quality? *Archives of Pediatric & Adolescent Medicine, 152,* 812–817.

Little, J., Bradley, L., Bray, M. S., Clyne, M., Dorman, J., Ellsworth, D. L., et al. (2002). Reporting, appraising and integrating data on genotype prevalence and gene-disease associations. *American Journal of Epidemiology, 156*(4), 300–310.

McGowan, J., & Sampson, M. (2005). Systematic reviews need systematic searchers. *Journal of the Medical Library Association, 93,* 74–80.

Muellerleile, P., & Mullen, B. (2006). Efficiency and stability of evidence for public health interventions using cumulative meta-analysis. *American Journal of Public Health, 96,* 515–522.

Mullen, P. D., & Ramírez, G. (2006). The promise and pitfalls of systematic reviews. *Annual Review of Public Health, 27,* 81–102.

Petitti, D. B. (1994). *Meta-analysis, decision analysis, and cost-effectiveness analysis: Methods for quantitative synthesis in medicine.* New York: Oxford University Press.

Stroup, D. F., Berlin, J. A., Morton, S. C., Olkin, I., Williamson, G. D., Rennie, D., et al. (2000). Meta-analysis of observational studies in epidemiology: A proposal for reporting. *Journal of American Medical Association, 283,* 2008–2012.

Sutton, A. J., & Abrams, K. R. (2001). Bayesian methods in meta-analysis and evidence synthesis. *Statistical Methods in Medical Research, 10,* 277–303.

Sutton, A. J., Abrams, K. R., Jones, D. R., Sheldon, T. A., & Song, F. (2000). *Methods for meta-analysis in medical research.* Chichester, UK: Wiley.

Truman, B. I., Smith-Akin, C. K., & Hinman, A. R. (2000). Developing the guide to community preventive services: Overview and rationale. *American Journal of Preventive Medicine, 18*(Suppl. 1), 18–26.

Web Sites

The Community Guide: http://www.thecommunityguide.org/.

Human Genome Epidemiology Network, Centers for Disease Control and Prevention: http://www.cdc.gov/genomics/hugenet/default.htm.

MIGRANT STUDIES

Migrant studies are an extension of the ecologic study design, which compares disease rates in different locations. In migrant studies, the disease rate among persons who have migrated from one location to another is compared with the disease rate in persons who did not migrate. Ideally, the rate for migrants is compared both with persons remaining in the country of origin and with lifelong residents of the destination or host country. Migrants share their genetic makeup and early life environment with persons remaining in the country of origin. They share recent environmental exposures with residents of the host country. Thus, the comparison of disease rates between the migrants and the nonmigrating populations is used to generate hypotheses about the relative importance of genetics and environment in determining disease risk. Migrant disease rates that remain similar to those in the country of origin suggest that genetic factors play a role in geographic variation. Migrant disease rates that converge on that of the host country suggest an important role for the environment. Comparisons between persons migrating at different ages, or between migrants and their offspring, may identify a critical age of exposure for environmental factors.

Migrant studies are likely to be informative when there is marked geographic variation in disease and little is known about the etiologic factors responsible for the variation. The diseases most extensively studied with migrant populations are multiple sclerosis and cancer. Multiple sclerosis has an unusual geographic pattern, with prevalence generally higher with increasing distance from the equator, in both hemispheres. Migrants from higher to lower risk areas, such as Europeans to Israel, South Africa, or Australia, or internal migrants from higher to lower latitudes within the United States, have disease risk intermediate between their place of origin and destination. However, there is little change in risk for migrants moving from lower to higher risk areas, such as Africa to Israel or southern to northern United States. Studies able to ascertain age at migration suggest disease risk is largely determined by age 15 or 20. These studies have been interpreted as most compatible with an environmental exposure in childhood being an important etiologic factor, such as a protective effect from early infection by an agent endemic in areas closer to the equator.

Most cancers show significant geographic variations. Breast and stomach cancers offer two contrasting patterns. Breast cancer rates are highest in the most developed Western countries. Rates for white migrants to the United States converge to rates for U.S.-born whites within 20 years of migration. However, although breast cancer rates for Asian migrants to the United States and their U.S.-born daughters are higher than rates for women in Asia, they are not as high as U.S.-born whites. This suggests the importance of environmental factors in breast cancer risk, but it does not exclude the possibility that there might be genetic differences in risk for Asian women, since even U.S.-born Asian women have lower rates of breast cancer than whites.

The international pattern for stomach cancer is quite different: Japan has one of the highest rates and the United States one of the lowest. Migrant studies, including those of Japanese migrants to Hawaii and their offspring, found that migrants had rates somewhat lower than persons remaining in Japan, while their offspring had much lower stomach cancer rates. This pattern suggests the importance of environmental factors, both in childhood and adulthood.

In addition to estimating change in disease risk at the population level, migrant populations also offer the opportunity to investigate the etiologic role of environmental factors that change dramatically with immigration, such as diet. For such studies, migrants are recruited to participate in case-control or cohort studies, and risk factors are directly assessed at the individual level.

Limitations of Migrant Studies

The two most serious limitations to migrant studies are data quality and selection bias. Migrant studies often use data routinely collected for surveillance, and this raises concerns about data quality and the comparability of data from different countries. Diagnostic criteria and the completeness of disease ascertainment may vary between countries. When death certificates are used to identify migrants, place of birth may be incomplete. Neither year of migration nor parents' birthplaces are generally recorded. Thus, death certificate studies are limited to first-generation migrants. Sample sizes of migrants with a particular disease may be small, limiting analyses to standardized mortality ratios or standardized incidence ratios. Ethnic identification may be inconsistent between sources of numerator data, such as death certificates or cancer registries, and denominator sources, usually a census.

International migration is not a random event, and the opportunity to carry out migrant studies depends on historical circumstances. Frequent migration destinations such as the United States, Australia, and Israel are usually the study settings, although there are also migration studies within a country, often from rural to urban areas. A fundamental limitation of migrant studies is that persons who migrate are different from persons who do not. They may differ systematically by religion, education, ethnicity, or social class. International migration is often a difficult process, and successful migrants are likely to be persons with intellectual, emotional, health, and financial resources. For these reasons, it is impossible to know whether the migrants would have experienced the same disease risk as persons remaining in the country of origin had they not migrated. Studies have often observed that migrants experience generally good health, which is sometimes called the "healthy immigrant" effect. In some cases, such as migrants to Israel, there may be no ethnically similar people remaining in the country of origin for comparison. If migrants systematically differ from nonmigrants with respect to underlying disease risk, even in the absence of the migration experience, then migrant studies are subject to selection bias.

—*Diane Sperling Lauderdale*

See also Asian American/Pacific Islander Health Issues; Bias; Immigrant and Refugee Health Issues; Latino Health Issues; Secondary Data

Further Readings

Gale, C. R., & Martyn, C. N. (1995). Migrant studies in multiple sclerosis. *Progress in Neurobiology, 47,* 425–448.

Haenszel, W., Kurihara, M., Segi, M., & Lee, R. K. (1972). Stomach cancer among Japanese in Hawaii. *Journal of the National Cancer Institute, 49,* 969–988.

Parkin, D. M., & Khlat, M. (1996). Studies of cancer in migrants: Rationale and methodology. *European Journal of Cancer, 32A,* 761–771.

Thomas, D. B., & Karaga, M. R. (1996). Migrant studies. In D. Schottenfeld & J. F. Fraumeni Jr. (Eds.), *Cancer epidemiology and prevention* (2nd ed., pp. 236–254). New York: Oxford University Press.

MISSING DATA METHODS

Virtually all epidemiologic studies suffer from some degree of missing or incomplete data. This means that some of the cases have data missing on some (but not all) of the variables. For example, one patient in a study may have values present for all variables except age. Another may have missing data on blood pressure and years of schooling. Missing data create problems for most statistical methods because they presume that every case has measured values on all variables in whatever model is being estimated. This entry surveys some of the many methods that have been developed to deal with these problems.

The most common method for handling missing data is complete case analysis (also known as listwise or casewise deletion). In this method, cases are deleted from the analysis if they have missing data on any of the variables under consideration, thereby using only complete cases. Because of its simplicity and because it can be used with any kind of statistical analysis, complete case analysis is the default in nearly all statistical packages. Unfortunately, complete case analysis can also result in the deletion of a very large fraction of the original data set, leading to wide confidence intervals and low power for hypothesis tests. It can also lead to biased estimates if data are not missing completely at random (to be defined below).

To avoid these difficulties and to salvage at least some of the discarded information, many different methods have been developed. Most of these methods are crude, ad hoc, and may only make things worse. Although more principled and effective methods have appeared in the past 20 years, they are still woefully underutilized.

Assumptions

Before examining various missing data methods, it is important to explain some key assumptions that are often used to justify the methods. The definitions given here are intended to be informal and heuristic.

Missing Completely at Random (MCAR)

Many missing data methods are valid only if the data are missing completely at random. Suppose that only one variable Y has missing data and that there are other variables (represented by the vector X) that are always observed. We say that data on Y are missing completely at random if the probability of missing data on Y is completely unrelated either to X or to Y itself. Symbolically, this is expressed as

$$Pr(Y \text{ missing } |X, Y) = Pr(Y \text{ missing}).$$

Note that missingness on Y can depend on other *unobserved* variables. It just can't depend on variables that are observed for the model under consideration. This definition can easily be extended to situations in which more than one variable has missing data, but the representation gets more complicated. Note also that MCAR is not violated if missingness on one variable is related to missingness in another variable. In an extreme but common situation, two variables may be always missing together or always present together; this does not violate MCAR.

Missing at Random (MAR)

MCAR is a very strong assumption. Some of the newer missing data methods are valid under the weaker assumption of missing at random. Again, let's suppose that only one variable Y has missing data, and that there are other variables X that are always observed. We say that data on Y are missing at random if the probability of missingness on Y may depend on X, but does not depend on Y itself after adjusting or controlling for X. In symbols, we say $\Pr(Y \text{ missing}|X, Y) = \Pr(Y \text{ missing}|X)$. Here's an example of a violation of this assumption: People with high income may be less likely to report their income, even after adjusting for other observed variables.

Although the MAR assumption is still fairly strong, it's much weaker than MCAR because it allows missingness to be related to anything that's observed. It's also an untestable assumption because a test would require that we know the values that are missing. If the data are MAR and if the parameters governing the missing data mechanism are distinct from the parameters in the model to be estimated, the missing data mechanism is said to be *ignorable*. That means that one can make valid inferences without explicitly modeling the mechanism that produces the missing data. Because the distinctness requirement is almost always satisfied, the terms *missing at random* and *ignorability* are often used interchangeably.

Goals for Missing Data Methods

To compare missing data methods, we need some criteria for evaluating them. Nowadays, most experts stress the quality of parameter estimates that are obtained when using a missing data method. In that regard, the goals for missing data methods are just the usual goals for good estimation:

1. Minimize bias.

2. Minimize sampling variability, that is, make the true standard errors as small as possible.

3. Get good estimates of uncertainty, that is, estimated standard errors and confidence intervals.

Most conventional methods fail to accomplish one or another of these goals. Nearly all of them (except for complete case analysis) are deficient in the estimation of standard errors and confidence intervals.

Conventional Methods

Here is a brief look at some conventional missing data methods and how they stack up on the three goals.

Complete Case Analysis

If the data are MCAR, the subset of the cases that are complete can be regarded as a simple random sample from the target sample. It follows that complete case analysis will not introduce any bias into parameter estimates, and the standard error estimates will be accurate estimates of the true standard errors. On the other hand, the standard errors may be much larger than necessary because much usable data have been discarded. Furthermore, depending on the analytic method and the parameters to be estimated, complete case estimates may be severely biased if the data are MAR but not MCAR. Surprisingly, however, neither MCAR nor MAR is required for complete case analysis when data are missing only on predictor variables in any kind of regression analysis.

Available Case Analysis

For linear models, a popular missing data method is available case analysis (also known as pairwise deletion). This method rests on the fact that, in most applications, the parameters in linear models can be expressed as functions of means, variances, and covariances. The basic idea is to estimate these "moments" by conventional methods, using all available data (so different numbers of cases might be used to estimate different moments), then substitute these estimates into formulas for the parameters of interest. If the data are MCAR, this method produces estimates that are consistent and, hence, approximately unbiased. However, the method may break down completely for some patterns of missing data. More important, there is no good way to get accurate estimates of standard errors using this method.

Dummy Variable Adjustment

For regression analysis with missing data on a predictor variable, a popular method is to substitute some constant for the missing data (e.g., the mean or 0) and then include in the regression an indicator (dummy) variable for whether or not the data are missing. For categorical predictors, a related method is to create an additional category for missing data. Unfortunately, these methods have been shown to produce biased estimates, even when the data are MCAR.

Imputation

A wide variety of missing data methods fall under the general heading of imputation, which simply means to fill in some reasonable guesses for the missing values, based on other available information. There are many ways to do this, the simplest of which is to replace missing values with the means of the observed values. Once all the missing data have been imputed, the analysis is done with standard statistical methods.

Virtually all conventional methods of imputation suffer from two problems. First, variances tend to be underestimated, leading to biases in any parameters that depend on variances (e.g., regression coefficients). Second, and arguably more serious, standard errors tend to be underestimated, leading to confidence intervals that are too narrow and *p* values that are too low. The reason for this should be intuitively obvious. Imputation substitutes "made up" data for real data, but standard software has no way of distinguishing imputed from real data. Consequently, standard error estimates assume more information than is really present.

Maximum Likelihood

One of the most general and effective methods for handling missing data is maximum likelihood estimation (MLE). Of course, MLE is widely used for all sorts of applications that do not involve missing data, for example, logistic regression. What makes it so attractive for missing data applications is that it satisfies all the three goals mentioned above. Estimates are approximately unbiased; all the available information is used to produce estimates that have minimum sampling variability; and standard errors are consistent estimates of the true standard errors.

Most software for MLE with missing data is based on the assumption that the data are missing at random. To do MLE, one first needs a probability model for the joint distribution of all the variables in the model of interest. For categorical variables, for example, one might specify a log-linear model. For continuous variables, a multivariate normal model is commonly assumed. Next, one must construct the likelihood function, which expresses the probability of the data as a function of the unknown parameters. Once the likelihood function is constructed, the final step is to find values of the parameters that maximize the likelihood.

If the missing data mechanism is ignorable (and therefore MAR) the construction of the likelihood function is fairly simple. When observations are independent, the likelihood for the whole sample is just the product of the probabilities of observing each of the observations. Suppose the model of interest has three variables X, Y, and Z. Suppose, further, that a particular observation has observed values of X and Y but is missing a value on Z. Let $p(x, y, z)$ be the probability function for all three variables. Then, if Z is discrete, the likelihood for that observation is found by summing $p(x, y, z)$ over all possible values of z. If Z is continuous, one integrates over the full range of values for z. If data are missing on that observation for both Y and Z, one integrates or sums over both variables.

Once the likelihood function has been constructed, maximization usually requires some numerical algorithm. For missing data applications, one popular maximization method is known as the expectation-maximization (EM) algorithm. This method involves iteration between two steps until convergence. The E-step consists of calculating the expected value of the log-likelihood, where the expectation is taken over variables with missing data, given the current values of the parameters. The M-step consists of maximizing this expected log-likelihood to get new values of the parameters. Most of the better-known statistical packages contain procedures for applying the EM algorithm under the multivariate normal model. The output of these procedures consists of ML estimates of the means, variances, and covariances.

Although the EM algorithm has its attractions, there are many other numerical methods that will yield the same ML estimates. For estimating the parameters of log-linear models with missing data, there are several freeware and commercial software packages available. For estimating linear models, it is a common practice to first estimate the means and covariance matrix by the EM algorithm and then use those statistics as input to a linear modeling program. Although this two-step procedure will give the correct parameter estimates, it will not yield correct standard errors, confidence intervals, or test statistics. To get correct values of these statistics, one must use "direct maximum likelihood" for the specified model. This method is currently available in many structural equation modeling programs.

Multiple Imputation

When feasible, MLE is an excellent method for handling missing data. Unfortunately, for many applications either the theory or the software is lacking. For example, it's not easy to find MLE software for doing logistic regression or Cox regression. In such cases, multiple imputation is an attractive alternative. Like ML, the estimates produced by multiple imputation are approximately unbiased with accurate standard errors. The statistical efficiency is *almost* at the maximum level achieved by MLE, but not quite.

The advantages of multiple imputation over MLE are that (a) it can be used with virtually any kind of data or model and (b) conventional software can be used for estimation. There are two disadvantages, however. First, there are many different ways to do multiple imputation, leading to some uncertainty and confusion. Second, every time you use it, you get a (slightly) different result, because a random element is deliberately introduced into the imputation process.

A fundamental principle of multiple imputation is that imputed values should be random draws from the predictive distribution of the variable with missing data, conditional on the values of the observed variables. For example, if imputations are based on linear regression (one of the more popular approaches to multiple imputation), the imputed values are generated by, first, calculating predicted values as one usually does with linear regression and, second, adding a random draw from the residual distribution for the regression equation. Introduction of this random element avoids the biases that typically occur with deterministic imputation.

The other key principle of multiple imputation is that more than one randomly imputed value should be generated for each missing datum. How many? Three is the minimum, and many multiple imputation software programs use a default of five. More is always better, but the returns diminish rapidly. Two things are accomplished by making the imputations multiple: (a) parameter estimates are considerably more efficient (i.e., have less sampling variability) and (b) having multiple imputations makes it possible to get good standard error estimates that accurately reflect the uncertainty introduced by the imputation process.

In practice, the multiple imputations are used to construct multiple data sets, and each data set contains different imputed values for the missing data. Conventional software is then applied to each data set to estimate the parameters (and their standard errors) for the model of interest. Using a few simple rules, these multiple estimates are then combined to get a single set of parameter estimates, standard errors, and test statistics. For the parameter estimates themselves, a simple average of the multiple estimates is sufficient. Combination of the standard errors requires the following steps: (a) square the estimated standard errors (producing variance estimates) and average them across the data sets; (b) calculate the variance of the parameter estimates across the multiple data sets; (c) add the results of (a) and (b) (applying a small correction factor to the variance); and (d) take the square root of that sum.

As noted, the most popular method for generating the imputed values is linear regression with random draws from the residual distribution. This is straightforward when there is only a single variable with missing data, but typically runs into difficulty when several variables have missing data. One solution, based on Bayesian principles, is an iterative Markov chain Monte Carlo (MCMC) algorithm that involves long sequences of repeated iterations.

Of course, many variables with missing data are categorical, and linear regression may not be a plausible method of imputation in those cases. Although ad hoc fix-ups of the linear model often work well for such variables, imputation can alternatively be based on logistic regression, Poisson regression, log-linear models, and other semi- or nonparametric approaches. The downside is that the MCMC algorithm may be difficult or impossible to implement for such models. Consequently, software based on these approaches typically use iterative methods that have no theoretical foundation.

Nonignorable Missing Data

As with ML, most methods and software for doing multiple imputation are based on the assumption that the missing data mechanism is ignorable and, hence, that the data are MAR. It's important to stress, however, that both multiple imputation and ML estimation can handle applications where the data are *not* MAR. Because there are often reasons to suspect that the data are not MAR (e.g., sicker patients may be more likely to drop out of a study than healthier patients), there has been no shortage of attempts to develop specialized models and methods for the nonignorable case. But doing this successfully requires a correct mathematical model for the missing data mechanism, and that is something that is usually quite difficult to come by. An incorrect choice can produce highly misleading results, and there is no way to test the fit of the model. For those who want to pursue such approaches, it is strongly advised that one try out several different missing data models to determine whether the results and conclusions are sensitive to the model choice.

—Paul D. Allison

See also Confidence Interval; Cox Model; Dummy Variable; Logistic Regression; Regression

Further Readings

Allison, P. D. (2001). *Missing data.* Thousand Oaks, CA: Sage.

Little, R. J. A., & Rubin, D. B. (2002). *Statistical analysis with missing data* (2nd ed.). Hoboken, NJ: Wiley.

Schafer, J. L. (1997). *Analysis of incomplete multivariate data.* New York: CRC Press.

Molecular Epidemiology

Although the recognition of molecular epidemiology as an epidemiology subspecialty is relatively recent, laboratory methods have long been used to classify disease and determine exposure in epidemiologic studies. For example, the ability to detect and identify bacteria was essential to the success of studies illuminating the epidemiology of typhoid by Wade Hampton Frost and others, as was the ability to measure blood lipids in the identification of an association between cholesterol and heart disease risk in the Framingham study. The distinction implied in the term *molecular epidemiology* arises from the challenges and opportunities of applying the rapidly expanding array of modern molecular techniques to studies of health and disease in populations. Modern molecular techniques include the ability to directly study genes (genomics), gene expression (transcriptomics), proteins (proteomics), and metabolites left behind by cell processes (metabolomics). These

techniques are applied in the rapidly expanding number of epidemiology specialties, most notably genetic, cancer, environmental, and infectious disease epidemiology.

The application of molecular techniques to epidemiology gives epidemiologists the tools to move beyond risk factor epidemiology and gain insight into the overall system of the disease. For infectious diseases, the system includes the transmission system, pathogenesis, and virulence of the agent. The inclusion of molecular tools has the potential to enhance diagnosis of outcome, and to detect low levels of exposure or markers of previous exposure, decreasing misclassification of outcome and exposure. Molecular epidemiologic studies can identify previously undetectable agents, enhance outbreak investigation, help describe disease transmission systems, and give insight into pathogen gene function and host-agent interaction. When applied in combination with appropriate epidemiologic methods, modern molecular techniques allow us to identify novel methods of disease prevention and control, markers of disease diagnosis and prognosis, and fertile research areas for potential new therapeutics and/or vaccines. However, the success of these studies depends not only on the molecular measure chosen, but also on whether the strengths and limitations of the chosen measure are considered in the design, conduct, and analysis, and interpretation of the study results.

Examples in this entry focus on applications in infectious disease epidemiology, which provide the additional challenges and opportunities of at least two genomes (sets of transcripts, proteins, and metabolites), that of the infectious agent and that of the host(s). However, the general principles described are applicable to all epidemiologic studies that incorporate molecular techniques.

Opportunities

The potential of modern molecular techniques in epidemiologic studies has been best explored with genomics. The promise of transcriptomics, proteomics, and metabolomics for increasing understanding of the distribution of health and disease in human populations is great, but at this writing, not much realized for infectious diseases. Thus, the opportunities for applying molecular tools to epidemiologic studies in infectious diseases described below involve primarily the use of genomic techniques.

Gaining Insight Into Gene Importance and Function

Many major human pathogens have been genetically sequenced, and hundreds of genomes will be sequenced in the near future. Unlike genes from multicelled organisms, single-celled organisms often vary greatly in genetic content and expression—that is, genes may be present or absent as well as expressed or silent. Once a single strain of an infectious agent has been sequenced, the sequence can be used as a reference for comparison with others in the same species, providing insight into the heterogeneity of the species. Sequence information can also be mined to identify risk factor genes of unknown function that are structurally similar to genes whose function is known, thereby giving insight into the function of these risk factor genes. Epidemiologic screening of collections of infectious agents for the prevalence of genes that alter the transmission, pathogenesis, and virulence of the agent can provide important insights into the potential importance and putative function of those genes. For example, a gene found more frequently in strains causing severe disease (virulent strains) than among strains that colonize without causing symptoms (commensal strains) suggests that the gene is worthy of more detailed laboratory analyses of its function.

Transcriptomics extends and refines this concept by enabling the identification of genes that are expressed rather than genes that are simply present in the genome. These technologies may be used to identify which genes an infectious agent expresses at different stages of pathogenesis. Expression profiling adds to our knowledge of disease pathology by separating the mechanisms associated with initiation of infection from those associated with disease progression. Furthermore, transcriptomics has the potential to greatly enhance our understanding of interactions between the infectious agent and the human host. For example, in a model system, we can identify which genes are expressed in response to infection. Understanding how virulence is regulated in vivo can point to new targets for therapeutics or vaccines.

Determining a Molecular "Fingerprint"

Infectious agents can be classified into unique groups based on direct or indirect measures of genetic sequence, yielding what is known as a *molecular fingerprint*. Molecular fingerprints for infectious agents are less subject to misclassification than typing systems based on phenotype, which may vary with growth conditions. For example, bacteria that are genetically identical may have different appearance ("morphology") depending on growth conditions. Furthermore, extrachromosomal material, such as plasmids, that code for antibiotic resistance or other characteristics used in typing may be gained or lost during storage and handling. Typing systems based on chromosomal material often focus on genetic regions that are less likely to develop mutations, known as highly conserved regions.

Several molecular typing techniques for infectious agents are based on genetic sequence. Techniques range from gel-based methods such pulsed-field gel electrophoresis (PFGE) used by the Centers for Disease Control and Prevention in PulseNET, PCR-based methods based on repeated elements, to sequencing conserved areas of the genome, such as multilocus sequence typing, to comparing entire genomes with that of a reference sequenced strain, known as genomotyping. These methods vary in cost, reliability, and adaptability to high throughput formats. When properly applied, molecular typing allows the investigator to confirm that strains are identical at the genetic level, generate hypotheses about epidemiologic relationships between strains in the absence of epidemiologic data, and describe distribution of strain types and identify the determinants of that distribution.

A primary application of molecular fingerprinting is in outbreak investigations. Molecular fingerprints confirm or refute epidemiologic hypotheses, for example, confirming that a particular food item is the common source for a widely disseminated foodborne outbreak. Molecular techniques also are used to confirm transmission events, particularly when epidemiologic data suggest limited contact, thus giving us new information about potential transmission modes. As part of a surveillance system, the identification of common molecular fingerprints can suggest potential epidemiologic linkages requiring further investigation. For example, there are sporadic cases of *Escherichia coli* O157:H7 that can occur in space-time clusters. If these cases share a common molecular fingerprint, an outbreak investigation is in order. Isolates from multiple clusters in different areas occurring in the same time period with a common molecular fingerprint can suggest a common source outbreak from a widely disseminated vehicle, such as occurred with spinach in 2006. Molecular fingerprints can distinguish between new infection and recurrence of existing infection, such as studies that confirmed exogenous reinfections with tuberculosis. Comparing the distribution of transposable genetic elements among different strain types can provide insight into whether the spread of factors coded for by genes in the transposable elements is primarily clonal or due to horizontal gene transfer. Understanding these types of evolutionary relationships is key to designing effective prevention and control strategies.

Identifying Previously Unknown or Uncultivable Infectious Agents

The vast majority of infectious agents cannot be cultured using standard laboratory techniques; thus, we have only limited knowledge about the numbers and types of bacteria, viruses, and fungi that live with us and in us. The ability to make a copy of genetic material and determine the genetic sequence, which can then be compared with known genetic sequence, has led to a radical reassessment of the amount of life around us, and has facilitated the identification of previously unknown infectious agents. The identification of the causative agent of HIV and Kaposi's sarcoma are attributable to the use of modern molecular techniques combined with epidemiologic principles. A great triumph of this technique was the identification of human papillomavirus as the cause of cervical cancer, leading ultimately to the development of an effective vaccine.

Understanding Host-Agent Interactions

Infectious diseases are often classified into those that primarily affect humans and those that primarily affect nonhumans. As we have increased our understanding of the genetics of human pathogens, there is increasing evidence that subsets of a particular human pathogen may be better adapted to human hosts with certain genetic characteristics. For example, there is some evidence that variants of tuberculosis from particular geographic areas spread more easily among persons from the same geographic area. Strains of human papillomavirus seem to persist longer among individuals whose genetic origin is the same as the origin of the virus: Variants of African origin persist longer among African Americans, and variants of European origin persist longer among European Americans. As we refine our understanding of both human and pathogenic genomes, we might discover answers to why some individuals suffer chronic, recurring infections and others are apparently resistant. These answers will provide important insights for the development of prevention and control strategies.

Implications of Adding Molecular Techniques to Epidemiologic Studies

The choice of a molecular technique should not be made lightly, because the choice not only affects study conduct and analysis but also can profoundly affect study design efficacy. A technique might be a direct or indirect measure of the exposure or outcome of interest. It might be able to characterize disease stage or history of exposure. Each molecular technique has its own reliability, validity, sensitivity to specimen collection and processing, and cost, which affect its suitability for a particular project. Furthermore, one must consider the ability of the molecular technique to capture the desired level of variance within and between individuals. For example, some hormone levels may vary greatly throughout the day in one individual, while levels of another biological marker may vary little between individuals over long periods of time.

General Comments on Selecting a Molecular Tool

In some ways, selecting a molecular measuring tool is no different from choosing the appropriate way to measure any item of interest in an epidemiologic context. A list of considerations is shown in Table 1. Because many molecular tools are sensitive to variance in technique, instruments, reagents used, and technician skill, the reliability and validity of any selected molecular tool will be different in different laboratories and should be determined prior to beginning any studies. If there is more than one laboratory, the investigator should also assess interlaboratory variation in addition to intralaboratory variation.

Some methods, such as gel-based typing methods, can be so sensitive to individual laboratory conditions that gel-to-gel variation makes it difficult to compare gel results between gels from the same laboratory, much less between different laboratories. Although running standards and using software that normalizes to those standards increase comparability, assessments

Table 1 Considerations When Choosing Between Molecular Typing Systems

Validity	High sensitivity (the probability that test is positive given that the sample is truly positive) and high specificity (the probability that test is negative given that the sample is truly negative)
Reliability	The assay is both repeatable: (same result in the same laboratory under conditions) and reproducible: same result in different laboratory
Transportability	Results are easily transported and compared between laboratories
Level of Discrimination	The number of categories that result from testing. Whether categories have biologic rationale such that categories can be collapsed in an interpretable meaningful way
Rapidity	The results will be available in a timely manner for the desired investigation
Cost	The resulting measures answer the question for a reasonable cost

of identity of bacterial strains using even gold-standard, gel-based typing methods such as PFGE are best made by running the strains on the same gel. This is true for all methods based on comparing visual band patterns. In contrast, sequence information can be ascertained with extremely high reliability and validity. Furthermore, sequence information is easily recorded and compared.

Other methods can be sensitive to how a specimen is collected, the media in which the specimen is stored, the time since collection, and the length and temperature of storage. The sensitivity may be a function of the specimen itself, as some molecules can degrade quickly, such as bacterial RNA. The specimen may include other material that interferes with the assay or degrades the substance of interest, so that considerable processing may be necessary prior to testing and/or storage. Some bacteria grow, albeit slowly, even when frozen, such as *Listeria* species. Therefore, a pilot study of all laboratory procedures is essential to identify any such problems prior to implementing the study.

Even valid and reliable methods vary in their level of discrimination, that is, the number of categories that result from a measurement. The same tool can be more or less discriminatory depending on how it is applied. For example, PFGE is not very discriminatory if the chosen restriction enzyme cuts the DNA into only one or two bands, but it is highly discriminatory if 30 bands result. The investigator needs to decide what level of information is required to answer the research question. While it may be attractive to use the most recently developed technique, a simpler

technique may give the answer at the level required at a much cheaper cost. Furthermore, the type of inferences the investigator wishes to make is an important consideration. Multilocus sequence typing was developed to study genetic lineages, which occur over thousands of years; thus, it may not be appropriate for determining genetic linkage in an outbreak, where genetic changes not captured by multilocus sequence typing may distinguish outbreak from nonoutbreak strains.

The investigator should also consider whether there is a biologic rationale for collapsing the separate categories derived from a highly discriminatory technique. A change in number of bands in a gel based method may result from a variety of different events, some of which are relevant to the question at hand, some of which are not. For example, band patterns in PFGE may be the same but the genetic content of the bands may vary. Whether categories can be collapsed may depend on epidemiologic information. For example, a one- or two-band difference in PFGE pattern may be considered the same organism in the context of an outbreak investigation, but not when comparing a large collection of organisms collected over time and space. Any technique based on band patterns, such as PFGE, can exhibit homoplasia, meaning that the same pattern can evolve by chance in two different groups. The probability of homoplasia increases as larger geographical and temporal frames are sampled, which becomes important when examining international or long-standing databases.

Results may be recorded on different types of scales that give the investigator more or less power in the analysis. The results may be qualitative (a simple positive/negative), nominal (putting results into groups but there is no order to groups), ordinal (putting results into groups where there is an implied order), or ratio (where the distances between points are equidistant and there is a meaningful zero point). Ratio scales give most power for the analysis. Ordinal and ratio scales are preferred, as categories might be reasonably collapsed in the analysis. Collapsing of categories is problematic for nominal variables, such as those that occur with gel-based typing techniques based on band patterns.

The investigator also needs to consider the timeliness of the results. In an outbreak investigation, having a timely answer may be essential, whereas in research settings, a more definitive but less timely answer might be desirable. Finally, cost is an important consideration. The investigator often must trade off the added precision and power that might be gained from using a more expensive test, with the loss of power from enrolling fewer participants.

Study Design

Obtaining biological specimens—especially those that require needle sticks or other procedures that are uncomfortable—often decreases response rates, thus increasing the potential for selection bias, and adversely affecting the study validity and generalizability. Investigators need to stick to sound epidemiologic principles for identifying, recruiting, and following study participants, and for determining sample size, and avoid being seduced by the latest laboratory method. The gain in power from decreased misclassification afforded by using a newer molecular technique can be rapidly offset by the increased cost per unit of the new technique, resulting in a need to reduce sample size.

After these basic design considerations, the investigator should consider how the choice of molecular tool might affect the study design. For example, if a test must be conducted on fresh samples, the sampling of cases and controls in a case-control study should be done such that the groups are sampled and tested in similar time periods to minimize potential biases resulting from assay drift, which is where a method gives increasingly higher or lower results with time. For nested case-control studies, how specimens are collected may determine whether controls can be sampled from the base population (case-based,

also called case-cohort, sampling) or at time of incidence disease (incidence density sampling).

Study Conduct

Molecular epidemiologic studies have added complexities associated with the collection and handling of specimens that may contain infectious agents. Study personnel must be protected from infection by vaccination and proper training, and appropriate precautions must be followed at all stages to minimize risk of infecting study personnel or others. There are substantial regulations about shipping and handling of diagnostic specimens and infectious agents; investigators should acquaint themselves with these prior to any data collection. Information about these regulations is available from the Centers for Disease Control and Prevention Web site (www.cdc.gov). Laboratories and facilities must be inspected and appropriate certifications obtained from the appropriate institutional biosafety committee.

Biological Versus Technical Variability

Prior to testing specimens, any assays or techniques should be tested and the reliability and validity in the hands of the investigators' team determined. Assays should be perfected so that any technical variation is minimized. The objective is to minimize variability in results stemming from technical issues so that the true biological variability will be measured. Sometimes, there is substantial diurnal biological variability. In this case, the investigator should consider strategies to minimize the effects of this variability, such as collecting all specimens at the same time of day or pooling specimens over the course of the day. For example, if testing urine for a metabolite, the investigators might use the first urine void of the day, or pool all urine from an individual over the course of a single day.

Quality Control and Quality Assurance

Study protocols should include ongoing quality control and quality assurance procedures to detect any problems with the protocol as the study proceeds, for example, including specimens with known values and/or duplicate specimens when material is shipped as a check that proper shipping procedures are followed. Laboratory personnel should be blinded to which specimens are standards or duplicates. Assays should be run in duplicate and positive and negative controls included in each run. Equipment needs to be calibrated frequently, and the reliability within and between technicians assessed.

Specimen Collection, Handling, and Storage

Tracking and logging of specimens is essential. The tracking must continue as long as specimens are stored, and items that might affect future assays noted, such as the number of times frozen specimens are thawed. Ideally, specimens are divided into separate vials (aliquoted) and stored in different locations. Aliquoting minimizes contaminations and problems with freezing and thawing. Storage in different locations helps minimize loss from untoward events such as equipment failure due to power losses. Specimen handling should be meticulous to avoid contamination. If testing infectious agents, the investigator should determine if the agent might change following successive cultures or under certain storage conditions. If specimens are to be frozen at low temperatures, it is essential to use labels that will not fall off on extended freezing. The labels should include all information that may help the laboratory technician to minimize error. Alternatively, the investigator can use bar codes linked to a database with all required information.

Recording Data

Specimens may be tested for several different substances, or several different specimens may be obtained from the same individual. If cultured for infectious agents, multiple isolates may be recovered from the same individual. The development of a study identifier that allows linkage to questionnaire information, but also includes information useful about the assay, is essential. For example, the identification number used in the laboratory might also include an indicator of when the specimen was collected, or if separated into components or tested for different substances, an additional indicator of the substance. For example, the first three numbers might indicate the individual, and the fourth number the site of collection (567-2, where 567 is study identification number and 2 indicates collected from urine). The investigator should consider how the data would be used in the

analysis, so the various databases can be merged with minimal amounts of data management.

Data Analysis

Epidemiologists are used to using either an individual or person-time as the denominator for estimating rates and proportions. However, individuals may be colonized with multiple strains of a single infection agent or at multiple sites that may or may not be independent. Depending on what relationship(s) the investigator intends to demonstrate, the strain of the infectious agent may be used as the unit of analysis. For example, if the outcome is transmission between couples, the denominator might be couples or the number of isolated organisms, some of which are and some of which are not transmitted.

The investigator might also wish to determine if an individual can be colonized with multiple strains of a single species or if host or agent factors inhibit colonization by multiple strains. For these analyses, the investigator must be aware of sampling errors, that is, the potential that a strain might truly be present and have been missed because of laboratory procedures. If culturing bacteria, an investigator might choose to test only the most common isolate, which precludes testing whether colonization inhibits coinfection with other strains ("super infection"). Multiple viral strains might also be cultured from a single individual, but only if the laboratory procedures are set up accordingly. Potential sampling errors and sensitivity of chosen technique to low levels of the organism of interest should also be taken into account when interpreting prevalence and incidence estimates.

In outbreak investigations, molecular evidence is often used to support or refute epidemiologic evidence gathered via questionnaire or medical records. Thus, the investigators need to be certain that the laboratory technique is appropriately classifying organisms into related groups. If an infectious organism changes rapidly—for example, if it uptakes or loses genetic material that codes for antibiotic resistance—it may still be part of the same chain of infection but may show a remarkably different molecular type depending on the typing system used. The speed of change depends on the characteristics of the organism itself; thus, investigators should take care to understand the molecular biology of the organism under study, as well as the strengths and limitations of any typing system when drawing inferences.

Future Opportunities and Challenges

As researchers gain experience in the application of molecular tools to epidemiologic studies of human pathogens, there is tremendous opportunity to increase understanding of the transmission, pathogenesis and evolution of human pathogens, and the interaction of human and pathogen genes. But many challenges lie ahead before this potential will be fully realized.

First, we will need to increase our understanding of the ecology of microorganisms that are normal inhabitants of the human bowel, skin, vaginal cavity, nose, and throat. Although we generally consider human pathogens in isolation, transmission and pathogenesis are not solely a function of a particular pathogen but are often modified by the presence of other pathogens. For example, the presence of genital ulcer disease increases transmission of HIV. A less obvious example is that bacterial vaginosis also increases transmission of HIV. Bacterial vaginosis is a disruption of the vaginal ecology that may or may not cause clinical symptoms. Similar disruptions of the ecology of other human microflora may be associated with increased disease risk. However, as of this writing, our understanding of the ecology of the human microflora is limited.

Second, current analytic methods are inadequate to deal with the complicated interactions inherent in molecular epidemiologic studies of agent-host interactions. We have the capacity to generate large amounts of data on the genetics of infectious agents, the expression of these genes during different aspects of the infection process, and the expression of human genes in response to infection. Thus, description is the order of the day. However, to truly advance the field, we will need to develop more complete theories to explain our observations. Molecular epidemiology of infectious diseases is one area of epidemiology that has obvious ties to evolutionary theory. Evolutionary theory is highly developed and there are associated analytic methods that we have just begun to apply in an epidemiologic context.

The second problem is tied to a final problem: Our understanding of the system is so limited that we fail to collect the correct data. This challenge can be addressed by the development of appropriate mathematical models. Even a simple conceptual model forces the investigator to explicitly specify the relationships between various aspects of the system, providing insight into what we do and do not know, and what additional data are lacking. Mathematical models also provide insight into the relative importance of various aspects of the system, and can take into account known theories and thus help develop new theories to explain the transmission, pathogenesis, and evolution of infectious diseases.

—Betsy Foxman

See also Genetic Epidemiology;Genomics; Outbreak Investigation

Further Readings

Bender, J. B., Hedberg, C. W., Besser, J. M., Boxrud, D. J., MacDonald, K. L., & Osterholm, M. T. (1997). Surveillance by molecular subtype for *Escherichia coli* O157:H7 infections in Minnesota by molecular subtyping. *New England Journal of Medicine, 337*(6), 388–394.

Blahna, M., Zalewski, C., Reuer, J., Kahlmeter, G., Foxman, B., & Marrs, C. F. (2006). The role of horizontal gene transfer in the spread of trimethoprim-sulfamethoxazole resistance among uropathogenic *Escherichia coli* in Europe and Canada. *Journal of Antimicrobial Chemotherapy, 57*(4), 666–672.

DeRiemer, K., & Daley, C. L. (2004). Tuberculosis transmission based on molecular epidemiologic research. *Seminars in Respiratory and Critical Care Medicine, 25*(3), 297–306.

Foxman, B., Manning, S. D., Tallman, P., Bauer, R., Zhang, L., Koopman, J. S., et al. (2002). Uropathogenic *Escherichia coli* are more likely than commensal *E. coli* to be shared between heterosexual sex partners. *American Journal of Epidemiology, 156*(12), 1133–1140.

Foxman, B., Zhang, L., Koopman, J. S., Manning, S. D., & Marrs, C. F. (2005). Choosing an appropriate bacterial typing technique for epidemiologic studies. *Epidemiologic Perspectives & Innovations, 2*, 10.

Gagneux, S., DeRiemer, K., Van, T., Kato-Maeda, M., de Jong, B. C., Narayanan, S., et al. (2006). Variable host-pathogen compatibility in *Mycobacterium tuberculosis*. *Proceedings of the National Academy of Sciences of the United States of America, 103*(8), 2869–2873.

Gerner-Smidt, P., Hise, K., Kincaid, J., Hunter, S., Rolando, S., Hyytia Trees, E., et al. (2006). PulseNet USA: A five-year update. *Foodborne Pathogens and Disease, 3*(1), 9–19.

Graham, M. R., Virtaneva, K., Porcella, S. F., Gardner, D. J., Long, R. D., Welty, D. M., et al. (2006). Analysis of the transcriptome of Group A *Streptococcus* in mouse soft tissue infection. *American Journal of Pathology, 169*(3), 927–942.

Manning, S. D., Tallman, P., Baker, C. J., Gillespie, B., Marrs, C. F., & Foxman, B. (2002). Determinants of co-colonization with group B streptococcus among heterosexual college couples. *Epidemiology, 13*(5), 533–539.

Porta, M., Malats, N., Vioque, J., Carrato, A., Soler, M., Ruiz, L., et al. (2002). Incomplete overlapping of biological, clinical, and environmental information in molecular epidemiological studies: A variety of causes and a cascade of consequences. *Journal of Epidemiology and Community Health, 56*, 734–738.

Rundle, A., Vineis, P., & Ashsan, H. (2005). Design options for molecular epidemiology research within cohort studies. *Cancer Epidemiology, Biomarkers, & Prevention, 14*(8), 1899–1907.

Tenover, F. C., McDougal, L. K., Goering, R. V., Killgore, G., Projan, S. J., Patel, J. B., et al. (2006). Characterization of a strain of community-associated methicillin-resistant *Staphylococcus aureus* widely disseminated in the United States. *Journal of Clinical Microbiology, 44*(1), 108–118.

Trottier, H., & Franco, E. (2006). The epidemiology of genital human papillomavirus infection. *Vaccine, 24*(Suppl. 1), S1–S15.

Vineis, P., Schulte, P., & Vogt, R. (1993). Technical variability in laboratory data. In P. Schulte & F. Perera (Eds.), *Molecular epidemiology. Principles and practices.* San Diego, CA: Academic Press.

Zhang, L., Foxman, B., Manning, S. D., Tallman, P., & Marrs, C. F. (2000). Molecular epidemiologic approaches to urinary tract infection gene discovery in uropathogenic *Escherichia coli. Infection and Immunity, 68*(4), 2009–2015.

MONITORING THE FUTURE SURVEY

Monitoring the Future (MTF) is an annual survey of the attitudes, values, and behaviors of a nationally representative sample of 15,000 to 19,000 American high school students and young adults. It is conducted by the Survey Research Center of the University of Michigan, with funding from the National Institute on Drug Abuse of the National Institutes of Health. MTF began collecting data, originally on 12th graders only, in 1975; since 1991, 8th and 10th graders have also been surveyed. Currently, approximately 50,000 students in the 8th, 10th, and 12th grades are surveyed each year. Participation rate has been 66% to 85% over all years of the study. In addition, follow-up mail questionnaires are sent biannually to a randomly selected sample from each senior class.

The primary focus of MTF is the use and abuse of tobacco, alcohol, and drugs by young adults and their perceptions and attitudes toward these substances. The MTF consists of two parts: core questions that include demographic information and basic questions about substance use, which are asked of every respondent, and ancillary questions on a variety of topics such as social and political attitudes, health behaviors, and educational aspirations, which are administered to different subsamples of respondents through the use of different questionnaire forms. MTF data, documentation, and supporting materials are available from the ICPSR and Monitoring the Future Web sites listed below.

Most MTF data are gathered through an annual cross-sectional survey of students currently attending school in the 8th, 10th, or 12th grades. These data are collected through self-administered questionnaires filled out by individual students, usually during a normal class period at their school. The survey administration is supervised by University of Michigan staff members and data are not shared with either the students' parents or school officials. Questionnaire forms are optically scanned and stored as an electronic data file.

MTF uses a probability sample design with three selection stages:

1. Broad geographic area (Northeast, North central, South, or West)

2. Schools or linked groups of schools within a geographic area

3. Students within schools—if a school has less than 350 students in the relevant grade, all are selected; if there are more than 350, participants are randomly selected

Schools who decline to participate are replaced with schools similar in type (public, Catholic or private/non-Catholic), geographic location, and size. Specific questionnaire forms (six were used in 2004) are administered in an ordered sequence so a nearly identical subsample of students completes each form.

A longitudinal component was added to the MTF in 1976: Since then, a random sample of about 2,400 students from that year's 12th-grade participants has been selected to participate in follow-up surveys. These participants are divided into two groups, who are mailed questionnaires in alternating years (so half the participants receive a questionnaire in odd-numbered years following 12th grade, i.e., Years 1, 3, 5, and so on, while half receive follow-up questionnaires in even-numbered years. Retention for the first year of follow-up averages 77%.

The greatest strength of MTF is the availability of data on the same questions over multiple years and the use of scientific sampling procedures to allow the computation of nationally valid estimates of responses. This allows researchers to address questions such as the prevalence of tobacco use among 12th graders and how that number has changed over the years. The large number of questions included in each survey, the extremely detailed examination of substance use, and the inclusion of a range of other types of questions also increases its usefulness. The most obvious limitation is that the MTF sample is not representative of all young Americans in the age groups included, only of those attending school: Young people who are home schooled, have dropped out, or are not attending school for some other reason (such as health problems or incarceration) are not included in the sample, and there is every reason to believe that they would differ systematically from young people attending conventional schools.

—*Sarah Boslaugh*

See also Alcohol Use; Child and Adolescent Health; Drug Abuse and Dependence, Epidemiology of; Tobacco

Further Readings

Johnston, L. D., O'Malley, P. M., Bachman, J. G., & Schulenberg, J. E. (2006). *Monitoring the future national results on adolescent drug use: Overview of key findings, 2005* (NIH Publication No. 06-5882). Bethesda, MD: National Institute on Drug Abuse.

Web Sites

Monitoring the Future (MTF) Series: http://webapp .icpsr.umich.edu/cocoon/ICPSR-SERIES/00035.xml.
Monitoring the Future: A Continuing Study of American Youth: http://www.monitoringthefuture.org

MORBIDITY AND MORTALITY WEEKLY REPORTS

See CENTERS FOR DISEASE CONTROL AND PREVENTION

MORTALITY RATES

Mortality rates (synonym: death rates) are used to quantify the tendency to die in a population during a given time period. Since death can be considered as the utmost form of "unhealthiness" or "disease," mortality rates are major (inverse) health indicators. Because measuring morbidity is often difficult, mortality rates or mortality-based indicators like life expectancy remain the major indicators used to ascertain the level of health in a society or social group.

Mortality rates always refer to a time period, usually 1 year, though monthly or even daily mortality rates are sometimes calculated for particular situations or processes—a war, epidemics, and so on. The annual crude death rate (m) can be thought as the proportion of the population dying during 1 year—presently not much above or below 1% throughout the world—and is computed by dividing the count of deaths during the year, d, by the total population or "population at risk," p, generally approximated by the population at mid year, and expressing the result per thousand or, more generally, per some power of 10. Therefore, $m = (d/p) \times 10^k$, and $k = 3$, if the rate is expressed per 1,000.

Mortality rates can be conceptualized as an approximate measure of the probability of death during a given period of time in members of the group for which the rate is calculated, or as a special type of incidence rate, where the "disease" is death. If we know that 48,700 deaths occurred over 2 years in a population of 2.1 million people, we can estimate the annual mortality rate during that period as approximately 11.6 per 1,000, since $(48,700/2)/2,100,000 = 0.011595$. However, when computing death rates for small groups, for instance, in a longitudinal study or a clinical trial, it is usually needed to consider properly the exact period of observation, expressing the rate per person-time units, and taking into account that those who die are no longer "at risk" for death. If 100 persons at the start of the observation period were followed for 3 years, during which 5 persons died, 2 at the end of the first year, and other 3 when 1.3, 2.2, and 2.6 years had passed, we have exactly

$$1.0 \times 2 + 1.3 \times 1 + 2.2 \times 1 + 2.6 \times 1 + 3 \times 95$$
$$= 293.1 \text{ person-years of observation.}$$

$$1 \times 2 = 2 + 1.3 = 3.3 \times 1 = 3.3 \times 1 = 3.3 + 2.2$$
$$= 5.5 \times 1 = 5.5 + 2.6 = 8.1 \times 1 = 8.1 + 3$$
$$= 11.1 \times 95 = 1054.5.$$

Since $5/293.1 = 0.0171$, the mortality rate can be expressed as 0.0171 deaths per person-year, or 17.1 deaths per 1,000 person-years, or as an annual death rate of 17.1 per 1,000.

An age-specific mortality rate is a death rate in a given age stratum. If the subindex i refers to the particular age stratum, the age-specific mortality rate will be $m_i = 10^k \times d_i/p_i$, where m_i is age-specific mortality in the age stratum i, d_i are total deaths in the age stratum i, and p_i is the population in that age.

Since the total death count in a population is the sum of all deaths in all age strata,

$$m = d/p = [d_1 + d_2 + d_3 + \cdots + d_k]/p$$
$$= [p_1 m_1 + p_2 m_2 + p_3 m_3 + \cdots + p_k m_k]/p$$
$$= [p_1/p]m_1 + [p_2/p]m_2 + [p_3/p]m_3$$
$$+ \cdots + [p_k/p]m_k$$
$$= s_1 m_1 + s_2 m_2 + s_3 m_3 + \cdots + s_k m_k,$$

where s_i is the proportion of the whole population living in the age stratum i and, therefore, $s_1 + s_2 + s_3 + \cdots + s_k = 1$. In compact notation,

$$m = \sum_{i=1}^{k} s_i \cdot m_i.$$

This means that the crude death rate is a weighted average of the age-specific death rates, with the weights being the shares of each age stratum in the whole population.

Since the probability of death is much higher during the first year of life than during the other years of childhood and then grows exponentially with age (Table 1), the crude death rate is strongly affected by the age structure of the population (the weights s_i), and will be large in societies with excellent health conditions but a high proportion of elderly in the population. For this reason, the crude mortality rate is not a good health indicator.

Age-specific, sex-specific, or age-and-sex-specific mortality rates are often computed to gauge health conditions in specific demographic groups. For instance, in 1990, 2,573 females aged 55 to 64 died in Sweden, out of a total of 429,914 females in this age

Table 1 Age-and-Sex-Specific Death Rates (per 1,000) in the United States in 1995

Ages	Males	Females
Below 1	8.44	6.90
5 to 14	0.27	0.18
15 to 24	1.41	0.48
25 to 34	2.10	0.80
55 to 64	14.17	8.41
75 to 84	73.77	48.83

Source: U.S. Census Bureau (2005).

group, which makes for a specific mortality rate of 6.0 deaths per 1,000 females aged 55 to 64, compared with 11.2 deaths per 1,000 males in the same age group. Save exceptional circumstances, male mortality is larger than female mortality in each age stratum (Table 1). Since differences in age-specific or age-and-sex-specific mortality rates cannot be caused by differences in age distribution, they can be used to compare health conditions across time in a given geographical region or across geographical regions in the same point in time. For example, mortality rates in females and males aged 55 to 64 in the United States were in 1990, 8.8 and 15.6 per 1,000, respectively, compared with much lower rates, 6.0 and 11.2, observed for females and males in that same age stratum in Sweden.

When mortality levels of entire populations across time or across regions need to be compared, the influence of the age-structure of the population is excluded through age-adjustment (synonym: age-standardization). Two methods of age-adjustment are used, direct and indirect adjustment. In the direct method, the most commonly used, the age-specific mortality rates of population and year of interest are applied to the age structure of a standard population (Figure 1).

If population A has the age-specific mortality rates $m_1, m_2, m_3, \ldots, m_k$, and the population proportions $s_1, s_2, s_3, \ldots, s_k$ in k age intervals, and population B has the age-specific mortality rates $\rho_1, \rho_2, \rho_3, \ldots, \rho_k$, and the population proportions $\sigma_1, \sigma_2, \sigma_3, \ldots, \sigma_k$, then the age-adjusted mortality rate of population A with population B as standard is

$$m_1 \sigma_1 + m_2 \sigma_2 + m_3 \sigma_3 + \cdots m_k \sigma_k,$$

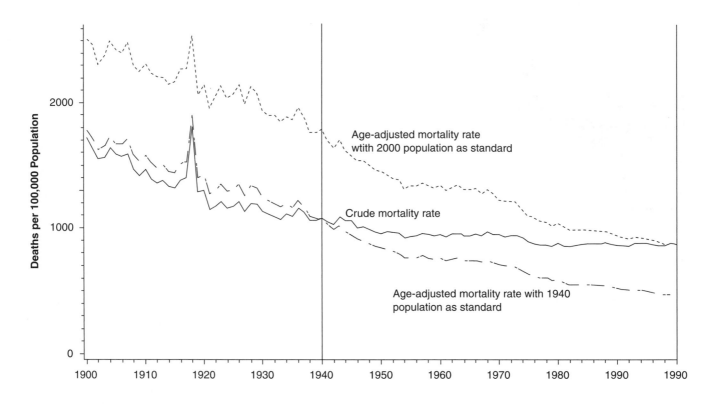

Figure 1   Mortality Rates in the United States Throughout the 20th Century

Source: U.S. Census Bureau (2007).

that is, $\sum_{i=1}^{k} m_i \cdot \sigma_i$.   Using the 1940 U.S. population as a standard, in 1990 the age-adjusted mortality rate was 5.2 per 1,000 for the general population of the United States, and 4.9 and 6.9 per 1,000 for whites and nonwhites, respectively. Age-adjusted mortality rates are often used to compare health conditions between different nations, regions, ethnic groups, or social classes. In every country in which age-adjusted or age-specific mortality has been compared among social classes, a gradient has been found with mortality increasing when going from high to low levels of income, wealth, education, or other social class indicator.

Since estimating the number of infants (and even children in poor countries) is difficult, the infant mortality rate is computed by dividing the annual death count of infants (children less than 1 year old) by the annual count of live births, and multiplying the result by 1,000, so that infant mortality is expressed usually as a rate of infant deaths per 1,000 live births. A similar rationale applies to the under-5 mortality rate, often called child mortality rate, computed as deaths below 5 per 1,000 live births. Neither the infant

mortality rate nor under-5 mortality rate are age-specific death rates in a strict sense, since the denominator of the rate is not a population count. However, both infant mortality and child mortality are good summary indicators of population health.

Cause-specific mortality rates are computed by dividing counts of deaths attributed to specific causes by the size of the specific group considered. Therefore, they can be age specific, sex specific, age-and-sex specific, and so on. A particular type of cause-and-sex-specific mortality rates is maternal mortality rates, which are referred to "all deaths ascribed to deliveries and conditions of pregnancy, childbirth, and the puerperium." Maternal mortality is much higher in poor countries and is usually sensitive to the availability of obstetric care, as well as the legal status of abortion and the social condition of women.

Because of the strong decline in deaths caused by infectious disease at all ages and mostly in infancy and childhood, age-specific mortality rates secularly declined in all countries in the world. This process started about one and a half or two centuries ago in Western Europe, a little bit later in North America

(Figure 1) and the rest of the industrialized world, and only in the past century in most countries of Latin America, Asia, and Africa. Except in very poor countries where infectious diseases such as malaria, tuberculosis, and AIDS are presently major killers, in most countries of the world the major causes of death and, therefore, the largest cause-specific death rates are presently illnesses of the heart and the circulatory system, malignancies, and injuries, mostly related to traffic.

—*José A. Tapia Granados*

See also Incidence; Life Expectancy; Person-Time Units; Prevalence; Rate; Ratio

Further Readings

Division of Health Statistics, World Health Organization. (1980). *Manual of mortality analysis: A manual on methods of analysis of national mortality statistics for public health purposes.* Geneva, Switzerland: Author.

Gordis, L. (2000). *Epidemiology* (2nd ed., pp. 42–56). Philadelphia: Saunders.

Lilienfeld, A. M., Lilienfeld, D. E., & Stolley, P. D. (1994). *Foundations of epidemiology* (3rd ed., chaps. 4 and 5). New York: Oxford University Press.

U.S. Census Bureau. (2005). *Statistical abstract of the United States.* Retrieved July 26, 2007, from http://www.census.gov/prod/www/statistical-abstract-1995_2000.html.

U.S. Census Bureau. (2007). *Statistical abstracts.* Retrieved July 26, 2007, from http://www.census.gov/prod/www/abs/statab.html.

MULTIFACTORIAL DISORDERS

See GENETIC DISORDERS

MULTIFACTORIAL INHERITANCE

The multifactorial inheritance model applies to diseases that depend on multiple genetic loci (polygenic) and the additional contribution of environmental factors. Multifactorial diseases are the result of the interplay of multiple environmental risk factors with more than one gene, where these multiple genes are viewed as susceptibility genes. In this model, genes may increase an individual's susceptibility to a particular disease, but the actual expression of the disease depends on the extent to which the individual encounters certain environmental exposures during embryogenesis or throughout his or her life.

Multifactorial diseases include birth defects such as neural tube defects, developmental disabilities such as autism and common adult-onset diseases such as cancer, diabetes mellitus, hypertension, and heart disease. In fact, most geneticists and epidemiologists today believe that the vast majority of diseases are inherited in a multifactorial fashion or their outcomes are influenced by multiple genetic and environmental factors. For example, the phenotypic outcomes in seemingly straightforward single gene or monogenic disorders (such as the classic autosomal recessive disorder, phenylketonuria, or PKU) are increasingly viewed from a multifactorial perspective as a result of new evidence of the complex relationship between genotype and phenotype in PKU.

Multifactorial diseases are labeled non-Mendelian because they do not exhibit the typical pedigree patterns we observe in Mendelian or monogenic disorders that depend on genotypic expression at one genetic locus (e.g., a recessive disorder such as sickle cell disease). An individual is at an increased risk for developing a multifactorial disease if one or more of his or her relatives are affected as well. This risk is greatest among first-degree relatives. However, patterns of multifactorial conditions are less predictable than diseases that are caused by single gene mutations. For example, multifactorial diseases such as asthma, coronary heart disease, and diabetes mellitus are heterogeneous in their etiology. This means that while the final phenotypic outcome of each disease is similar among individuals, each disease is really a group of diseases, with each subtype having variable genetic and environmental causes.

The complex etiology of multifactorial diseases cannot be discussed without a basic understanding of polygenic inheritance. Also known as quantitative inheritance, polygenic inheritance refers to an inheritance pattern in which traits are controlled by two or more genes, each having a small effect on phenotypic expression. These genes contribute some cumulative effect on the phenotype. These effects may be simple, as in a specific gene adding or subtracting from the measured value of the phenotype, or more complex when other genes or environmental factors influence the phenotype. Unlike basic Mendelian traits, polygenic traits show a continuous distribution of phenotypic values in a population and display a bell-shaped, or Gaussian, curve when their frequency distribution is plotted on a graph. Polygenic characteristics in humans include height, skin color, dermatoglyphics, blood pressure, head circumference, and intelligence. For continuous traits such as height and head circumference, abnormality is defined arbitrarily (usually 2 *SD* over or below the mean).

The polygenic threshold theory attempts to explain how the inheritance of continuous traits may be used to conceptualize the occurrence of dichotomous characters such as the presence or absence of a birth defect. According to the polygenic threshold theory, an individual has a certain degree of polygenic susceptibility, or genetic liability, for a particular disease. Theoretically, this susceptibility is normally distributed within populations, with individuals displaying varying degrees of genetic susceptibility. Individuals who exceed the critical threshold value for susceptibility to a disease will develop it, while those below this value will not.

The polygenic threshold theory is applied in genetic counseling to explain the observed patterns of recurrence risk for multifactorial diseases among family members. Individuals who are affected with a multifactorial condition have genotypes composed of many high-susceptibility alleles. Because they share more genes in common with the affected individual, close relatives will be more likely to fall above the threshold of susceptibility than unrelated individuals, and hence will be more likely to develop the disease themselves.

As mentioned previously, the recurrence risk for multifactorial diseases does not follow basic Mendelian patterns. For example, among parents who are carriers for a recessive disorder such as sickle cell disease, the risk of having an affected pregnancy is 1 in 4, or 25%. On the other hand, the recurrence risk for parents who have a child with a multifactorial disease typically falls around 3% to 5%. While data among populations and families vary, this risk generally increases if more than one member of the family is affected with the multifactorial disease in question.

For multifactorial diseases to develop, genetic predispositions must interact with some environmental exposure or trigger, or perhaps an array of environmental factors over the entire course of an individual's life. In addition to genetic liability, an individual's environmental liability must also be taken into account when attempting to explain the etiology of multifactorial diseases. In theory, genetically susceptible individuals will not develop a multifactorial disease until they exceed the threshold values for exposure to environmental risk factors. For example, specific genes have been identified as risk factors for many birth defects in infants. However, the vast majority of, if not all, birth defects are now thought to result from the combination of both genetic and environmental factors. The most well-documented environmental factor in the etiology of birth defects is the role of maternal folic acid intake in the risk of neural tube defects (NTDs). Studies have shown specific genes in the developing infant that increase the risk of developing an NTD. Nevertheless, women can significantly reduce the risk of occurrence of a child with an NTD by consuming adequate amounts of folic acid both prior to conception and during pregnancy.

There are no tests to determine the genetic predispositions of individuals to most multifactorial diseases. The best approach for combating multifactorial diseases is to identify and modify the environmental factors that interact with susceptible genotypes. As of yet, the environmental risk factors for many multifactorial diseases are still unknown. In addition, it is unclear how environmental factors interact with specific genes to cause disease. Clearly, future research is needed to identify (1) the underlying genes that predispose individuals or populations to multifactorial diseases, (2) the environmental factors that increase or decrease the expression of predisposing genotypes, and (3) the complex mechanisms by which gene-gene and gene-environment interactions result in multifactorial diseases.

—Cynthia Taylor and F. John Meaney

See also Gene; Gene-Environment Interaction; Genetic Counseling; Genetic Epidemiology; Phenotype

Further Readings

King, Richard, A., Rotter, Jerome, I., & Motulsky, A. G. (2002). *The genetic basis of common diseases* (2nd ed.). New York: Oxford University Press.

Strachan, T., & Read, A. P. (2004). *Human molecular genetics 3* (3rd ed.). New York: Garland Science.

Turnpenny, P., & Ellard, S. (2004). Polygenic and multifactorial inheritance. In *Emery's elements of medical genetics* (12th ed., pp. 137–146). London: Churchill Livingstone.

MULTILEVEL MODELING

Multilevel modeling is the simultaneous use of more than one source of data in a hierarchical structure of units and is useful for analysis of clustered or longitudinal data. Single-level models are unable to accommodate the characteristics of hierarchical data structures, such as unit of analysis, aggregation bias, state dependency, and within-group and between-group heterogeneity, resulting in misestimations. By accommodating these characteristics, multilevel modeling allows researchers to use data more fully and efficiently and to assess the direction and magnitude of relationships within and between contextual and individual factors.

In the past few years, multilevel modeling, also known as hierarchical linear models, mixed-effects models, random-effects models, and random-coefficient models, has become increasingly common in public health research, partly due to growing interest in social determinants of health and partly due to the growing availability of multilevel statistical methods and software.

Multilevel modeling is a powerful research method that promises to complicate and explicate the field of epidemiology. The inclusion of multiple levels of data in simultaneous analysis models allows for more efficient use of data and provides greater information about within-group and between-group effects and relationships. However, attention must be paid to group-level measurement issues and complex data structures, and better social epidemiology theoretical models are needed to guide empirical research.

With the development of research into social inequalities in health in the late 20th century came an interest in social epidemiology that sought to draw focus away from decontextualized individual characteristics and toward their social or ecological context. Such research can be thought of as encompassing multiple layers surrounding and intersecting with the individual, as illustrated by the multiple layers or levels of the ecological model, including intrapersonal, interpersonal, institutional, community, and policy. At the same time, significant contributions to statistical theory for multilevel methods were being made by Dennis V. Lindley and Adrian F. M. Smith, Arthur P. Dempster, Nan M. Laird, and Donald B. Rubin, and others.

Statistical Model

As in other research fields, notably education in which children are clustered within classrooms and classrooms are clustered within schools, data for epidemiologic analysis are not limited to measurements of the individual, but can include measurements within or outside of individuals. For example, blood pressure and heart rate can be measured within an individual, individuals measured within a family, families measured within neighborhoods, and neighborhoods measured within geographic regions. Similarly, repeated observations are measurements nested or clustered within individuals over time, and also produce a measurement hierarchy. Such hierarchies or clusters, even if random in origin, mean that except at the highest level of measurement there will be subgroups of observations that are similar to each other, because they come from the same group. For example, individuals within families are likely to be more similar to each other on observable and unobservable characteristics than are individuals across families. Such correlations violate the assumption of independence on which most traditional statistical techniques are based, and can result in incorrect standard errors and inefficient parameter estimates. While group level characteristics can be included in single-level contextual analyses of individual outcomes, this method requires group characteristics to be fixed, or averaged, within and between groups. Within-group and between-group heterogeneity are the hallmark of hierarchically structured data and require specialized statistical methods to simultaneously compute within-group and between-group variances.

The mathematical equation for a multilevel model can be thought of as separate equations for each level of measurement. For example, in a two-level analysis of a normally distributed individual outcome predicted by one independent variable measured at the individual level (Level 1), and one independent variable measured at a group level (Level 2), one can write first a single-level equation for individuals in groups (e.g., neighborhoods), and then write a single-level equation for the group effect, as follows:

$$Y_{ij} = b_{0j} + b_{1j}X_{ij} + \varepsilon_{ij}, \varepsilon_{ij} \sim N(0, \sigma^2),$$

where $i = 1,\ldots,n$ individuals, $j = 1,\ldots,n$ groups, Y_{ij} is the individual outcome for the ith individual in the jth group and X_{ij} is the individual (Level 1) independent variable measurement for ith individual in the jth group. Individual-level errors within each group (ε_{ij}) are assumed to be normally distributed with a mean of zero and a variance of σ^2. Regression coefficient b_{0j} is the group-specific intercept and b_{1j} is the group-specific effect of the individual-level variable(s); these vary across groups j.

Next, equations for these group-specific (Level 2) regression coefficients are written using a group-level measurement as the independent variable, as follows:

$$b_{0j} = \gamma_{00} + \gamma_{01}C_j + U_{0j}, U_{0j} \sim N(0, \tau_{00}),$$
$$b_{1j} = \gamma_{10} + \gamma_{11}C_j + U_{1j}, U_{1j} \sim N(0, \tau_{11}),$$

where C_j is the group-level independent variable. The common intercept across groups is γ_{00}, and γ_{01} is the effect of the group-level independent variable on the group-specific intercepts. Similarly, γ_{10} is the common slope associated with the individual-level variable across groups, and γ_{11} is the effect of the group-level independent variable on the group-specific slopes. U_{0j} and U_{1j} are the random error terms for the Level 2 equations, and are assumed to be normally distributed with a mean of zero and variances of τ_{00} and τ_{11}. The Level 2 random error terms allow for the assumption that the group-specific intercepts and slopes are actually random samples from a larger, normally distributed population of group-specific values. Without the random effects, this model becomes a one-level model with averaged fixed group-level effects. Finally, these equations can be combined into one multilevel equation by replacing the regression coefficients in the Level 1 model with the Level 2 equations, as follows:

$$Y_{ij} = \gamma_{00} + \gamma_{01}C_j + \gamma_{10}X_{ij} + \gamma_{11}C_jX_{ij} + U_{0j} + U_{1j}X_{ij} + \varepsilon_{ij}.$$

The parameter estimates resulting from this equation can address questions such as the following: Are individual and group variables related to outcomes when tested simultaneously? Do individual characteristics associated with outcomes vary across groups? How much variation is explained at each level? Estimation of group-level effects and between-group differences depends on the number of groups included at Level 2. Statistical inferences have generally been based on the method of maximum likelihood. More recently, Bayesian methods of inference have been applied to multilevel models. The intraclass correlation provides a measure of the similarity among Level 1 measurements within each Level 2 group.

Multilevel models can be applied to various and complex data structures as dictated by the data or conceptual models. Multilevel models can incorporate multiple independent variables at different levels as well as interaction terms. Models can be expanded to three or more levels, such as repeated blood pressure measures (Level 1) in individuals (Level 2) in clinics (Level 3). The relationships between levels, known as cross-level effects, can be various, including linear, quadratic, or nonexistent in either or both directions. Some hierarchical data are complicated by cross-classification, such that lower-level measures get classified in unexpected or multiple higher-level groups. For example, students may be in multiple classes within the same school, individuals may attend clinics outside their neighborhoods, or people may move or change experimental assignment in the course of a longitudinal study.

The linear random-effects model can be transformed for nonnormal response data, including binary, count, ordinal, multinomial data, and survival analysis. Multilevel models also have been applied to the analysis of latent variables and meta-analytic data. Software commonly used for multilevel analysis includes HLM, MIX, MLWIN, MPLUS, SAS, and recent versions of SPSS.

An Example From Psychiatric Epidemiology

Twentieth-century epidemiologic research in the United States has consistently shown that people who live with mental illness are far more likely to live in poverty than the general population. In 1969, Barbara and Bruce Dohrenwend published a review of available studies of psychiatric epidemiology, *Social Status and Psychological Disorder: A Causal Inquiry*, and reported that the only consistent correlation with severe mental illness they found across different cultures and times was low socioeconomic status. In the 1980s, the National Institute of Mental Health's Epidemiologic Catchment Area (ECA) study conducted psychiatric diagnostic interviews with approximately 20,000 adult respondents (anyone above age 18) in five cities: New Haven, Connecticut; Baltimore, Maryland; St. Louis, Missouri; Durham, North Carolina; and Los Angeles, California. The ECA found that about 20% of respondents had an active mental disorder, with a lifetime reported prevalence of 32%. In this study, higher prevalence of active mental disorder was associated with being African American, being unemployed, and other measures of social class. Bruce, Takeuchi, and Leaf (1991) used a measurement of individual poverty status in a multivariate logistic regression analysis of the 12-month incidence of mental disorders. They found individual poverty to be associated with greater likelihood of any mental disorder, adjusted odds ratio (95% confidence interval) = 1.92 (1.12, 3.28); and greater likelihood of major depression, adjusted odds ratio (95% confidence interval) = 2.29 (1.19, 4.43).

Over a decade later, Goldsmith, Holzer, and Manderscheid (1998) analyzed ECA data in conjunction with the neighborhood data from the 1980 decennial census. In addition to individual characteristics, their one-level logistic regression models included what they called social area dimensions of neighborhoods. These dimensions were social rank or economic status (median household income of census tract), family status (percentage of households with husband-wife families), residential lifestyle (percentage of single dwelling units), and ethnicity (90% or more white, mixed, and 90% or more minority). Individual risk factors included age, gender, marital status, race, and education. They found that controlling for individual characteristics, only living in a low economic status neighborhood (compared with medium or high status) was statistically significantly associated with greater likelihood of having a 12-month mental disorder (prevalence), adjusted odds ratio (95% confidence interval) = 1.43 (1.18, 1.74); living in a majority ethnic minority neighborhood (compared with mixed or majority nonminority) was associated with greater likelihood of having a past mental disorder. By assessing the magnitude of statistically significant odds ratios and changes in model fit, Goldsmith and colleagues posited that with the exception of economic status, inclusion of neighborhood characteristics contributed little to individual-level explanations of psychiatric epidemiology.

Like Goldsmith et al., Silver, Mulvey, and Swanson (2002) combined ECA and census data to develop a multilevel model of the 12-month prevalence of specific mental disorders, including schizophrenia and major depression. In this analysis, nine census tract measures of neighborhood structure were selected: (1) percentage of persons living below the poverty line; (2) percentage of husband-wife families; (3) percentage of families with children that are female-headed; (4) percentage of households with public assistance income; (5) adult unemployment rate in the tract; (6) percentage of families with income above $30,000; (7) percentage of adults employed in executive or managerial jobs; (8) percentage of housing units that are rentals; and (9) percentage of persons above 5 years old who did not live at that address 5 years earlier.

A factor analysis of these measures was used to derive two variables: neighborhood disadvantage and neighborhood residential mobility. Finally, neighborhoods were coded as either racially homogeneous (90% or greater of one race) or heterogeneous. In multivariate logistic regression models including both individual and neighborhood characteristics, neighborhood mobility was associated with greater likelihood of schizophrenia, adjusted odds ratio (95% confidence interval) = 1.27 (1.02, 1.59) and greater likelihood of major depression, adjusted odds ratio (95% confidence interval) = 1.16 (1.03, 1.29). The index of neighborhood disadvantage was also associated with greater likelihood of major depression, adjusted odds ratio (95% confidence interval) = 1.14 (1.01, 1.31). In these models, individual-level poverty (household income less than $10,000 per year) was associated with greater likelihood of schizophrenia, adjusted odds ratio (95% confidence interval) = 2.66 (1.30, 5.42), and major depression, adjusted odds ratio (95% confidence interval) = 1.69 (1.20, 2.36). In their analysis, they used the multilevel equation $y_{ti} = \alpha + \beta' \chi_{ti} + v_{ti}$, where t indexes census tracts and i indexes individuals within tracts, and $v_{ti} = \varepsilon_t + v_{ti}$. The authors report that when the analyses were reestimated using hierarchical linear regression, there was no significant census tract level variation in the distribution of mental disorders after the individual- and neighborhood-level variables were added to the model, and therefore argue that Level 2 variance (tract level) does not warrant use of multilevel levels with these data.

In a multilevel model of incident cases of schizophrenia in 35 neighborhoods in Maastricht, the Netherlands, Van Os, Driessen, Gunther, and Delespaul (2000) found that controlling for individual characteristics, deprived neighborhoods (characterized by relatively high unemployment and welfare dependence) were associated with greater incidence of schizophrenia, with relative risk and 95% confidence interval of 1.07 (1.01, 1.14) and 1.04 (1.00, 1.08), respectively. They also report that the Level 2 (neighborhood) variance is not statistically significant at 0.14 (95% confidence interval 0.00, 0.29; $p = 0.055$), yet still constitutes about 12% of the total observed variance. Unlike Silver et al. (2002), they argue that this level of random neighborhood variance is not a chance finding and is an argument in support of using multilevel methods.

A number of other researchers have used multilevel models to examine effects of neighborhood deprivation or disorder on symptoms of depression or psychological distress and identified significant associations. There has been a lack of consistency in the application of theoretical frameworks and operationalization of measures, which may have detracted from the usefulness of multilevel measures in psychiatric epidemiology thus far.

Theoretical and Measurement Challenges

Multilevel modeling allows researchers to use powerful statistical techniques to incorporate multiple measurement levels of data. However, there is concern that the theoretical and conceptual developments are lagging behind computational abilities. To date, more multilevel empirical research has been conducted than theoretical models of contextual influence have been developed. As a result, epidemiologists have used theories from other fields such as sociology and community psychology for explanatory models. However, given the potential complexity of multilevel relationships as described above, more specific theories and hypotheses may be needed for epidemiologic models. For example, the appropriate size or scope of a group is debatable: Overly large group identities, such as cities or states, may be too large to detect between-group variation, but very small identities, such as census block or family may lack variation at the individual level. Choice of group size should be dictated by theory or hypothesis rather than empirically.

Group-level definition and measurement are other challenges to multilevel modeling. For example, neighborhood can be defined geographically or as an abstract concept based on dynamic interaction. These types of group characteristics have been called derived variables and integral variables. Derived variables, also known as analytical, aggregate, or compositional variables, summarize the characteristics of the individuals in the group (mean proportions, or measures of dispersions), such as median household income or proportion of household members with a high school education. A special type of derived variable is the average of the dependent variable within the group, for example, prevalence of infection or prevalence of a behavior. Integral variables, also known as primary or global variables, describe characteristics of the group that are not derived from characteristics of individuals, such as availability of services, certain regulations, or political systems. A special type of integral variable refers to patterns and networks of contacts or interactions among individuals within groups. Although distinct, derived and integral variables are closely related. For example, the composition of a group may influence the predominant types of interpersonal contacts, values, and norms or may shape organizations or regulations within the group that affect all members.

Traditional psychometric methods of evaluating scale reliability and validity are inadequate for the assessment of nonindividual neighborhood, or ecological, measures. Raudenbush and Sampson (1999) have proposed a methodology for understanding the psychometric properties of ecological measures, called ecometrics. For example, in developing a neighborhood-level measure from a survey of individual residents, an individual's item responses are aggregated to create a single scale, and then all individuals' scales are aggregated into a neighborhood measure. In this case, unlike in traditional psychometrics, scale reliability depends not only on the number of items in a scale and item consistency within a respondent but also on the number of respondents and the scale consistency with respondents, or intersubjective agreement. Furthermore, ecometric assessment of a neighborhood measure requires examination of potential sources of bias, such as nonrepresentative sampling, which should be adjusted for statistically. Similar techniques can be applied to assessing the reliability of observational data, where the unit of observation is aggregated, rather than individuals' survey responses, interrater agreement can be calculated, and biases arising from the sample (e.g., time of day of observations) adjusted. In addition to reliability analyses, ecometrics includes methodologies for other aspects of scale construction, including analysis of ecological scale dimensionality and validity, although use of these techniques is not often reported.

—Jane K. Burke-Miller

See also Geographical and Social Influences on Health; Geographical and Spatial Analysis; Social Capital and Health; Social Epidemiology; Social Hierarchy and Health

Further Readings

Bruce, M. L., Takeuchi, D. T., & Leaf, P. J. (1991). Poverty and psychiatric status. *Archives of General Psychiatry*, *48*, 470–474.

Dempster, A., Laird, N., & Rubin, D. (1977). Maximum likelihood from incomplete data via the EM algorithm.

Journal of the Royal Statistical Society, Series B, 39, 1–38.

Diez-Roux, A. V. (2000). Multilevel analysis in public health research. *Annual Review of Public Health, 21,* 171–192.

Diez-Roux, A. V. (2002). A glossary for multilevel analysis. *Journal of Epidemiology & Community Health, 56,* 588–594.

Diez-Roux, A. V. (2003). The examination of neighborhood effects on health: Conceptual and methodological issues related to the presences of multiple levels of organization. In I. Kawachi & L. F. Berkman (Eds.), *Neighborhoods and health* (pp. 45–64). New York: Oxford University Press.

Dohrenwend, B. P., & Dohrenwend, B. S. (1969). *Social status and psychological disorder: A causal inquiry.* New York: Wiley-Interscience.

Duncan, C., Jones, K., & Moon, G. (1998). Context, composition, and heterogeneity: Using multilevel models in health research. *Social Science & Medicine, 46,* 97–117.

Goldsmith, H. F., Holzer, C. E., & Manderscheid, R. W. (1998). Neighborhood characteristics and mental illness. *Evaluation and Program Planning, 21,* 211–225.

Goldstein, H. (2003). *Multilevel statistical models* (3rd ed.). London: Arnold.

Lindley, D., & Smith, A. (1972). Bayes estimates for the linear model. *Journal of the Royal Statistical Society Series B (Methodological), 34*(1), 1–41.

O'Campo, P. (2003). Invited commentary: Advancing theory and methods for multilevel models of residential neighborhoods and health. *American Journal of Epidemiology, 157*(1), 9–13.

Raudenbush, S. W., & Bryk, A. S. (2002). *Hierarchical linear models: Applications and data analysis methods* (2nd ed.). Thousand Oaks, CA: Sage.

Raudenbush, S. W., & Sampson, R. J. (1999). Ecometrics: Toward a science of assessing ecological settings, with application to the systematic social observation of neighborhoods. *Sociological Methodology, 29,* 1–41.

Silver, E., Mulvey, E. P., & Swanson, J. W. (2002). Neighborhood structural characteristics and mental disorder: Faris and Dunham revisited. *Social Science & Medicine, 55,* 1457–1470.

Subramanian, S. V., Jones, K., & Duncan, C. (2003). Multilevel methods for public health research. In I. Kawachi & L. F. Berkman (Eds.), *Neighborhoods and health* (pp. 65–111). New York: Oxford University Press.

Van Os, J., Driessen, G., Gunther, N., & Delespaul, P. (2000). Neighborhood variation in incidence of schizophrenia. *British Journal of Psychiatry, 176,* 243–248.

MULTIPLE COMPARISON PROCEDURES

The issue of multiple comparisons has created considerable controversy within epidemiology. The fundamental questions are which procedure to use and whether probabilities associated with multiple tests should be adjusted to control Type I errors. The latter topic appears the most contentious.

It is helpful to make a distinction between *multiple comparisons*, which usually involve comparison of multiple groups or treatment arms on one dependent variable, and *multiple testing*, which usually involves the comparison of two (or more) groups on multiple dependent variables. Although both procedures raise many of the same questions, they differ in some important ways. Multiple comparison procedures are more formalized than those for multiple testing.

A Type I error, also referred to as alpha or by the Greek letter α, refers to the probability that a statistical test will incorrectly reject a true null hypothesis (H_0). In most cases, α is set at .05 or .01. When we test multiple differences (whether between groups or for different dependent variables), we can talk about Type I errors in two different ways. The *per comparison* error rate is the probability of an error on each of our comparisons, taken separately. Alternatively, the *experiment-wise* or *family-wise* error rate is the probability of making at least one Type I error in a whole set, or family, of comparisons. An important argument in epidemiology is which of these error rates is the appropriate one.

Multiple Comparisons

One approach to making multiple comparisons is to define a set of linear contrasts that focus specifically on important questions of interest. Normally, these questions are defined before the start of an experiment and relate directly to its purpose. For a clinical trial with two control groups and several treatment groups, we might, for example, create a contrast of the mean of the control groups versus the mean of the combined treatment groups. Or we might ask whether the mean of the most invasive medical procedure is significantly different from the mean of the least invasive procedure. We usually test only a few contrasts, both to control the family-wise error rate and because other potential contrasts are not central to our analysis. Generally, though not always, researchers will use some variant of a Bonferroni procedure (described below) to control the family-wise error rate over the several contrasts.

An alternative approach to multiple comparisons is to use a procedure such as the Tukey HSD ("honestly significant difference") test. (There are many such tests, but the Tukey is a convenient stand-in for the others. These tests are discussed in any text on statistical methods and can be computed by most software programs.) The Tukey is a range test and is based on the Studentized range statistic. It modifies the critical value of the test statistic depending on the number of levels of the dependent variable. Other tests differ in how that critical value is determined, often in a sequential manner. The Tukey procedure performs all possible comparisons between pairs of groups and places the groups into homogeneous subsets based on some characteristic, in this example their mean. For instance, in an experiment with six groups there might be three homogeneous subsets, such that within each subset the mean values of each group do not differ significantly from each other. These homogeneous subsets may overlap; for instance, $\mu_1 = \mu_2 = \mu_3$; $\mu_3 = \mu_4 = \mu_5$; $\mu_5 = \mu_6$. The presence of overlapping sets is often confusing to users, but is inherent in the test. In addition, detection of homogeneous, but overlapping, subsets is seldom the goal of a statistical analysis, and it may be difficult to use this information. A third difficulty is posed by multiple outcomes; in fact, most researchers using multiple comparison procedures either do not measure more than one dependent variable, or they consider different dependent variables to be distinct and treat them separately. The final way of making comparisons among groups is to use some sort of Bonferroni correction. The Bonferroni inequality states that the probability of the occurrence of one or more events cannot exceed the sum of their individual probabilities. If the probability of a Type I error for one contrast is α, and we create k contrasts, the probability of *at least* one Type I error cannot exceed $k\alpha$. So if we run each contrast at $\alpha' = \alpha/k$, then the family-wise error rate will never exceed α. The Bonferroni procedure and the sequential tests based on it are widely applicable.

Multiple Testing

The more tests you do, the more likely you are, purely by chance, to find a significant difference when the null hypothesis is actually true. That was the rationale behind the development of multiple comparison procedures, and it is the rationale behind the current debate over how to treat the comparison of two groups on multiple dependent variables. This is a situation in which Bonferroni corrections are often advocated.

It should be apparent that the Bonferroni correction is applicable to any set of multiple tests, whether they be multiple comparisons on k means, multiple t tests on k different dependent variables, or tests on correlations in a matrix. We can hold the family-wise error rate at .05 for two contrasts by evaluating each test at $\alpha = .05/2 = .025$, and we can do the same thing when we have two t tests on two dependent variables. The big question is whether we should.

When Should We Adjust Probabilities?

Given that we have good methods for controlling the family-wise error rate, when should we employ them—and when should we not do so? When computing pairwise comparisons of each mean against each other mean, there is not much of an argument. The Tukey, or one of its variants, should be used, and the family-wise error rate should be set at α. However, when the researcher is running only a few very specific contrasts that derive directly from the nature of the study, and that were identified before the data were analyzed and were not chosen simply because they were the largest difference, then a good case can be made for running each one at α per comparison, although some would argue for a corrected α.

There is certainly room for debate here, but there is nothing sacred about $\alpha = .05$. If there are three contrasts and one person adjusts α and another does not, they are simply working at different significance levels. It is no different from the general case where one person may prefer $\alpha = .01$, while another chooses $\alpha = .05$ for a single t test. However, it is easier to find significant results at a higher α level, so sometimes the discussion becomes contentious because results that are significant without Bonferroni adjustment become nonsignificant when the adjustment is applied.

When it comes to multiple outcome measures, things are somewhat less clear. Consider a psychologist who compares two groups in differentially stressful environments using a symptom checklist having multiple subtest scores. That researcher could use Hotelling's T^2 test, treating all dependent variables simultaneously. However, this will not yield specific information about the variables that are affected. Alternatively, he or she could run an unadjusted t test on each variable, but that would strike most people as a fishing expedition, and the associated Type I error rate would be high. Finally, he or she could run those *t* tests but adjust the significance levels with a Bonferroni adjustment. In this example, the last option would seem to make the most sense.

Next, consider a study of cancer treatments with two dependent variables—tumor reduction and survival. These are two quite different outcome measures, and there is no obvious reason why they should be treated together, so an adjustment does not seem necessary. As others have pointed out, a treatment that reduces tumors but has no effect on survival is quite different from a treatment that has no effect on tumors but increases survival. As a general rule, when a clinical trial is designed to look at two or three different questions, especially if those questions lead to different outcome behaviors on the part of a researcher or physician, then it makes sense to treat those separately. If there is no clear hierarchy of questions, or no obvious measure of outcome (as in the case of a symptom checklist with multiple subscales), then the prudent thing to do would be to control family-wise error.

It is extremely rare for a study to exist on its own without a context. Choices about corrections for multiple comparisons should take into account the following facts: (1) Studies are designed for specific reasons against a background literature that is relevant to subsequent actions. (2) The fact that a particular treatment is effective may be trumped by the fact that it is outrageously expensive. (3) Not every statistically significant difference will lead to future implementation of the procedure. (4) A single study is not likely to change medical practice. In that context, it is often reasonable to take a more liberal approach and not restrict the study to a family-wise error rate.

—*David C. Howell*

See also Analysis of Variance; Clinical Trials; Hypothesis Testing; *p* Value; Significance Testing

Further Readings

Cook, R. J., & Farewell, V. T. (1996). Multiplicity considerations in the design and analysis of clinical trials. *Journal of the Royal Statistical Society, Series A, 159*(Pt. 1), 93–110.

Holm, S. (1979). A simple sequentially rejective multiple test procedure. *Scandinavian Journal of Statistics, 6*, 65–70.

Savitz, D. A., & Olshan, A. F. (1995). Multiple comparisons and related issues in the interpretation of epidemiologic data. *American Journal of Epidemiology, 142*, 904–908.

Thompson, J. R. (1998). Invited commentary: Re: "Multiple comparisons and related issues in the interpretation of epidemiologic data." *American Journal of Epidemiology, 147*, 801–806.

MULTIVARIATE ANALYSIS OF VARIANCE

Multivariate analysis of variance (MANOVA) is a statistical technique used extensively in all types of research. It is the same thing as an analysis of variance (ANOVA), except that there is more than one dependent or response variable. The mathematical methods and assumptions of MANOVA are simply expansions of ANOVA from the univariate case to the multivariate case.

A situation in which MANOVA is appropriate is when a researcher conducts an experiment where several responses are measured on each experimental unit (subject) and experimental units have been randomly assigned to experimental conditions (treatments). For example, in a double-blind study systolic and diastolic blood pressures are measured on subjects who have been randomly assigned to one of two treatment groups. One group receives a new medication to treat high blood pressure, and the other group receives a placebo. The group that receives the placebo is considered a control group. The researcher wants to know whether the new medication is effective at lowering blood pressure.

There are several compelling reasons for conducting a MANOVA instead of an ANOVA. First, it is more efficient and economical in the long run to measure more than one response variable during the course of an experiment. If only one response is measured, there is the risk that another important response has been ignored. The measurement of several response variables provides a more thorough understanding of the nature of group differences given the response variables.

Another good reason to use MANOVA is that analyzing multiple responses simultaneously with a multivariate test is more powerful than analyzing the individual responses separately with multiple univariate tests. The chances of incorrectly rejecting the null hypothesis are inflated with multiple univariate tests, because the Type I error rate (α) increases with each additional test. For instance, the overall Type I error rate for two univariate tests each with α set at .05 is .10 $(1 - (.95)^2)$ rather than .05.

Finally, the correlation between the response variables is taken into account in a multivariate test. The result is that differences between groups that are not detected by multiple univariate analyses may become obvious. Figure 1 illustrates the hypothetical univariate distributions of two response variables, X_1 and X_2, for two study groups. The distributions appear to overlap such that no significant difference in means between groups is expected. In Figure 2, the multivariate distributions for the same response variables are illustrated with 95% confidence ellipses drawn about the group means. The figure shows that the two groups do not overlap as much as might be expected given the univariate distributions. Figure 3 illustrates the same multivariate distributions, except that the response variables are negatively correlated rather than positively correlated as in Figure 2. Given the degree to which the ellipses overlap in Figure 3, the null hypotheses may not be rejected.

When conducting a MANOVA, several assumptions are made about the data. When these assumptions do not hold, conclusions based on the analysis may be erroneous. The assumptions are as follows:

- The experimental units are random samples of target populations.
- The observations are independent of each other.
- The response variables are distributed multivariate normal. There is no test for multivariate normality commonly available. Generally, multivariate normality can be assumed when the individual variables are normally distributed; however, it is not guaranteed. Additionally, MANOVA is particularly sensitive to outliers so it is important to check for them prior to analysis. Outliers should be transformed or

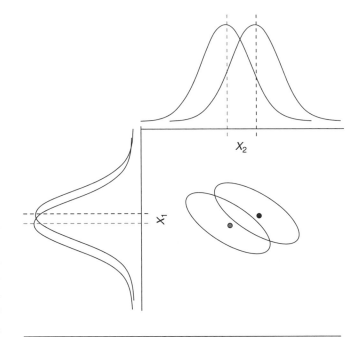

Figure 2   Multivariate Distribution for Two Populations, Two Positively Correlated Responses

omitted from the analysis. Deviation from multivariate normality has less impact in larger samples.
- All populations have the same covariance matrix (homogeneity of covariance). This assumption is made because the error sums of squares are computed by adding the treatment sums of squares weighted by $(n_i - 1)$, where n_i is the number of experimental units in each treatment. Otherwise, adding the treatment sums of squares would be inappropriate.

In the blood pressure experiment, there is one factor; medication type. The number of factor levels or treatments (k) for medication type is two, medication and placebo. The number of responses (p) is two, systolic blood pressure and diastolic blood pressure. The appropriate model for this experiment is a one-way MANOVA. The model is constructed as follows:

$$x_{ij} = \mu + \tau_i + e_{ij}$$

where

x_{ij} are observations randomly sampled from p-variate populations representing the ith treatment on the jth unit, $j = 1, 2, \ldots, n_i$ and $i = 1, 2, \ldots, k$.

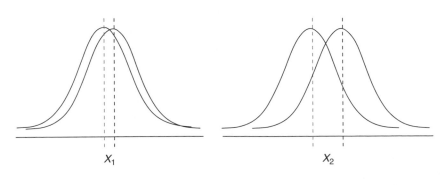

Figure 1   Univariate Distributions for Two Populations, Two Responses

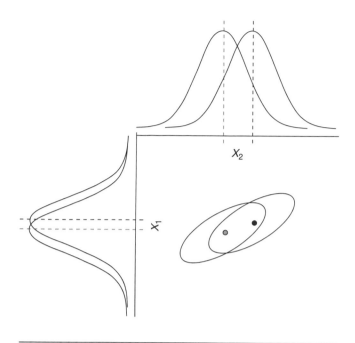

Figure 3   Multivariate Distribution for Two Populations, Two Positively Correlated Responses

e_{ij} are independent random variables with mean $\mathbf{0}$ and variance $\mathbf{\Sigma}$. $N_p(\mathbf{0}, \mathbf{\Sigma})$.

$\boldsymbol{\mu}$ is a vector of overall means.

$\boldsymbol{\tau}_i$ represents the main effect of the ith treatment subject to the following restriction: $\sum_{i=1}^{k} n_i \tau_i = 0$.

All the vectors are $p \times 1$.

The null hypothesis is that there are no differences in treatment means for either response due to the main effect of medication type.

Suppose there was another factor in the blood pressure example, say gender. In addition to the parameters for $\boldsymbol{\mu}$ and the main effect of medication type, $\boldsymbol{\tau}_i$, there would be a parameter for the main effect of gender, $\boldsymbol{\beta}_l$, and a parameter for the interaction effect of the two factors, $\boldsymbol{\gamma}_{il}$, where $i = 1, \ldots, k, l = 1, \ldots, b$. The error parameter becomes e_{ilj}, where $j = 1, \ldots, n$ and n is the number of experimental units in each treatment. The model is subject to the following restriction:

$$\sum_{i=1}^{k} \tau_i = \sum_{l=1}^{b} \beta_l = \sum_{i=1}^{k} \gamma_{il} = \sum_{l=1}^{b} \gamma_{il} = 0.$$

Now, the three null hypotheses are that there are no differences in treatment means for either factor

due to (1) the main effect of treatment type, (2) the main effect of gender, or (3) the interaction between treatment type and gender.

The goal of MANOVA, as in ANOVA, is to test for differences between treatment means. However, instead of testing the equality of means for one response variable as in ANOVA, the means for all response variables are tested for equality simultaneously. Suppose there are k treatments and p response variables. The null hypothesis is

$$H_0 : \boldsymbol{\mu}_1 = \boldsymbol{\mu}_2 = \ldots = \boldsymbol{\mu}_k,$$

where $\boldsymbol{\mu}_i$ is a $p \times 1$ vector, $i = 1, \ldots, k$.

In ANOVA, the overall test of significance is based on the ratio of the between-subject sums of squares to the within-subject sums of squares (SS_B/SS_W) adjusted for degrees of freedom. The multivariate case is more complex, because there is information for p variables that must be considered jointly to obtain an overall test of significance. There are four overall multivariate tests of significance designed specifically for this purpose: Wilks's lambda, Pillai's trace, Roy's greatest characteristic root, and Hotelling's T.

Overall MANOVA tests are conducted for the main effect of each factor on the response variables. When there is more than one independent variable, overall MANOVA tests are conducted for the effect of the interaction of the factors on the response variables. If the mean vector for at least one treatment is not equal to all the others, then the null hypothesis that there is no difference between mean vectors is rejected.

To decide whether to reject the null hypothesis, the overall MANOVA test statistics are transformed into an approximate F distribution. Most statistical analysis computer programs execute the transformations specific to each test and output the results. The null hypothesis can be rejected if the p value of the observed F statistic is less than the set α level. The results of these four tests will disagree as to whether to reject the null hypothesis at the set α level, except in the case where $k = 2$ or $p = 1$. It is not always easy to know which test to use. While Wilks's lambda is used the most often, researchers have studied each test under conditions violating one or more assumptions. They have found that the tests are generally robust to departures from multivariate normality. They have also found that the tests are not robust to departures from homogeneity of variance/covariance when there are unequal sample sizes. When there are equal sample sizes, Pillai's trace was found to be the most robust against violation of assumptions than any of the other tests.

When a MANOVA has produced a significant main effect, there are two approaches to exploring differences between groups to determine the source. One approach is to interpret the contributions of the response variables. There are several ways of doing this, but the two most common are interpreting univariate *F* tests on each of the response variables and interpreting the coefficients of the discriminant function. Univariate *F* tests may indicate which response is causing the significance. Discriminant functions are linear combinations of the *p* original variables designed to maximize the differences between groups. The magnitude of the coefficients indicates the importance of the variable to the separation of groups relative to the other variables. In a multivariate environment, the discriminant function approach is preferable; however, caution must be exercised when using these methods of interpretation. The univariate *F* tests do not take the correlation between the response variables into account. The magnitude of the discriminant function coefficients may be misleading if the original variables are highly correlated.

The other approach to exploring group differences is to perform contrasts on the response variables. Multivariate contrasts are performed on the vector of responses. There are several multivariate statistics available to test for mean differences between the two groups. Univariate contrasts are performed on each variable individually as in ANOVA. The same contrasts used in ANOVA are appropriate in this application. Univariate contrasts can be used to further explore significant multivariate contrasts.

—*Mary Earick Godby*

See also Analysis of Variance; Discriminant Analysis

Further Readings

Bray, J. H., & Maxwell, S. E. (1985). *Multivariate analysis of variance.* Beverley Hills, CA: Sage.
Hand, D. J., & Taylor, C. C. (1987). *Multivariate analysis of variance and repeated measures: A practical approach for behavioral scientists.* New York: Chapman & Hall.
Johnson, R. A., & Wichern, D. W. (2002). *Applied multivariate statistical analysis.* Englewood Cliffs, NJ: Prentice Hall.
Mardia, K. V., Kent, J. T., & Bibby, J. M. (1979). *Multivariate analysis.* San Diego, CA: Academic Press.
Wickens, T. D. (1995). *The geometry of multivariate statistics.* Hillsdale, NJ: Lawrence Erlbaum.

MUTATION

A mutation is a transmissible or heritable change in the nucleotide sequence of the genetic material of a cell or virus. Mutations are either spontaneous, occurring naturally due to errors in DNA or RNA replication, or induced by external agents. When identifying the etiology of a disease and the factors that alter a person's risk for disease, epidemiologists must often determine the unique contributions of environmental and genetic factors. Increasingly, we are made aware of the importance of mutations in the development of disease and the evolution of pathogens.

Mutations are often involved in the etiology of diseases attributed to host genetic factors. Mutations of the breast cancer susceptibility genes *BRCA1* or *BRCA2* result in an increased risk of developing breast cancer or ovarian cancer and account for up to half of hereditary breast cancers. It is believed that these genes normally play a role in repairing breaks in double-stranded DNA induced by radiation and that mutations in these genes hinder this mechanism, resulting in DNA replication errors and cancer. The effect of host mutations need not be deleterious as certain mutations confer protection from disease. A mutant variant of the chemokine receptor 5 resulting from a 32 base pair deletion (CCR5Δ32) is associated with nearly complete resistance to HIV-1 infection in homozygous individuals and partial resistance with delayed disease progression in heterozygous individuals. CCR5 is a necessary coreceptor for HIV-1 infection; individuals with at least one mutant allele do not express the receptor on their cell surfaces and are thereby protected.

Mutations acquired by pathogens may alter infectivity and virulence, and therefore, affect disease in the host. Influenza virus lacks a proofreading mechanism and thus allows errors during replication to remain undetected and uncorrected, resulting in an accumulation of point mutations and the ultimate emergence of a new antigenic variant. This process is referred to as *antigenic drift* and is the reason why the human influenza vaccine must be updated on an annual basis. Avian influenza viruses undergo limited antigenic drift in their aquatic bird reservoirs; however, the accumulation of mutations becomes more pronounced when the virus spreads through domestic poultry, and continued accumulation could support human-to-human transmission as witnessed with the 1918 Spanish influenza pandemic.

Epidemiologists are recognizing with increasing frequency the contributions of genetic factors such as mutations in the development of both chronic and communicable diseases.

—Margaret Chorazy

See also Association, Genetic; Gene; Gene-Environment Interaction; Genetic Epidemiology; Genetic Markers

Further Readings

Andersen, W. R., & Fairbanks, D. J. (1999). Mutation. In *Genetics: The continuity of life* (pp. 124–155). Pacific Grove, CA: Brooks/Cole.

Blanpain, C., Libert, F., Vassart, G., & Parmentier, M. (2002). CCR5 and HIV infection. *Receptors and Channels, 8,* 19–31.

National Library of Medicine, National Center for Biotechnology Information. (n.d.). Cancers. In *Genes and disease.* Retrieved January 31, 2007, from http://www.ncbi.nlm.nih.gov/books/bv.fcgi?rid=gnd.chapter.10.

Webster, R. G., & Hulse, D. J. (2004). Microbial adaptation and change: Avian influenza. *Revue Scientifique et Technique (International Office of Epizootics), 23*(2), 453–465.

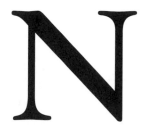

NATIONAL AMBULATORY MEDICAL CARE SURVEY

The National Ambulatory Medical Care Survey (NAMCS) is a national survey that provides information about the delivery and use of ambulatory medical care services provided by nonfederal, office-based physicians in the United States. The NAMCS captures information about patient demographics, sources of payment, the reason for visit, and diagnosis and drug information. Epidemiologists, physician associations, and policymakers frequently use the gathered data to identify patterns of care in the United States, discover emerging trends and issues, or support and inform decision making.

Since 1989, the NAMCS has been conducted annually; prior to that, it was conducted annually from 1973 to 1981 and also in 1985. Each year approximately 3,000 physicians are randomly selected to provide information on approximately 30 patient visits seen at their practice over a 1-week period.

Included within the scope of the NAMCS are physician services provided in locations such as free-standing clinics or urgent care centers, neighborhood mental health centers, or a health maintenance organization. Services provided in locations such as hospital emergency departments, institutional settings such as schools or prisons, and locations that specialize in laser vision surgery are not included in the survey. Physicians specializing in anesthesiology, pathology, or radiology services are also excluded. The NAMCS

data are collected by the National Center for Health Statistics of the Centers for Disease Control and Prevention.

Physicians complete the questionnaires that are used to compile the NAMCS data, and their participation is entirely voluntary. The NAMCS data are *de-identified*, meaning all personal identifying information is removed to protect the confidentiality of the respondents and their patients. During the past 10 years, participation rates have varied between 65% and 75%. Various strategies have been attempted to improve response rates such as publicity campaigns and eliminating questions with high item nonresponse. Physicians are not remunerated for their participation in the survey, but are motivated to take part so that their practice and others that are similar will be represented in the data.

When conducting analyses on the NAMCS, it should be noted that it is a record-based survey that captures information about episodes of care. The unit of analysis is therefore episodes of care, that is, patient visits, not number of patients. Hence, population incidence and prevalence rates cannot be calculated from the NAMCS data. However, it is possible to compute estimates for things such as the most common reasons patients visit their doctors or the percentage of office visits that include mention of particular pharmaceuticals. Estimates that are based on at least 30 individual records and also have a relative standard error less than 30% are considered reliable. To improve reliability, data from the NAMCS can be combined with data from its sister survey the National Hospital Ambulatory Medical Care Survey. Because of the sampling design, the survey should be used primarily to determine national estimates: Meaningful assessments cannot be made at lower levels of geography such as states or counties. The sample data must be weighted to produce national estimates.

—Alexia Campbell

See also Centers for Disease Control and Prevention; Health Care Services Utilization; National Center for Health Statistics

Web Sites

Centers for Disease Control and Prevention, Ambulatory Health Care Data: http://www.cdc.gov/nchs/about/major/ahcd/namcsdes.htm.

NATIONAL CENTER FOR HEALTH STATISTICS

The National Center for Health Statistics (NCHS) is the principal U.S. Federal agency responsible for collecting, analyzing, and disseminating statistical information relevant to the health and well-being of the American public. The purpose of the NCHS is to provide information that may be used to guide actions and policies to improve the health of Americans. It is a center within the Centers for Disease Control and Prevention, which is located within the Department of Health and Human Services. The NCHS, along with nine other federal statistical agencies, is represented on the Interagency Council on Statistical Policy (ICSP), part of the Office of Management and Budget (OMB). The purpose of the ICSP is to coordinate statistical work and provide advice and counsel to the OMB.

The NCHS conducts a wide range of annual, periodic, and longitudinal sample surveys and administers the National Vital Statistics Systems. Among the best known of the NCHS surveys are the National Health and Nutritional Examination Survey, the National Health Interview Survey, the National Immunization Survey, the Longitudinal Studies on Aging, and the National Survey of Family Growth. Through the National Vital Statistics System, the NCHS collects information on vital events from the vital registration systems of the jurisdictions responsible for collecting them, that is, the systems within each of the 50 states, Washington, D.C., New York City, and the territories of Puerto Rico, the U.S. Virgin Islands, Guam, American Samoa, and the Commonwealth of the Northern Mariana Islands. The NCHS then compiles and analyzes this information and in some cases links it to other NCHS data sets. As a rule, the NCHS does not release information about individuals and does not provide copies of birth and death certificates, a responsibility that remains with the local jurisdiction.

The NCHS produces a number of publications and reports, ranging from simple one-page fact sheets about particular health topics to detailed descriptions of the NCHS surveys and analyses of data from those surveys. The *Advance Data* report series provides timely analyses of data from current survey, usually focused on a narrow topic such as HIV risk in young adults and are relatively brief (20 to 40 pages). The *National Vital Statistics Reports* series, which replaces the *Monthly Vital Statistics Reports*, provides timely reports of birth, death, marriage, and divorce statistics, and includes four to six special issues per year that focus on specialized topics such as trends in Cesarean birth rates or births to women aged between 10 and 14 years. The *Vital Health and Statistics Series* produces reports in 24 different series, which cover a range of topics from technical descriptions of the survey design and data collection methods of the NCHS surveys to analysis of data from those surveys and vital statistics data. Often, *Advance Data* reports are followed up by a more detailed report in the *Vital Health and Statistics Series*. Most of these publications are available for free download from the NCHS Web site.

Much of the data collected by the NCHS are available for download through the NCHS Web page or may be requested on CD or tape. Some of the NCHS data that are not publicly accessible due to confidentiality restrictions are available through the NCHS Research Data Center (RDC). To gain access to restricted data, which includes NCHS survey data at lower levels of geographic aggregation or which include more contextual information than can be included in publicly released files, researchers must submit a proposal to the RDC and agree to follow specified procedures to protect the confidentiality of survey respondents.

—Sarah Boslaugh

See also Centers for Disease Control and Prevention; Governmental Role in Public Health; National Health and Nutrition Examination Survey; National Health Interview Survey; National Survey of Family Growth; Public Health Surveillance

Further Readings

Hetzel, A. M. (1997). *U.S. Vital statistics system: Major activities and developments, 1950–95.* Hyattsville, MD: National Center for Health Statistics. Retrieved November 24, 2006, from http://www.cdc.gov/nchs/products/pubs/pubd/other/miscpub/vsushist.htm.

Web Sites

National Center for Health Statistics: www.cdc.gov/nchs

NATIONAL DEATH INDEX

The National Death Index (NDI) is a computerized index of information compiled by the National Center for Health Statistics (NCHS) from death record information submitted to the NCHS by the state offices of vital statistics. This national file of death records contains a standard set of identifying information for each decedent, which includes first and last names, middle initial, father's surname, social security number, sex, race, date of birth, state of birth, state of residence, marital status, and age at death.

The NDI enables investigators to ascertain if the participants in their studies have died by matching the identifying information for an individual with the NDI database. The NDI Retrieval Program searches the NDI file to identify possible matches between a particular NDI death record and a particular user record. An NDI match can identify the state in which death occurred, the date of death, and the death certificate number. To qualify as a possible match, both records must satisfy at least one of seven criteria. The complete social security number alone would provide a match; the other six matching criteria consist of various combinations of birth date, name, and father's surname. When a user record matches one or more NDI records, an NDI Retrieval Report is generated, listing all the identifying information for each of the possible matches, and indicating items that match exactly, items that do not match, and items that possibly match. However, it is up to the users to determine whether NDI records match the individuals in their studies.

In designing a study in which ascertaining death might be important, investigators should collect as many of the NDI data items as possible to optimize the assistance available through the NDI. Using NDI-Plus, investigators can obtain the ICD-9 codes for the cause of death (underlying cause and multiple causes). The NDI does not provide copies of death certificates.

The NDI database contains death record information (beginning with 1979 deaths) for all 50 states, the District of Columbia, Puerto Rico, and the Virgin Islands. Death records are added to the NDI file annually, about 12 months after the end of each calendar year. Approximately 2 million death records are added each year. Deaths during the 2005 calendar year will be available for the NDI search in April 2007.

Use of the NDI is restricted to statistical purposes involving medical and health research. Investigators planning to use the NDI must complete an application and review process, which usually takes 2 to 3 months. Users must meet confidentiality requirements and must submit data on study subjects in a manner that meets the NCHS technical specifications. The fees for routine NDI searches, as of June 2007, consist of a $350 service charge, plus $0.21 per study subject for each year of death searched if vital status of subject is unknown, and $5.00 per decedent if subjects are known to be deceased. Fees for the optional NDI-Plus are slightly higher. A free user's manual can be requested from the NDI; it includes a sample application form.

—Judith Marie Bezy

See also Death Certificate; International Classification of Diseases; National Center for Health Statistics

Further Readings

National Center for Health Statistics. (1997). *National Death Index user's manual* (Publication No. 7–0810). Hyattsville, MD: U.S. Department of Health and Human Services, Centers for Disease Control and Prevention.
National Center for Health Statistics. (1999 revised). *National Death Index Plus: Coded causes of death, supplement to the NDI user's manual* (Publication No. 0–0190). Hyattsville, MD: U.S. Department of Health and Human Services, Centers for Disease Control and Prevention.

Web Sites

National Death Index, National Center for Health Statistics: www.cdc.gov/nchs/ndi.htm.

NATIONAL HEALTH AND NUTRITION EXAMINATION SURVEY

The National Health and Nutrition Examination Survey (NHANES) is a series of cross-sectional, nationally representative surveys conducted by the National Center for Health Statistics. The NHANES uniquely combines in-person interviews with physical examinations and is the authoritative source of objective information on the health and nutritional status of the U.S. population. In 2002, the Continuing Survey of Food Intakes by Individuals (CSFII) of the Department of Agriculture was incorporated into the NHANES. The integrated dietary component is now called *What We Eat in America.*

Findings from the survey provide estimates of important health conditions and risk factors in the U.S. children and adults, such as blood-lead levels, obesity, oral health, sexually transmitted diseases, and smoking. Survey data are also used to assess rates of previously undiagnosed conditions, monitor trends in risk behaviors and environmental exposures in the overall population and subgroups, analyze risk factors for selected disease, explore emerging public health issues, and develop appropriate public health policies and interventions related to health and nutrition.

Survey History

The NHANES resulted in the late 1960s from the addition of a nutritional component to the Health Examination Survey, established by the National Health Survey Act of 1956. While the NHANES was conducted on a periodic basis from 1971 to 1994, the current survey has been carried out continuously since 1999. The data are now released for public use in 2-year increments.

In the current survey, approximately 7,000 individuals of all ages are interviewed in their homes each year. Of these, approximately 5,000 also complete a health examination component. Fifteen primary sampling units (PSUs), which are counties or small groups of counties, are visited annually. To ensure reliable estimates for important population subgroups, the current survey includes oversamples of low-income persons, adolescents between 12 and 19 years of age, persons 60+ years of age, African Americans, and Mexican Americans. The current continuous design of the NHANES allows annual estimates to be calculated for some health indicators. However, data combined over several years are often necessary to produce reliable statistics in the overall sample or in subgroups.

Previous surveys in the NHANES series included the NHANES I (1971–1975), the NHANES II (1976–1980), the NHANES III (1988–1994), the Hispanic HANES (1982–1984), and the NHANES I Epidemiologic Follow-Up Study (NHEFS) (1982–1984, 1986, 1987, and 1992). The NHANES I interviewed a sample of 31,973 persons aged between 1 and 74 years, 23,808 of whom were also given a health examination. The sample was selected to include oversampling of population subgroups thought to be at high risk of malnutrition, including low-income persons, preschool children, women of childbearing age, and the elderly. The NHANES II included a sample of 25,286 persons aged between 6 months and 74 years who were interviewed and 20,322 who were also examined. Children and persons living at or below the poverty level were oversampled. The NHANES III further expanded the age range to include infants as young as 2 months of age, with no upper age limit on adults. Information was collected on 33,994 persons, of whom 31,311 were examined. Younger and older age groups, as well as blacks and Hispanics, were oversampled during the NHANES III. The Hispanic HANES (HHANES) was conducted to obtain reliable estimates of the health and nutritional status of Puerto Ricans, Mexican Americans, and Cuban Americans residing in the United States. The survey included 7,462 Mexican Americans from Texas, Colorado, New Mexico, Arizona, and California; 1,357 Cuban Americans from Dade County, Florida; and 2,834 Cuban Americans from the New York area, including parts of New Jersey and Connecticut.

The NHEFS is a longitudinal study designed to investigate the relationships between clinical, nutritional, and behavioral factors assessed in the NHANES I and subsequent morbidity, mortality, and hospital utilization, as well as changes in risk factors, functional limitations, and institutionalization. The NHEFS cohort includes all 14,407 persons aged between 25 and 74 years who completed a medical examination for the NHANES I. Four follow-up studies have been conducted, and mortality data collection is scheduled to continue indefinitely.

Data Collection

The NHANES employs a stratified, multistage probability sample of the civilian noninstitutionalized U.S. population. Four sampling stages are used to produce a nationally representative sample: PSUs, which are counties or small groups of counties; area segments of PSUs such as a block or group of blocks containing a cluster of households; households within segments; and finally, one or more persons within households.

The data are collected from two primary sources, an initial household interview and a standardized health examination conducted by trained medical personnel. The household interview includes demographic, socioeconomic, dietary, and health-related questions. Health examinations for eligible participants usually occur in mobile examination centers, which are tractor trailers specially outfitted for physical and dental examinations and laboratory tests.

Data Uses

The data from the NHANES have been used in a large number of epidemiological studies and health-related research. An electronic search conducted using the National Library of Medicine Pub Med on July 17, 2006, produced 10,499 scientific journal articles identified with the search term *NHANES*. Findings from the NHANES have contributed directly to the U.S. public health policies and health services. The data from NHANES documented the considerable increase in obesity in the United States since 1980 and substantiate the current national effort aimed at addressing this epidemic in adults and children. When nutrition data from the NHANES I and II indicated that many Americans were consuming inadequate amounts of iron, the government responded by fortifying grain and cereal with iron. The NHANES has also contributed to other health-related guidelines and reforms such as folate fortification of grain, reduction of lead in gasoline, and development of growth charts for children.

—*Helen L. Kwon and Luisa N. Borrell*

See also National Center for Health Statistics; Nutritional Epidemiology; Prevalence; Probability Sample

Further Readings

National Center for Health Statistics. (n.d.). *National health and nutrition examination survey*. Retrieved September 7, 2006, from www.cdc.gov/nchs/nhanes.htm.
National Center for Health Statistics. (1963). Origin, program, and operation of the U.S. National Health Survey. *Vital Health Statistics, 1*, 1–41.
National Center for Health Statistics. (1994). Plan and operation of the Third National Health and Nutrition Examination Survey, 1988–94. *Vital Health Statistics, 1*, 1–39.
National Research Council. (2005). Federal data sets on food and nutrition. In *Improving data to analyze food and nutrition policies* (pp. 26–52). Washington, DC: National Academies Press. Retrieved September 7, 2006, from http://www.nap.edu/catalog/11428.html.

NATIONAL HEALTH CARE SURVEY

The National Health Care Survey (NHCS) is a group of eight related surveys conducted under the auspices of the National Center for Health Statistics (NCHS). Each collects data from health care providers or establishments (such as hospitals) or their records, rather than from patients, and each is based on a multistage sampling plan that allows the computation of valid national estimates of different aspects of health care utilization. These surveys gather information about patients, caregivers, and institutions, as well as on health care events such as physician office visits, hospitalizations, and surgeries. The data for many of the surveys included in the NHCS are available for public use and may be downloaded from the NHCS Web site.

The four original parts of NHCS were the National Hospital Discharge Survey (NHDS), the National Ambulatory Medical Care Survey (NAMCS), the National Nursing Home Survey (NNHS), and the National Health Provider Inventory (NHPI). Later surveys added to the NHCS are the National Survey of Ambulatory Surgery (NSAS), the National Hospital Ambulatory Medical Care Survey (NHAMCS), the National Home and Hospice Care Survey (NHHCS), and the National Employer Health Insurance Survey (NEHIS).

The NAMCS and NHAMCS gather information about ambulatory care: visits to physician's offices in the case of the NAMCS and to hospital outpatient departments (OPDs) and emergency departments (EDs) in the case of the NHAMCS. The NAMCS began collecting data in 1973 and has been conducted annually since, except for the years 1982 to 1984 and 1986 to 1988. The information collected by the NAMCS, which is reported by physicians, includes patient demographics, expected payment source, patient's complaint, procedures and services performed, and medications. The NHAMCS has been conducted annually since 1992; it was begun in recognition of the fact that an increasing number of physician visits took place in OPDs and EDs rather than physician offices. It collects similar information to the NAMCS plus information about characteristics of the hospital, such as type of ownership. The NHAMCS information is reported by hospital staff, and slightly different forms are used for ED and OPD visits.

The NHDS, which has been conducted annually since 1965, was one of the first facility-based surveys conducted by the NCHS. It collects data from a sample of inpatient records from a national sample of about 500 hospitals: Federal, military, institutional, and Veteran's Affairs hospitals are excluded from the sample, as are hospitals with fewer than six beds or with an average length of stay longer than 30 days. The data collected include patient demographics, diagnoses, procedures and discharge status, and admission and discharge dates.

The NNHS was first conducted in 1973 to 1974 and has since been conducted for the years 1977, 1985, 1995, 1997 and 1999, and 2003. It collects data on both facilities, such as size, ownership, and occupancy rate, and on the residents (current and discharged), such as demographics, health status, and services received.

The NHPI, as the name suggests, is an inventory rather than a survey. It was conducted once, in 1991, and provides a comprehensive national listing of health care providers as of that year. The data were collected via mail questionnaires, and two different forms were used, for the two types of providers included. Nursing homes and board and care homes were sent Facility questionnaires, while home health agencies and hospices were sent Agency questionnaires. The information collected includes location, staff, total number of clients served in 1990, age and sex of residents (Facility questionnaire only), and number of current and discharged clients. The NHPI has served as a sampling frame for other health care provider inventories as well as a source of data.

The NSAS was conducted in 1994, 1995, and 1996, to supplement information about inpatient

medical and surgical care collected through the NHDS, largely in response to the dramatic growth of ambulatory surgery facilities in the 1980s. The data were abstracted from medical records and included patient demographic information, expected source of payment, time spent in different phases of care, type of anesthesia used, final diagnoses, and surgical and diagnostic procedures performed.

The NHHCS was conducted in 1992, 1993, 1994, 1996, 1998, and 2000 through interviews with administrators and staff at home health agencies (who provide care in an individual's place of residence, for the purpose of restoring or maintaining health or minimizing the effects of illness or disability) and hospices (who provide palliative and supportive care services, for a dying person and their families, in either the person's home or in a specialized facility); the staff member was directed to refer to the patient's medical record to answer questions about current and discharged patients. The data collected about agencies included ownership, certification, number of patients seen, and number and types of staff members. The data collected on current and discharged patients included demographic characteristics, functional status, health status, payment information, and services used.

The NEHIS was the first federal survey to collect data about employer-sponsored health insurance that represented all employers in the United States and all health plans offered by those employers. The NEHIS was conducted only once, in 1994: Due to confidentiality concerns, the data have not been released to the general public but may be accessed through application to the Research Data Center of the NCHS. The NEHIS conducted a probability sample of business establishments (e.g., a single General Motors plant in a specific geographic location), governments, and self-employed individuals; for employers who offered a large number of insurance plans to their employees, a random sample of plans offered was also taken. This methodology allows valid estimates to be computed at the level of the individual state as well as at the national level. Information collected by the NEHIS includes availability of employer-sponsored health insurance, characteristics of plans offered, benefits, and costs.

—*Sarah Boslaugh*

See also Health Care Delivery; Health Care Services Utilization; Health Economics; National Ambulatory Medical Care Survey; National Center for Health Statistics

Further Readings

Dennison, C., & Pokras, R. (2000). Design and operation of the National Hospital Discharge Survey: 1988 Redesign. National Center for Health Statistics. *Vital Health Statistics*, *1*(39), 1–42.

Gottfried, I. B., Bush, M. A., & Madans, J. H. (1993). Plan and operation: National Nursing Home Survey Followup, 1987, 1988, 1990. National Center for Health Statistics. *Vital Health Statistics*, *1*(30), 1–65.

Haupt, B. J. (1994). Development of the National Home and Hospice Care Survey. National Center for Health Statistics. *Vital Health Statistics*, *1*(33).

Kovar, M. G. (1989). Data systems of the National Center for Health Statistics. National Center for Health Statistics. *Vital Health Statistics*, *1*(23).

McCaig, L. F., & McLemore, T. (1994). Plan and operation of the National Hospital Ambulatory Medical Care Survey. National Center for Health Statistics. *Vital Health Statistics*, *1*(34).

McLemore, T., & Lawrence, L. (1997). Plan and operation of the National Survey of ambulatory surgery. National Center for Health Statistics. *Vital Health Statistics*, *1*(37).

Web Sites

National Health Care Survey: http://www.cdc.gov/nchs/nhcs.htm.

NATIONAL HEALTH INTERVIEW SURVEY

The National Health Interview Survey (NHIS) is the principal source of national information about the health of the civilian noninstitutionalized U.S. population. The NHIS began collecting data in 1957 and has been conducted by the National Center for Health Statistics (NCHS) since 1960, when the NCHS was formed by combining the National Vital Statistics Division and the National Health Survey. Content covered by the NHIS has been updated every 10 to 15 years since its inception and was substantially revised for the surveys beginning in 1997.

The NHIS was authorized by the National Health Survey Act of 1956, which provided for a continuing survey to collect accurate and up-to-date information on the health of the U.S. population. The topics covered by the 2005 NHIS include demographics, specific medical conditions, activity limitations, general mental and physical health, physical activity, alcohol use, access to health care, health services utilization, health-related knowledge, blood donation, and HIV testing. The data drawn from the NHIS are used to monitor trends in illness and disability, to track progress toward achieving national health objectives, for epidemiologic and policy analysis, and for evaluating the effectiveness of Federal health programs.

The NHIS gathers data through personal interviews conducted in the respondent's household by employees of the U.S. Census Bureau following procedures specified by the NCHS. Within a household (defined as the people living within an occupied living unit and often synonymous with "family"), one adult is selected to provide data on all household members. In addition, one randomly selected adult and one randomly selected child (if available) are selected for further data collection; the adult provides information for both himself or herself and the child. The NHIS data are collected using a sampling plan that allows for the creation of national but not state-level estimates of the topics covered: Detailed information about the sampling plans used in different years is available from the NHIS Web site. Oversampling of African Americans and Hispanics has been included in the NHIS sampling plan since 1995 to allow more accurate estimates for those subgroups. In 2004, the NHIS collected data from 94,460 individuals in 36,579 households, with a response rate of 86.9%. The NHIS data, questionnaires, and ancillary information including documentation and syntax files to process the data are available from the NHIS Web page, as are tables and reports drawn from the NHIS summarizing different aspects of the health of the U.S. population.

—*Sarah Boslaugh*

See also Centers for Disease Control and Prevention; Governmental Role in Public Health; Health Behavior; National Center for Health Statistics; Public Health Surveillance

Further Readings

Adams, P. F., & Schoenborn, C. A. (2006). Health behaviors of adults: United States, 2002–2004. *Vital Health Statistics*, *10*(230), 1–140.

Bloom, B., & Dey, A. N. (2006). Summary health statistics for U.S. children: National Health Interview Survey, 2004. *Vital Health Statistics*, *10*(227), 1–85.

Web Sites

National Health Interview Survey (NHIS): http://www.cdc.gov/nchs/nhis.htm.

NATIONAL IMMUNIZATION SURVEY

The National Immunization Survey (NIS) began collecting data in 1994 for the purpose of establishing estimates of up-to-date immunization levels in each state, the District of Columbia, and 27 large urban areas. The NIS is conducted by the National Opinion Research Center for the Centers for Disease Control and Prevention; it is jointly sponsored by the National Immunization Program and the National Center for Health Statistics. Children between the ages of 19 and 35 months living in the United States at the time of the survey are the target population for the NIS: Data about their immunizations are collected from a parent or other adult from the child's household who is knowledgeable about their immunization record. If possible, this information is confirmed with the child's immunization providers.

The vaccinations included in the NIS are those recommended by the Advisory Committee on Immunization Practices, which are currently 4 doses of diphtheria, tetanus, and acellular pertussis vaccine (DTaP); 3 doses of polio vaccine; 1 dose of measles/mumps/rubella (MMR) vaccine; Haemophilus influenzae Type b vaccine (Hib); hepatitis A vaccine (Hep A); 3 doses of hepatitis B vaccine (Hep B); 1 dose of varicella zoster vaccine (chicken pox); 4 doses of pneumococcal conjugate vaccine (PCV); and influenza vaccine. Hepatitis A is recommended only in selected states with a high incidence of the disease. All vaccines except varicella, influenza, and pneumococcal have been included in the NIS since its inception: Pneumococcal was added in 2002, and influenza and hepatitis A were added in 2003.

The NIS collects data in two ways: through telephone interviews with households selected through random-digit dialing and through a mail survey of physicians and other vaccination providers; the latter is called the Provider Record Check Study. The telephone interview collects information from parents of eligible children about the immunizations each child has received, the dates of the immunizations, and the demographic and socioeconomic information about the household. If the parent grants permission, the child's vaccination providers are contacted to verify the child's vaccination record. The state and local estimates of vaccination coverage are calculated every quarter using NIS data and are used to evaluate progress toward national and local immunization goals. The coverage for series of vaccines is also reported, including the 4:3:1:3:3 series (4+ DTaP, 3+ polio, 1+ MMR, 3+ Hib, and 3+ Hep B).

—Sarah Boslaugh

See also Centers for Disease Control and Prevention; Child and Adolescent Health; National Center for Health Statistics; Survey Research Methods; Vaccination

Further Readings

Smith, P. J., Hoaglin, D. C., Battaglia, M. P., Barker, L. E., & Khare, M. (2005). Statistical methodology of the National Immunization Survey, 1994–2002. National Center for Health Statistics. *Vital and Health Statistics*, 2(138).

Web Sites

National Immunization Survey (NIS) data and documentation are available for download from the NIS Web site: http://www.cdc.gov/nis/datafiles.htm. (Currently data for the years 1995–2004 are available.)

NATIONAL INSTITUTES OF HEALTH

The National Institutes of Health (NIH) is a U.S. Federal government agency, located in a suburb of Washington, D.C., that disburses more than $28 billion annually to fund biomedical research. The extramural, or granting, program, distributes 80% of the funds to universities and foundations in the United States and across the world. The scientists in the intramural, or on-campus, program conduct basic and clinical research based in 27 institutes and centers, including a brand-new (2004) 242-bed research hospital.

The NIH traces its origins to 1887 and a one-room laboratory in Staten Island, New York. Originally conceived of as the research division of the Marine Hospital Service (MHS), the NIH, then known as the Hygienic Laboratory, was an experiment. The MHS had been charged with preventing people with cholera, yellow fever, and other infectious diseases from entering the United States: Perhaps a laboratory could help public health officials understand these diseases better to prevent future epidemics.

The experiment worked. Within 5 years, the Congress deemed the laboratory worthy of expansion and moved its facilities to Washington, D.C., to be closer to the seat of the Federal government. Its first director, Joseph Kinyoun, was charged with tasks such as cleaning up the city's water supply and reducing its air pollution. In 1901, the Congress authorized $35,000. The next year, the divisions of the new laboratories were formalized. The Division of Pathology and Bacteriology was joined by the Divisions of Chemistry, Pharmacology, and Zoology. The professional staff was filled out with scientists with doctoral degrees rather than physicians, emphasizing the importance of basic research.

In its initial years, epidemiological studies made up much of the work of the agency. In 1906, Hygienic Laboratory workers pursued a landmark study of typhoid in Washington, D.C., in which they identified the milk supply as the culprit in spreading the disease. In the next decade, new diseases were elucidated, such as tularemia, and old diseases were explored. For example, groundbreaking use of epidemiological techniques allowed Joseph Goldberger to prove that pellagra was caused by a vitamin deficiency and was not an infectious disease as had been previously assumed. In the next few decades, NIH scientists pursued studies of diseases in varied communities, from endemic and epidemic typhus in the South to Rocky Mountain spotted fever in the West. They identified and confirmed the vectors (spreaders) of diseases, such as showing, for example, that the body louse was responsible for spreading epidemic typhus fever.

The early decades of the 20th century brought other scientific advances in the area of public health. The Hygienic Laboratory, in charge of regulating biologics before the 1971 creation of the Food and Drug Administration, established the standards for antitoxins. Working to prevent diseases as well as to understand them, scientists studied water pollution and sewage, with important results in the creation of pure water systems. Evans, studying undulant fever, helped officials decide to call for the pasteurization of milk to prevent this and other illnesses. And in the 1920s, Hygienic Laboratory scientists studied the relationship between canning and food poisoning. This type of research led to better public health guidelines.

In 1930, major changes came to NIH. The Congress renamed the Hygienic Laboratory the National Institute (singular) of Health and authorized the payout of fellowship money for basic research. These fellowships form the majority of the NIH's research program today. In 1937, with the founding of the National Cancer Institute, the Congress began a several-decade process of opening new institutes at NIH to deal with specific diseases. Cancer, a chronic disease, marked an important switch away from the agency's long focus on infectious diseases. Institutes would often be formed around a single disease, such as heart disease, mental health, and diabetes. In the late 1930s, the NIH campus moved to its current location in suburban Bethesda, Maryland, where the operation expanded into several buildings specially equipped with up-to-date facilities.

During World War II, the scientists at NIH worked with the military to analyze the reasons why so many potential inductees were unfit for general military service. The two common causes of rejection were defective teeth and venereal disease. These realizations led to new funding for research into these areas. Other divisions worked on issues such as dangers in war-related industries. Research into vaccines expanded during the war years, and scientists worked on vaccines for yellow fever and typhus, specifically for military forces. The researchers at the NIH campus in Bethesda teamed up to find an alternative to quinine for prevention and treatment of malaria, a major scourge for American troops overseas.

In the post–World War II era, the NIH became more recognizable as the agency that it is today. When the grants program was expanded to the entire agency, the total budget expanded from $8 million in 1947 to more than $1 billion in 1966. In these years, the Congress designated more institutes to focus on specific diseases: lifecycle research on childhood and aging and drug and alcohol abuse. By 1960, there were 10 components. By 1970, this number increased to 15, and in 2006 the NIH had 27 institutes and centers.

Epidemiological work in the mid-20th century done by the NIH was spread around the world. Using data obtained from local neighborhoods and from infants and children housed at an institution in Washington, D.C., Robert Huebner and his colleagues identified new viruses. An expanded vaccine research program helped find methods to combat them. The Nobel Laureate Carleton Gadjusek identified the kuru virus prevalent among the South Fore people of New Guinea as stemming from a particular funerary practice. Kuru was later identified as a prion disease. Baruch Blumberg and others discovered the Australian antigen during their work in the 1950s and 1960s. This led to a test to screen donated blood for hepatitis B, greatly reducing the risk of transfusion hepatitis. One of the NIH's most famous long-term epidemiological studies was the Heart Disease Epidemiology study at Framingham, Massachusetts, which started in 1949 and followed subjects for many years while recording notes about their diet and lifestyles. After 1946, the Centers for Disease Control in Atlanta took over much of the NIH's epidemiology work, especially in terms of identifying the causes of epidemics.

A major asset was the opening of a hospital to the NIH main campus in Bethesda. The Clinical Center, which opened in 1953 and expanded into a state-of-the-art new building in 2004, was specially designed to bring research laboratories into close proximity with hospital wards to promote productive collaboration between laboratory scientists and clinicians.

The NIH budget slowed down considerably in the 1960s and 1970s. This was due in part to wariness on the part of the Congress and the public about the efficacy of basic research in solving major health crises. However, the HIV/AIDS crisis in the 1980s highlighted the need for basic research in immunology and other disciplines. The important NIH research in the late 20th century also included studies that helped demonstrate that recombinant DNA research did not pose great risk of unleashing deadly novel organisms, leading to a rapid increase in molecular studies of disease. In the late 1980s, the NIH and the Department of Energy launched the Human Genome Project with the goal of mapping and sequencing the entire collection of human genes. The 1990s saw an emphasis in research on women's health with the Women's Health Initiative. And there have been many other successes: More than 100 NIH-funded scientists have won the Nobel Prize, including 5 who did their prize-winning work in the intramural program.

The turn of the 21st century has been a period of regrowth. The NIH Director Elias Zerhouni started the Road Map Initiative to direct monies to research problems that needed the attention of the entire agency rather than just one institute. The doubling of the NIH budget between 1998 and 2003 was meant to jump-start research: With an FY06 budget of more than $28 billion, the NIH today would barely be recognizable to Joseph Kinyoun and his staff of the one-room laboratory more than a century earlier.

—*Sarah A. Leavitt*

See also Centers for Disease Control and Prevention; Food and Drug Administration; Framingham Heart Study; Goldberger, Joseph; Governmental Role in Public Health

Further Readings

Farreras, I. G., Hannaway, C., & Harden, V. A. (Eds.). (2004). *Mind, brain, body, and behavior: Foundations of neuroscience and behavioral research at the National Institutes of Health.* Amsterdam: IOS Press.

Hannaway, C., Harden, V. A., & Parascandola, J. (Eds.). (1995). *AIDS and the public debate: Historical and contemporary perspectives.* Amsterdam: IOS Press.

Harden, V. A. (1986). *Inventing the NIH: Federal Biomedical Research Policy, 1887–1937.* Baltimore: Johns Hopkins University Press.

Harden, V. A. (1990). *Rocky Mountain spotted fever: History of a twentieth-century disease.* Baltimore: Johns Hopkins University Press.

Kraut, A. M. (2003). *Goldberger's War: The life and work of a public health crusader.* Boston: Hill & Wang.

Web Sites

National Institutes of Health: www.nih.gov.
Office of NIH History: www.history.nih.gov.

NATIONAL MATERNAL AND INFANT HEALTH SURVEY

The National Maternal and Infant Health Survey (NMIHS) was a longitudinal study of factors related to adverse pregnancy outcomes. Conducted by the National Center for Health Statistics in 1988 and 1991, the latter is often referred to as the Longitudinal Follow-Up. The NMIHS was conducted to augment data available in vital statistics records, collecting information on maternal sociodemographic characteristics, pregnancy history, health status, and health care types and sources. The vital statistics records included birth, fetal death, and infant death records. The NMIHS was the first national survey conducted in the United States to collect data simultaneously on births, fetal deaths, and infant deaths.

The NMIHS data were collected by questionnaires mailed to a nationally representative survey sample of women who gave birth or had a fetal or infant death in 1988. The data were collected from 9,953 women who gave birth, 3,309 who had fetal deaths, and 5,532 who had infant deaths. The NMIHS data are weighted to be representative of all births, fetal deaths, and infant deaths in 1988. Additionally, 93% of mothers consented to have their health care providers contacted. Questionnaires were administered to physicians, hospitals, and other health care providers linked to the outcomes, and this information was added to that collected from the individual mothers.

The mother's questionnaire was 35 pages long and included detailed questions on prenatal care; health during pregnancy; use of birth control; breastfeeding; desire for the pregnancy; use of tobacco, alcohol, and drugs; and demographic and socioeconomic characteristics of the mother and father. The provider questionnaire included questions about prenatal and postpartum care, medication use, diagnostic and other procedures performed, and infant health status.

The data from the NMIHS have been used by researchers to study a range of issues related to maternal and child health and well-being. The findings include the following:

- High income inequality was associated with an increased risk of depression and poor physical health, especially for the poorest fifth of women with young children.
- Low birthweight and early-childhood asthma were strongly and independently linked, with an estimated 4,000 excess asthma cases ascribed to low birthweight.
- Women with depressive symptoms after delivery were significantly more likely to report child behavior problems, including temper tantrums and difficulties interacting with other children, than those who did not report depressive symptoms.

The data from the NMIHS are publicly available. The data from the 1988 and 1991 surveys are available separately; however, to protect the confidentiality of respondents, the data sets can be linked only at the Research Data Center of the National Center for Health Statistics in Hyattsville, Maryland.

—*Anu Manchikanti*

See also Child and Adolescent Health; Maternal and Child Health Epidemiology; Pregnancy Risk Assessment and Monitoring System; Preterm Birth

Further Readings

National Center for Health Statistics. (2005). *National Maternal and Infant Health Survey*. Retrieved August 15, 2005, from http://www.cdc.gov/nchs/about/major/nmihs/abnmihs.htm.
Sanderson, M., & Gonzalez, J. F. (1998). 1988 National Maternal and Infant Health Survey: Methods and response characteristics. *Vital and Health Statistics. Series 2, Data Evaluation and Methods Research, 125*, 1–39.

NATIONAL MORTALITY FOLLOWBACK SURVEY

The National Mortality Followback Survey (NMFS) has been conducted sporadically since 1961 by the National Center for Health Statistics (NCHS) to collect information on various specific topics related to mortality in the United States, including the events and circumstances that preceded death, and relevant characteristics of the decedent. The NMFS has been conducted six times: four times in the 1960s, in 1986, and most recently, in 1993.

The main national database for the United States mortality statistics (the National Death Index) is maintained by the NCHS and is compiled from the official death certificate registries maintained by individual states. The NMFS was created to enrich the national mortality database by collecting information not available from death certificates. Each of the six surveys has been unique; each has focused on different topics and has used a variety of survey instruments and sources. The objective has been to focus on specific topics of current interest to public health researchers and policymakers, using instruments designed to fit the purposes of the individual survey rather than using a uniform instrument to gather data on a consistent group of topics.

All the surveys have obtained information from persons identified on the death certificates as informants (next of kin or a person familiar with the decedent). The surveys have collected information by means of mail questionnaires, personal interviews, and/or telephone interviews. The sample for each survey has been drawn from the Current Mortality Sample, a systematic 10% of the states' death certificates.

The topics covered have varied from survey to survey. The 1961 survey sought information on the use of hospital and institutional care during the last year of life. The 1962 to 1963 survey focused on socioeconomic factors. The 1964 to 1965 survey obtained data on health care expenditures during the last year of life, sources of payment, and health insurance coverage. The 1966 to 1968 survey focused on the link between smoking and cancer mortality.

The two most recent surveys have been more comprehensive (covering a larger sample and more information items and sources) than the surveys conducted in the 1960s, and they have attempted to provide comparability with the data obtained by previous surveys.

The 1986 survey covered three topics: socioeconomic factors, risk factors related to premature death, and health care provided in the last year of life. Brief questionnaires were mailed to all hospitals, nursing homes, and other health care facilities reportedly used by decedents in their last year of life. The sample (18,733) was an approximate 1% sample of all deaths of adults over age 25 in 1986.

The 1993 survey included the 1986 topics and added a fourth topic, disability in the last year of life. The 1993 survey sought information from medical examiner/coroner offices if death was due to homicide, suicide, or accidental injury. The 1993 sample included 22,957 deaths in 1993 of persons aged 15 and older.

Both the 1986 and 1993 surveys examined the reliability of information reported on the death certificate by comparing it with the information reported by the survey respondent. The comparable items included age, race, gender, veteran status, education, occupation, and industry.

The two most recent surveys each included all states except one. In 1986, Oregon was not represented, and in 1993, South Dakota was not sampled, due to state restrictions on the use of death certificate information. Public use data files from the 1986 and 1993 NMFS surveys are available for purchase through the National Technical Information Service. The reports based on the surveys have been published by the National Center for Health Statistics.

—Judith Marie Bezy

See also Death Certificate; National Center for Health Statistics; National Death Index

Further Readings

National Center for Health Statistics. (n.d.). *National Mortality Followback Survey (NMFS) Public-Use Data Files.* Retrieved September 7, 2006, from http://www.cdc.gov/nchs/products/elec_prods/subject/nmfs.htm.

Seeman, I. (1992). National Mortality Followback Survey: 1986 Summary, United States. *Vital and Health Statistics, 20*(19).

Seeman, I., Poe, S., & Powell-Griner, E. (1993). Development, methods, and response characteristics of the 1986 National Mortality Followback Survey. Hyattsville, MD: National Center for Health Statistics. *Vital and Health Statistics, 1*(29).

NATIONAL SURVEY OF FAMILY GROWTH

The National Survey of Family Growth (NSFG) is a nationally representative survey of adults in the United States that collects data on topics related to sexual behavior, fertility, infant health, marriage, and family life. It has been conducted periodically since 1973, and the first five administrations of the NSFG (1973, 1976, 1982, 1988, and 1995) collected information from women aged between 15 and 44 years only (considered the age range most likely to give birth); the most recent NSFG, conducted in 2002, collected information from both men and women and included more questions about sexual behavior than the previous surveys. Although the NSFG sample is nationally representative, it is not sufficiently large to allow analyses at geographic levels smaller than the four census regions (Northeast, Midwest, South, and West); metropolitan area versus nonmetropolitan area analyses are also supported.

The NSFG data are collected through in-person home interviews. For the 2002 administration, responses to particularly sensitive questions on topics such as sexual orientation, number of sexual partners, safe sex practices, and pregnancy terminations were collected through Audio Computer-Assisted Self-Interviewing (ACASI). This is an interview technique in which the respondent enters answers to questions directly into the computer rather than responding verbally to questions posed by the interviewer; the purpose of this technique is to gather more honest responses to sensitive questions by freeing the respondent from discussing personal issues in front of another person. The survey sample for each of the first five administrations of the NSFG included about 8,000 to 10,000 women, sampled from the civilian, non-institutionalized population of women aged between 15 and 44 years living in the 48 contiguous United States; all 50 states were included beginning with the fourth administration. The 2002 NSFG survey sample included 7,643 women and 4,928 men.

For the first five administrations of the NSFG, data were collected into two types of files: an *interval*, or *pregnancy*, file and a *respondent* file. The data collected have varied somewhat in each administration, but in general the *pregnancy* file contains information about topics such as contraceptive use, prenatal care, pregnancies, and births, and the *respondent* file includes personal and demographic information about the women surveyed, such as education, race, employment, marital status, living arrangements, family size, number of pregnancies and adoptions, health insurance coverage, and child care arrangement. The 2002 NSFG collected data in three types of files: a *female respondent* file, a *male respondent* file, and a *female pregnancy* file. The *female respondent* and *male respondent* files contain information similar to the respondent file of the first five administrations, while the *female pregnancy* file includes the woman's pregnancy history.

Most NSFG data are available on CD-ROM from the National Center for Health Statistics Web site and on data tapes from the National Technical Information Service. The sensitive data collected by ACASI are not included in these sources: Due to confidentiality concerns, access to these data requires a special application to the NSFG.

—*Sarah Boslaugh*

See also Interview Techniques; Reproductive Epidemiology; Sexually Transmitted Diseases; Sexual Risk Behavior; Women's Health Issues

Further Readings

Lepkowski, J. M., Mosher, W. D., Davis, K. E., Groves, R. M., van Hoewyk, J., & Willem, J. (2006). National Survey of Family Growth, Cycle 6: Sample design, weighting, imputation, and variance estimation. *Vital Health Statistics, 2*(142), 1–82.

Web Sites

National Survey of Family Growth: http://www.cdc.gov/nchs/nsfg.htm.

NATIVE AMERICAN HEALTH ISSUES

See AMERICAN INDIAN HEALTH ISSUES

NATURAL EXPERIMENT

A natural experiment is an observational study that takes advantage of a naturally occurring event or situation that can be exploited by a researcher to answer a particular question. Natural experiments are often used to study situations in which a true experiment is not possible, for instance, if the exposure of interest cannot be practically or ethically assigned to research subjects. Situations that may create appropriate circumstances for a natural experiment include policy changes, weather events, or natural disasters. This entry describes natural experiments, examines the limitations to such experiments that exist as a result of confounding, and discusses the use of instrumental variables to control confounding.

The key features of experimental study designs are manipulation and control. Manipulation, in this context, means that the experimenter can control which research subjects receive which exposures: For instance, those randomized to the treatment arm of an experiment typically receive treatment from the drug or therapy that is the focus of the experiment, while those in the control group receive no treatment or a different treatment. Control is most readily accomplished through random assignment, which means that the procedures by which participants are assigned to a treatment and control condition ensure that each has equal probability of assignment to either group. Random assignment ensures that individual characteristics or experiences that might confound the treatment results are, on average, evenly distributed between the two groups. In summary, then, an experiment is a study in which at least one variable is manipulated and units are randomly assigned to the different levels or categories of the manipulated variables.

Although the gold standard for epidemiologic research is often considered to be the randomized control trial, this design can answer only certain types of epidemiologic questions, and it is not useful in the investigation of questions for which random assignment is either impracticable or unethical. The bulk of epidemiologic research relies on observational data, which raises issues in drawing causal inferences from the results. A core assumption for drawing causal inference is that the average outcome of the group exposed to one treatment regimen represents the average outcome the other group would have had if they had been exposed to the same treatment regimen. If treatment is not randomly assigned, as in case of observational studies, the assumption that the two groups are exchangeable (on both known and unknown confounders) cannot simply be assumed to be true.

For instance, suppose an investigator is interested in the effect of poor housing on health. Because it is neither practical nor ethical to randomize people to variable housing conditions, this subject is difficult to study using an experimental approach. However, if a housing policy change such as a lottery for subsidized mortgages was enacted that enabled some people to move to more desirable housing while leaving other similar people in their previous substandard housing, it might be possible to use that policy change to study the effect of housing change on health outcomes. One well-known natural experiment occurred in Helena, Montana, where smoking was banned from all public places for a 6-month period. The investigators reported a 60% drop in heart attacks for study area during the time the ban was in effect.

Because natural experiments do not randomize participants into exposure groups, the assumptions and analytical techniques customarily applied to experimental designs are not valid for them. Rather, natural experiments are quasi experiments and need to be thought about and analyzed as such. The lack of random assignment means multiple threats to causal inference, including attrition, history, testing, regression, instrumentation, and maturation, may influence observed study outcomes. For this reason, natural experiments will never unequivocally determine causation in a given situation. Nevertheless, they are a useful method for researchers and if used with care can provide additional data that may help with a research question and that may not be obtainable in any other way.

Instrumental Variables

The major limitation in inferring causation from natural experiments is the presence of unmeasured confounding. One class of methods designed to control confounding and measurement error is based on instrumental variables (IV). Although these variables have been used in economics for decades, they are little known in epidemiology. While useful in a variety of applications, the validity and interpretation of IV estimates depend on strong assumptions, the plausibility of which must be considered with regard to the causal relation in question.

If we are interested in the causal effect of X (exposure) on Y (outcome), and we can observe their relation to a third variable Z (IV or instrument) that is associated with X but not with Y (except through its association with X), then under certain conditions we can write the $Z - Y$ association as the product of $Z - X$ and $X - Y$ associations as follows:

$$\text{Assoc } ZY = \text{Assoc } ZX \times \text{Assoc} XY$$

and solve this equation for the XY association.

This equation is particularly useful when (1) the XY relationship is confounded by unmeasured covariates (but the ZX and ZY relationships are not) or (2) the XY relationship cannot be directly observed, but Z is an observable surrogate, or instrument, for X.

IV analyses use data from researcher-randomized or natural experiments to estimate the effect of an exposure on those exposed. IV analyses depend on the assumption that subjects were effectively randomized, even if the randomization was accidental (in the case of an administrative policy change or exposure to a natural disaster) and/or adherence to random assignment was low. IV methods can be used to control for confounding in observational studies, control for confounding due to noncompliance, and correct for misclassification.

Confounding in Observational Studies

Administrative policies, government legislation, and other external forces often create natural or quasi experiments in which an individual's probability of exposure is affected by forces uncorrelated with individual-level health outcomes. Such policies could be used as an instrument in epidemiologic analysis. For instance, if we are interested in the causal effect of X (income) on Y (self-rated health), and we can observe their relation to a third variable Z (an IV or instrument, in this case, a state-level increase in the minimum wage), and we know the relation between X and Y is confounded by U (unobserved or unmeasured variables, such as race, wealth, area-level economic health, etc.), then we can use Z to estimate the relationship between X and Y provided it meets both the following assumptions:

1. Z is associated with X.
2. Z is not associated with Y.

We cannot use Z to estimate the relationship between X and Y if any of the following is true:

1. Z is associated with Y.
2. Z is associated with U.
3. U is associated with Z.

Characteristics of a Good Instrument

To even consider a potential instrument for use in IV, it must meet the following three assumptions: (1) the instrument (Z) must be associated (in known and measurable ways) with the exposure (X), (2) the instrument (Z) cannot be associated with outcome (Y), and (3) the deviation of the instrument (Z) from the exposure (X) is independent of other variables or errors. Furthermore, to interpret IV effect estimates as causal parameters, we need to further assume that the direction of the effect of Z on X is the same for everyone in the sample (the monotonicity assumption). Any instrument not meeting these assumptions for the causal contrast in question is not appropriate for use in analysis.

Limitations of IV Analysis

IV analysis is limited, particularly in light of the assumptions imposed on the relationship between the instrument and the exposure and outcome. Even a small association between the instrument and the outcome, which is not solely mediated by the exposure of interest, can produce serious biases in IV effect estimates. It can also be difficult to identify the particular subpopulation to which the causal effect IV estimate applies (those whose exposure would be affected by the instrument if offered). If the relationship between the instrument and the exposure is weak, IV analysis can add considerable imprecision to causal effect estimates. The multiple instruments can be useful both to improve the statistical power of an IV analysis and, if power is adequate, to test the validity of instruments against one another. Some instruments may be valid only after conditioning on

a measured covariate. A common prior cause of the instrument and the outcome renders the instrument invalid unless that confounder can be measured and statistically controlled. Small sample size poses an additional challenge in applying IV methods.

—Lynne C. Messer

See also Causal Diagrams; Causation and Causal inference; Quasi Experiments; Study Design

Further Readings

Glymour, M. (2006). Natural experiments and instrumental variable analysis in social epidemiology. In J. M. Oakes & J. S. Kaufman (Eds.), *Methods in social epidemiology* (pp. 429–460). San Francisco, CA: Jossey-Bass.

Greenland, S. (2000). An introduction to instrumental variables for epidemiologists. *International Journal of Epidemiology, 29,* 722–729.

Sargent, R. P., Shepard, R. M., & Glantz, S. A. (2004). Reduced incidence of admissions for myocardial infarction associated with public smoking ban: Before and after study. *British Medical Journal, 328*(7446), 977–980.

NEGATIVE BINOMIAL REGRESSION

See REGRESSION

NEGATIVE PREDICTIVE VALUE

See CLINICAL EPIDEMIOLOGY

NETWORK ANALYSIS

Over the past two decades, the epidemic of HIV has challenged the epidemiological community to rethink the framework for understanding the risk of infectious disease transmission, both at the individual level and at the level of population transmission dynamics. Research has rapidly converged on the central importance of partnership networks. Systematic patterns in social networks have always served to channel infectious diseases—from the sequence of plagues in

Europe and the introduction of European childhood infections into the Native American populations to the polio epidemics of the early 20th century and the contemporary outbreaks of cholera and typhoid that attend mass movements of refugees. The methodology for network data collection and analysis in epidemiology, however, is only now being developed. This entry examines the role of networks in disease transmission, as well as the origins of network analysis in social science and epidemiology. The entry focuses on the role of social networks in sexually transmitted infections (STIs), where networks determine the level of individual exposure, the population dynamics of spread, and the interactional context that constrains behavioral change. Network analysis has had the largest impact in this field, and it represents a paradigm shift in the study of STI.

Types of Transmission Via Social Networks

Like the movement of exchangeable goods, the diffusion of pathogens through a human population traces the structure of social networks. The pattern of spread is jointly determined by the biology of the pathogen and the social structure that can support it, so different kinds of diseases travel along different structural routes. The plague, for example, is spread by a mobile vector of rats and fleas that makes for an efficient, long-lasting infectious vehicle. The disease can travel via long-distance transportation and trade routes even when travel is slow paced, with macroeconomic relations helping to structure the diffusion path. For influenza and measles, in contrast, transmission requires casual or indirect personal contact in a relatively short period of time. The spread of these infections is structured by locations of frequent collective activity, such as schools and supermarkets today, with transportation networks serving as potential bridges between communities and sparsely settled or less traveled routes serving as buffers. Finally, there are infections spread only by intimate or prolonged contact; STIs are a classic example. These diseases travel along the most selective forms of social networks, operating on what is comparatively a very sparse microstructure, with a typically modest duration of infection. The structure of sexual networks varies within and between societies, governed by local norms, power differentials, and oppositional subcultures. Here, as with other infectious diseases, the transmission network determines the potential for epidemics and the opportunities for prevention.

Network Epidemiology and Sexually Transmitted Infections

Network epidemiology offers a comprehensive way of thinking about individual sexual behavior and its consequences for STI transmission. Unlike other health-related behaviors (e.g., smoking) and safety-related behavior (e.g., using seat belts), behaviors that transmit STIs directly involve at least two people, as well as other persons to whom they may be linked. Understanding this process requires moving beyond the standard, individual-centered research paradigm. This has important implications for the analytic framework, data collection, and intervention planning.

The analytic framework must take a relational approach, integrating individual behavior into partnership contexts, and aggregating partnership configurations into networks. This is a marked departure from the standard approach to behavioral research that seeks to link individual attributes to individual outcomes. The data collection and statistical analysis need to be revised accordingly, making the partnership—rather than the individual—the primary sampling unit. While we know a lot about sampling individuals, we know much less about sampling partnerships and networks. Finally, analyzing the network data that are collected requires different statistical methods, since the defining property of such data is that the units are not independent. The methods for analyzing dependent data are not unknown—spatial statistics, time series, and multilevel models provide a starting point—but the statistical tools needed to analyze networks have only recently been developed.

Given these difficulties, why bother taking a network approach? Why not simply focus on individual risk factors for acquisition of disease? The answer is that network epidemiology succeeds where more traditional epidemiological approaches have failed: explaining differentials in risk behavior, epidemic potential in low-risk populations, and the persistent and substantial prevalence differentials across populations.

In one sense, a network explanation is almost tautological: Individuals are infected by their partners, who are in turn infected by their partners—*networks* is just a term that describes this process. But the concept also has explanatory power and prevention implications, as it changes the focus from "what you do" to "whom you do it with." This allows for behaviors to vary within as well as between persons, and for the same individual behavior to lead to different infection outcomes in different contexts.

As a result, the network perspective changes the way we think about targeting concepts such as "risk groups" and "risk behaviors." The inadequacy of these concepts became clear as HIV prevalence rose among groups that do not engage in individually risky behavior, for example, monogamous married women. By the same token, a group of persons with extremely "risky" individual behavior may have little actual risk of STI exposure if their partners are uninfected and are not linked to the rest of the partnership network. It is not only individuals' behavior that defines their risk but also the behavior of their partners and (ultimately) their position in a network.

The network perspective also changes the way we think about the population-level risk factors. The key issue is not simply the mean number of partners but the connectivity of the network, and connectivity can be established even in low-density networks. One of the primary ways in which this happens is through concurrent partnerships. Serial monogamy in sexual partnerships creates a highly segmented network with no links between each pair of persons at any moment in time. If this constraint is relaxed, allowing people to have more than one partner concurrently, the network can become much more connected. The result is a large increase in the potential spread of STIs, even at low levels of partnership formation.

Finally, the network perspective changes the way we think about behavior change. Because the relevant behavior occurs in the context of a partnership, individual knowledge, attitudes, and beliefs do not affect behavior directly. Instead, the impact of these individual-level variables is mediated by the relationship between the partners. A young woman who knows that condoms help prevent the sexual spread of HIV may be unable to convince her male partner to use one. It is not her knowledge that is deficient, but her control over joint behavior.

Origins of the Field

The analysis of network structures has a relatively long history in the social sciences, which is where the most comprehensive methodology has been developed, and the study of diffusion through structured populations in epidemiology is also long standing. In recent years, physicists have also begun to work on the epidemiology of diseases on networks.

Social Science Roots

Social network analysis is an established subfield in the social sciences, with a professional organization (the International Network for Social Network Analysis [INSNA]), an annual meeting (the "Sunbelt" social network conference, now in its 26th year), and several journals (*Social Networks, Connections*). It is an interdisciplinary field, and it has developed a unique set of methodological tools.

For the past 25 years, social network analysts have been developing quantitative tools for empirical studies. There are several distinct approaches, defined by the type of data collected. The first is based on a network census—data collected on every node and link for a (typically small) population. The current textbooks and most popular computer packages for social network analysis have these methods at their core. The second approach is based on sampled network data. The most well-known of these is the local network (or egocentric) sample design: a sample of the nodes (egos), with a "name generator" in the questionnaire to obtain a roster of their partners (alters), and "name interpreters" to collect information on these partners (for a good example and discussion). With this simple study design, no attempt is made to identify or enroll the partners. Local network data collection costs about the same as a standard survey, is relatively easy to implement, and is less intrusive than complete network data collection. In between these two approaches lies a range of link-tracing designs for collecting network data—snowball samples, random walks, and most recently, respondent-driven sampling. The absence of methods for analyzing such data previously limited the use of this approach, but new methods are now available and are becoming more common.

Rapid progress is being made now in the development of methodology for network analysis. Methods have been developed to handle networks sampled with egocentric and link-tracing designs. Statistical theory is being developed for estimation and inference, which is complicated for networks given the dependent data and nonlinear threshold effects. The class of models being developed not only can represent an arbitrarily complex network structure but can also test the goodness of fit of simple parsimonious models to data. A computer package (statnet) has been released that allows researchers to use these methods for network analysis. The algorithm used for network estimation in this package can also be used for simulation. So, for the first time, researchers can simulate networks using models and parameters that have been derived from data and statistically evaluated for goodness of fit.

Roots in Epidemiology

Epidemiologists had a tradition of modeling infectious disease spread through "structured populations" well before the explicit connection was made to social network analysis. The spatial spread of infections was an early focus, with models for the dynamics of childhood disease transmission among families, neighborhoods, schools and playgroups, epidemics on islands, and pandemics spreading through the network of airline routes. The models for wildlife disease transmission, especially rabies, were built around small interacting subgroups connected by occasional long jump migrations, anticipating the "small world" models in the recent physics literature.

Simple network-like models for sexually transmitted pathogens began to be developed in the late 1970s and early 1980s when, despite the relative availability of penicillin, gonorrhea and syphilis rates rose precipitously in the United States. The surveys of STI clinic patients in the late 1970s found that repeat cases contributed disproportionately to the total caseload: A total of 3% to 7% of the infected persons accounted for about 30% of the cases. Simulation studies showed that this group can act as a "reservoir," allowing an infection to persist in a population where the average level of activity is otherwise too low to allow for sustained transmission. This research led to the "core group" theory: If endemic persistence is due to this small core group, then all cases are caused directly or indirectly by the core. The core group thus came to be seen as the primary driving force in STIs, and also as the locus for highly effective intervention targeting. But concerns began to be raised about the limitations of the core group concept with the emergence of generalized HIV epidemics in the countries of sub-Saharan Africa.

The first explicit link between social network methods and STI dynamics was made by Alden Klovdahl in 1985. His paper was written before the virus that causes AIDS had been identified, and the mechanism of transmission had not been conclusively demonstrated. A large number of theoretical and empirical studies have since followed that use network concepts and methods to help understand the different patterns of HIV spread in different countries, the disparities in infection prevalence within countries, the behaviors that increase exposure risk, and the opportunities for prevention. At their best, network models help us understand the population-level implications of individual behavior: How the choices that individuals make link together and aggregate up to create the partnership network that either inhibits or facilitates transmission.

What Have We Learned?

Network methods are beginning to be used in a number of communicable disease contexts, including studies of the most effective intervention strategies for containing the spread of pandemic influenza (H5N1, the "avian (bird) flu"), containing the impact of bioterrorist attacks with agents such as smallpox, and reducing the spread of bovine spongiform encephalitis across farms. The most intensive use of the methods, however, is in the field of STI, and that is where the most detailed lessons have been learned.

Using network analysis, researchers have identified two basic behavioral patterns that have a large impact on the STI transmission network: selective mixing and partnership timing. Both are guided by norms that influence individual behavior, which in turn create partnership network structures that leave distinctive signatures on transmission dynamics and prevalence. Selective mixing is about how we choose partners: How many partnerships form within and between groups defined by things such as age, race, and sexual orientation. Assortative mixing leads to segregated networks that channel infection and can sustain long-term prevalence differentials, such as the persistent racial differentials observed in the United States. Partnership timing is about the dynamics of relationships: Monogamy requires partnerships to be strictly sequential, concurrency allows a new partnership to begin while an existing partnership is still active. Long-term monogamous pair formation slows down the rate of disease transmission, as concordant pairs provide no opportunity for spread, and discordant pairs remain together after transmission has occurred. Concurrent partnerships, in contrast, can dramatically amplify the speed of transmission.

Partnership networks also have other structural features that can be important for STI spread, including closed cycles (e.g., the triangles and odd-numbered cycles that can emerge in same-sex networks, and larger even-numbered cycles for heterosexual networks) and highly skewed distributions for the number of sexual partners.

Small differences in the pattern of contacts can have huge effects on the transmission network structure. An average increase of only 0.2 concurrent partners can be enough to fundamentally change the connectivity of a network and create a robust connected network core. This is important to remember when evaluating the significance of empirical differences in sample data. Most samples are not large enough to detect a difference this small as statistically significant, but the difference may still be substantively important. The good news is that, just as small changes may be enough to push transmission above the epidemic threshold in some groups, small changes may be all that are needed to bring transmission down below the threshold.

Persistent prevalence disparities across populations for a wide range of infectious diseases are a signal that the underlying transmission network is probably the cause. A combination of processes may be at work: assortative mixing (which segregates populations) and small variations in concurrent partnerships (which differentially raises the spread in some groups). The disparities that can be sustained in such networks can be surprisingly large, even when the behaviors do not appear to differ much by group. For this reason, it is important that we have an accurate empirical picture of the key aspects of the transmission network. We need to know what behavior needs to change, who needs to change it, and the relevant cultural contexts, so that our intervention efforts can be properly targeted and maximally effective.

—*Martina Morris*

See also Outbreak Investigation; Partner Notification; Sexually Transmitted Diseases

Further Readings

Borgatti, S., Everett, M., & Freeman, L. (1999). *UCINET (Version 5)*. Harvard, MA: Analytic Technologies.
Fischer, C. S. (1982). *To dwell among friends: Personal networks in town and city*. Chicago: University of Chicago Press.
Handcock, M. S., Hunter, D. R., Butts, C. T., Goodreau, S. M., & Morris, M. (2003). *Statnet: Software tools for the representation, visualization, analysis and simulation of social network data (Version 1.11)*. Seattle, WA: Center for Studies in Demography and Ecology, University of Washington.
Hethcote, H., & Yorke, J. A. (1984). *Gonorrhea transmission dynamics and control*. Berlin, Germany: Springer Verlag.
Kaplan, E. H., Craft, D. L., & Wein, D. L. (2003). Emergency response to a smallpox attack: The case for mass vaccination. *Proceedings of the National Academy Sciences, 99*, 10395–10440.
Klovdahl, A. S. (1985). Social networks and the spread of infectious diseases: The AIDS example. *Social Science & Medicine, 21*(11), 1203–1216.
Koehly, L., Goodreau, S., & Morris, M. (2004). Exponential family models for sampled and census network data. *Sociological Methodology, 34*, 241–270.
Longini, I. M., Jr., Nizam, A., Xu, S., Ungchusak, K., Hanshaoworakul, W., Cummings, D. A., et al. (2005). Containing pandemic influenza at the source. *Science, 309*(5737), 1083–1087.
Morris, M. (Ed.). (2004). *Network epidemiology: A handbook for survey design and data collection*. Oxford, UK: Oxford University Press.
Snijders, T. A. B. (2002). Markov Chain Monte Carlo estimation of exponential random graph models [Electronic version]. *Journal of Social Structure, 3*(2). Retrieved from http://citeseer.ist.psu.edu/snijders02markov.html.
St. John, R., & Curran, J. (1978). Epidemiology of gonorrhea. *Sexually transmitted diseases, 5*, 81–82.
Thomas, J. C., & Tucker, M. J. (1996). The development and use of the concept of a sexually transmitted disease core. *Journal of Infectious Diseases, 174*(Suppl. 2), S134–S143.
Thompson, S. K., & Frank, O. (2000). Model-based estimation with link-tracing sampling designs. *Survey Methodology, 26*(1), 87–98.
Wasserman, S., & Faust, K. (1994). *Social network analysis: Methods and applications*. Cambridge, UK: Cambridge University Press.

NEUROEPIDEMIOLOGY

Neuroepidemiology is the application of the methods of epidemiology to the problems of clinical neurology, to study the frequency of neurologic disorders, their risk factors, and their treatments. In addressing the distribution and determinants of neurologic disease in the population, the end goal of neuroepidemiology is to prevent or improve the outcomes of neurologic disease. According to World Health Organization (WHO) data, neuropsychiatric disorders account for more than 10% of the global burden of disease. This entry discusses the unique issues one must address in neuroepidemiological studies; considers neurologic disorders either infectious in nature or common enough to have implications for public health, as well as uncommon disorders that offer important lessons in the study of such conditions; outlines the process of events that must occur for case identification for inclusion in neuroepidemiological studies; and considers important outcome measures evolving in this field.

Special Aspects of Neurologic Conditions

The human nervous system comprises the brain, spinal cord, and peripheral nerves. The brain and spinal cord constitute the central nervous system (CNS) while the remainder of the nervous system, including the lumbosacral and brachial plexus, constitute the peripheral nervous system (PNS). Virtually all bodily functions are controlled or regulated by the nervous system, including motor function, sensation perception, memory, thought, consciousness, and basic survival mechanisms such as regulation of heart rate and rhythms and respirations. As such, dysfunction in the nervous system can present with a vast spectrum of physical signs and symptoms, and the potential to misattribute neurologic disorders to other organ system is considerable.

To understand the complexities of neurologic investigations and disorders one must recognize that CNS tissue does not, as a general rule, regenerate or repair particularly well after insult or injury. Recovery is more likely to be mediated by plasticity in the system that allows alternate pathways to assume functions previously held by dead or damaged regions, and such plasticity is most abundant in infants and children, declining substantially with age. Unlike other organ systems, the CNS relies almost exclusively on glucose for metabolic function. The metabolic rate of the brain is extremely high and very vulnerable to injury if nutrients, such as glucose or oxygen, provided through blood flow are disrupted. Anatomically, the nervous system exists in a separate compartment from the rest of the body, being protected from traumatic injury by bony encasement (skull and spinal column) and from exogenous exposures by the blood-brain barrier and the blood-nerve

barrier. Anatomic localization of injury or dysfunction in the nervous system is the most critical element in determining symptomatology—"Where is the lesion?" is the key mantra physicians address when first assessing a patient with potential neurologic disease, lesion location being one of the most important aspects for the development of a differential diagnosis and ultimately a clinical diagnosis leading to treatment.

Given the nervous system's poor capacity for regeneration, limited plasticity, and anatomic isolation (i.e., encased in the skull and/or spinal column), access to CNS tissue for pathologic diagnosis is often not possible. Since a vast array of physical signs and clinical symptoms can occur as a result of nervous system dysfunction and there is limited opportunity for pathologic diagnosis, expert physician evaluation and/or careful application by trained personnel using validated diagnostic criteria are the most crucial tools for case identification. A worldwide survey of available resources for neurological diagnosis and care conducted by the WHO and the World Federation of Neurology clearly illustrate the devastating lack of health care providers with neurologic expertise in most of the developing world, although developing regions suffer disproportionately from such conditions. Hence, lack of experts either to make the diagnosis or to develop appropriate diagnostic tools for population-based assessment remains a major barrier to neuroepidemiological studies in many regions of the world.

Barriers to Neuroepidemiological Studies

In their excellent textbook on neuroepidemiology, Nelson, Tanner, Van Den Eeden, and McGuire (2003) carefully outline the particular challenges to studying neurologic disorders from an epidemiologic perspective. These include the following:

- The diagnostic criteria vary across studies and over time. The resources-limited settings, particularly those without access to imaging or neurophysiologic studies, will be limited in their application of diagnostic criteria using such technologies.
- The definitive diagnosis may require postmortem examination by a qualified neuropathologist. The proportion of deaths with associated autopsy completion is declining in developed countries, and neuropathologists are nonexistent or very limited in less developed countries.
- The diagnosis during life may require an expert (e.g., neurologist).

- Many neurologic diseases, including infectious disorders with important public health implications, are relatively rare.
- The precise time of disease onset may be uncertain given the insidious onset of some symptoms such as memory loss or weakness.
- There is a long latent period before diagnosis in some diseases, and the duration of this may vary based on the clinical expertise and diagnostic technologies accessible to a person with the condition. Under some circumstances, diagnosis never occurs.
- Intermittent symptoms and signs occur in some diseases.
- Most neurologic diseases are not reportable, even in developed countries, and there are very few neurologic disease registries.

Neurologic Disorders of Particular Relevance to Neuroepidemiology

Some neurologic disorders and their particular relevance to neuroepidemiology are listed in Tables 1, 2, and 3.

Case Identification

Neurologic Symptoms and Patient Interpretation

For case identification to occur during life, persons with the disorder and/or their family members must recognize the symptoms as abnormal and seek care. This may seem trivial, but cultural interpretation of the

Table 1   Neurologic Disorders That Contribute Substantially to the Global Burden of Disease

Disorder	Relevance
Cerebrovascular disease (stroke)	This is responsible for > 10% of the global burden of disease with incidence increasing.
Cerebral palsy	This is a common, chronic disorder originating in childhood with associated motor problems resulting in lifelong disability (Nelson, 2002).
Bacterial meningitis	This is infectious and a common killer of children, especially in Africa's meningitis belt. Many types are preventable with vaccination.
Epilepsy	This is the most common, chronic neurologic disorder in many regions of the world. Despite available treatments, the treatment gap remains > 85% in most of the developing countries. Stigma-mediated morbidity is particularly problematic.
Dementia	This increases substantially in prevalence in developed regions as the average age of the population increases. The improved survival results in longer duration of disability. This is an emerging economic crisis for the United States.
Cognitive impairment from malnutrition	Chronic micronutrient deficiency and protein malnutrition in infancy and early childhood appears to place children at risk for permanent cognitive impairment. The loss of human capital related to lack of basic goods is likely staggering, though poorly quantified.
Cerebral malaria	It kills more than 1 million children annually, most of whom are in Africa. The emerging data confirm that survivors are at risk of neuropsychiatric, neurologic, and cognitive impairments.
Traumatic brain/spinal cord injury	It represents preventable cause of neurologic morbidity and mortality, often among young adults, for most regions of the world.
Headache disorders	These are an important cause for short-term, recurrent disability resulting in loss of productivity and absenteeism from work and/or school. It is associated with substantial decline in health-related quality of life for many affected individuals.

Table 2 Potentially Infectious Disorders With Implications for Public Health

Disorder	Relevance
Bacterial meningitis	This is infectious and a common killer of children, especially in Africa's meningitis belt. Many types are preventable with vaccination.
Epilepsy	This is the most common, chronic neurologic disorder in many regions of the world. Despite available treatments, the treatment gap remains >85% in most of the developing countries. Stigma-mediated morbidity is particularly problematic.
Cerebral malaria	This kills more than 1 million children annually, most of whom are in Africa. The emerging data confirm that survivors are at risk of neuropsychiatric, neurologic, and cognitive impairments.
Tetanus	This is common in developing countries due to unvaccinated mothers and inappropriate care of the umbilical cord in the neonate. This is a potentially preventable cause of mortality for those under 5 years of age.
New variant Creutzfeldt Jacob Disease (nvCJD)	This is a fatal neurodegenerative disorder, primarily among young adults related to ingestion of infected meat—a human illness resulting from the bovine epidemic of "mad cow disease." This is a prion-related infection.
Amyolateral sclerosis Parkinsonism dementia (ALS/PD) complex of Guam	This is an epidemic of fatal neurodegenerative disease not previously described that occurred in the Chamorro population of Guam. The etiology remains unclear, and the epidemic appears to be resolving or evolving (Wiederholt, 1999).
Kuru	This is a prion-medicated infectious disorder identified among the tribes of Papua New Guinea. Intense epidemiologic and anthropologic investigations identified traditional burial preparations involving aspects of cannibalism as the cause of this epidemic. Reviewing the history of the kuru epidemic and the associated investigations offers many "lessons" for neuroepidemiologists today.
CJD	This is a rapidly progressive neurodegenerative dementia with variable other features that may be genetic and/or infectious in nature. Rare but with the potential to spread through inappropriate sterilization of biopsy equipment or tissue handling.

symptoms of events such as seizures may affect where care is sought. In developing regions, seizures may be interpreted as the result of witchcraft or spiritual possession and care may be sought from traditional healers and/or clerics. Partial seizures with psychic phenomena (e.g., intense fear) that are not accompanied by generalized tonic-clonic seizures may be misinterpreted as psychiatric symptoms. Individuals with recurrent severe headaches may self-treat with over-the-counter medications and never seek formal medical care, particularly if the patient has limited access to medical treatment. Care for intermittent symptoms from conditions such as multiple sclerosis (MS) may be deferred or delayed until disability occurs, and this will result in prevalence skewed toward individuals with better access to care and a prognosis that is apparently worse for those from a lower socioeconomic status or regions geographically distant from advanced diagnostic services. When reviewing neuroepidemiologic data for different subpopulations, one should consider how early symptoms might be interpreted (or misinterpreted) by the population under study.

Health Care Provider Expertise

Even if someone suffering from nervous system dysfunction seeks physician-level care, the neurologic knowledge and expertise of the physician may determine whether or how rapidly a diagnosis is made. In the United States, many medical schools do not require graduating students to complete a rotation in clinical neurology. In developing regions, there may be no neurologist available to train medical students and postgraduates in training. The level of health care

Table 3 Conditions Often Under Epidemiologic Study for Etiologic and Prognostic Data

Condition	Relevance
Traumatic brain/spinal cord injury	This represents preventable cause of neurologic morbidity and mortality, often among young adults, for most regions of the world.
Parkinson's complex of Guam	This is an epidemic of fatal neurodegenerative disease not previously described that occurred in the Chamorro population of Guam. The etiology remains unclear, and the epidemic appears to be resolving or evolving.
Kuru	This is a prion-medicated infectious disorder identified among the tribes of Papua New Guinea. Intense epidemiologic and anthropologic investigations identified traditional burial preparations involving aspects of cannibalism as the cause of this epidemic. Reviewing the history of the kuru epidemic and the associated investigations offers many "lessons" for neuroepidemiologists today.
CJD	This is a rapidly progressive neurodegenerative dementia with variable other features that may be genetic and/or infectious in nature. Rare but with the potential to spread through inappropriate sterilization of biopsy equipment or tissue handling.
Multiple sclerosis	This is a chronic inflammatory disorder involving demyelination of the CNS. It is common among neurologic disorders. Usually nonfatal, but may result in substantial disability among people during their biologically and economically productive lifetime. The etiology remains unclear.
Parkinson's disease	This is a chronic, progressive neurodegenerative disorder characterized by motor abnormalities, including tremor. It is relatively common among neurologic disorders. The etiology remains unclear.
Amyolateral sclerosis (ALS)	This results in progressive loss of motor neurons resulting in progressive weakness with bulbar and respiratory weakness, usually resulting in death within ~1 year unless ventilatory support is provided. The etiology remains unclear.
Primary brain tumors	Tumor type and location are generally age dependent. Data are available through cancer registries. The etiology usually is unknown.

provider expertise is likely especially important in diagnosing uncommon conditions (e.g., Creutzfeldt-Jakob disease [CJD]) or uncommon presentations of common conditions (e.g., partial seizure disorder without secondary generalization).

Diagnostic Testing

The array of diagnostic testing available to provide supportive and confirmatory data of neurologic disorders is substantial, but these cannot be used as a substitute for clinical expertise. The conduct and interpretation of such studies requires additional expertise and are subject to misapplication in the wrong hands. Common diagnostic tests used in more developed regions are noted below. Further details are available on the Web site listed at the end of this entry.

Neuroimaging

The anatomic details of abnormalities in the CNS can often be identified by computed axial tomography—the CT scan. The CT scans offer good clarity for acute blood and bone pathology, but imaging of the lower brain (i.e., the brainstem region) and acute ischemia cannot be seen. The CT scan has the advantage of being rapid and relatively inexpensive compared with magnetic resonance imaging (MRI). MRI provides much more detailed information regarding the state of soft tissue and is the preferred imaging modality for cord lesions and acute stroke. Vascular anatomy, based on blood flow, can also be viewed. Vascular anatomy can also be assessed with Doppler technology. The WHO atlas provides details as to the availability of these imaging modalities in various regions of the world.

Electrophysiologic Tests

Brain function and the potential propensity for seizure activity as well as subtyping of seizure disorders into various syndromes may be facilitated with the use of electroencephalography (EEG). An EEG involves placement of recording electrodes on the scalp with amplifiers used to record brain activity in the cortical neurons accessible to this surface. This is a relatively cheap and noninvasive test, but requires substantial expertise for interpretation, especially among children. Inexperienced physicians have a propensity to report false-positive abnormalities in normal records.

The function of peripheral nerves, the spinal cord, and brain stem function can be assessed by various methods in which stimuli (electrical, visual, or auditory) are provided peripherally and a more central/proximal response to the stimuli is recorded. Examples include visual evoked responses, bilateral auditory evoked responses, and somatosensory evoked potentials. The peripheral nerve function is also assessed through nerve conduction velocities measured along the peripheral neuroaxis.

Muscle abnormalities may be investigated by electromyography, which involves the insertion of very fine needles into muscle and recording the background activity and activity changes that occur with activation. The clinical and epidemiological values of essentially all neurophysiologic studies heavily depend on the expertise of the technician and the interpreting clinician.

Cerebrospinal Fluid and Other Laboratory Analysis

The presence of the blood-brain and blood-nerve barriers limit the capacity of routine serum and blood work to provide information on the state of the nervous system. Cerebrospinal fluid (CSF) can be obtained, however, through a relatively noninvasive and generally safe procedure—the lumbar puncture (sometimes referred to as a spinal tap). Theoretically, most physicians should be able to perform a spinal tap but patient reluctance to undergo the procedure and physician inexperience can result in limited CSF data or delayed diagnoses. Basic laboratory tests, such as a Gram stain or cell count are almost universally available in laboratories, even in developing regions. More sophisticated tests, for example, the 14-3-3 protein used in the diagnosis of CJD, usually have to be sent to central research or university laboratories. The stability of assessments on CSF samples that have been stored and shipped is often unknown.

Complex Diagnostic Criteria

For research purposes, clear diagnostic criteria are necessary and many neurologic disorders use fairly complex clinical diagnostic criteria. The application of such complex criteria will depend on the expertise of the assessor as well as availability of diagnostic tests. For population-based studies, screening instruments are often used to identify potential cases that are then referred on to more advanced expertise for second-level assessment. In such cases, the screening tool should be designed to provide a low false negative, high false positive rate (i.e., more sensitive, less specific). The validity of such screens, and of the associated diagnostic criteria against the "gold standard," ideally should be available. Screens and assessments that include patient reports of symptoms (i.e., most screens and assessments) should be validated in the culture and language in use.

Other Outcome Measures

Mortality

For some neurologic disorders, simply "counting" bodies is probably sufficient for understanding the incidence of the disease. Rapidly progressive, fatal conditions such as CJD exemplify this. But if progression is very rapid, and/or autopsy data are limited, the diagnosis of rapidly progressive, fatal neurologic conditions is likely to be missed, especially in regions with limited resources and expertise.

Functional Status

For chronic and disabling conditions, such as MS, mortality data will provide little information about the epidemiology of the disease. The measures of disability such as the Barthel Index or Kurtkze's Disability Scale are more useful for this purpose. An array of neurological scales are available for use within both pediatric and adult populations and have been detailed in Herndon's textbook of neurological rating scales.

Health-Related Quality of Life (HRQOL)

The trends in more patient-oriented outcome measures (i.e., outcomes that matter to the patient!) have led to the development of various instruments to assess HRQOL based on patient-reported data of symptoms and impact of symptoms on their lives. Generic measures applicable to most conditions include the SF-36® (short form 36), a 36-item questionnaire. Many neurologic disorders also have a disease-specific instrument already developed and validated in many populations. For example, the QOLIE-89 (quality of life in epilepsy) includes the SF-36® plus 53 additional, epilepsy-specific items. Although HRQOL measures are not often used as the primary outcome in clinical trials, these measures provide important additional data regarding disease severity, treatment effects, and prognosis among people with chronic neurologic disorders and should be of substantial interest to those working in neuroepidemiology.

—Gretchen L. Birbeck

See also Psychiatric Epidemiology; Quality of Life, Quantification of; Screening; SF-36® Health Survey

Further Readings

Batchelor, T., & Cudkowicz, M. (Eds.). (2001). *Principles of neuroepidemiology*. Woburn, MA: Butterworth-Heinemann.

Bergen, D. C. (1998). Preventable neurological diseases worldwide. *Neuroepidemiology, 17*(2), 67–73.

Herndon, R. (2006). *Handbook of neurologic rating scales* (2nd ed.). New York: Demos Medical.

Nelson, K. B. (2002). The epidemiology of cerebral palsy in term infants. *Mental Retardation and Developmental Disabilities Research Reviews, 8*(3), 146–150.

Nelson, L. M., Tanner, C. M., Van Den Eeden, S., & McGuire, V. M. (Eds.). (2003). *Neuroepidemiology: From principles to practice*. Oxford, UK: Oxford University Press.

World Health Organization. (2004). *Atlas: Country resources for neurological disorders 2004*. Geneva: Author.

Wiederholt, W. C. (1999). Neuroepidemiologic research initiatives on Guam: Past and present. *Neuroepidemiology, 18*(6), 279–291.

Web Sites

Details on common diagnostic tests used in more developed regions can be accessed at http://www.merck.com/mrkshared/mmanual/section14/chapter165/165d.jsp.

NEWBORN SCREENING PROGRAMS

Newborn screening for disease is a highly effective public health effort to prevent the consequences of certain diseases in affected newborns. Through testing of blood samples from and administration of hearing tests to newborn infants, targeted diseases are detected very early, often before manifestations of diseases are evident, enabling rapid initiation of treatment of these diseases. This entry summarizes the mechanism of screening, the diseases screened, and the treatment of some of these diseases and highlights the potential of newborn screening for identification and control of other health problems.

Newborn screening comprises a system through which a laboratory, public or private, processes a newborn blood specimen to detect the possible presence of a disease in the infant. The newborn screen blood sample is usually obtained by a health care provider, typically a hospital nurse. The blood sample is placed on a special newborn screening card, the blood is dried, and the card is then transported to the testing laboratory. If the test is normal, the results are sent to the infant's health care provider and the testing is complete; if the test is abnormal, newborn screening programs follow-up measures ensure that the infant with a positive result enters into treatment for the disease. These steps include notification of the infant's physician and family of the positive screening result; obtaining a specimen for a second screening test; and, if the second screen is positive, a visit to a clinical specialist for diagnostic testing (the laboratory screening test typically detects an elevation in a substance that can occasionally be temporary and not indicative of actual disease). Finally, if the diagnostic test indicates the presence of a disease, the infant undergoes the therapeutic treatment recommended by existing clinical standards for the specific disease typically by a specialist trained to care for the specific disorder.

All 50 states and the territories perform screening tests of newborn blood specimens to detect diseases for which a treatment prevents the medical complications of untreated disease. With improvements in testing technology, most newborn screening programs are now expanding the number of disorders for which screening is done. This entry discusses the development of newborn screening, the current expansion of the programs, and the potential for future newborn screening.

Historical Background

Following the rediscovery of Mendel's genetic principles at the beginning of the 20th century, medical practitioners began to recognize that many human diseases are genetic. Throughout the early part of the century, an understanding of the principles of genetics advanced. Subsequent advances included the identification of deoxyribonucleic acid (DNA) as the genetic material; the delineation of the molecular structure of DNA by Watson and Crick in 1953; and, at the end of the century, completion of the draft sequence of the human genome.

Hand in hand with these advances in genetics were advances in biochemistry. It became clear that while DNA contained the information for life, biochemical pathways and molecules produced from genetic material were the engine of this information. If there is an alteration in genetic information, this typically results in a biochemical disturbance.

In 1902, Sir Archibald Garrod noticed that patients with a disease he called alkaptonuria excreted excessive amounts of alkapton (a urinary chemical that turned the urine to a dark color that was later identified as homogentisic acid) into the urine. Based on the pattern of inheritance Garrod recognized as Mendelian (in this case, recessive), he correctly concluded that this disorder represented a genetic alteration in metabolism. The term *inborn errors of metabolism* eventually was coined to describe collectively the diseases of patients with genetic defects in biochemical pathways.

Enzymes perform most of the biochemical reactions in cells. They are proteins whose function is to perform a chemical reaction in which one chemical substance is converted into another. The original chemical is called a substrate, and the end chemical is the product. Research over the century has identified thousands of chemical reactions, and these reactions are mediated by thousands of enzymes. If an enzyme does not function, then the reaction does not occur and substrates for the reaction accumulate and products become deficient. As all enzymes are the products of genes, the presence of defective enzymes usually means an alteration in the genetic information present in the patient.

Following Garrod's initial description, additional inborn errors were identified based on analyses of patient samples. Typically, the substrate for a defective enzymatic reaction accumulates in tissues and blood and is excreted into urine and/or stool where the elevations can be detected by testing. Phenylketonuria (PKU) was recognized as an inborn error in 1934 and determined to be due to elevations of the amino acid phenylalanine due to defective function of the enzyme phenylalanine hydroxylase. Analysis of institutionalized, mentally retarded patients revealed that many of them had PKU. In the 1950s, Dr. Horst Bickel and associates showed that blood levels of phenylalanine could be reduced in PKU patients by a diet low in protein (and, thus, phenylalanine). With reduction of blood phenylalanine levels, many medical symptoms improved. These observations set the stage for newborn screening.

In the early 1960s, motivated in part by a family history of mental retardation, in a son, and phenylketonuria, in a niece, Dr. Robert Guthrie described a method for the detection of elevated blood phenylalanine in blood samples obtained from newborns. He deduced that placement of affected infants on infant formula low in protein would reduce their blood levels of phenylalanine and prevent development of mental retardation. The problem was to identify infants affected with PKU before the onset of symptoms. Guthrie approached public health officials, and policies to screen all newborn infants for PKU were implemented. This effort rapidly spread throughout the United States, and soon all states were screening infants for PKU. Dr. Guthrie's hypothesis regarding early treatment of PKU by a phenylalanine (protein) restricted diet was correct and highly successful in preventing the devastating complications of untreated disease.

Building on the PKU experience, it was soon recognized that other inborn errors could be detected by assays of accumulated compounds or of enzymes in newborn blood and that many of these additional diseases had effective treatments. From the 1960s to the present, the number of disorders identified through newborn screening programs has slowly increased.

Current Screening Procedures

Typically, a newborn screen is obtained from an infant at approximately 24 to 48 hr of age. The heel of the infant is warmed, and a lancet is used to puncture the skin and obtain capillary blood. The drops of blood are placed onto a special filter paper card, and the blood spot is dried. Demographic information is recorded on the card, and it is sent to the screening laboratory.

Once at the laboratory, small circular punches of the dried blood are obtained and processed for analysis. The sample may be tested for chemicals that accumulate due to an enzymatic defect, the activity of a specific enzyme can be assayed, or a protein can be analyzed by biochemical means.

Full testing of the sample usually takes about 2 to 3 days. The results are then compared with laboratory-generated normal values and the result reported to the infant's physician. Typically, the result of the newborn screen is complete when the infant is 7 to 10 days of age. This rapid analysis is necessary as some of the disorders for which screening is done can cause critical illness in the first 2 weeks of life. If there is an abnormality, the physician may need to repeat the newborn screen or move to more definitive testing.

Disorders Detected in Newborn Screening

Within the past decade, the application of tandem mass spectrometry to newborn screening has enabled significant expansion of the number of disorders that can be detected. This has led organizations such as the American College of Medical Genetics and the March of Dimes to propose a panel of disorders in an attempt to expand and unify newborn screening programs in all states. The recommended panel includes 29 disorders, including congenital hearing loss. These 29 disorders are thought to represent disorders for which a favorable treatment exists. They can be broadly grouped into amino acid disorders, organic acid disorders, fatty acid oxidation defects, hormonal disorders, hemoglobinopathies, vitamin disorders, carbohydrate disorders, pulmonary disorders, and congenital hearing loss. Tandem mass spectrometry does enable testing for other disorders for which effective treatments do not yet exist and leaves the decision for testing of these additional disorders to individual states.

Amino Acid Disorders

These disorders include some of the first to be part of routine newborn screening programs. PKU is due to a functional defect in the enzyme phenylalanine hydroxylase. As a result, phenylalanine, which derives from dietary protein, accumulates to high levels and, with time, can cause neurologic damage and ultimately mental retardation. Treatment with a low-protein/phenylalanine diet prevents development of these symptoms.

Maple syrup urine disease is due to a functional defect in the enzyme branched chain α-ketoacid dehydrogenase. Accumulation of the branched chain amino acids leucine, isoleucine, and valine and their respective ketoacids is rapidly damaging to the nervous system. Rapid treatment with a low-protein diet reduces these levels and prevents neurologic damage.

Homocystinuria is due to defective function of the enzyme cystathionine-β-synthase. Elevation of methionine and homocysteine occur and, with time, can damage the eye and blood vessels. A low-protein/methionine diet reduces blood levels and the risk of these complications.

Tyrosinemia Type I is due to dysfunction of the enzyme fumarylacetoacetic acid hydrolase. Damage to the liver occurs within 4 to 6 months and can be prevented with medications and a low-tyrosine diet.

Citrullinemia and argininosuccinic acidemia are urea cycle disorders due to defective function of argininosuccinic acid synthase and lyase, respectively. Severe elevations in blood levels of ammonia result and can damage the nervous system. Institution of a low-protein diet helps lower blood ammonia levels and prevent damage.

Organic Acid Disorders

Organic acid disorders comprise the group providing the largest increase in the number of diseases included in expanded newborn screening programs. Included in the recommended 29 disorders are the following: isovaleric acidemia, glutaric acidemia Type I, 3-hydroxy-3-methylglutaric acidemia, multiple carboxylase deficiency, methymalonic acidemia due to mutase deficiency, cblA and cblB deficiency, 3-methylcrotonyl-CoA carboxylase deficiency, propionic acidemia, and β-ketothiolase deficiency. As a group, they typically present with severe acidosis and neurologic dysfunction. Treatment is effected through institution of a low-protein diet and disease-specific medications.

Fatty Acid Oxidation Defects

The fatty acid oxidation defects are due to defective functioning of enzymes involved in the breakdown of stored fat used for energy production. Typically, they cause symptoms during times of insufficient food intake, but some also cause liver or heart damage without fasting. There are many enzymes in these metabolic processes, including medium chain acyl-CoA dehydrogenase, very long chain acyl-CoA dehydrogenase, long chain 3-hydroxy acyl-CoA dehydrogenase, trifunctional protein, and others. Treatment varies with the individual disorder but in general includes avoidance of fasting and limitation of fat intake.

Hormonal Disorders

Congenital hypothyroidism is one of the most common disorders detected by newborn screening and was the second disorder (following PKU) to be included on a routine basis in newborn screening programs. Insufficient thyroid hormone production by the thyroid gland, whether due to failure of formation of the gland or due to an enzyme defect in the synthesis of hormone, results in mental retardation and poor growth. Treatment with replacement of thyroid hormone is effective in preventing these symptoms.

Congenital adrenal hyperplasia, due to adrenal 21-hydroxylase deficiency, can cause loss of body salts and masculinization of female genitalia. The loss of body salt can be life threatening. Treatment by hormone replacement can reverse the loss of body salt. Treatment of masculinization of the female genitalia may require surgery.

Hemoglobinopathies

Hemoglobin is the oxygen-transporting protein present in red blood cells. Genetic alterations in the structure of hemoglobin may alter its function. One of the most common of these defects, that as a group are called hemoglobinopathies, is sickle-cell anemia. This disorder is common in populations of individuals of African American ancestry and causes anemia and a predisposition to bacterial infection that can be prevented with antibiotics. The newborn screen will also detect other clinically significant hemoglobinopathies such as thalassemia and hemoglobin E.

Vitamin Disorders

Biotinidase is an enzyme involved in preserving the body's levels of the important vitamin biotin. When biotinidase function is defective, the body gradually becomes deficient in biotin, and this deficiency disrupts function of biotin-requiring enzymes. The

symptoms include skin rash, hair loss, seizures, and neurologic damage. Supplementation with biotin prevents these symptoms.

Carbohydrate Disorders

Classic galactosemia is due to a defect in the function of the enzyme galactose-1-phosphate uridyltransferase. Galactose is a sugar found in a variety of foods, especially in dairy foods containing the disaccharide lactose. Defective functioning of galactose-1-phosphate uridyltransferase causes accumulation of galactose, which can damage the liver and the eyes. Restriction of dietary lactose reduces blood levels and prevents this damage.

Pulmonary Disorders

Cystic fibrosis is one of the most common genetic diseases in populations of European ancestry. It is due to a defective function of the cystic fibrosis membrane transconductance regulator. Abnormal movement of water and salts within internal body ducts results in abnormally thick mucous. This thick mucous plugs the ducts of the respiratory, reproduction, and gastrointestinal tracts. This causes damage to the pancreas and the lungs. Identification of affected infants allows early treatment for nutritional and growth problems.

Hearing Loss

Congenital hearing loss is very common, and identification of infants enables interventions to improve speech development. There are many genetic and nongenetic causes of hearing loss in the newborn. Early treatment with speech therapy helps hearing impaired children improve communication skills.

The Future of Newborn Screening

The 29 disorders were recommended for screening because each has some therapeutic intervention that helps prevent development of medical complications. There are, however, many other disorders that could be detected in the newborn screen sample. It is highly likely that testing will be expanded beyond 29 disorders in the future.

The newborn blood sample can contain antibodies that indicate exposure to infectious diseases such as toxoplasmosis, cytomegalovirus, and human immunodeficiency virus. While not genetic diseases, these infectious diseases have important public health considerations that make early identification important. The blood spot may contain substances such as methamphetamine, heroin, and cocaine that would indicate the use of these substances by the mother shortly before delivery. Importantly, the blood sample also contains DNA, the genetic material of the human body. Tests for genetic diseases by analysis of DNA continue to expand at an exponential pace. Potential diseases for testing include certain cancers, Huntington disease, fragile X syndrome, and many other inherited diseases.

Such testing does, however, have ethical and legal risks. Because of public health and legal considerations beyond the medical effects on the infant, such testing would likely require parental informed consent. Additionally, psychological harm may result from knowing in childhood that one is going to develop an untreatable disease in the future, and identification of individuals with a genetic disease may result in discrimination in obtaining health insurance. These are important issues that will need to be resolved by future debate and policy but highlight the testing potential offered by the newborn screen.

—*Randall A. Heidenreich*

See also Genetic Counseling; Genetic Disorders; Mutation; Screening

Further Readings

Guthrie, R. (1992). The origin of newborn screening. *Screening, 1*, 5–15.

Marsden, D., Larson, C., & Levy, H. L. (2006). Newborn screening for metabolic disorders. *Journal of Pediatrics, 148*, 577–584.

Therrell, B. L., Panny, S. R., Davidson, A., Eckman, J., Hannon, W. H., Henson, M. A., et al. (1992). U.S. newborn screening guidelines: Statement of the Council of Regional Networks for Genetic Services. *Screening, 1*, 135–147.

NIGHTINGALE, FLORENCE

(1820–1910)

In the 19th century, Florence Nightingale played a key role in the areas of public health policy, medical statistics, hospital design, and patient care. Stepping over gender stereotypes, she reached beyond the typical role of a nurse by studying statistics, hospital management, philosophy, and sanitation. She was a fan of Edwin Chadwick, a sanitary reformer who was influential in passing England's Public Health Act of 1848. Chadwick's premise was that filth, poor ventilation, and unclean water were the causes of disease development. Each of these factors was present in Scutari (the Greek name for Istanbul, Turkey) during the Crimean War. Nightingale's statistical abilities were apparent in her work there; according to historical documents, approximately a year after her arrival at Scutari in 1854, survival rates improved significantly.

Nightingale was never mentioned in a voluminous post–Crimean War report written by the surgeons who served in the war. Historians attribute their refusal to grant her credit for her accomplishments to their resentment of her obtained power. They argued that her statement that providing hygiene, clean air, and nourishment had beneficial effects on mortality rates was inaccurate; instead, they claimed decreased mortality rates were a consequence of lower nurse-patient ratio after she arrived with more nurses. In spite of her critics, her successes were acknowledged by the creation of the Nightingale Fund as a "thank you" offering from the people of England. The first nonsectarian nursing school was established as a result of the fund. Furthermore, Nightingale is credited for using statistical graphs effectively to make changes in hospitals. She became a Fellow of the Royal Statistical Society in 1858 and an honorary member of the American Statistical Association in 1874. Nightingale's contributions to health statistics and epidemiology are clearly outlined in Table 1.

Nightingale's words reflect the challenge for health care researchers worldwide:

> You can see the power of careful, accurate, statistical information from the way that I used them in my pleas to Government to improve the conditions of ordinary soldiers and of ordinary people. I collected my figures with a purpose in mind, with the idea that they could be used to argue for change. Of what use are statistics if we do not know what to make of them? What we wanted at that time was not so much an accumulation of facts, as to teach the men who are to govern the country the use of statistical facts. (Maindonald & Richardson, 2004, unpaginated)

—*Anne P. Odell*

See also Epidemiology, History of; Public Health, History of; War

Table 1   Modern Hospital Epidemiology Versus 19th Century Hospital Epidemiology

Modern Hospital Epidemiology

Observational Studies	Analytical Studies	Interventional Epidemiology	Prevalence Studies	Results
Frequency of infections in relation to person, time, and place	Cohort studies trials	Random clinical trials	Snapshot in time of infections clinically active	Prevention of catheter-related bloodstream infection
Hypothesis about source, reservoir, mode, and route of transmission	Case-control trials	Evidence-based trials	Efficacy of infection control practices—measured by repeated prevalence studies	Prevention of pneumonia
	Quantifies attributes, morbidity, mortality, and costs			Prevention of surgical site infections
	For future projections and prevention			Control of multiresistant microorganisms

Note: This chart demonstrates the influence of Nightingale's work on modern hospital statistics from the National Center for Nursing Research (1992). The highlighted areas are stemmed from Nightingale's work.

Further Readings

Gill, C. J., & Gill, G. C. (2005). Nightingale in Scutari: Her legacy reexamined. *Clinical Infectious Diseases, 40*(12), 1799–1805.

Maindonald, J., & Richardson, A. M. (2004). This passionate study: A dialogue with Florence Nightingale. [Electronic version]. *Journal of Statistics Education, 12*(1). Retrieved July 19, 2006, from http://www.amstat.org/publications/jse/v12n1/maindonald.html.

Nightingale, F. (with contributions by Mundinger, M. O.), et al. (1999). *Florence Nightingale : Measuring hospital care outcomes.* (Excerpts from the books Notes on matters affecting the health, efficiency, and hospital administration of the British Army founded chiefly on the experience of the late war, and Notes on hospitals.) Oakbrook Terrace, IL: Joint Commission on Accreditation of Healthcare Organizations.

NONPARAMETRIC STATISTICS

Some of the most popular statistical inferential techniques in epidemiological research are those that focus on specific parameters of the population such as the mean and variance. These *parametric statistics* share a number of common assumptions:

- There is independence of observations except when data are paired.
- The set of observations for the outcome (i.e., dependent) variable of interest has been randomly drawn from a normally distributed or bell-shaped population of values.
- The dependent variable is measured on at least an interval-level scale of measurement (i.e., it is rank ordered and has equidistant numbers that share similar meaning).
- The data are drawn from populations having equal variances or spread of scores.
- Hypotheses are formulated about parameters in the population, especially the mean.
- Additional requirements include nominal- or interval-level independent variables, homoscedasticity, and equal cell sizes of at least 30 observations per group.

Examples of commonly used parametric statistical tests include the independent *t* test, the Pearson product-moment correlation, and analysis of variance (ANOVA). These techniques have frequently been used even when the data being analyzed do not adequately meet the assumptions of the given parametric test.

While some parametric tests (e.g., the *t* test) are *robust* in that they can withstand some violations of their assumptions, other tests (e.g., ANCOVA and Repeated Measures ANOVA) are not so flexible. It is extremely important, therefore, that the researchers carefully examine the extent to which their data meet the assumptions of the tests that they are considering. When those assumptions are not met, one option is to use nonparametric statistics instead.

Characteristics of Nonparametric Statistics

There are alternative statistical tests that make fewer assumptions concerning the data being examined. These techniques have been called *distribution free-er* (because many are not entirely free of distributional assumptions) or *nonparametric tests.* Common assumptions for non-parametric tests include the following:

- Like parametric tests, nonparametric tests assume independence of randomly selected observations except when the data are paired.
- Unlike parametric tests, the distribution of values for the dependent variable is not limited to the bell-shaped normal distribution; skewed and unusual distributions are easily accommodated with nonparametric tests.
- When comparing two or more groups using rank tests, the distribution of values within each group should have similar shapes except for their central tendency (e.g., medians).
- There are no restrictions as to the scale of measurement of the dependent variable. Categorical and rank-ordered (ordinal) outcome variables are acceptable.
- The major focus of analysis in nonparametric statistics is on either the rank ordering or frequencies of data; hypotheses, therefore, are most often posed regarding ranks, medians, or frequencies of data.
- The sample sizes are often smaller (e.g., $n \leq 20$).

Types of Nonparametric Tests

There are a wide variety of nonparametric statistical tests that are available in user-friendly computer packages for use in epidemiology. Table 1 summarizes the most commonly used nonparametric tests, their purposes, the type of data suitable for their use, and their parametric equivalents, if any. The following is a brief overview of these statistics. For more details on these and other nonparametric tests as well as instructions on how to generate these statistics in various statistical packages, the interested reader is

Table 1 Commonly Used Nonparametric Tests, Their Purpose, Types of Data Required, and Their Parametric Equivalents

Tests	Nonparametric Test	Level of Measurement of Data		Parametric Equivalent
		Independent Variable	Dependent Variable	
1. *Goodness-of-fit tests* (To determine if the distribution of a data set is similar to that of a hypothesized target population)	Binomial test	—	Nominal (dichotomous)	None
	Chi-square goodness-of–fit test	—	Nominal	None
	Kolmogorov-Smirnov one-sample test	—	Ordinal, interval, or ratio	One-sample *t* test
	Kolmogorov-Smirnov two-sample test	Nominal (dichotomous)	Ordinal, interval, or ratio	Independent *t* test
2. *Tests for two related samples, pretest-posttest measures for single samples* (To identify differences in paired data, e.g., pre-post data for same group of subjects, or subjects matched according to defined criteria)	McNemar test	Paired nominal (dichotomous) data		None
	Wilcoxon signed ranks test	Paired ordinal, interval, or ratio data		Paired *t* test
3. *Repeated measures for more than two time periods or matched conditions* (To evaluate differences in paired data repeated across more than two time periods or matched conditions)	Cochran's *Q* test	Paired nominal (dichotomous) data		None
	Friedman test	Paired ordinal, interval, or ratio data		Within-subjects repeated measures ANOVA

Category	Statistical test			
4. *Tests for differences between two independent groups* (To examine differences between two independent groups)	Fisher exact test	Nominal	Nominal	None
	Chi-square test of independence	Nominal	Nominal	None
	Mann-Whitney U test	Nominal	Ordinal, interval, or ratio	Independent t test
5. *Tests for differences among more than two independent groups* (To compare more than two independent groups)	Chi-square test for independent samples	Nominal	Nominal	None
	Mantel-Haenszel chi-square test for trends	Nominal	Nominal	None
	Kruskal-Wallis one-way ANOVA by ranks test	Nominal	Ordinal, interval, or ratio	One-way ANOVA
6. *Tests of association* (To examine the degree of association, or correlation, between two variables)	Phi coefficient	Nominal (dichotomous)	Nominal (dichotomous)	None
	Cramér's V coefficient	Nominal	Nominal	None
	Point biserial correlation	Ordinal, interval, or ratio	Nominal	None
	Spearman rho rank order correlation	Ordinal, interval, or ratio	Ordinal, interval, or ratio	Pearson r

referred to the texts on nonparametric statistics cited at the end of this entry.

Goodness-of-Fit Tests

Goodness-of-fit tests are used when a researcher has obtained a set of data from a sample and wants to know if this set of data is similar to that of a specified target population. For example, we might want to know whether the distribution of smokers and nonsmokers in a given sample is similar to previously published national norms. We might also be interested in comparing rates of specific cancers from one country with that of another. These types of tests are goodness-of-fit tests because they compare the results obtained from a given sample with a prespecified distribution. Three nonparametric goodness-of-fit tests that are frequently used in epidemiology are the binomial test, the chi-square goodness-of-fit test, and the Kolmogorov-Smirnov one- and two-sample tests.

Binomial Tests

The binomial test uses the binomial distribution to determine the probability that a sample of data with dichotomous outcomes (e.g., smokers vs. nonsmokers) could have come from a population with a prespecified binomial distribution. This test is especially useful when sample sizes are small. All that is required is (1) a dichotomous outcome variable whose values are frequencies, not scores, and (2) knowledge about the expected proportions in the population. There is no parametric alternative to this test.

Chi-Square Goodness-of-Fit Tests

Not all nominal-level variables are dichotomous. For example, the researcher may be interested in comparing the frequencies of different types of cancer in a given sample with what would have been expected given what is known or hypothesized about a target population. The chi-square goodness-of-fit test allows for comparison of actual frequencies of categorical data with those of a population of interest. This very flexible test of frequencies has few assumptions, and because it evaluates nominal-level data, there is no parametric alternative.

Kolmogorov-Smirnov One- and Two-Sample Tests

The Kolmogorov-Smirnov (K-S) one- and two-sample tests allow the researcher to examine whether a set of continuous outcome data (i.e., at least ordinal level of measurement) is similar to a hypothesized set of continuous data with a prespecified distribution (e.g., normal, Poisson, or uniform distributions). To do this, the K-S statistic compares the cumulative distribution of a sample variable with that which would have been expected to occur had the sample been obtained from a theoretical parent distribution (e.g., a Poisson distribution). The one-sample K-S test focuses on a continuous outcome variable (e.g., time to recovery from chemotherapy) and the two-sample test allows for a comparison of the continuous variable between two independent groups (e.g., gender). Technically, the parametric counterparts to the one- and two-sample K-S tests are the one- and two-sample t tests. However, the K-S statistics have the advantage of comparing the cumulative distribution of the sample data with that of a prespecified distribution, not just the measure of central tendency.

Tests for Two Related Samples

In epidemiology, the researcher is often interested in evaluating data that have been collected from a single sample that have been paired through using subjects as their own controls (e.g., pretest, posttest data) or as matched pairs (e.g., subjects matched on age and then randomly assigned to an intervention/control group). The two commonly used nonparametric tests for two related samples are the McNemar and Wilcoxon signed ranks tests.

McNemar Tests

The McNemar test is useful when the researcher has a pretest-posttest design in which subjects are used as their own controls, and the dependent variable is dichotomous. This versatile statistic can be used to determine whether the distribution of a dichotomous outcome variable (e.g., willingness to undergo a colonoscopy: yes or no) changes following an intervention (a colon cancer prevention program). Because the McNemar test is used with dichotomous data, there is no parametric counterpart to this test.

Wilcoxon Signed Ranks Tests

The McNemar test can only determine whether or not a change has occurred from one time period to another; it cannot be used to evaluate the extent of change in a variable. The Wilcoxon signed ranks test is a commonly used statistical test that enables the researcher to assess the extent of change in a continuous variable (e.g., self-efficacy regarding ability to undergo a colonoscopy) across two time periods (e.g., prior to and following a colon cancer prevention program).

The assumptions of the Wilcoxon signed ranks test are fairly liberal. The major requirement is that the continuous data being examined be paired observations that are at least ordinal level of measurement both within and between pairs of observations. The parametric alternative to the Wilcoxon signed ranks test is the paired t test.

Repeated Measures for More Than Two Time Periods

In epidemiological research, we are often interested in repeated observations across more than two time periods, for example, preintervention, postintervention, and follow-up. Two nonparametric tests that can be used to evaluate differences in paired data repeated across more than two time periods or matched conditions are the Cochran's Q test and the Friedman test.

Cochran's Q Tests

Cochran's Q test extends the McNemar test to examine change in a dichotomous variable across more than two observation periods. It is especially appropriate when subjects are used as their own controls and the dichotomous outcome variable (e.g., smoking cessation, yes or no) is measured across multiple time periods or under several types of conditions. Like the McNemar test, Cochran's Q test can only detect whether or not a change has occurred across time, not the extent of that change. It also focuses on change in a single group across time (e.g., the intervention group). Group × time interactions cannot be evaluated using this statistic. There is no parametric alternative to this test.

Friedman Tests

The Friedman test is the preferred nonparametric statistic when the outcome data being evaluated across multiple time periods are continuous (e.g., body weight). This test can also be used to evaluate differences among matched sets of subjects who have been randomly assigned to one of three or more conditions. The Friedman test examines the ranks of the data generated during each time period or condition to determine whether the variables share the same underlying continuous distribution and median. When significant differences are found with this statistic, post hoc tests (e.g., the Wilcoxon signed ranks test) are needed to determine where the specific time differences lie. Because this is a within-subjects test, the Friedman test is not useful for evaluating between-group differences. The parametric equivalent to this test is the within-subjects repeated-measures ANOVA without a comparison group.

Tests for Differences Between Two Independent Groups

In epidemiology, we are often interested in comparing outcomes obtained among groups that are independent of one another, such as an intervention and control group, smokers and nonsmokers, persons with or without cancer. Three nonparametric tests that are available when the independent variable is nominal level of measurement with two mutually exclusive levels are the Fisher exact test, the chi-square test of independence, and the Mann-Whitney U test.

Fisher's Exact Tests

Fisher's exact test is used to evaluate the degree of association between a dichotomous independent and dependent variable (e.g., gender and smoking status). It is especially useful when sample sizes are small (e.g., $n \leq 15$). Because the Fisher exact test deals exclusively with variables that are measured at the nominal level, there is no parametric equivalent to this test. When the sample size is sufficiently large, the chi-square test of independence is typically used.

Chi-Square Test of Independence

The chi-square test of independence (χ^2) is one of the most commonly used nonparametric statistics in epidemiology. It is an easily understood statistic that is used to evaluate the association between two categorical variables that have two or more levels. Because the generated chi-square statistic is an overall test of association, additional tests (e.g., the phi and Cramér's V statistics) are used to evaluate the strength of the relationship between the two categorical variables. Since both the independent and the dependent variables are nominal level of measurement, there is no parametric equivalent to this chi-square test.

Mann-Whitney U Tests

The Mann-Whitney U test is useful when the independent variable is dichotomous, and the continuous dependent variable is measured on at least an ordinal scale. Like its parametric counterpart, the independent *t* test, the Mann-Whitney test compares measures of central tendency between two independent groups (e.g., perceived quality of life in smokers and non-smokers). Unlike the *t* test, the Mann-Whitney test uses medians for comparison, not means. The Mann-Whitney test is almost as powerful as the *t* test, especially when the sample size is small and the outcome data being analyzed are not normally distributed.

Tests for Differences Among More Than Two Independent Groups

In epidemiology, there are often more than two independent groups that are being compared. Subjects may be assigned randomly to more than two intervention conditions, or three or more patient groups having different diagnoses (e.g., type of cancer) may be compared with regard to an outcome variable (e.g., level of fatigue). Three nonparametric tests that may be used given these conditions will be briefly examined below: the chi-square test for *k* independent samples, the Mantel-Haenszel chi-square test, and the Kruskal-Wallis one-way ANOVA by ranks test.

Chi-Square Tests for k Independent Samples

The chi-square test for *k* independent samples (χ^2) is an extension of the chi-square test for two independent samples discussed above except that, with this chi-square statistic, both the independent and the dependent variables are categorical with more than two levels (e.g., the relationship between five levels of racial/ethnic status and four stages of cancer among women with breast cancer). Similar to the previous chi-square statistic, the data consist of frequencies, not scores, and there are no repeated observations or multiple response categories. Once a significant association is determined, the Cramér's *V* statistic is used to assess the strength of the relationship between the two categorical variables. Because it is insensitive to order, this test is not the one of choice when either of the categorical variables has ordered levels. There is no parametric alternative to this test.

Mantel-Haenszel Chi-Square Tests for Trends

It often happens in epidemiological research that the categorical variables being examined have a natural order (e.g., stages of disease, where 1 is the least serious and 4 the most serious) yet are not sufficiently ordinal to be considered continuous variables. Unlike the previous chi-square tests, the Mantel-Haenszel chi-square test for trends takes order into account. It has been used, for example, in case control studies in which there are stratified 2×2 tables, and the researcher is interested in comparing the likelihood of the occurrence of an event (e.g., contracting cancer) given two groups that have been exposed or not exposed to a risk factor (e.g., cigarette smoking) and who have been matched or paired with regard to certain characteristics (e.g., gender or age). Because the variables being examined with this test statistic are categorical, there is no parametric equivalent to this test.

Kruskal-Wallis One-Way ANOVA by Ranks Tests

The Kruskal-Wallis (K-W) one-way ANOVA by ranks is a test that can be used to determine whether *k* independent samples (e.g., stage of cancer) are similar to each other with regard to a continuous outcome variable (e.g., level of fatigue). The K-W test is an extension of the two-sample Mann-Whitney test and is used when the independent variable is categorical with more than two levels and the dependent variable is continuous. When a significant finding is obtained, post hoc tests (e.g., the Mann-Whitney *U* test) are used to determine group differences. The parametric equivalent to the K-W test is the one-way ANOVA. While the ANOVA is more powerful than the K-W test when the assumptions of the ANOVA are met, the K-W test is reported to be more powerful than the ANOVA when the data are skewed or when there are unequal variances.

Tests of Association Between Variables

It frequently occurs in epidemiological research that we are interested in measuring the degree of association or correlation between two variables. Depending on the level of measurement of the two variables being examined, there are a number of nonparametric tests that can provide information about the extent of their relationship. The four commonly used measures of association in epidemiology are the phi and Cramér's *V* coefficients for nominal-level variables, the point biserial correlation for examining the relationship between a dichotomous and a continuous variable, and the Spearman rho rank order correlation coefficient for two continuous variables.

Phi and Cramér's V Coefficients

The phi and Cramér's *V* coefficients are used to evaluate the strength of relationship between two nominal-level variables when the chi-square statistic has been found to be significant. The phi is used when the two nominal-level variables are dichotomous; the Cramér's *V* coefficient is used with nominal-level variables with more than two levels.

Because both statistics take into account sample size, the researcher is able to compare strengths of association across studies. Both coefficients typically range in values between 0 and 1.00 with higher values indicating greater strength of association. Because both coefficients are calculated from the chi-square statistic, the requirements for these coefficients are similar to those for the chi-square statistic. If the contingency table being examined is 2 × 2 and the categories are coded "0" and "1," both coefficients have the same value and are similar to the absolute value of a Pearson correlation. If that is not the case, there is no parametric alternative to these useful tests.

Point Biserial Correlation

Sometimes the researcher is interested in assessing the strength of relationship between an independent variable that is continuous (e.g., number of cigarettes smoked) and a dependent variable that is dichotomous (disease state: lung cancer, no lung cancer). The point biserial correlation is a special case of the parametric Pearson product-moment correlation. It is considered to be nonparametric because one of the variables being assessed is dichotomous. Like the Pearson *r*, the point biserial correlation coefficient can range between −1.0 and +1.0 with higher absolute values indicating a greater strength of relationship between the two variables.

Spearman Rank-Order Correlation

The Spearman rank-order correlation coefficient (also known as *Spearman's rho* or r_s) is one of the best-known and most frequently used nonparametric statistics. It is used to examine the relationship between two continuous variables (e.g., age and level of depression). Its parametric alternative is the Pearson product-moment correlation coefficient.

Like the point biserial correlation, Spearman's rho is a special case of the Pearson *r* but is based on the ranking of observations, not their actual values. This test statistic can range in value between −1.0 and +1.0 with higher absolute values indicating a stronger relationship. The squared values of Spearman's rho offer a reasonable estimate of the strength of the relationship between the two continuous variables of interest.

Conclusion

When making a decision as to whether to use a parametric or nonparametric test, the researcher needs to be aware of the assumptions underlying each test being considered and assess the extent to which the data meet those assumptions. No statistical test is powerful if its assumptions have been seriously violated. Nonparametric statistics are extremely useful analytic tools given their ability to accommodate small sample sizes, categorical and ordinal level data, and unusual sampling distributions. As a result, they offer feasible and potentially powerful solutions to problematic situations.

—*Marjorie A. Pett*

See also Chi-Square Test; Fisher's Exact Test; Logistic Regression; Measures of Association

Further Readings

Conover, W. J. (2003). *Practical nonparametric statistics* (3rd ed.). New York: Wiley.
Daniel, W. W. (2000). *Applied nonparametric statistics.* Boston: PWS-Kent.
Green, S. B., & Salkind, N. J. (2007). *Using SPSS for Windows and Macintosh: Analyzing and understanding data* (5th ed.). Upper Saddle River, NJ: Prentice Hall.
Munro, B. H. (2005). *Statistical methods for health care research* (5th ed.). Philadelphia: Lippincott.
Pett, M. A. (1997). *Nonparametric statistics for health care research: Statistics for small samples and unusual distributions.* Thousand Oaks, CA: Sage.
Sheskin, D. J. (2007). *Handbook of parametric and nonparametric statistical procedures* (4th ed.). New York: Chapman & Hall.
Siegel, S., & Castellan, N. J. (1988). *Nonparametric statistics for the behavioral sciences* (2nd ed.). New York: McGraw-Hill.

Normal Distribution

The normal distribution, also known as Gaussian distribution or "bell-shaped" distribution, is the most widely used distribution in statistical work for both theoretical and practical reasons. It was first introduced by French mathematician Abraham de Moivre in an article in 1734. The name *Gaussian distribution* refers to the German mathematician and scientist Carl Friedrich Gauss, who rigorously applied the distribution to real-life data. This distribution was used in the analysis of errors of experiments during the early 19th century.

The normal distribution is the cornerstone of most statistical estimation and hypothesis testing procedures, and statistical methods used in epidemiology are no exception. Many important random variables in epidemiology and health sciences, such as distribution of birthweights, blood pressure, or cholesterol levels in the general population, tend to approximately follow a normal distribution. Moreover, the central limit theorem provides a theoretical basis for its wide applicability. Many random variables do not have a normal distribution themselves; however, the sample mean of the variable has an approximate normal distribution when the sample size is large enough, and the sampling distribution of the mean is centered at the population mean. The normal distribution is generally more convenient to work with than any other distribution, particularly in hypothesis testing and confidence interval estimation. For example, in linear and nonlinear regression, the error term is often assumed to follow a normal distribution.

Characterization of the Normal Distribution

The normal distribution is fully defined by two parameters, μ and σ^2, through its probability density function as

$$f(x) = \frac{1}{\sqrt{2\pi}\sigma} \exp\left(-\frac{(x-\mu)^2}{2\sigma^2}\right), \quad -\infty < x < +\infty, \quad [1]$$

where μ is the mean parameter and could take any real value and parameter σ^2 is the variance of the normal distribution (equivalently, σ is standard deviation) with $\sigma > 0$. For example, for diastolic blood pressure, the parameters might be $\mu = 80$ mmHg, $\sigma = 10$ mmHg; for birthweight, they might be $\mu = 120$ oz, $\sigma = 20$ oz. Figure 1 shows the plot of the probability density function for a normal distribution with $\mu = 80$ and $\sigma = 10$.

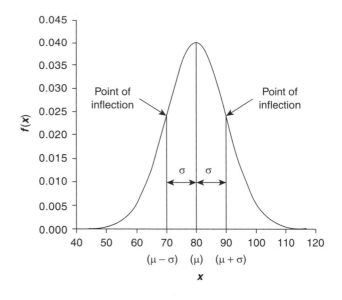

Figure 1   Graphical Illustration of Probability Density Function of Normal Distribution $N(80, 100)$

The density function of the normal distribution resembles a bell-shaped curve, with the mode at μ and the most frequently occurring values around μ. The curve is unimodal and symmetric around μ, and for normal distribution, the mean, median, and mode all equal to μ. The curve has an inflection point on each side of μ at $\mu - \sigma$ and $\mu + \sigma$, respectively. A point of inflection is a point where the slope of the curve changes direction. The distances from μ to points of inflection provide a good visual sense of the magnitude of the parameter σ.

To indicate that a random variable X is normally distributed with mean μ and variable σ^2, we write $X \sim N(\mu, \sigma^2)$. The symbol $\sim$ indicates "is distributed as." The entire shape of the normal distribution is determined by μ and σ^2. The mean μ is a measure of central tendency, while the standard deviation σ is a measure of spread of the distribution. The parameter μ is called the location parameter, and σ^2 is the scale parameter. To see how these parameters affect location and scale, density functions of normal distribution with different means or variances can be compared. For instance, if two normal distributions have different means μ_1 and μ_2 but the same variance σ^2, where $\mu_1 > \mu_2$, then the two density functions will have same shape but the curve with larger mean (μ_1) will be shifted to the right relative to the curve with the smaller mean (μ_2). Figure 2 shows the comparison of

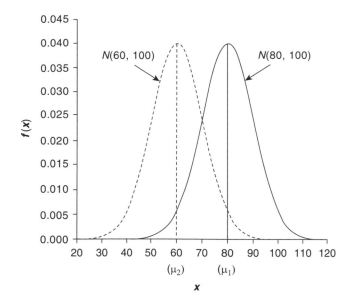

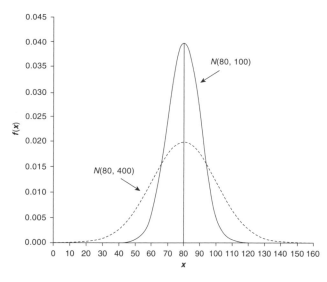

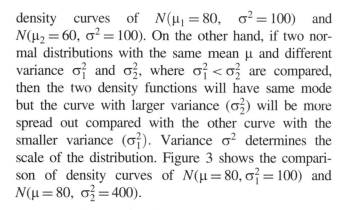

Figure 2 Comparison of Probability Density Function of Normal Distributions $N(80, 100)$ and $N(60, 100)$

Figure 3 Comparison of Probability Density Function of Normal Distributions $N(80, 100)$ and $N(80, 400)$

density curves of $N(\mu_1 = 80, \sigma^2 = 100)$ and $N(\mu_2 = 60, \sigma^2 = 100)$. On the other hand, if two normal distributions with the same mean μ and different variance σ_1^2 and σ_2^2, where $\sigma_1^2 < \sigma_2^2$ are compared, then the two density functions will have same mode but the curve with larger variance (σ_2^2) will be more spread out compared with the other curve with the smaller variance (σ_1^2). Variance σ^2 determines the scale of the distribution. Figure 3 shows the comparison of density curves of $N(\mu = 80, \sigma_1^2 = 100)$ and $N(\mu = 80, \sigma_2^2 = 400)$.

Standard Normal Distribution

A normal distribution with mean 0 and variable 1 is called a standard normal distribution and denoted as $N(0, 1)$. The probability density function in this case reduces to

$$f(x) = \frac{1}{\sqrt{2\pi}} \exp\left(-\frac{x^2}{2}\right), \quad -\infty < x < +\infty. \quad [2]$$

The standard normal distribution is symmetric around 0. The importance of the standard normal distribution is that any normal distribution can be transformed into a standard normal distribution, and tables

for the standard normal distribution are widely available for calculating cumulative probabilities or p values for a Z test. Any normal distribution may be transformed into a standard normal distribution as given by

$$\text{If } X \sim N(\mu, \sigma^2) \text{ and } Z = (X - \mu)/\sigma,$$
$$\text{then } Z \sim N(0, 1). \quad [3]$$

The procedure in Equation 3 is known as standardization of a normal variable.

Cumulative Distribution Function

For a given normal distribution, it is often of interest to calculate the proportion of data falling within a certain range. For example, suppose that in a population, diastolic blood pressure follows a normal distribution with $\mu = 80$ mmHg and $\sigma = 10$ mmHg. People with diastolic blood pressure between 80 and 90 are categorized as prehypertensive; we may want to find the proportion of people in a given population with prehypertension based on diastolic blood pressure. Such proportion is calculated by using the cumulative distribution function (cdf).

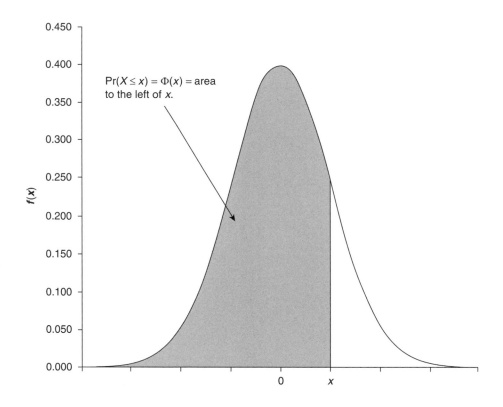

Figure 4   Graphical Illustration of Cumulative Distribution Function $\Phi(x)$ for a Standard Normal Distribution

The cdf for a standard normal distribution is denoted as

$$\Phi(x) = \Pr(X \leq x),   [4]$$

where $X \sim N(0, 1)$, and this function is shown as in Figure 4. Φo$x$pgs the shaded area under the curve, to the left of x. The whole area under the curve is 1. For example, $\Phi(1, 96) = \Pr(X \leq 1.96) = 0.975$. That is, if X follows a standard normal distribution, then 97.5% of the values from this distribution will be less or equal than 1.96. A table for the standard normal distribution is provided in most statistics books, which allows calculation of this type of probability. Many software packages also provide a function to calculate the cdf. For example, $\Pr(X \leq 1.96)$ could be evaluated using function NORMSDIST in EXCEL 2003 as NORMSDIST(1.96) = 0.975.

From the symmetric properties of standard normal distribution, the following relationship exists for cdf (Figure 5):

$$\Phi(-x) = \Pr(X \leq -x) = \Pr(X \geq x)$$
$$= 1 - \Pr(X \leq x) = 1 - \Phi(x).   [5]$$

Furthermore,

$$\Pr(a \leq X \leq b) = \Pr(X \leq b) - \Pr(X \leq a)$$
$$\text{for any values } a < b.   [6]$$

The above formulas provide means to evaluate the probabilities of the standard normal distribution. For any normal distribution $N(\mu, \sigma^2)$, the probabilities would be evaluated by first transforming $N(\mu, \sigma^2)$ into a standard normal distribution. Note that as stated in Equation 3 above, if $X \sim N(\mu, \sigma^2)$, then $Z = (X - \mu)/\sigma \sim N(0, 1)$. Therefore, to find the probability of values between a and b with $a < b$ from the distribution $X \sim N(\mu, \sigma^2)$, use

$$\Pr(a \leq X \leq b) = \Pr\left(\frac{a - \mu}{\sigma} \leq Z \leq \frac{b - \mu}{\sigma}\right)$$
$$= \Pr\left(Z \leq \frac{b - \mu}{\sigma}\right) - \Pr\left(Z \leq \frac{a - \mu}{\sigma}\right).   [7]$$

Recall that the area under the curve is 1 no matter what values μ and σ^2 take on for a given normal distribution. Now, let's go back to the blood pressure example. In a population, diastolic blood pressure

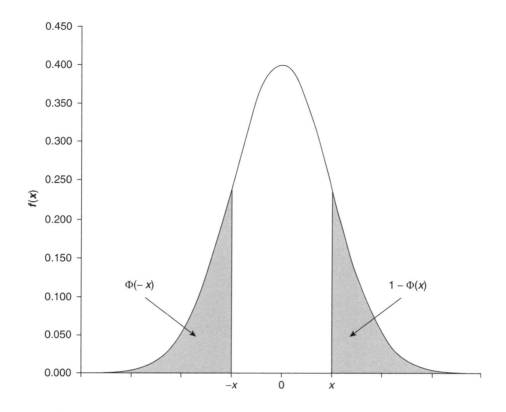

Figure 5   Graphical Illustration of the Symmetry in Cumulative Distribution Function Φ (x) for a Standard Normal Distribution

follows $N(80, 10)$. To calculate the proportion of prehypertensive individuals in this population, use the formula

$$\Pr(80 \leq X < 90) = \Pr\left(\frac{80-80}{10} \leq Z < \frac{90-80}{10}\right)$$
$$= \Pr(0 \leq Z < 1)$$
$$= \Pr(Z < 1) - \Pr(Z \leq 0)$$
$$= 0.50 - 0.16 = 0.34.$$

So about 34% of people are prehypertensive based on diastolic blood pressure with a value between 80 and 90. Note that for any continuous distribution, $\Pr(X \leq x) = \Pr(X < x)$ because the probability of any point is 0.

The cdf can be used to precisely calculate the probability of data falling into any range, given the mean and standard deviation of a data set that follows the normal distribution. But there is an empirical rule that is particularly useful in dealing with normal distributions:

- Approximately 68% of the data will fall within a standard deviation of the mean.
- Approximately 95% of the data will fall within 2 standard deviations of the mean.
- About 99% and 99.7% of the data will fall within 2.5 and 3 standard deviations of the mean.

The above empirical rule provides a handy quick estimate of the spread of the data and is quite useful in practice.

—*Rongwei (Rochelle) Fu*

See also Central Limit Theorem; Confidence Interval; Hypothesis Testing; Sampling Distribution

Further Readings

Casella, G., & Berger, R. L. (2001). *Statistical inference* (2nd ed.). Belmont, CA: Duxbury Press.

Krishnamoorthy, K. (2006). *Handbook of statistical distributions with applications.* Boca Raton, FL: Chapman & Hall.

Patel, J. K., & Read, C. B. (1996). *Handbook of the normal distribution* (2nd ed.). New York: Marcel Dekker.

Rosner, B. (2006). *Fundamentals of biostatistics* (6th ed.). Belmont, CA: Thomson Brooks/Cole.

NOTIFIABLE DISEASE

Notifiable diseases are those for which regular collection of case information is deemed necessary in preventing and controlling the spread of disease among the population. State and local officials have the authority to mandate diseases reporting within their jurisdictions. Nationally notifiable diseases are suggested by the Council of State and Territorial Epidemiologists (CSTE); participation by states and territories in the National Notifiable Disease Surveillance System (NNDSS) is voluntary.

History

To prevent the introduction and subsequent spread of cholera, smallpox, plague, and yellow fever in the United States, in 1887 the Congress authorized the U.S. Marine Hospital Service, now the Public Health Service (PHS), to collect case data from overseas consuls. The collection of information on these first four notifiable diseases was expanded to include cases in the Unites States in 1893. Until the 1950s, state and territorial health authorities worked with the PHS to designate additional notifiable diseases. The first annual summary of notifiable disease, published in 1912, included reports from 19 states, the District of Columbia, and Hawaii for 10 infectious diseases.

By 1928, 29 diseases were being reported by all states, the District of Columbia, Hawaii, and Puerto Rico. In 1951, the CSTE was formed and became responsible for designating diseases to be included in the NNDSS. That year, 41 infectious diseases were nationally notifiable.

Traditionally, notifiable diseases were infectious diseases. However, in 1995 the first noninfectious condition, elevated blood-lead levels, was added to the NNDSS. The following year the first risk factor, cigarette smoking, was added. In 2006, more than 60 diseases and conditions were nationally notifiable.

Local, National, and International Notifiable Diseases

While CSTE suggests nationally notifiable diseases, it does not have the authority to require states' participation in the NNDSS. Within its jurisdictions, states and territories have the authority to designate which diseases must be reported. Based on the needs and resources of each region, local notifiable diseases lists may exclude diseases included in the NNDSS and include diseases not surveilled nationally. Notifiable disease lists are not static; diseases are added or removed based on current public health needs. Notifiable diseases may be classified on the urgency of reporting and assigned varying time requirements. Generally, physicians and diagnostic laboratories are responsible for reporting cases to local health authorities who, in additional to immediate control and prevention activities, report cases to the state health departments.

All states and territories are required to report cases of cholera, plague, yellow fever, and other quarantinable diseases of international concern. Internationally reportable diseases are dictated by the International Health Regulations set forth by the World Health Organization.

—*Michelle Kirian*

See also Centers for Disease Control and Prevention; Council of State and Territorial Epidemiologists; Public Health Surveillance

Further Readings

Centers for Disease Control and Prevention. (2006, January). *National Notifiable Diseases Surveillance System.* Retrieved November 6, 2006, from http://www.cdc.gov/EPO/DPHSI/nndsshis.htm.
World Health Organization. (2006). *Epidemic and Pandemic Alert and Response (EPR): International Health Regulations (IHR).* Retrieved November 8, 2006, from http://www.who.int/csr/ihr/en.

Web Sites

Council of State and Territorial Epidemiologists: http://www.cste.org.

NULL AND ALTERNATIVE HYPOTHESES

Stating null and alternative hypotheses has become one of the basic cornerstones of conducting epidemiological research. A hypothesis is typically defined as a tentative proposal or statement that explains certain observations or facts and is testable by further investigation. Testing hypotheses allows researchers to assess scientifically whether the explanation in question can be falsified. Critical to this process is the idea that, in research, it can never be directly proven that a proposition is true. To do so would imply that the results of a single study would hold across all time, all persons, and all cultures. Therefore, falsification of the null hypothesis has become the basis of scientific investigation as currently practiced.

Researchers approach the idea of "truth" indirectly by developing and testing null and alternative hypotheses. Typically, null and alternative hypotheses are stated so that they are mutually exclusive and exhaustive. The null hypothesis, written as H_0, is the statement that the researcher hopes to reject. Specifically, it is a claim about a population parameter that is assumed to be true until it is declared false. Many times, but not always, the null hypothesis represents a null effect (i.e., there is no relationship between the independent and dependent variable). For example, in a cohort study examining tobacco use and lung cancer, the H_0 might be that smoking status is *not* significantly associated with the development of lung cancer. The alternative hypothesis, denoted as H_A or H_1, is the basic statement that is tested in the research; in the tobacco study example, the H_A might be that smoking status *is* significantly associated with the development of lung cancer. After stating the null and alternative hypotheses, researchers aim to find evidence to reject the null hypothesis; otherwise, they would state that they "failed to reject" the null. If researchers do find enough evidence to reject the null hypothesis, they still might not be able to theoretically "accept" the alternative hypothesis. This is because, in theory, the methods of hypothesis testing are probabilistic, and by definition, probability includes some level of uncertainty. This idea is similar to the guilty/not guilty decision in our judicial system. In finding a defendant not guilty, the jury determines that there is insufficient evidence to find the person guilty; this is not the same as claiming that he or she is innocent. However, in practice, when researchers reject the null hypothesis in their study, they generally do "accept" the alternative at least under the conditions of their specific experiment.

Because hypotheses are developed to be testable, they must be stated in a clear, unambiguous manner. The alternative hypothesis might describe a relationship with a specific direction (e.g., $\mu \geq 100$ or "smoking status is positively associated with the development of lung cancer") or could relate to the statistical test being employed (e.g., the odds ratio $\neq 1$ or $\beta \neq 0$).

Conversely, the null hypothesis could indicate no effect (e.g., smoking status is not associated with the development of lung cancer or $\beta = 0$) or could describe the opposite direction of what researchers are investigating (e.g., $\mu < 100$). It is important to note that when writing null or alternative hypotheses, the population parameters (e.g., μ or p) are used instead of the sample statistics (e.g., $\bar{x}$ or $\hat{p}$) since researchers aim to make inferences to the population level.

History of Hypothesis Testing

The concept of hypothesis testing became institutionalized in research in the mid-1950s. In addition to being influenced by philosophers of science such as Karl Popper, the current hypothesis testing process has incorporated two approaches, the Fisher approach to null hypothesis testing and Neyman-Pearson decision theory. The original Fisher approach calls for the researcher to set a statistical null hypothesis and to report the exact level of significance (e.g., $p = .05$). This approach does not state a specific alternative hypothesis and was suggested only when researchers know little about the problem at hand. Building off Fisher's approach, the Neyman-Pearson theory indicates that two hypotheses are created and a choice must be made. In this approach, two statistical hypotheses are developed and α, β, and sample size are decided before the study begins. If study findings fall into the rejection region of the first hypothesis, then there appears to be more solid evidence to support the second hypothesis. The problem is that this approach puts the researcher at risk for making two types of error solely on the basis of the data. The first—and most egregious—is a Type I or an α (alpha) error, which occurs when the researcher decides to reject the null hypothesis when it is actually true. The value of α represents the probability of committing this type of error. The other type of error—a Type II or β (beta) error—occurs when the null hypothesis should be rejected but is not.

Critiques of Hypothesis Testing

While hypothesis testing remains an essential component of epidemiologic research, there are several criticisms of the method. Depending on how the hypotheses are stated, hypothesis testing may not provide any information on the magnitude or direction of the relationship. Evidence for whether to reject or not reject the null hypothesis may also be highly sensitive to sample size and significance level (α) that was set. Most important, researchers should never use statistics mechanically. Past literature, clinical meaningfulness, and study rigor should all be carefully considered when conducting studies to test hypotheses. Additionally, to minimize problems in hypothesis testing, researchers should develop clear, testable hypotheses and report effect size and confidence intervals when discussing study results.

—*Lisa S. Wolff*

See also Significance Testing; Study Design; Type I and Type II Errors

Further Readings

Bohrnstedt, G. W., & Knoke, D. (1988). *Statistics for social data analysis.* Itasca, IL: F. E. Peacock.

Goodman, S. N. (1999). Toward evidence-based medical statistics. 1: The *P* value fallacy. *Annals of Internal Medicine, 130*(12), 995–1004.

Mann, P. S. (2001). *Introductory statistics.* New York: Wiley.

Nickerson, R. S. (2000). Null hypothesis significance testing: A review of an old and continuing controversy. *Psychological Methods, 5*(2), 241–301.

Rothman, K. J. (2002). *Epidemiology: An introduction.* New York: Oxford University Press.

NUTRITIONAL EPIDEMIOLOGY

Although observations on relationships between diet and health have always been recognized, the systematic science of nutritional epidemiology in populations is relatively recent. Important observations propelling the field of nutrition forward were numerous in the 18th and 19th centuries, as it was recognized that deficiencies in certain classes of foods led to important diseases such as scurvy, rickets, pellagra, and beriberi. This was followed by the rapid sequential discovery of the vitamins in the early 20th century. Since then, the focus of diet and health has shifted to include the problems of obesity and the role of diet on chronic disease risk. Just as the parent field of epidemiology is defined as the investigation of the frequency, distribution, and risk factors influencing disease in populations, nutritional epidemiology may be defined as the frequency and distribution of nutrition-related diseases

as well as the relation of nutritional intake and status to disease outcomes.

Nutrition Monitoring and Surveillance

The systematic quantification of nutritional status with population surveys has been done only relatively recently. Early surveys in the United States, such as the Ten-State Nutrition Survey released by the U.S. Centers for Disease Control in 1971, identified stunted growth associated with insufficient food in low-income groups. Such results led President Johnson to declare a "War on Hunger" in the United States in 1966. In the relatively short time since then, food availability has changed rapidly with associated changes in nutritional risk, such that we have gone from substantial undernutrition to a current epidemic of obesity in all income categories. At the same time, heart disease and cancer have escalated as the major diseases contributing to mortality as we have made progress against deficiency and infectious disease. Fortunately, these changes have been well documented at the national level with the representative U.S. Department of Agriculture Continuous Survey of Food Intake of Individuals and the U.S. Department of Health and Human Services National Health and Nutrition Examination Surveys (NHANES) that have been conducted periodically since 1970. These have now been combined into the Continuous NHANES, which is released for public use in 2-year cycles.

With the encouragement of the World Health Organization, nutritional surveillance activities are now also implemented in many developing countries. These include organized community weighing programs, school entry height measurements, and the addition of nutrition modules to existing national surveys to provide data that document trends in nutritional status and support policy decisions to target and improve identified nutrition problems.

Diet and Health

A central focus of nutritional epidemiology is to inform dietary recommendations by clarifying the role of food and nutrient intake to the risk of health outcomes. Early work in this area began from ecological observations that there were large differences in the prevalence of differing chronic diseases across countries with differing food patterns. For example, death rates from heart disease or colon cancer have been shown to be positively associated with higher-than-average fat intakes across countries. However, such an association does not necessarily imply a causal relationship—particularly in such ecologic observations, as numerous other exposures differ across countries. Migration studies, documenting change in risk associated with the movement of groups from their native country to a new environment, provide further evidence of the importance of environmental exposures, as opposed to genetic variation, in disease risk. Central among these are changes in diets, adding more evidence for several diet and health relationships.

However, the relationship between behavior and nutritional status or nutrition and health is complex—chronic diseases, in particular, are due to a constellation of factors. The omnipresent possibility of alternative explanations precludes the ability to prove causality in observational nutritional epidemiology. To infer likelihood of causality, the criteria developed by Austin Bradford Hill (1897–1991), a British statistician, are followed. They include temporal relationship (a risk factor must precede the onset of disease), strength of statistical association, evidence of dose-response, consistency of the relationship across studies and population groups, biological plausibility, and careful consideration of possible alternative explanations.

Several of these criteria are challenging to fulfill in studies of diet and disease. For rare diseases, such as most cancers, the case-control design is usually used. Dietary intake and other exposures must be recalled by patients and/or their proxies as well as by matched controls. Although these studies have provided considerable information on likely dietary risk factors, concern about the likelihood of recall bias must always be considered. Longitudinal cohort studies offer several benefits in that the exposure—diet and nutritional status—may be measured prior to the development of the disease, providing evidence of temporality and avoiding much of the reporting bias. Such studies, including the Harvard University Nurses and Male Health Professionals Health Studies and the Framingham Heart Study, among others, have provided a tremendous amount of information that has improved our understanding of the central role that dietary intake plays in protecting health and preventing chronic disease. Although such large studies are few because of their high cost, they continue to provide exciting results.

Collinearity across foods and nutrients is another limitation in identifying causal associations between specific nutrients and disease outcomes. For example, diets that are high in fat are often also low in fruit and vegetables and associated nutrients. Therefore, it becomes difficult to tease out the effects of any single nutrient. Furthermore, the discovery of the importance of numerous chemical constituents in food and of interactions across nutrients, in combination with the failure of several large vitamin supplementation trials to show benefit, has increased the understanding that whole foods rather than single nutrients appear to be most protective. In response to this, dietary patterns research, looking at the total diet defined by computer algorithms based either on the correlation matrix of individual food group intakes (factor analysis) or the spatial distance across food group intakes (cluster analysis) has emerged as a complementary way of confirming the importance of diet on health.

All dietary methods suffer from random error due to day-to-day variation and imprecision in reporting. This has the tendency to attenuate correlations and relative risk estimates in relation to the true associations. Advances in assessment methodology and in statistical approach, including improved understanding of measurement error, have improved the ability to estimate associations and to adjust for alternative explanations.

Although nutritional epidemiology holds much in common with other branches of epidemiology, it poses unique challenges. In particular, the measurement and interpretation of dietary exposures require careful consideration in the design, implementation, and analysis. Much work during recent decades has been devoted to the measurement, validation, and interpretation of error in dietary assessment.

Dietary Exposures

Dietary intake is a complex exposure that includes a nearly infinite mix of foods, portion sizes, and preparations. Exposures of interest may include foods themselves, or more commonly, nutrients. These include total energy; macronutrients such as total fat, saturated fat, and carbohydrate; micronutrients such as vitamins and minerals; and more recently, a variety of phytochemicals in foods. The validity of any of these measures depends on the quality and availability of a precise nutrition database of food composition. The U.S. Department of Agriculture provides this information based on chemical analysis of foods.

However, constant changes in the food supply and demand for additional nutrients mean that this must be continually updated, and database inadequacies remain an important limitation for work in nutritional epidemiology in many countries.

The methods of dietary assessment in common use each have advantages and disadvantages. Short-term methods include weighed dietary records, where individuals are either observed or asked to record their own food intakes, using dietary scales to weigh portions before and any waste after consumption to get accurate quantitative measures of actual intake. This method provides good quantitative data, but it requires either that researchers observe intakes or that participants themselves record detailed intake data, and this may lead to selection bias. In addition, the attention given to food intake during the implementation of this method has shown that individuals tend to consume less than they usually do—either because of the work involved in the measurement itself or because of their heightened awareness of their intake. A second popular method is the 24-hr dietary recall. Either in person or by telephone, a trained interviewer asks individuals to recall what they ate and drank the previous day. The studies comparing reported with observed intakes have shown good validity for this method, although a tendency to underreporting persists, due to some forgotten foods and underestimation of portion sizes. Improvements in the method include the use of portion-size visuals to improve quantity estimation, and a multiple pass approach to improve completeness. Using the multiple pass approach, individuals are asked to recall their intake in a series of steps that begins with a quick list of foods consumed, followed by reviews that probe for forgotten foods, define eating occasion and time, and complete detailed information on preparation and portion size.

These methods provide valuable data for population intakes, including detailed information on specific foods used, preparation methods, meal patterns, the times of day that foods are consumed, and how foods are consumed together. As such, they continue to be used in national surveys for the purpose of nutrition monitoring and comparison of intakes by population subgroups. However, they have the distinct disadvantage of misclassifying individuals in relation to their usual intake, thereby attenuating the ability to relate dietary intake to health outcomes at the individual level. Because individuals consume differing types and quantities of foods on any given day relative to another, a single day, or even a few days, of intake may misrepresent usual exposure. The likelihood of misclassification varies by nutrient and by the complexity in the diet. The random error associated with this day-to-day variation has been quantified in numerous studies. Based on the ratio of within- (day-to-day) to between-person variation in intake, the number of days of intake needed for a stable estimate can be calculated. For energy and macronutrients, where habit and individual regulation of intake are more direct, a few days may be sufficient. The same is true for micronutrients or food substances present in specific foods that tend to be consumed (or not) regularly in the dietary pattern of the population, such as calcium from milk or caffeine from coffee. On the other hand, obtaining information on consumption of micronutrients that are irregularly distributed in foods that are consumed less frequently, such as vitamin A (very high in liver, and green leafy vegetables, but low in most foods) may require so large a number of days as to be practically infeasible.

For this reason, longer-term methods of usual intake tend to be favored in nutritional epidemiology. Food frequency questionnaires consist of a detailed food list. Subjects are asked to respond to a set of frequency options for each food-line item, which may include groups of foods that are nutritionally similar (such as "green leafy vegetables such as spinach, kale, and collard greens"). Frequency options generally range from never or less than once per month to more than once per day. By linking these responses to a specially designed nutrient database, nutrient intakes can be calculated. Some food frequency questionnaires rely only on frequency responses to calculate nutrients, while others add questions on usual portion size to further quantify exposures. Additional refinements—such as added questions on low fat versus regular versions of specific foods or specific type of breakfast cereal used—are often added to further improve estimation. It has been recognized that certain categories of foods, such as fruits and vegetables, may be overestimated when a long list of items is presented. Therefore, most questionnaires calibrate total fruit and vegetable intake with a summary question on the number of servings of these foods typically consumed per day. Statistical adjustment for total energy intake is generally conducted when examining nutrient intake to outcome measures. This realigns the ranked data on individual foods or nutrients to partially adjust for differences in total food intake due to differing individual energy requirements, and also tends to correct some of the distortion that may otherwise occur by assuming standard portion sizes.

Validation work comparing such questionnaires with multiple dietary recalls and, more recently, to biomarkers, has generally supported their utility in nutritional epidemiologic research. They have been shown to rank individuals reasonably well with respect to comparison measures of intake—either multiple dietary records or recalls, or biomarkers. Their great advantage is their relatively low cost. However, they also have important limitations. Because of the grouping of foods and lack of information on specific preparations, as well as on actual portion size, the resulting estimation of nutrient intake is only semiquantitative and depends on assumptions included in the associated nutrient database. Recent comparisons with recovery biomarkers—which accurately capture the body's processing of energy or specific nutrients, and thus serve as objective measures of intake—have questioned the validity of food frequency questionnaires for estimating total energy and protein intakes. Furthermore, the food list and assumed preparation of foods will be valid only for the general population for which it was developed. As such, subgroups in the population or other populations with differing dietary patterns may be seriously misrepresented by standard instruments.

Anthropometric Measures

Nutritional status itself may be either an outcome or an exposure in nutritional epidemiology. Stunting and wasting in children and wasting in adults under conditions of severe food shortages remain important outcomes in nutritional epidemiology in underdeveloped countries, and these continue to be studied in relation to the proximal risk factors, food intake and infectious disease, as well as more distal economic and social factors. Measures of undernutrition have been defined for children by the World Health Organization based on growth standards developed with a healthy U.S. population. In addition to measures of relative weight for age, weight for height, and height for age, measures of upper arm circumference and head circumference are frequently used as indicators of inadequate growth and nutritional status.

On the other hand, the prevalence of obesity is increasing rapidly throughout the world. Accepted measures of obesity are based on body mass index (BMI; height in meters/square of weight in kilograms; m/kg^2)

of > 30 for adults. BMI cutoff values for children have been published by the U.S. Centers for Disease Control and Prevention, based on data from U.S. children, by age and sex group, as measured in national surveys prior to the recent increase in childhood obesity. Obesity is used both as an outcome measure of concern on its own and as a risk factor for many additional health outcomes. Numerous studies have identified obesity as a risk factor for type 2 diabetes, heart disease, and several cancers. There has also been an increasing understanding that fat deposited in the abdomen may pose greater health risks than fat deposited elsewhere in the body, because these fat cells are more metabolically active, releasing inflammatory hormones and fatty acids that negatively affect glucose metabolism, blood pressure regulation, and triglyceride production. Waist circumference has, therefore, emerged as an important measure of disease risk, with current cutoff values for risk as >88 cm for women and >102 cm for men.

Biochemical Indicators

Nutritional status may also be measured with biochemical indicators, or biomarkers, from body tissues—most frequently from plasma, serum, or urine. Iron status, for example, is a common nutrient for which laboratory tests provide accurate assessments. Biomarkers may also be used as indicators of dietary intake and, as such, are used to validate dietary methods. However, the translation of dietary intake into biomarkers is affected by several factors unique to each nutrient, including absorption and conditions of metabolism and homeostatic regulation, and it may be further affected by other factors such as medications, nutrient interactions, and smoking. For some nutrients, such as folate, there is usually a clear relationship between dietary intake and blood concentration, suggesting that either measure may be used to assess status. Others, such as calcium, are tightly regulated by homeostatic mechanisms that maintain blood concentrations within a narrow band. Therefore, usual dietary intake will be a better measure than blood measures. Some nutrients, such as plasma vitamins K, are metabolized rapidly in the blood and represent only recent intake, while others, such as serum ferritin, represent long-term stores.

Unfortunately, reliable biomarkers of dietary intake do not currently exist for most nutrients. Recovery biomarkers that have made important contributions to advancing the field include doubly labeled water for energy intake and urinary nitrogen for protein intake. Several blood nutrient measures correlate well with intake. These include folate, vitamin B_6, K, C, E, and carotenoids. The blood concentrations of others, such as vitamin A, are regulated and therefore show insufficient variation to relate to diet except at the extremes. Another, vitamin B_{12}, often does not relate well to dietary intake, due to large individual variation in absorption. For some nutrients, functional indicators rather than direct indicators may be more useful. For example, methylmalonic acid—a product of a metabolic reaction that requires vitamin B_{12}—provides a useful measure of vitamin B_{12} status.

The wealth of information that has resulted from nutritional epidemiology studies over recent decades has made major contributions to our understanding of the central importance of good dietary intake patterns to our health—influencing national dietary guidelines and policy, food industry regulation and product formulation, and individual behavior. The field continues to evolve, with improved methodology. Emerging work highlights the important role of genetic variation in defining effects of dietary exposures on individual disease risk with the promise of exciting new findings and more specific individual dietary prescriptions for health—nutritgenomics—in the relatively near future.

—Katherine L. Tucker

See also Gene-Environment Interaction; Hill's Considerations for Causal Inference; Malnutrition, Measurement of; Obesity; Study Design

Further Readings

Bingham, S. A. (2002). Biomarkers in nutritional epidemiology. *Public Health Nutrition, 5,* 821–827.

Briefel, R. R. (1994). Assessment of the U.S. diet in national nutrition surveys: National collaborative efforts and NHANES. *American Journal of Clinical Nutrition, 59,* 164S–167S.

Flegal, K. M., Wei, R., & Ogden, C. (2002). Weight-for-stature compared with body mass index-for-age growth charts for the United States from the Centers for Disease Control and Prevention. *American Journal of Clinical Nutrition, 75,* 761–766.

Frasier, G. E. (2003). A search for truth in dietary epidemiology. *American Journal of Clinical Nutrition, 78,* 521S–525S.

Gibson, R. (2005). *Principles of nutritional assessment.* New York: Oxford University Press.

Jacques, P. F., & Tucker, K. L. (2001). Are dietary patterns useful for understanding the role of diet in chronic disease? *American Journal of Clinical Nutrition, 73,* 1–2.

Kaaks, R., Ferrari, P., Ciampi, A., Plummer, M., & Riboli, E. (2002). Uses and limitations of statistical accounting for random error correlations in the validation of dietary questionnaire assessments. *Public Health Nutrition, 5,* 969–976.

Margetts, B. M., & Nelson, M. (Eds.). (1991). *Design concepts in nutritional epidemiology.* New York: Oxford University Press.

Mason, J. B., & Mitchel, J. T. (1983). Nutritional surveillance. *Bulletin of the World Health Organization, 61,* 745–755.

Ordovas, J. (2006). The quest for cardiovascular health in the genomic era: Nutrigenetics and plasma lipoproteins. *Proceedings of the Nutrition Society, 63,* 145–152.

Willett, W. (1998). *Nutritional epidemiology.* New York: Oxford University Press.

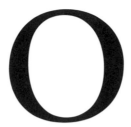

OBESITY

During the final two decades of the 20th century, a dramatic increase in the prevalence of obesity occurred in the United States and in many developed and developing countries throughout the world. By the end of the 20th century, there were more than 1 billion overweight adults worldwide, among whom more than 300 million were obese. Obesity had become a significant contributor to the global burden of chronic disease and disability and a major public health issue. The rising rates among children were a particular concern. This entry considers the definition and epidemiology of obesity, its health consequences, the causes of obesity, and efforts to address it through public policy.

Definition

Obesity is defined as increased body weight related to excess accumulation of body fat. The term commonly refers to a range of weight above that which is considered healthy for a given height. A simple and widely used method for estimating body fat, the body mass index (BMI), or Quetelet index, is calculated by dividing weight in kilograms by the square of height in meters (BMI = kg/m^2). BMI does not measure body fat directly but correlates with direct measures of body fat, such as underwater weighing and dual-energy X-ray absorptiometry (DXA).

The current BMI categories for adults 20 years and older published by the U.S. National Heart, Lung, and Blood Institute (NHLBI) of the National Institutes of Health is similar to the classification used by the World Health Organization (WHO) (see Table 1). The primary BMI cutoff points for excess weight occur at 25, 30, and 40 kg/m^2. Obesity is defined as a BMI of 30 or more.

For children and adolescents, BMI is plotted on national growth charts developed by the U.S. Centers for Disease Control and Prevention (CDC) to obtain percentile rankings among children of the same sex and age in the United States. The CDC and the American Academy of Pediatrics (AAP) recommend the use of BMI to screen for overweight in children and adolescents aged 2 to 19 years. Health advocates prefer the term *overweight* over *obese* to avoid the potential stigma of the label in this age group. The CDC BMI-for-age weight status categories for children and adolescents are provided in Table 2.

As a simple and inexpensive method for measuring relative weight, BMI cannot distinguish between

Table 1 Weight Status Categories for Adults Aged 20 Years and Older

Weight Status	Obesity Class	BMI (kg/m²)
Underweight		<18.5
Healthy weight		18.5–24.9
Overweight		25.0–29.9
Obesity	I	30.0–34.9
	II	35.0–39.9
Extreme obesity	III	≥40.0

Source: U.S. National Institutes of Health.

Table 2   Weight Status Categories for Children and Adolescents Aged 2 to 19

Weight Status	Percentile Range
Underweight	Less than the 5th percentile
Healthy weight	5th percentile to less than the 85th percentile
At risk of overweight	85th to less than the 95th percentile
Overweight	Equal to or greater than the 95th percentile

Source: U.S. Centers for Disease Control and Prevention.

increased weight for height due to body fat from that attributable to fat-free mass (muscle, bone, and fluids). Thus, BMI may lead to overestimates of adiposity in athletes, for example. More direct methods of estimating body fat include skinfold thickness, ultrasound, computed tomography, and magnetic resonance imaging (MRI).

Among adults, the NHLBI guidelines recommend assessing two additional predictors of potential health risks associated with overweight and obesity, in addition to BMI. These are waist circumference, as abdominal fat is associated with greater health risk, and also other risk factors and comorbidities associated with obesity, such as high blood pressure and physical inactivity. Both absolute waist circumference and waist-to-hip ratio are used to assess central obesity, also known as "apple-shaped" or "masculine" obesity, in which the main fat deposits are stored around the abdomen and upper body.

Epidemiology

Obesity became a leading global public health concern by the end of the 20th century. In the United States, obesity prevalence among adults aged 20 years or older doubled between 1980 and 2002. By 2003 to 2004, an estimated 66.3% of U.S. adults were either overweight or obese, including 32.2% who were classified as obese. During the final two decades of the 20th century, obesity rates among adults increased threefold or more in parts of the United Kingdom, Eastern Europe, the Middle East, the Pacific Islands, Australasia, and China. In developing countries, excess body fat may often paradoxically coexist with undernutrition. While global recognition of the growing public health problem did not occur until the end of the 20th century, by 2002, obesity was considered the sixth most important risk factor contributing to the overall burden of disease worldwide. At least 1.1 billion adults worldwide were classified as overweight or obese, including 312 million who were obese.

The burden of obesity is not evenly distributed throughout populations. Obesity tends to be higher among women, the poor, and racial/ethnic minorities. Regional differences may also be observed. For example, some Asian countries have low overall rates of obesity but relatively high rates of central obesity, with the accompanying excess risks of diabetes and cardiovascular disease.

Among children and adolescents aged 6 to 19 years in the United States, obesity prevalence tripled between 1980 and 2002. By 2003 to 2004, an estimated 33.6% of U.S. children and adolescents aged 2 to 19 years were at risk of overweight or overweight, including 17.1% who were overweight. Globally, 10% of children were at risk of overweight or overweight by 2002.

Health Risks and Consequences

The growing rates of overweight and obesity became a major public health concern because of the elevated health risks associated with excess body weight. Obesity is related to a higher prevalence of intermediate metabolic consequences and risk factors, such as high blood pressure, elevated triglycerides (blood fat), decreased HDL cholesterol ("good cholesterol"), and the so-called metabolic syndrome, defined in the United States as three of five features: large waist circumference, abnormal concentrations of triglycerides, HDL cholesterol, fasting glucose, and hypertension. Obesity is also associated with several health outcomes, including type 2 diabetes, coronary heart disease, stroke, osteoarthritis, sleep apnea and respiratory problems, and some cancers, including endometrial, colon, gall bladder, prostate, kidney, and postmenopausal breast cancer.

Overweight and obesity are also associated with premature deaths. In the United States, an estimated 300,000 deaths per year can reportedly be attributed to obesity, which would make it second only to smoking as the main preventable cause of illness and premature death. Mortality appears to increase on a continuum with increasing body weight, with a small increase in risk in those with a low BMI (below 20 or 22 kg/m^2) and a greater increase in those with a BMI above 30 kg/m^2.

Among children and adolescents, weight-related health consequences are expected to continue to increase in the coming years. Cardiovascular risk factors, such as high blood pressure and high cholesterol, are becoming increasingly common in this group, while "adult" diseases, such as type 2 diabetes, have increased dramatically among overweight adolescents. Other health conditions related to overweight among children and adolescents include asthma, sleep apnea, and nonalcoholic fatty liver disease. The most immediate consequences for overweight children are probably psychosocial, including social discrimination, decreased self-esteem, and decreased quality of life. Overweight children have an increased chance of becoming overweight or obese adults, with the accompanying health risks.

Causes and Solutions

Obesity is a consequence of excess energy (caloric) intake over total daily energy expenditure. While genes are important determinants of individuals' susceptibility to weight gain, energy balance results from the complex interactions between genetic, biological, psychological, behavioral, sociocultural, and environmental factors that affect both energy intake and expenditure.

While the exact causes remain uncertain for the increase in obesity rates among U.S. children, adolescents, and adults, several societal trends may be implicated. Nutritional patterns changed in recent decades as both parents entered the workforce, more meals were eaten outside the home, and marketing by the food industry increased the consumption of take-out foods and larger portion sizes. Levels of physical activity declined as the use of automobiles, television, computers, and mechanical aids increased. Changes to the physical design of communities, such as the increase in urban sprawl, created further barriers to physical activity. In poor communities and nonwhite communities, neighborhood safety and the lack of recreational facilities, supermarkets, and healthy food outlets present additional barriers to physical activity and healthy eating.

Likewise, the increase in obesity in other parts of the world may have been fueled by modernization, urbanization, and the globalization of food markets.

Many developing countries are undergoing the nutrition transition toward increased consumption of energy-dense foods high in saturated fats and sugars, coupled with reduced physical activity. Fetal undernutrition followed by rapid childhood weight gain may contribute to the development of insulin resistance and the metabolic syndrome, a pattern observable in developing countries such as India and China.

Growing concern over the rising prevalence of obesity in the population overall and in children, in particular, has prompted increasing programmatic and policy responses at the local, national, and international levels. Government initiatives have included funding programs for after-school activities, removal of vending machines in schools, nutritional labeling of food products, and walking initiatives. Further efforts that engage multiple sectors, including government, industry, media, health systems, workplaces, schools, communities, and families will be needed to stem the tide of the obesity epidemic.

—*Helen L. Kwon*

See also Body Mass Index (BMI); Cardiovascular Disease; Chronic Disease Epidemiology; Diabetes; Urban Sprawl

Further Readings

Hedley, A. A., Ogden, C. L., Johnson, C. J., Carroll, M. D., Curtin, L. R., Flegal, K. M. (2004). Prevalence of overweight and obesity among US children, adolescents, and adults, 1999–2002. *Journal of the American Medical Association, 291*(23), 2847–2850.

Institute of Medicine. (2005). *Preventing childhood obesity: Health in the balance.* Washington, DC: National Academies Press.

U.S. Centers for Disease Control and Prevention. (n.d.). *Overweight and obesity.* Retrieved September 22, 2005, from http://www.cdc.gov/nccdphp/dnpa/obesity/index.htm.

U.S. Department of Health and Human Services. (2001). *The Surgeon General's call to action to prevent and decrease overweight and obesity.* Rockville, MD: Author.

World Health Organization. (2003). Diet, nutrition and the prevention of chronic diseases. In *Technical report series 916.* Geneva, Switzerland: Author.

OBSERVATIONAL STUDIES

Observational epidemiology refers to the branch of epidemiology devoted to using nonexperimental studies to describe the health status of populations and generate evidence about determinants of health outcomes. Experimental designs in epidemiology, generally referred to as clinical trials, involve assignment of the principal independent variable, the "treatment," to subjects. Often this assignment is randomly allocated, which offers profound advantages for making causal inferences, but it can also be nonrandom. In observational studies, the investigators do not assign treatment to subjects. The principal independent variable is some endogenous or exogenous exposure observed as it naturally occurred. When observational epidemiologic studies are designed to draw inferences about health outcome across different exposure groups, they are considered "analytic." When they are intended only to describe the frequency of a risk factor or disease in a population, they are considered "descriptive." However, the line between descriptive and analytic observational epidemiologic studies is often blurred as descriptive studies typically contrast disease frequency endpoints across population subgroups, and analytic studies can also report on the absolute frequency of disease or exposure in the population sample under study. This entry describes cohort studies, case-control studies, cross-sectional studies, and ecologic studies and discusses the problem of confounding and ways in which it can be addressed.

There are fundamental challenges in making causal inferences about associations between exposures and diseases based on evidence from observational epidemiologic studies. In any analytic epidemiologic study, the goal is to estimate average causal effects in groups (i.e., we do not scrutinize individual participants, subject by subject, to see if in each case there is biological evidence linking exposure and disease). Because there is no way to observe the average disease experience of the exposed group under conditions of no-exposure (the "counterfactual" condition), estimating the average causal effect of exposure is done by comparing the disease experience of the exposed group with that of a different group of individuals without exposure. Consequently, the fundamental challenge to valid estimation of these effects is the similarity of these groups (or their "exchangeability"). Here, randomization is a great help because study groups that are randomly assigned to exposed versus unexposed status will, on average, be similar. However, when exposed and unexposed groups are merely observed as they occur

in nature, it is extremely unlikely that they will be similar. If the groups differ on factors other than exposure that are associated with disease risk, estimated associations between exposure and disease will be confounded. Minimization of the influence of confounding is, consequently, critical to success in observational epidemiologic studies.

Types of Observational Studies

Analytic observational studies with individuals as the unit of analysis are generally categorized into three types: cohort studies, case-control studies, and cross-sectional studies. Observational studies correlating only group-level information on risk factors and outcomes are ecologic studies.

Cohort Studies

Cohort studies entail the follow-up of populations or population samples for incident disease endpoints. Exposure status is characterized at baseline and is commonly also tracked for change over time. Follow-up can occur coincident with calendar time (prospective or concurrent cohort studies) or, retrospectively, where disease status on the cohort members is known at the time the study is initiated and available data sources are used to "assemble" and characterize exposure in the cohort at baseline and is followed forward to the present (retrospective or nonconcurrent cohort studies). In cohort studies, analyses are based on contrasting disease experience in exposure groups. The approach of contrasting disease experience can be based on cumulative incidence, incidence rates, or time-to-event. Methods have been developed and are widely available to account for censoring—the loss of the ability to follow study subjects either at the start (late-entry or left censoring) or end (right censoring) of follow-up. Similarly, analyses of cohort data can be based on current or cumulative exposure at baseline and can consider time-varying exposure over the course of follow-up.

Case-Control Studies

Case-control studies are retrospective studies that involve sampling conditional on disease status. A sample of cases, typically incident cases, is selected, as is a sample of noncases (controls) drawn from the same population giving rise to cases. Matching of controls to cases on potential confounders is a commonly used design feature in case-control studies. The measure of association between exposure and disease is based on a comparison of the odds of exposure in cases and controls. Because the case-control design is retrospective and involves sampling of controls, it tends to be less resource intensive than the cohort design that involves follow-up of large number of subjects. However, the process of selection of the case and control groups can introduce bias, as can any misclassification arising from the retrospective nature of exposure assessment. Cohort studies are by no means immune to selection and information biases but, because of their design, case-control studies typically require extra efforts to protect against bias.

The case-control design has been adapted for implementation within prospective cohort studies. Here, cases that arise during follow-up of the cohort make up the case group, and controls are either a sample of noncases matched on time of case diagnosis (the nested case-control study) or a sample of the entire cohort enrolled at the start of the study (the case-cohort design). These approaches take advantage of the prospective data collection and follow-up of the cohort design and economize by requiring exposure assessment only on cases and controls as opposed to the entire cohort. This is particularly useful in investigations involving costly biomarkers of exposure. Nested case-control studies are analyzed with conventional matched methods, and a range of more specialized techniques has been developed for case-cohort studies. Other adaptations of the case-control design also exist, with the most notable being the case-crossover study. This design is particularly well-suited for the study of trigger exposures—that is, those exposures occurring proximate to disease such as car phone use prior to automobile accidents or physical exertion prior to myocardial infarction. In the case-crossover study, exposure in cases is assessed during a short time window preceding disease onset. Rather than comparing this exposure experience with that of an independent control group as one would do in a conventional case-control study, it is contrasted with the exposure experience during a different time window within each case. Under this design, each case essentially serves as its own control, thus limiting the possibility of confounding by factors that are fixed or change slowly over time.

Cross-Sectional Studies

A cross-sectional study is based on a study sample taken at a particular point in time, with outcome and exposure data assessed simultaneously. This design is distinct from a case-control design in that there is no sampling conditional on disease status and no focus on incident disease, and there tends to be less effort to develop retrospective data on exposures. The cross-sectional study is most appropriately used in descriptive epidemiology to generate estimates of prevalence of health outcomes and risk factors in the population. Causal inference based on correlation of these cross-sectional measures is vulnerable not only to confounding but to a number of other major biases (e.g., incidence prevalence bias, reverse causation bias).

Ecologic Studies

Finally, observational studies that correlate data on risk factors and outcomes measured only at the group level are referred to as ecologic studies. Because the actual outcome status of individuals with particular exposure status is not known in these designs, they have been criticized as being subject to bias (referred to as ecologic fallacy) in making inferences about individual-level associations between risk factors and outcomes. However, associations between group-level variables can be important tools in evaluating community health. For example, there can be a true negative association between socioeconomic status and a disease occurrence at the individual level within communities, but across communities the group-level association between average socioeconomic status and average disease risk can be positive. If the individual-level data were used to anticipate the direction of the group-level association, inference would be biased (the atomistic or individualistic fallacy). Understanding the mechanisms behind individual and group-level associations can be quite informative in the planning of public health interventions. Multilevel analysis is the approach taken in studies designed to simultaneously assess the effect of both individual and group-level variables on individual outcomes.

The Challenge of Confounding

As mentioned, the principal threat to validity of causal inference in analytic observational epidemiology studies conducted at the individual level is confounding.

When designing observational studies, considerable attention needs to be placed on strategies for confounder control. This process should begin with careful consideration of the causal model underlying the outcome under study. Directed acyclic graphs, diagrams linking variables by arrows representing direct causal effects that also illustrate the underlying causal determinants of observed statistical associations, are being used increasingly by epidemiologists as a tool to help understand the fairly complex confounding structures that can arise even when as few as two or three potential confounders are under consideration. Options available for confounder control in the design phase of a study include restriction and matching, while stratification and multivariable methods are options during the data analysis phase of the study. Propensity scores are being considered more and more as an efficient means of controlling for multiple measured confounders through both matching and adjustment. A better understanding of the potential impact of unmeasured confounders can be gained through formal sensitivity analyses. Periodically, epidemiologists also debate the merits and applicability of instrumental variable model approaches, commonly used in econometrics, for control of unmeasured confounders, but the assumptions involved in these models have, to this point, limited their use in observational epidemiology.

Given the substantive challenges posed by confounding in observational epidemiology and the ability of randomization to address these, the randomized controlled trial (RCT) is viewed as the superior study design. In instances where conflicting evidence is generated by RCTs and observational epidemiologic studies, the temptation is to presume that the RCT results are more valid. However, there are a number of points to consider when comparing observational epidemiology with RCTs. First, there are a large number of risk factors that can never be evaluated in RCTs because it would be unethical or impossible to randomize. Next, RCTs are often conducted on select population subgroups, for example, those of a certain age or background risk level. While results from these trials may have superior internal validity for the subgroup studied, findings from observational studies on broader population groups can have more generalizability. Finally, all observational studies are not by definition of equal quality. In a number of research areas, findings from well-designed prospective cohort studies generate findings that agree with RCTs. In these situations, the discrepancies across the bodies of

observational and experimental evidence have been driven by findings from case-control, cross-sectional, or ecologic studies.

—*Craig Newschaffer*

See also Bias; Causation and Causal Inference; Confounding; Descriptive and Analytic Epidemiology; Study Design

Further Readings

Concato, J. (2004). Observational versus experimental studies: What's the evidence for a hierarchy? *NeuroRx, 1*, 341–347.

D'Agostino, R. B., Jr., & D'Agostino, R. B., Sr. (2007). Estimating treatment effects using observational data. *Journal of the American Medical Association, 297*, 314–316.

Hernan, M. A. (2004). A definition of causal effect for epidemiological research. *Journal of Epidemiology and Community Health, 58*, 265–271.

Lash, T. L. (2007). Heuristic thinking and inference from observational epidemiology. *Epidemiology, 18*, 67–72.

Lawler, D. A., Smith, G. D., & Ebrahim, S. (2004). Commentary: The hormone replacement-coronary heart disease conundrum: Is this the death of observational epidemiology? *International Journal of Epidemiology, 33*, 464–467.

ORAL CONTRACEPTIVES

Oral contraceptives, commonly referred to as "the pill," provide a hormonal method for women to prevent pregnancy. The two basic types are combination pills, which contain both estrogen and progestin (a synthetic version of progesterone), and progestin-only pills. Since their introduction in 1960, oral contraceptives have become the most popular form of reversible birth control in the United States. More than 100 million women use this method worldwide, although its use varies substantially by country.

History

In 1951, activist Margaret Sanger began to work with Dr. Gregory Pincus to develop a birth control pill. In less than a year, Pincus was able to demonstrate that progesterone inhibits ovulation in rabbits and rats, but he lacked the funding necessary to continue his research. Simultaneously, an orally effective form of synthetic progesterone was created by Carl Djerassi, a chemist working in Mexico City, and Frank Colton, the chief chemist at the pharmaceutical company G.D. Searle. In 1953, philanthropist Katharine McCormick agreed to provide Pincus with funding for further research. Pincus collaborated with Dr. John Rock for the first human trials in 1954 and submitted the formulation developed by G.D. Searle and Company, called Enovid, for FDA approval in 1956. The FDA approved Enovid for treatment of severe menstrual disorders the following year. Searle received FDA permission in 1960 to sell a lower dose formula of Enovid as a contraceptive. In 1962, the drug company Syntex released another oral contraceptive, Ortho Novum, using the formula developed by Djerassi. The progestin-only pill was developed in the early 1970s in response to concerns about the relationship between estrogen and thrombo-embolic disease. In the 1980s, multiphasic oral contraceptives were developed that contain varying levels of progestin and estrogen throughout the standard 21-day cycle. Emergency contraception, a high dose of an oral contraceptive used by women after intercourse to prevent unwanted pregnancy, became more accessible beginning in the mid-1990s. In 2006, the FDA approved one option, Plan B, for use without a prescription for women aged 18 and older. Current oral contraceptives typically contain less than 1/10 the amount of progestin and 1/4 of the estrogen as found in the early versions.

Mechanism of Action

The hormones in combined oral contraceptives suppress both follicular development and ovulation. They also alter cervical mucus to make it more hostile toward sperm in case ovulation does occur. Progestin-only pills work by reducing and thickening cervical mucus to prevent sperm from reaching an egg. This type also inhibits the thickening of the uterine lining, which prevents a fertilized egg from implantation in the uterus.

The exact mechanism of action with emergency contraceptives is uncertain and may depend on the time in a woman's cycle that they are used. If taken at the beginning of a cycle, they may prevent or delay ovulation. If ovulation has already occurred, they may interfere with fertilization or implantation. The effectiveness of emergency contraceptives decreases as the length of time after unprotected intercourse increases.

Benefits

The most significant benefit of oral contraceptives is the decreased risk of pregnancy and pregnancy-related complications, including ectopic pregnancy. Among "perfect" users who do not miss any pills, approximately 1 woman in 1,000 become pregnant during the first year of use. Typical users have a pregnancy rate of 60 to 80 per 1,000 women during the first year. A World Health Organization (WHO) study found no significant difference in effectiveness when comparing six brands of combined pills. Progestin-only pills have slightly lower effectiveness.

Non-pregnancy-related benefits include less iron deficiency anemia due to lighter menstrual bleeding, more regular menstrual cycles, less severe premenstrual symptoms, and less dysmenorrhea. Oral contraceptives reduce the risk of epithelial ovarian cancer and endometrial cancer and prevent ovarian cysts. They may also protect against bone density loss, benign breast disease, pelvic inflammatory disease, and colorectal cancer.

Health Risks

Older women who use oral contraceptives and have hypertension or smoke have an increased risk of heart attack and stroke. A multicountry study by the WHO found that the relative risk for myocardial infarction increases substantially among users who also have other risk factors for heart disease such as smoking, hypertension, and diabetes. Among women without these additional risk factors, the study found no increased risk among current or past users.

The risk for other circulatory diseases, particularly venous thromboembolism, is also increased. Several studies have found a small increase in blood pressure among users, and one cohort study of 68,000 nurses in the United States reported that users were twice as likely to develop hypertension compared with nonusers, though this risk decreased after discontinuation. Additional health risks include the accelerated development of gallbladder disease among already susceptible women and rare, noncancerous liver tumors.

The relationship between oral contraceptives and the development of cervical cancer remains uncertain. While recent studies have found an increased association of cervical cancer and preinvasive lesions, the epidemiologic evidence cannot conclusively determine if this is due to biological or behavioral factors. Women also have an elevated risk of diagnosis of early occurring breast cancer, which may be partially attributable to more frequent breast exams. The risks of both cervical neoplasia and breast cancer disappear within 10 years after discontinuation of use.

Common side effects of oral contraceptives include nausea, breast tenderness, irregular bleeding, and depression. These often subside after several months of use.

—*Martha Decker*

See also Reproductive Epidemiology; Women's Health Issues

Further Readings

ACOG Practice Bulletin. (2005). Clinical Management Guidelines for Obstetrician-Gynecologists, Number 69, December 2005 (replaces Practice Bulletin Number 25, March 2001). Emergency contraception. *Obstetrics and Gynecology, 106*(6), 1443–1452.

Asbell, B. (1995). *The pill: A biography of the drug that changed the world.* New York: Random House.

Beral, V., Hermon, C., Kay, C., Hannaford, P., Darby, S., & Reeves, G. (1999). Mortality associated with oral contraceptive use: 25 year follow up of cohort of 46,000 women from Royal College of General Practitioners' oral contraception study. *British Medical Journal, 318*(7176), 96–100.

Blackburn, R. D., Cunkelman, J. A., & Zlidar, V. M. (2000). *Oral contraceptives: An update. Population Reports,* Series A, No. 9. Baltimore: Johns Hopkins University School of Public Health, Population Information Program.

Chasan-Taber, L., Willett, W. C., Manson, J. E., Spiegelman, D., Hunter, D. J., Curhan, G., et al. (1996). Prospective study of oral contraceptives and hypertension among women in the United States. *Circulation, 94*(3), 483–489.

Connell, E. B. (2002). *The contraception sourcebook.* New York: McGraw-Hill.

Gazit, C. (2002). *The pill: American experience.* Boston: WGBH. Retrieved October 1, 2006, from http://www.pbs.org/wgbh/amex/pill.

World Health Organization. (1997). Acute myocardial infarction and combined oral contraceptives: Results of an international multicentre case-control study. *Lancet, 349*(9060), 1202–1209.

ORAL HEALTH

Oral health conditions include a number of congenital or developmental anomalies, such as clefts and tumors. But the most common oral health problem is tooth decay, known medically as dental caries. Although dental caries is largely preventable, more than half of all adults above age 18 present early signs of this disease and, at some point in life, about three out of four adults will develop the disease. In older adults, tooth decay and periodontal disease are the leading causes of tooth loss. Tooth decay is also common among children as young as 5 years and remains the most common chronic disease of children aged 5 to 17 years. It is estimated that tooth decay is four times more prevalent than asthma in childhood. Poor oral health has been related to decreased school performance, poor social relationships, and less success later in life. It is estimated that about 51 million school hours per year are lost in the United States alone because of dental-related illness. In adults, dental caries and, eventually, tooth loss can reduce chewing ability that leads to detrimental changes in food selection. This, in turn, may increase the risk of particular systemic diseases such as cardiovascular diseases.

Despite numerous epidemiologic studies currently available to assess the pattern of dental caries in oral health, there are still some fundamental questions that remain unanswered. As an example, many dentists believe that there are spatial symmetries in the mouth with respect to caries development, but this has never been demonstrated statistically. Although many dental studies provide detailed tooth-level data on caries activity, most analyses still rely on the decayed, missing, and filled (DMF) index introduced in the 1930s. This approach operates at the mouth level, that is, it counts the number of decayed teeth within a person's mouth without including information on which specific teeth are decayed; therefore, it may not be relevant in assessing the spatial distribution of the dental caries in a mouth. A more useful way to study oral health may be to collect data at the tooth level. Models that summarize tooth-level data can be used to answer questions related to tooth surface susceptibility to caries experience, symmetries in the mouth with respect to dental caries, and differences in surface susceptibility according to caries risk groups. Use of tooth-level models should improve our ability to analyze and interpret complex dependent data generated from clinical trials and epidemiologic studies in dental research.

Tooth Decay and Measurement

Tooth decay is ubiquitous and is one of the most prevalent oral diseases. It is a localized, progressive demineralization of the hard tissues of the crown (coronal enamel, dentine) and root (cementum, dentine) surfaces of teeth. The demineralization is caused by acids produced by bacteria, particularly *mutans Streptococci* and possibly *Lactobacilli* that ferment dietary carbohydrates. This occurs within a bacteria-laden gelatinous material called dental plaque that adheres to tooth surfaces and becomes colonized by bacteria. Thus, caries results from the interplay of three main factors over time: dietary carbohydrates, cariogenic bacteria within dental plaque, and susceptible hard tooth surfaces. Dental caries is a dynamic process since periods of demineralization alternate with periods of remineralization through the action of fluoride, calcium, and phosphorous contained in oral fluids.

According to the World Health Organization, both the shape and the depth of a carious lesion at the tooth level can be scored on a 4-point scale, D_1 to D_4. Level D_1 refers to clinically detectable enamel lesions with noncavitated surfaces; D_2 to clinically detectable cavities limited to the enamel; D_3 to clinically detectable lesions in dentin; and, finally, D_4 to lesions into the pulp. The threshold traditionally used in epidemiologic studies is based on D_3, which ignores all signs of lesions less severe than clinically detectable lesions. In the past, it has been argued that enamel lesions could not be included in epidemiologic studies because the reproducibility achieved was lower and insufficient. However, as reported by Marisol Tellez, studies have shown excellent reproducibility with kappa coefficients around .80 using the D_1 threshold in survey settings as well as clinical trials.

Despite these detailed tooth-level data, the methods for analyzing dental caries outcomes in human populations still rely on the calculation of the DMF index, developed in the 1930s. This index is applied to all the teeth (DMFT) or to all surfaces (DMFS). These scores are typically analyzed as counts using Poisson models or negative binomial models to account for overdispersion as a result of mixtures in the data. Other approaches consist of dichotomizing or constructing ordered levels according to a graded scale using some threshold values. Despite an extensive use of these indexes and related models, they have some recognized limitations. These scores are not very informative in studying tooth-specific problems. Different types of teeth (incisors, canine, and molars in primary dentition) and tooth surfaces (facial, lingual, occlusal, mesial, distal, and incisal surfaces) are not equally susceptible to dental caries. For example, the different morphology of the pit-and-fissure surfaces of teeth makes them more susceptible to decay than the smooth surfaces. Thus, it is no surprise to find that the posterior molar and premolar teeth that have pit-and-fissure surfaces are more susceptible than the anterior teeth. The application of the traditional DMF index to the skewed data on caries that frequently emerge today is one of the factors contributing to the underestimation of the prevalence of caries and the overestimation of the temporal change. Thus, it places limitations on the population strategy to be used in caries prevention, and it contributes to a lack of discrimination between individuals with differences in caries activities. A tooth- and surface-level analysis can give a better understanding of the pattern of dental caries over time.

In addition, most research on dental caries is based on cross-sectional studies or surveillance data. For example, G. D. Slade and colleagues reported a cross-sectional dental study involving 9,690 Australian schoolchildren aged 5 to 15 years. However, like most caries surveys, this study is limited in its ability to examine questions involving duration of time, for example, the period between tooth eruption and caries development, and to investigate the interrelationship among teeth and tooth surfaces within the mouth in terms of caries development. Yet most interesting scientific questions in dentistry deal with the development of caries over time, determinants of oral hygiene in general, and the intra-oral distribution of the disease in the mouth across time. Therefore, in addition to cross-sectional studies and surveillance data, these questions beg for high-quality longitudinal studies. Most of the inconsistencies in the dental oral literature may be the result of the inability of cross-sectional studies to accurately describe the etiology of dental caries.

Statistical Models for Highly Correlated Dental Data

A tooth-surface and tooth-level analysis in dental research poses a number of difficulties due to inherent spatial association of tooth surfaces and teeth in the mouth. This then necessitates the use of multivariate methods for correlated data. These multivariate models consist of (1) a parameter vector that accounts for the effects the independent variables have on the location parameter of each tooth-surface and tooth-level outcome and (2) an association component that corrects these location parameters for potential correlation among all outcomes from the same mouth. When the emergence times of dental caries of different teeth are to be compared, a multivariate model is needed to accommodate the multiplicity of outcomes from the same mouth. A popular model choice would be frailty models, which are basically random effects survival models. These models are enormously popular in the analysis of clustered time-to-event data. Such models account for correlations between survival rates in neighboring spatial regions such as tooth surfaces. In longitudinal studies that aim at studying the dynamics of caries across time, another important issue is the serial association induced by measurements taken on the same tooth or tooth surface over time. A good model for the covariance function of a stationary process in space and time should then accurately describe the variances and correlations of all linear combinations of the processes. In particular, it does not suffice to find a model that describes the purely temporal covariances and the purely spatial covariances accurately. Rather, it is critical to capture the spatiotemporal interactions as well. A great alternative to this class of models is the generalized estimating equations methodology where independent models are fitted to each tooth or tooth-surface outcome, and a sandwich estimator is used to adjust the model estimates' standard errors for association in the data.

In analyzing survival data in dental research, one is typically faced with the problem that the exact time of surface and tooth decay is typically unknown. This then imposes constraints on the model, rendering the approach based on the events (surface decay) themselves somewhat problematic. A simplistic approach to address these issues is to consider a survival approach where the outcome of interest is the emergence time of surface or tooth decay, which is an interval-censored observation. Compared with right-censored data, techniques for interval-censored data are less well developed, and their statistical properties are much more complex. For example, the convergence rate of nonparametric estimates of the survival curve for interval-censored data is known to be smaller than that of right-censored data. This then invalidates the use of the Wald approach to compute confidence intervals of the survival curve for interval-censored data. There is a common consensus from the current literature to use parametric models such as accelerated failure time models for interval-censored data. The widespread use of nonparametric methods for right-censored survival data has limited the use of parametric models with interval-censored data.

Future Research

Methods of identifying early carious lesions accurately and of identifying children at a high risk of dental caries are required. Also needed are studies to confirm the relation between the vulnerability of occlusal surfaces to caries and the time since tooth eruption. Prospective studies to examine all possible factors associated with nursing caries are also needed. For this, it is essential that we have effective and rigorous statistical methods to understand the etiology of dental caries. For this, it is recommended that regression models for spatial-temporal change data and models for multivariate failure time data with applications to caries on tooth surfaces be developed.

The use and acceptance of statistical models in dental research requires reliable and user-friendly software, readily available to perform regression analysis routinely. The software should be time-efficient, well-documented, and, most important, must have a friendly interface.

—David Todem

See also Child and Adolescent Health; Longitudinal Research Design; Regression; Study Design; Survival Analysis

Further Readings

Bogaerts, K., Leroy, R., Lesaffre, E., & Declerck, D. (2002). Modelling tooth emergence data based on multivariate interval-censored data. *Statistics in Medicine, 21,* 3775–3787.

Hougaard, P. (2000). *Analysis of multivariate survival data.* New York: Springer.

Slade, G. D., Spencer, A. J, Davies, M. J., & Stewart, J. F. (1996). Caries experience among children in fluoridated Townsville and unfluoridated Brisbane. *Australian and New Zealand Journal of Public Health Dentistry, 20,* 623–629.

Tellez, M., Sohn, W., Burt, B. A., & Ismail, A. I. (2006). Assessment of the relationship between neighborhood characteristics and dental caries severity among low-income African-Americans: A multilevel approach. *Journal of Public Health Dentistry, 66,* 30–36.

ORGAN DONATION

Organ donation has become the treatment of choice for end-stage renal disease (ESRD) in addition to other types of organ failure, notably heart, liver, and lung. By all accounts, the shortage of transplantable organs is a public health crisis with one person on the United Network of Organ sharing (UNOS) transplant waiting list dying approximately every 17 min. In 2005, there were more than 90,000 individuals awaiting transplantation.

There are two possible sources of organs for transplant: deceased organ donation that has provided the major source of transplantable organs and living donation usually, but not always, from the families of waiting recipients. Deceased donors are the only feasible source of heart donation and are by far the single most important source of livers, lungs, intestinal organs, and pancreata. Most living donation involves kidneys (92%) or liver segments (8%).

The number of deceased and living donors for all organs was 14,491 in 2004, with 7,593 deceased and 6,898 living donors. The number of all organ donors has increased at an average rate of 7% per year. Although the increase in living donors has been a major contributor in helping ameliorate the organ donor shortage in the United States, the numbers of persons on the waiting list is growing faster, with a net increase in the waiting list of 11% per year.

The other major change in the donor pool has been an inclusion of older donors and a change in the cause of death of donors. The average age of deceased donors rose by 2.1 years between 1996 and 2001 and is now in the mid-30s. Living donors are, on average, a year older than deceased donors. Living donors are more likely to be female (approximately 58%), while deceased donors are more frequently male (60%). A total of 79% to 82% of living donors are white, and deceased donors are also predominantly white (85%). Total minority donations increased by 56% from 1992 to 2001, while the number of white organ donors increased by 32% over the same period.

These trends in the organ donor profile reflect the continued shift away from the young adult who dies from a traumatic head injury to the older adult who dies from a cerebrovascular event. The progressive increase in the median age of deceased donors over the past 10 years has exceeded that of the general population since 1996.

In 2001, there were 695 donations resulting from anoxic brain deaths, up 12% from 2000 and up by 32% since 1995—the fastest rise among the causes of death for deceased donors. The rise in anoxic deaths resulted primarily from the increased frequency of drowning, drug intoxication, and cardiovascular events. Cerebrovascular deaths continue to lead as the primary cause for deceased donations (43% of all deceased donors in 2001).

Consent to organ donation by families of brain-dead patients has been a major barrier to maximizing the numbers of solid organs available for transplant in the United States. Despite public opinion polls reporting that more than 85% of the American public is willing to donate, fewer than half choose to donate a family member's organs when asked.

The Uniform Anatomical Gift Act (UAGA), drafted by the National Conference of Commissioners on Uniform State Laws in 1968 and modified in 1987, regulates organ donation in the United States. By 1973, it had been passed by all 50 states. Aimed at enabling individuals or their families to donate organs, UAGA also served to establish altruism and voluntariness as the bedrock of organ donation and procurement in the United States, while outlawing the sale of organs. This law recognizes the rights of individuals to donate by means of an organ donor card and gives the immediate family of a deceased person the option to donate. In 1973, the End-Stage Renal Disease Program provided federal financial support for organ transplantation by funding 100% of organ procurement costs through Medicare. Federal organization and oversight of organ procurement were further developed in 1984, when Congress passed the National Organ Transplantation Act (NOTA). This law created the Organ Procurement Transplant Network (OPTN), which has the responsibility for setting standards and rules regarding the distribution of human organs procured in this country and also outlaws the sale of organs.

Two key factors are responsible for the critical shortage of transplantable solid organs in the United States. First, it has been estimated that no more than 15,000 deceased brain-dead donors are available each year in the United States. In 2005, more than 90,000 individuals were waiting to receive a transplant. Second, the rate of consent for organ donation by next of kin has limited the number of organs available for transplant. On average, no more than 50% of those families from whom donation is requested agree to

donate. Increases in the total number of organs procured have resulted largely from an expansion of the
donor pool (e.g., accepting older patients as donors)
and from improvements in procedures for referring
and requesting organ donation from families of potential donor patients (living donation).

Major legislative efforts to encourage the donation
of organs have been undertaken since the 1970s. In
1986, Health Care Financing Administration (HCFA)
made it mandatory that hospitals request organ donation from donor-eligible families, and the Joint Commission on Accreditation of Health Care Organizations
(JCAHO) made it a requirement for hospital accreditation. These laws and regulations were not effective in
improving consent rates. Whereas surveys show that
99% of Americans are aware of transplantation, and at
least 85% say they would donate their organs if asked,
rates of consent to requests made for deceased patients'
organs continue to hover at 50%.

In 1998, HCFA required that hospitals notify their
local organ procurement organization (OPO) about
all deaths and imminent deaths, and that families
must be approached about donation in collaboration
with the local OPO. Underlying this regulation
(known as "required referral" or "routine notification") was the premise that health professionals
alone were not effectively communicating with families about donation. This regulation, too, has had
little impact on actual rates of consent to donation,
although some regions have seen an increase in
numbers of organs procured. A new legislative effort,
termed *donor designation* or *first-person consent*, now
makes it possible for donation to occur without family
permission if the deceased has a valid donor card or
driver's license designation.

Recent studies have emphasized the importance
of the process of asking for organ donation. This
process entails the identification of donation-eligible
patients and then making a request. It is first necessary to identify that someone is a potential organ
donor. Until recently, this process was almost completely in the hands of hospital health care providers.
Data showed that the ability of health care providers
to recognize a donor was variable, ranging from
70% to 100%. To address this problem, the 1998
HCFA regulations required that the local OPO be
called about each hospital death. Data indicate that
referral and request rates also vary widely, ranging
from 65% to 99%. Referral rates average 80%, and
requests are made in 84% of cases.

Different practices of discussing and obtaining
consent from families have been widely debated and
are the subject of some controversy. Factors such as
when the request should be made, who should request
organ donation, what should be discussed with the
family, and how (or if) families who initially refuse
organ donation should be reapproached have all
received attention. Some strategies, however, have
not proven fruitful or have not been confirmed. For
example, studies of timing of the donation request
conducted in the early 1990s suggested that "decou-
pling" the request from pronouncement of death
would create a significant rise in consent rates. However, studies that are more recent have revealed that
the issue is more complex, and that raising the issue
of organ donation with families earlier in the course
of the patient's hospitalization—especially once the
futility of treatment has been determined—may be the
most useful practice.

Families often refuse to consent to organ donation
because they are concerned about mutilation of the
body. A recent study found that families were more
likely to donate when this issue was discussed openly
rather than avoided. Additionally, spending more time
with families and discussing specific issues about
organ donation, such as the patient's wishes concerning donation, the choice concerning what organs to
donate, and the fact that there are no costs associated
with donation, are significantly associated with consent to donation. Families who spent more time and
discussed more donation-related issues are five times
more likely to donate.

The 1998 regulations also sought to guarantee
that experienced requesters speak with families.
Again, recent data indicate that this will be a fruitful
strategy if it can be successfully implemented. For
example, an earlier study found that health care providers who rated themselves as more uncomfortable
speaking with families about organ donation were
less likely to obtain consent than those who reported
themselves as comfortable with discussing the topic
and answering the family's questions.

Legislative efforts have yet to close the gap
between donor potential and organs procured. Studies now indicate that the process itself is of critical
importance. Appropriate training and hospital donation development are needed to improve performance in the procurement of organs from deceased
donors. Rates of living donation continue to rise in
the United States, contributing to the availability of

transplants for patients in need of kidney and liver transplantation.

—*Laura A. Siminoff*

See also Ethics in Health Care; Governmental Role in Public Health; Health Care Delivery; Health Communication; Informed Consent

Further Readings

Boulware, L. E., Ratner, L. E., Cooper, L. A., Sosa, J. A., LaVeist, T. A., Powe, N. R. (2002). Understanding disparities in donor behavior: Race and gender differences in willingness to donate blood and cadaveric organs. *Medical Care, 40*(2), 85–95.

Gallup Organization. (1993). *The American public's attitudes toward organ donation and transplantation.* Boston: Partnership for Organ Donation.

Institute of Medicine. (2006). *Organ donation: Opportunities for Action.* Washington, DC: Author.

Sheehy, E., Conrad, S. L., Brigham, L. E., Luskin, R., Weber, P., Eakin, M., et al. (2003. Estimating the number of potential organ donors in the United States. *New England Journal of Medicine, 349,* 667–674.

Siminoff, L. A., Gordon, N., Hewlett, J., & Arnold, R. M. (2001). Factors influencing families' consent for donation of solid organs for transplantation. *Journal of the American Medical Association, 286*(1), 71–77.

Siminoff, L. A., Lawrence, R. H., & Arnold, R. M. (2003). Comparison of black and white families' experiences and perceptions regarding organ donation requests. *Critical Care Medicine, 31*(1), 146–151.

Siminoff, L. A., & Mercer, M. B. (2001). Public policy, public opinion, and consent for organ donation. *Cambridge Quarterly of Healthcare Ethics, 10,* 377–386.

Sque, M., Long, T., & Payne, S. (2005). Organ donation: Key factors influencing families' decision-making. *Transplant Proceedings, 37,* 543–546.

OSTEOPOROSIS

Osteoporosis is a skeletal disorder characterized by low bone mass and deterioration of bone quality leading to bone fragility and increased risk of fracture. More than 10 million Americans above the age of 50 have osteoporosis. Women are two to three times as likely to be affected as men. Osteoporotic fractures lead to significant morbidity and excess mortality; of those experiencing a hip fracture, one out of five will die in the following year and less than one out of three will regain prefracture physical ability. The direct and indirect costs associated with all osteoporotic fractures in the United States exceed $20 billion dollars annually.

History

The term *osteoporosis*—Greek for porous bone— was first coined in the 1830s by French pathologist Georges Chretien Frederic Martin Lobstein in describing the larger than normal holes he noticed in some bones. At the time of the observation, no further significance was associated with the condition. A century later, in 1934, Yale anatomists discovered estrogen's role in bone formation while studying factors causing increased bone mass in female pigeons as compared with males. With the pigeon study in mind, six years later, Fuller Albright, a Massachusetts General Hospital physician, proposed estrogen to be important in controlling calcium concentrations in human bone and suggested that estrogen-related bone loss was responsible for the fractures afflicting his older women patients.

Etiology

Primary, *age-related osteoporosis* is the most common form of the disease, resulting largely from age- and hormone-related decreases in bone quality. Risk factors for osteoporosis and related fractures include physical inactivity, previous fractures, smoking, low body weight, low exposure to sunlight (in people above 50), tendency to fall, alcohol consumption, and impaired vision. Preliminary research also suggests an important role for genetic predisposition in the development of osteoporosis. Reduced bone quality due to diseases, disorders, medication use, and/or toxin exposure is referred to as secondary osteoporosis. Many who are diagnosed with osteoporosis have had exposures to secondary causes occurring earlier in life.

Pathogenesis

Bone is a living matrix comprised largely of crystals of calcium and phosphate, or hydroxyapatite, and the protein collagen. Throughout life, bones change in shape, size, and position through the processes of modeling and remodeling. Modeling allows bones to grow and shift in space by forming new bone at one site while removing it from another within the same bone. Remodeling is the removal and replacement of bone at the same site. Remodeling, which becomes the dominant process in both sexes around 20 years of age, is important in the repair of microdamage resulting from stresses on the skeleton, in the replacement of older bone tissue, and in the bioavailability of calcium and phosphate stored in bone for use in other bodily functions. Estrogen influences bone quality by directly and indirectly affecting the activity of osteoclasts, cells that break bone down, and osteoblasts, cells that build bone.

During menopause, a drastic reduction in estrogen production by the ovaries leads to remodeling imbalance and subsequent loss of bone mineral density (BMD). The sudden decrease in estrogen triggers an increase in osteoclast formation and recruitment, inhibits osteoclast apoptosis, and promotes osteoblast apoptosis. This acute phase of rapid bone loss lasts for 4 to 8 years.

Following the acute phase, a period of slow, continuous bone loss progresses throughout the rest of life. Age-related retarded bone formation, decreased calcium and vitamin D intake, decreased physical activity, and the loss of estrogen's effects on calcium absorption in the intestines and calcium conservation in the kidneys contribute to slow bone loss. Reduced dietary calcium intake and absorption further the disease process by increasing parathyroid hormone levels leading to calcium removal from the bones for use in other systems. Thinning of bone in itself is not a significant cause of morbidity and mortality; weakened bones are, however, more likely to suffer damage following trauma.

With aging, men suffer only a slow reduction in sex hormones and therefore osteoporosis develops through a slow, continuous process of bone loss similar to that in women. Up to 50% of elderly men are deficient in active sex steroids.

The disease processes associated with secondary osteoporosis are varied and include genetic disorders (e.g., cystic fibrosis), conditions leading to estrogen or testosterone deficiencies in adolescence or following development of peak bone density (e.g., anorexia nervosa, athletic amenorrhea, Turner's syndrome), excess production of or treatment with thyroid hormone or glucocorticoids (e.g., thyrotoxosis, Cushing's syndrome), diseases or conditions leading to reduced intestinal absorption of calcium or phosphate (e.g., celiac disease), conditions that disrupt vitamin D metabolism (e.g., cirrhosis due to hepatitis B or C), and rheumatic disorders (e.g., Lupus, rheumatoid arthritis).

Impact

While osteoporosis is associated with an increased risk for all types of fractures, the most common sites are the hip, spine, and wrist. Fractures, especially of the hip, can be painful and disfiguring, and often require hospitalization; most never regain prefracture physical functioning. Almost 10% of those experiencing any fracture and more than a quarter of those who suffer a hip fracture are physically impaired and unable to live without assistance. Fractures also have indirect consequences such as disrupted abdominal anatomy leading to constipation, distention, and reduced appetite. Psychological effects, including depression, anxiety, fear, and strained interpersonal relationships are common sequelae. Both hip and spine fractures are associated with excess mortality; one in five persons experiencing a hip fracture dies within the subsequent year due to comorbidities.

Epidemiology

Rates of osteoporosis and osteoporosis-related fractures vary by ethnicity, gender, and geography. Men, with higher peak bone densities than women, are less likely to suffer a primary osteoporotic fracture. In the United States, among Caucasians, 50% of women and 20% of men older than 50 will experience a fragility fracture in their remaining lifetime. Women are more likely to suffer hip and wrist fractures. Rates of vertebral fractures, which are more often associated with bending and lifting objects than with falls, are more similar between men and women.

Because of the lack of uniform availability of testing procedures, the incidence of hip fracture is often used as an international index for osteoporosis. Possibly due to genetic predisposition and/or environmental factors, fractures, especially those of the hip, are more likely to occur in Caucasian than in non-Caucasian populations. Generally, osteoporosis rates are highest in North American and European countries and lowest in African countries. By the year 2050, Asian populations are expected to account for more than half of all hip fractures. Fracture rates also vary within ethnic groups; for example, controlling for race/ethnicity, hip fracture rates are higher in urban areas. Secondary osteoporosis strikes both young and old and men and women equally.

Diagnosis

Osteoporosis is diagnosed by assessing BMD. While other bone parameters such as shape, geometry, type of bone (trabecular or cortical), degree of mineralization, microdamage accumulation, and rate of bone turnover are important in determining bone strength, these measures have yet to be incorporated into standard testing techniques. The World Health Organization has identified the following risk factors that, when measured in addition to BMD, give a more accurate prediction of future fracture risk: age, existence of previous fractures, glucocorticoid use, cigarette smoking, heavy alcohol consumption, and female low body weight.

Dual-energy X-ray absorptiometry is used to measure overall BMD and is the gold standard for osteoporosis diagnosis. According to the World Health Organization, someone with a BMD 2.5 or more standard deviations below that of the young adult mean is considered to have osteoporosis. Osteopenia, a precursor to osteoporosis, is diagnosed when BMD is between 1 and 2.5 standard deviations below the mean. Any fracture resulting from low trauma or due to a fall from standing height is also diagnostic of osteoporosis, regardless of BMD.

Prevention

Prevention of osteoporosis generally depends on increasing bone density and reducing the risk of falling, through exercises including walking, aerobics, weight bearing and resistance exercises, and balance training. Studies have shown reduced risk of fracture with smoking cessation and calcium supplementation. Pharmacologic treatments, such as bisphosphonates and hormone replacement therapy, have proven effective in increasing BMD and decreasing the risk of fractures, though recently characterized health risks associated with the latter have resulted in the discouragement of its use.

—*Michelle Kirian*

See also Aging, Epidemiology of; Injury Epidemiology; Vitamin Deficiency Diseases; Women's Health Issues

Further Readings

Fitzpatrick, L. A. (2002). Secondary causes of osteoporosis. *Mayo Clinic Proceedings, 77,* 453–468.

Johnell, O., & Hertzman, P. (2006). *What evidence is there for the prevention and screening of osteoporosis?* Health Evidence Network report. Copenhagen, Denmark: WHO Regional Office for Europe.

Patlak, M. (2001). Bone builders: The discoveries behind preventing and treating osteoporosis. *FASEB Journal, 10,* 1677E.

Sambrooke, P., & Cooper, C. (2006). Osteoporosis. *Lancet, 367,* 2010–2018.

U.S. Department of Health and Human Services, Office of the Surgeon General. (2004). *Bone health and osteoporosis: A report of the Surgeon General.* Rockville, MD: Author.

Weitzmann, M. N., & Pacifici, R. (2006). Estrogen deficiency and bone loss: An inflamatory tale. *Journal of Clinical Investigation, 116*(5), 1186–1194.

World Health Organization. (2003). *Prevention and management of osteoporosis.* WHO Technical Report Series 921. Geneva, Switzerland: Author.

OUTBREAK INVESTIGATION

Outbreak investigations are a subgroup of epidemiologic studies called "field investigations." When the numbers of persons affected by a particular disease, usually infectious, exceeds the number of cases expected in a given place during a given time period, it may be said that there is an outbreak of that disease. Epidemiologists may then conduct targeted investigations to (a) determine the cause and etiology of the disease, (b) to limit the spread and severity of illness of the disease, and (c) to prevent future outbreaks. In addition, investigations of this sort can serve to identify new modes of transmission of illnesses, identify new pathogens, and monitor the effectiveness of prevention activities. Collectively, these activities make up an outbreak investigation. Investigations of this type require epidemiologists to seek out and collect information (via interviews, lab studies, etc.) from persons affected by the disease.

Though the precise order may vary, most outbreak investigations share many steps and tasks in common. First, investigators must determine that an outbreak actually exists. The presence of a potential outbreak can be detected by any of several sources, including health care workers, laboratory workers, the general public, formal disease surveillance systems, or other health data. Investigators then compare the numbers of currently observed cases with historical data for the similar time period in previous years to determine that the observed cases represent an actual outbreak. Several sources of data adequate for this sort of comparison exist and may include disease surveillance records, birth certificates, death certificates, hospital discharge information, and so on. Changes in observed numbers of cases may be due to reasons other than the presence of an outbreak, for instance if there was an underlying change in case ascertainment or a change in the population at risk for the disease.

In addition to confirming the presence of an outbreak, investigators must also confirm the diagnosis and generate a case definition. The case definition, ideally consisting of the simplest, most concrete criteria possible, will help investigators and health care workers identify persons to be included in the investigation, and may be refined as new information about the illness and at-risk populations come to hand. Interviews with or surveys of cases will help place each case within the epidemiologic triad of person, place, and time, and can help refine ideas and initial hypotheses regarding who is at risk as well as beginning to address the issues of how and why the outbreak began. In an iterative process, investigators will continue to refine their case definition and explanatory hypotheses as new information comes to hand via interviews and surveys.

Once some of this preliminary descriptive work has been completed, investigators will plan and conduct an analytic study to further identify the source of the infection. Most commonly, case-control study designs are used, though cohort studies can also be used. As in more controlled study settings, both study designs have their advantages and disadvantages. Case-control studies are often used in the context of a large outbreak, where relative efficiency in both time and cost is important. In addition, in many outbreaks, the entire cohort is often not clearly defined, making a case-control study approach more appropriate. Case-control studies may also be nested within larger cohort studies, where testing a specific hypothesis on the entire larger cohort is not feasible. Cohort study designs have the advantages that investigators can evaluate multiple disease outcomes and can directly measure attack rates.

In an outbreak investigation, an investigator's work is not completed with the identification of the source of the outbreak. Investigators must also prepare a written report summarizing what they have learned about the outbreak, to guide future control and prevention efforts. Investigators must also implement those control and prevention methods, usually with some combination of (a) eliminating the source of the pathogen, (b) interrupting the spread from person to person, and/or (c) protecting individuals from consequences of exposure with methods such as vaccination, prophylactic medication, and so on.

Outbreak investigations differ from other epidemiologic studies in several ways, and they present unique challenges as well. The problem necessitating an outbreak investigation is usually unexpected and, thus, rapid response and immediate epidemiologist presence are required. The need for timely intervention also often means that outbreak investigations are more limited than other investigations. The aim is to conduct studies as scientifically rigorous as possible within these constraints. As with other studies, outbreak investigations are vulnerable to various kinds of bias, though perhaps in ways unique to these investigations. For example, most epidemiologic studies are vulnerable to sampling biases, but in an outbreak investigation, some or many of the people involved may be highly motivated to not cooperate with investigation for reasons such as protecting their own financial interests or reputation. In addition, cases may be distributed over a wide geographic area, making full characterization of the cases difficult. Outbreaks may also occur in areas with poor infrastructure, making optimal investigation difficult. In the instance of a relatively small outbreak, sample size may not be sufficient to detect small effects. And publicity about the outbreak or investigation may serve to communicate preconceived notions about the outbreak, resulting in biased information and potentially erroneous conclusions.

—*Annette L. Adams*

See also Epidemic; Field Epidemiology; Natural Experiment

Further Readings

Brownson, R. C. (1998). Outbreak and cluster investigations. In R. C. Brownson & D. B. Petitti (Eds.), *Applied epidemiology: Theory to practice* (pp. 71–104). New York: Oxford University Press.

Koehler, J., & Duchin, J. (2003). Outbreak investigation. In T. D. Koepsell & N. S. Weiss (Eds.), *Epidemiologic methods: Studying the occurrence of illness* (pp. 464–489). New York: Oxford University Press.

OVERMATCHING

To control for potential confounders or to enhance stratified analysis in observational studies, researchers may choose to match cases and controls or exposed and unexposed subjects on characteristics of interest. If matching is superfluous or erroneous, overmatching may occur. The three main effects of overmatching are a loss of statistical efficiency, introduction of bias, and loss of financial efficiency.

Background

To reduce confounding or to enhance stratified analysis, unexposed subjects in cohort studies or controls in case-control studies may be chosen to be identical or similar to exposed subjects or cases with respect to the distribution of one or more variables. Overmatching, sometimes referred to as overmatching bias, occurs when matching is done incorrectly or unnecessarily leading to reduced efficiency and biased results. Overmatching generally affects case-control studies.

Effects of Overmatching

Loss of Statistical Efficiency

In case-control studies, if cases and controls are matched on a variable that is associated to the exposure but not the disease, chosen controls are more similar to cases than the base population in respect to the exposure. The forced similarity between cases and controls in respect to the exposure obscures the relationship between the exposure and the disease. Matching on an exposure-associated variable will cause the crude odds ratio to be closer to 1—that is, to the null value. However, when stratified by the matching variable, stratum-specific odds ratios will be unbiased. If confounding is present, bias due to matching on an exposure-associated variable will cause the odds ratio to go toward the null regardless of the direction of the confounding. The degree of information loss due to overmatching depends on the absolute correlation between the matching variable and the exposure of interest. Matching on a nonconfounder necessitates

stratified analysis that would otherwise not be necessary, and it reduces study efficiency.

Introduction of Bias

If controls are matched to cases on a variable that is affected by both the exposure and the disease or is an intermediate between exposure and disease, both the crude and adjusted odds ratios will be biased. Like matching on exposure-only-associated variables, matching on an intermediate or variable affected by exposure and disease will force the odds ratios toward the null. However, unlike matching on an exposure-only-associated variable, it is not possible to get unbiased stratified measures of effect.

Loss of Financial Efficiency

Matching can lead to greater statistical efficiency by ensuring that cases will have one or more matched controls for comparison in stratified analysis. Also, matching may offer a cost benefit if the collection of exposure data from many people is very expensive. However, if the matching process is complicated and involves many matching variables, it may be difficult and costly to identify and recruit potential controls. Also, if matching is done unnecessarily, additional costs associated with recruiting further controls may incur. Potential statistical benefits and costs should be assessed prior to matching.

—*Michelle Kirian*

See also Bias; Confounding; Matching; Study Design

Further Readings

Agudo, C., & Gonzales, C. A. (1999). Secondary matching: A method for selecting controls in case control studies on environmental risk factors. *International Journal of Epidemiology, 28,* 1130–1133.

Rothman, K. J., & Greenland, S. (1998). Matching. In K. J. Rothman & S. Greenland (Eds.). *Modern epidemiology* (pp. 147–161). Philadelphia: Lippincott Williams & Wilkins.

Szklo, M., & Nieto, F. J. (2004). *Epidemiology: Beyond the basics.* Boston: Jones & Bartlett.

P

PAIN

Pain is a complex biopsychosocial phenomenon that most human beings experience at different times throughout their life span. This phenomenon has perplexed man for centuries, and for centuries pain has been poorly managed. Today, health care professionals are placed in a position where patients rely on them to provide pain control, and effective pain management is important in enabling patients to progress in their rehabilitation and to have an improved quality of life. This entry reviews definitions of pain, summarizes the demographics and epidemiology of pain, and describes the physiology of pain and its categorization. It also considers the interventions available, as well as some of the ethical issues that arise with respect to pain treatment.

Ancient civilizations, including early Mesopotamia, Egypt, China, Greece, and Rome, used various primitive approaches to treat pain. Via writings, carvings, and other documents, anthropologists have found evidence of pain interventions, including ancient pharmacopoeia such as the use of opium, scopolamine, ephedrine, ginseng, Siberian wort, snake venom, and various other treatments. Nonpharmacological interventions included prayer, dance rituals, music, bloodletting, hydrotherapy, and other cultural remedies.

The universally accepted definition of pain, according to the International Association for the Study of Pain (IASP) and the American Pain Society (APS), is "an unpleasant sensory and emotional experience associated with actual or potential tissue damage or described in terms of such damage" (Mersky, 1986, p. S217). This definition does not ask for organic proof that pain exists. A second definition coined by McCaffery (1968) says, "pain is whatever the experiencing person says it is, whenever the experiencing person says it is (p. 95)." This definition points to the subjectivity of pain. Pain is experienced differently by individuals based on their cultural background, upbringing, personal values, genetics, and the meaning they attribute to pain.

Pain is a protective mechanism that provides warning of assaults or damage to or within the body; however, if left untreated, this protective mechanism can become a chronic and destructive condition. Unrelieved pain remains a critical problem in all areas of health care. The most undertreated populations include children, the elderly, minorities, and women mostly due to myths and misconceptions related to the pain mechanism. Toward the end of the 20th century and the beginning of the current century, the undertreatment of pain became increasingly evident as interested health care professionals studied this problem. Several organizations, most notably the Joint Commission on Accreditation of Health Care Organizations (JCAHO), have developed standards, publications, and guidelines for practice related to the relief of pain and care at the end of life.

Demographics and Epidemiology

Algology is the study and science of pain phenomena, and an algologist is a student, investigator, or practitioner of algology. Pain studies conducted by pain organizations and algologists are tracked by the American Pain Foundation. According to APS, 50 million people are disabled by pain in the United States, and an estimated 9% of the U.S. adult population suffers from moderate to severe pain. Findings from studies conducted between 1996 and 2004 indicate that work to improve the relief of pain must continue.

Key findings include the following:

• More than two thirds of full-time employees (68%), the equivalent of more than 80 million full-time employees, suffer from pain-related conditions. Fourteen percent of all full-time employees—more than 17 million—took sick days in 1995 due to pain conditions, resulting in more than 50 million work days. Sixty-nine percent said they were compensated 100% of their salaries for sick days, which translates to a cost of more than $3 billion in wages for lost sick days. Furthermore, 80% of all pain sufferers have gone on short-term disability because of pain.

• One in five Americans above 60 years of age takes pain medication to control pain that lasts for 6 months or more; this represents 18% of Americans in this age group. Two out of three older Americans who take pain medications said pain still prevents them from performing routine tasks, engaging in hobbies, or doing things they enjoy.

• Despite people's use of medications, two thirds of chronic pain sufferers (13.6 million Americans) cannot perform routine tasks because of chronic pain. Portenoy breaks down the prevalence of cancer pain as follows: (a) at time of diagnosis, 30%, (b) during active treatment, 30% to 50%, and (c) with advanced disease, 70% to 90%. The APS reemphasizes the significance of undertreatment of pain as a public health problem with consequences that include increases in health care expenditures and worker absenteeism, as well as a decrease in quality of life.

Research findings by scientists and practitioners such as Bonica, Ferrell, Libeskind, Melzack, and Wall indicate that unrelieved pain can produce serious adverse immunological, psychological, and physical effects. The personal cost of unrelieved pain includes the eight Ds: depression, disease, distraction, drugs, doctor shopping, drinking, disability, and death. In recent years, there has been an increase of liability in relation to the undertreatment of pain, with successful lawsuits being waged under elder abuse laws on behalf of elderly clients whose pain was insufficiently treated.

The Agency for Health Care Research and Quality (AHRQ) affirms that "pain is a complex, physiological and subjective response with several quantifiable features, including intensity, time course, quality, impact, and personal meaning; and the single most reliable indicator of the existence and nature of pain is the patient's self-report" (p. 4). Several reasons are responsible for the undertreatment of pain, including myths and misconceptions, health professionals' lack of knowledge, patients' fears of addiction and overtreatment, and practitioners' fear of regulatory agencies.

In 2000, California recognized pain as a fifth vital sign. As a result, all health care agencies are required to include comfort assessment, and all medical schools are required to include pain management in their curriculum. It is believed that other states will soon follow with similar laws. Although there has been increased interest in the study of pain in recent years, there is still much that is not understood. In 2000, Congress declared 2000 to 2010 as the Decade of Pain control and Research, a mandate supported by the APS as the leading professional society in the field of pain management. In addition, the APS has developed and implemented the following core programs: (a) Public Awareness, (b) Professional Awareness, (c) Public Policy Agenda, and (d) Research Agenda.

Physiology

The oldest theory of pain that is still used today is the gate theory, which describes the mechanisms of pain. The flow of pain impulses from the peripheral nervous system and descending messages from the central nervous system can be increased or decreased by a neural "gating" mechanism in the dorsal horn (substantia gelatinosa). Endogenous opioids "dose" the gate and reduce transmission of pain. This mechanism, termed *nociception*, takes place in four stages.

1. *Transduction* begins in the periphery at the site of injury. Cell damage releases sensitizing substances: prostaglandin, bradykinin, serotonin, substance P, and histamine. An action potential results from the release of these substances (nociceptive pain) plus a change in the charge along the neuronal membrane or abnormal processing of stimuli by the nervous system (neuropathic pain). The change in the charge occurs when sodium moves into the cell and other ion transfers occur.

2. *Transmission* occurs in three phases. (a) The first phase is from the injury site to the spinal cord. Nociceptors terminate in the spinal cord. (b) The second phase is from the spinal cord to brain stem and thalamus. Release of substance P and other neurotransmitters continue the impulse across the synaptic cleft between the nociceptors and the dorsal horn neurons. From the dorsal horn of the spinal cord, neurons such as the spinothalamic tract ascend to the thalamus. Other tracts carry the message to different centers in the brain. (c) The third phase is from the thalamus to cortex. The thalamus acts as a relay station sending impulses to central structures for processing.

3. *Perception or the conscious experience of pain.*

4. *Modulation or the inhibition of nociceptive impulses.* Neurons originating in the brain stem descend to the spinal cord and release substances such as endogenous opioids, serotonin, and norepinephrine that inhibit the transmission of nociceptive impulses.

Pain Categories

Pain is broken down into categories based on the duration of pain (acute and chronic) and by physiology (cancer, nociceptive, and neuropathic).

Duration

Acute pain refers to pain that has a short life span. Once the cause, for instance, an injury, illness, or surgery, has resolved, the pain resolves. Postsurgical pain and procedural pain are subcategories of acute pain. Acute pain (also known as physiological pain) is usually somatic and/or visceral or nociceptive (e.g., surgical pain from traumatized skin, muscle, and visceral organs). Acute pain may be related to trauma, surgery, the inflammatory process, injury, or procedures. It is a short-term pain experience that demonstrates progressive resolution as the tissue heals, characterized by common physiologic responses (elevated heart rate, blood pressure, and respiratory rate; diaphoresis) and common behavioral responses (grimacing, crying, moaning, guarding). The cause is usually known and has a beginning and an end.

Chronic pain (also known as pathophysiological pain) persists longer than the usual course of an acute disease or a reasonable time for an injury to heal and may be associated with a chronic pathological process that causes continuous or intermittent pain for months or years. The cause of the pain may not be evident. Physiological and behavioral responses are not always evident in this group due to their return to baseline. Chronic pain serves no purpose and may have severe, intermittent exacerbations. The chronic pain patient population is increasing as a result of an increase in patient population of aging baby boomers and increased side effects from medical treatments, such as from antifungals or chemotherapies.

Physiology

Cancer pain results from three primary causes. It may be (1) related to tumor involvement, encroachment of surrounding tissues and organs by the tumor in 65% to 85% of cancer patients with pain; (2) a result of cancer treatment such as radiation or chemotherapy in 15% to 25% of cancer patients with pain; or (3) unrelated to cancer or its treatments in 3% to 10% of cancer patients with pain, resulting in structural and chemical alterations that affect the nature of the impulses. In some cases, these nerve endings remain hyperexcited, and normal touch is experienced as a severe painful burning sensation.

Neuropathic pain refers to an abnormal pain that outlasts the injury and is associated with nerve and/or central nervous system changes. Examples of this type of pain include neuropathies, postherpetic neuralgia, trigeminal neuralgia, complex regional pain syndrome, and others. Complex regional pain syndrome was previously termed *reflex sympathetic dystrophy*. During the Civil War, it was termed *causalgia*. Neuropathic pain is difficult to treat, but it can be done. This pain is described by patients as "hot, burning, prickly, needles and pins, electric-shock-like, shooting, lancinating etc."

Nociceptive pain emanates from damaged tissues, unlike neuropathic pain, which emanates from nerve damage. Examples of this include surgical pain, pain from fractures, burns, infections, lacerations, arthritis, organ (visceral) pain related to illness or organ damage, and so on. This pain is usually described using terms such as dull, deep, hard, bruised, sharp, aching, throbbing, or sore.

Pain Interventions

The most crucial part of managing pain is an appropriate pain assessment. This assessment consists of onset, location, duration, characteristics, aggravating/ alleviating factors, radiating, temporal factors, and severity. Several tools have been developed that are valid and reliable to measure pain. Examples of these tools include the 0 to 10 or 0 to 5 numerical scales, word descriptors, and Wong-Baker faces. The most commonly used scale is the 0 to 10 numerical scale. A behavior checklist has been designed for nonverbal or cognitively impaired patients. The list includes behaviors such as grimacing, moaning, guarding, and so on, and if the patient exhibits any or more of the behaviors on the list, it can be concluded that the patient is experiencing some form of discomfort.

Pharmacological interventions for pain include opioids, nonsteroidal antiinflammatory drugs (NSAIDS), and adjuvant analgesics. Nonpharmacological interventions include music, prayer, massage, acupuncture, cold, heat, relaxation exercises, and invasive procedures such as blocks, spinal cord stimulator implants, intrathecal pump implants, and others.

Research affirms that the best approach for the treatment of pain is multimodal. Treatment may include analgesics, physical therapy, cognitive approaches, mechanical interventions, complementary alternative approaches, and invasive procedures. Under the category of analgesics fall several medications that may be used independently of each other or in conjunction with each other. These analgesics include opioids, adjuvants, and NSAIDS.

Opioids are still the most important kind of analgesic. In the opioid category, there are two types: agonists and agonist-antagonist. Agonists are those opioids that bind to the mu receptors to produce analgesia. Agonist-antagonists are those opioids that presumably bind to the mu receptor but either exert no action (competitive agonist at the mu receptor) or exert only a limited action (partial agonist). Some medications such as nalorphine, cyclazosine, and nalbuphine block the mu receptor (competitive antagonists) but have a partial analgesic effect at other receptors. Analgesics mixed with other analgesic compounds—such as codeine and acetaminophen (Tylenol {#}3), hydrocodone and acetaminophen (Vicodin), or oxycodone and aspirin (Percodan)— are sometimes called weak opioids. Opioids do not have ceiling doses, meaning that the dose can be increased as much as needed until the patient achieves analgesia or experiences intolerable side effects. Mixed analgesics have ceilings based on the nonopioid. The maximum acetaminophen dose per 24 hr

is 4 g. Adjuvants comprise medications that are indicated for other conditions and are used to treat pain. Adjuvants include anticonvulsants, antidepressants, steroids, local anesthetics, antihypertensives, and muscle relaxants. The final group of analgesics is the NSAIDS and acetaminophen.

Ethics

Practitioners are at times confronted with ethical issues related to treatments. One such treatment is the placebo. Placebo use is considered unethical if it is used for reasons other than research and the patient has not signed an informed consent. End-of-life care includes managing pain and symptoms such as terminal agitation. Opioids, sedatives, and other analgesics are used to provide comfort to the dying. Other dilemmas arise when patients are suspected of "drug seeking" and practitioners refuse to provide analgesic interventions. Definitions have been provided to help guide practice. The problem with opioids is that to patients with addictive personalities, the step to drug abuse is very short. This causes clinicians to feel uncomfortable when prescribing opioids—thus the tendency to underprescribe.

In 2001, the American Academy of Pain Medicine, the American Pain Society, and the American Society of Addiction Medicine recognized the following definitions and recommended their use:

1. *Addiction* is a primary, chronic, neurobiological disease, with genetic, psychosocial, and environmental factors influencing its development and manifestations. It is characterized by behaviors that include one or more of the following: impaired control over drug use, compulsive use, continued use despite harm, and craving.

2. *Physical dependence* is a state of adaptation that is manifested by a drug class specific withdrawal syndrome that can be produced by abrupt cessation, rapid dose reduction, decreasing blood level of the drug, and/or administration of an antagonist.

3. *Tolerance* is a state of adaptation in which exposure to a drug induces changes that result in a diminution of one or more of the drug's effects over time.

4. *Pseudoaddiction* describes patient behaviors that may occur when pain is undertreated. Patients with unrelieved pain may become focused on obtaining medications, may "clock watch," and may otherwise seem inappropriately "drug seeking." Even

behaviors such as illicit drug use and deception can occur in the patient's efforts to obtain pain relief. Pseudoaddiction can be distinguished from true addiction in that the behaviors resolve when pain is effectively treated.

—Patti Shakhshir

See also Cancer; Drug Abuse and Dependence, Epidemiology of; Ethics in Health Care; Quality of Life, Quantification of

Further Readings

Agency for Health Care Research and Quality. (1994). *Clinical practice guideline: Management of cancer pain.* Rockville, MD: U.S. Department of Health and Human Services.

American Cancer Society. (2001). *Guide to pain control: Powerful methods to overcome cancer pain.* Atlanta, GA: Author.

American Pain Society. (2003). *Principles of analgesic use in the treatment of acute pain and cancer pain* (5th ed.). Glenview, IL: Author.

Doka, K. J. (2006). *Pain management at the end of life: Bridging the gap between knowledge and practice.* Washington, DC: Hospice Foundation of America.

Kuebler, K. K., Berry, P. H., & Heidrich, D. E. (Eds.). (2002). *End of life care: Clinical practice guidelines.* Philadelphia: W. B. Saunders.

McCaffery, M. (1968). *Nursing practice theories related to cognition, bodily pain, and man-environment interactions.* Los Angeles: University of California at Los Angeles Student's Store.

McCaffery, M., & Pasero, C. (1999). *Pain: Clinical manual* (2nd ed.). St. Louis, MO: Mosby.

Melzack, R., & Wall, P. D. (2003). *Handbook of pain management.* New York: Churchill Livingstone.

Mersky, H. (Ed.). (1986). Classification of chronic pain: Descriptions of chronic pain syndromes and definitions of pain terms. *Pain, 24*(Suppl. 1), S215–S221.

Portenoy, R. K., & Lesage, P. (1999). Management of cancer pain. *Lancet, 353*(9165), 1695–1700.

Raj, P. P. (2003). *Pain medicine: A comprehensive review* (2nd ed.). St. Louis, MO: Mosby.

Ross, E. L. (2004). *Hot topics: Pain management.* Philadelphia: Hanley & Belfus.

Schechter, N. L., Berde, C. B., & Yaster, M. (Eds.). (2003). *Pain in infants, children, and adolescents* (2nd ed.). Philadelphia: Lippincott Williams & Wilkins.

Smith, H. S. (2003). *Drugs for pain.* Philadelphia: Hanley & Belfus.

St. Marie, B. (2002). *American Society of Pain Management Nurses: Core curriculum for pain management nursing.* Philadelphia: W. B. Saunders.

Pan American Health Organization

The Pan American Health Organization (PAHO) is the oldest international public health agency in the world. Since 1902, it has worked to improve the health and living standards of the people of the Americas. PAHO is part of the United Nations system, serves as the Regional Office for the Americas of the World Health Organization, and is the health organization of the Inter-American System. The organization is not a financing agency but rather a technical cooperation agency, helping countries share technical information and mobilize health resources. From its headquarters in Washington, D.C., PAHO directs the scientific and technical efforts of experts in 27 country offices and in nine scientific centers. PAHO's annual budget for its core programs totals about $130 million, largely from assessed contributions paid by Member Governments. In addition, PAHO receives some support for health programs from other contributing countries, foundations, and the private sector.

PAHO refers to the regional cooperation among countries on health issues as Pan-Americanism, and the organization has helped countries work cooperatively, initiating multicountry health ventures in Central America, the Caribbean, the Andean Region, and the Southern Cone. Its field office on the U.S.-Mexico border works with states and counties on both sides of the border to solve common health problems.

PAHO's Mission, Vision, and Values

As stated on its Web site, PAHO's mission is to lead strategic collaborative efforts to promote equity in health, to combat disease, and to improve the quality and lengthen the lives of the peoples of the Americas. It works with the ministries of health of member nations and many other groups to improve the health of the peoples of the Americas and to strengthen health systems. PAHO promotes primary health care strategies to reach people in their communities and to extend health services equitably to all individuals, especially those who are vulnerable and impoverished. It supports programs to reduce the toll of chronic diseases and prevent transmission of communicable diseases, including old diseases that have reemerged—such as cholera, dengue, and tuberculosis—and new diseases such as HIV/AIDS, West Nile virus, and SARS.

PAHO's vision is to be the major catalyst for ensuring that all the peoples of the Americas enjoy optimal health and contribute to the well-being of their families and communities.

PAHO's values, as stated on its Web site ("About PAHO"), are the following:

- *Equity:* Striving for fairness and justice by eliminating differences in health that are unnecessary and avoidable
- *Excellence:* Achieving the highest quality in what [the organization] does
- *Solidarity:* Promoting shared interests and responsibilities and enabling collective efforts to achieve common goals
- *Respect:* Embracing the dignity and diversity of individuals, groups, and countries
- *Integrity:* Assuring transparent, ethical, and accountable performance

PAHO's Leadership

Dr. Mirta Roses Periago of Argentina became the new Director of the Pan American Health Organization on January 31, 2003. The Ministers of Health of the Americas elected her to a 5-year term. She is the fourth Latin American and the first woman to lead the world's oldest international health agency. Dr. Joxel García, a native of Puerto Rico and former commissioner of the Connecticut Department of Public Health, was PAHO's deputy director until October 31, 2006. Dr. Carissa Etienne, a former official of the Ministry of Health of Dominica and head of its National AIDS Program, is PAHO's assistant director.

PAHO's Activities

PAHO works with the countries in a variety of areas such as disease prevention and control, family and community health, sustainable development and environmental health, technology and health services delivery, information and knowledge management, health analysis and information systems, emergency preparedness and disaster relief, strategic analysis and partnerships, and strategic health development and public information, among others. PAHO is committed to the United Nations' Millennium Development

Goals and supports the drive to provide primary health care for all.

PAHO focuses on providing equal access to quality health care, safe drinking water and adequate sanitation to the most vulnerable groups, including mothers and children, laborers, the poor, the elderly, refugees, and displaced persons. PAHO also works to ensure that the countries' "have-nots" benefit from environmental protection against pollution, including toxic waste. Efforts are also directed at reducing pernicious gender inequity, reducing domestic abuse, and providing information on reproductive health.

A major priority for the Americas is to cut infant mortality, and PAHO is working to prevent infant deaths through the Integrated Management of Childhood Illness strategy, a simple and practical approach that teaches health workers a complete protocol for evaluating the health status of children brought to a health post or clinic. This helps reduce toll from diarrheal diseases, including cholera, and provides adequate diagnosis and treatment of acute respiratory infections, saving the lives of hundreds of thousands of children each year.

PAHO is committed to eliminating or controlling vaccine-preventable disease. One of the most notable successes was the eradication of smallpox from the Americas in 1973, a triumph that 5 years later led to global eradication of the dreaded disease. In 1994, PAHO led the eradication of polio from the Americas. Polio eradication is now a global goal. PAHO is on the way to eliminating measles from this hemisphere. Health officials have also agreed to seek to eradicate rubella and congenital rubella syndrome, responsible for many birth defects, and are pressing on with the introduction of new vaccines such as Haemophilus influenza B to reduce meningitis and respiratory infections.

PAHO also supports efforts to control malaria, Chagas' disease, dengue, urban rabies, leprosy, and other diseases that affect people in the Americas.

Action is ongoing to increase the supplies of safe blood by screening 100% of donated units of blood for disease and infection. Ensuring that volunteers free of disease donate all blood for transfusion is a critical goal for PAHO.

PAHO helps countries to identify and promote healthy lifestyles and to cope with issues of mental health, family health, reproductive health, and nutrition. It addresses major nutritional problems, including protein-energy malnutrition, and is working to eliminate iodine and vitamin A deficiencies. It also assists countries with health problems typically found in developed and urbanized cultures, such as cardiovascular diseases, cancer, accidents, smoking, addiction to drugs and alcohol, and others. PAHO's governing bodies have mandated PAHO to move aggressively in the fight to reduce the use of tobacco, emphasizing the negative health consequences and high costs of tobacco use.

PAHO disseminates scientific and technical information through publications, its Internet site, and networks of journalists, libraries, and documentation centers. It is a leader in the use of advanced communications technologies for health promotion, education, and a variety of specialized public health fields.

PAHO coordinates emergency humanitarian relief and technical assistance to regions struck by natural disasters and helps them prepare adequately to mitigate the effects of disasters.

—*Daniel Epstein*

See also Child and Adolescent Health; Epidemiology in Developing Countries; Maternal and Child Health; Vaccination; World Health Organization

Web Sites

Pan American Health Organization: http://www.paho.org.

PANEL DATA

Panel data, also known as longitudinal data, are important in many areas of research, including epidemiology, psychology, sociology, economics, and public health. Data from longitudinal studies in clinical trials and cohort studies with long-term follow-ups are a primary example of panel data. Unlike data from traditional cross-sectional studies, panel data consist of multiple snapshots or panels of a study group or a cohort of subjects over time and, thus, provide a unique opportunity to study changes in outcomes of interest over time, causal effects, and disease progression, in addition to providing more power for assessing treatment differences and associations of different outcomes. Such data also present many methodological challenges in study designs and data analyses, the most prominent being correlated responses and missing data. As a result,

classic models for cross-sectional data analysis such as multiple linear and logistic regressions do not apply to panel data.

Methodologic Issues for Panel Data Analysis

In cross-sectional studies, observations from study subjects are available only at a single time, whereas in longitudinal and cohort studies, individuals are assessed or observed repeatedly over time. By taking advantages of multiple assessments over time, panel data from longitudinal studies capture both between-individual differences and within-individual dynamics, offering the opportunity to study more complicated biological, psychological, and behavioral hypotheses than those that can be addressed using cross-sectional or time-series data. For example, if we want to test whether exposure to some chemical agent can cause a disease of interest such as cancer, the between-subject difference observed in cross-sectional data can provide evidence only for an association or correlation between the exposure and disease. The supplementary within-individual dynamics in panel data allows for inference of a causal nature for such a relationship.

Although panel data provide much richer information about the relationship among different outcomes, especially their causal nature, they raise challenging methodologic issues for study design, data analysis, and interpretation of analysis results. The two most important concerns are correlated responses and missing data. First, panel data create correlated responses because repeated assessments are collected from the same subject. For example, if we measure an individual's blood pressure twice, the two readings are correlated since they reflect the health condition of this particular individual; if he or she has high blood pressure, both readings tend to be higher than the normal range (positively correlated) despite the variations over repeated assessments. The existence of such within-subject correlations invalidates the independent sampling assumption required for most classic models, and as a result, statistical methods developed based on the independence of observations, such as the analysis of variance (ANOVA) and the multiple linear and logistic regression models, are not valid for panel data. In the blood pressure example, if we ignored the correlations between the two readings and modeled the mean blood pressure using ANOVA, then for a sample of n subjects, we would claim to have $2n$ independent observations. However, if the two readings were collected within a very short time span, say 5 s apart, they would be almost identical and would certainly not represent independent data comparable to blood pressure readings taken from two different people. In other words, the variation between two within-subject readings would be much smaller than any two between-subject observations, invalidating the model assumption of independent observations and yielding underestimated error variance in this case. Although assessments in most real studies are not spaced as closely as in this extreme example, the within-subject correlation still exists. Ignoring such correlations by applying classic models may yield incorrect inferences.

Missing data present a more serious challenge in the analysis of panel data. Because panel data are collected over time, frequently in studies of lengthy duration, missing data are inevitable and happens for a variety of reasons. For example, in clinical trial studies, subjects may simply quit the study or not return for follow-up visits because of problems with transportation, weather, deteriorated or improved health condition, relocation, accidental death, treatment complications, and so on. Because missing data can seriously bias model estimates for panel data analysis, they are characterized in terms of their impact on inference through statistical assumptions or missing data mechanisms, which allow statisticians to ignore the multitude of specific reasons for missing data when performing data analysis. The *missing completely at random* (MCAR) assumption refers to a class of missing data that do not affect inference on model parameters when completely ignored. MCAR corresponds to a layperson's notion of data missing at random and includes all types of missing data that are unrelated to study or treatment, such as relocation, transportation problems, and bad weather conditions. Another important class of missing data is called *missing at random* (MAR), which generalizes MCAR to deal with treatment-related missing data. In many clinical trials, missing data are often associated with the treatment interventions under study. For example, a patient may quit the study if he or she feels that the study treatment has deteriorated his or her health condition, and any further treatment would only worsen the medical or psychological problems. Or, a patient may feel that he or she has completely responded to

the treatment and does not see any additional benefit in continuing the treatment. In such cases, missing data do not follow the MCAR model since it is predicted by study or treatment-related responses. This class of reasons for missing data is modeled by the MAR assumption, which posits that the occurrence of a missing response depends on the response history or observed pattern. Thus, MAR postulates a plausible and applicable missing data condition that encompasses many treatment-related missing data and constitutes a sensible statistical approach to address bias in such situations. It is important to distinguish between these two common types of missing data, as some statistical models for panel data analysis only provide unbiased estimates under the stronger MCAR assumption, as we discuss next.

Modeling Approaches for Panel Data Analysis

As most classic models do not apply to panel data, specialized methods must be employed to address the within-subject correlation and missing data problems. The two most popular approaches for panel data analysis are the mixed-effects models (MM) and generalized estimating equations (GEE). MM is a general class of models that can be used for regression analysis with continuous, ordinal, categorical, and count responses. As panel data are common in an ever-widening variety of experimental and observational study designs in the biological, biomedical, behavioral, economic, epidemiological, and social sciences, various applications of MM have been found in these disciplines under different guises such as random coefficient models, random effects models, random regression, hierarchical linear models, latent variable models, mixed models, and multilevel linear models. Unlike the classic multivariate linear model, MM does not directly model the correlations among the repeated, within-subject responses but rather employs random effects (or latent variables) to account for such correlations. As a result, this approach enables one to model correlation structures without directly involving the within-subject responses, giving rise to a powerful and flexible way to deal with missing data as well as to address varying assessment times often found in cohort and longitudinal observational studies.

MM is a class of parametric models, requiring analytic distribution assumptions for both the response (observed) and the random effects (latent). A fundamental problem with using random effects to account for correlated responses is the difficulty in empirically validating the distribution assumption for the random effects since they are latent variables. Further exacerbating this problem, MM relies on the distribution assumption for the response for inference. If either set of assumptions is violated, estimates will be biased, laying the basis for spurious findings.

A remarkable breakthrough underlying GEE-based inference is the elimination of both sets of assumptions, leading to inference of model parameters that are robust to data distributions and within-cluster correlation structures. Like MM, GEE is a general class of regression models capable of accommodating all types of responses. However, unlike MM, which relies on parametric distributions for the random effects and response for inference, GEE models the marginal mean of the response and uses estimating equations for inference, eliminating both layers of assumptions and thereby providing unbiased estimates regardless of the complexity of the correlation structure and the data distribution. Thus, under GEE, neither the specification of random effect nor the distribution of response is required.

A major weakness of GEE is that it requires MCAR to provide unbiased estimation of model parameters. In this regard, MM is more robust as it guarantees valid inference under both MCAR and MAR, provided, of course, the model assumptions (particularly the distribution ones) are met. This limitation of GEE is addressed by the latest development on GEE-based inference and in particular, the weighted GEE (WGEE), which extends the GEE to provide valid inference under MAR. Thus, WGEE is robust against not only data distributions but also the missing data types.

MM, GEE, and WGEE are implemented in most popular statistical software such as SAS, Splus, and SPSS. For example, MM is implemented in the SAS NLMIXED procedure and GEE and WGEE in the GENMOD procedure.

Other Related Topics

There are several panel-data-related topics that are not covered in this entry. For example, measurement error may arise in panel data that cannot be addressed by classic measurement error models. Also, in clinical trials that involve higher mortality rates, it may be necessary to jointly model the patient's dropout process and outcome of interest to provide more information about the progression of disease. In addition to MM, GEE, and WGEE, multiple imputation (MI) may also be used to address missing data. A great advantage of MI is that it uses software for complete data analysis to provide inference in the presence of missing data. However, as the specialized methods such as MM and GEE are implemented in most major statistical packages, MI is not widely used for panel data analysis. Finally, causal inference involving multiple outcomes collected over time cannot be addressed by MM, GEE, or WGEE and requires more specialized methods such as the structural equation models. The list of further readings provides detailed discussions of these and other panel-data-related research topics.

—*Changyong Feng, Wan Tang, and Xin Tu*

See also Descriptive and Analytical Epidemiology; Missing Data Methods; Robust Statistics; Study Design

Further Readings

Diggle, P. J., Heagerty, P. J., Liang, K. Y., & Zeger, S. L. (2002). *Analysis of longitudinal data* (2nd ed.). Oxford, UK: Oxford University Press.

Dmitrienko, A., Molenberghs, G., Chuang-Stein, C., & Offen, W. (2005). *Analysis of clinical trials using SAS: A practical guide.* Cary, NC: SAS Institute.

Hanley, J. A., Negassa, A., Edwardes, M. D. deB., & Forrester, J. E. (2003). Statistical analysis of correlated data using generalized estimating equations: An orientation. *American Journal of Epidemiology, 157,* 364–375.

Hsiao, C. (2003). *Analysis of panel data* (2nd ed.). Cambridge, UK: Cambridge University Press.

Little, R. J., & Rubin, D. B. (1987). *Statistical analysis with missing data.* New York: Wiley.

Rotnizky, A., & Robins, J. M. (1997). Analysis of semi-parametric regression models with non-ignorable non-response. *Statistics in Medicine, 16,* 81–102.

Schafer, J. L. (1997). *Analysis of incomplete multivariate data.* New York: Chapman & Hall.

Tu, X. M., Kowalski, J., Zhang, J., Lynch, K., & Crits-Christoph, P. (2004). Power analyses for longitudinal trials and other clustered study design. *Statistics in Medicine, 23,* 2799–2815.

Parasitic Diseases

Parasites can be defined as organisms that live in or on another organism called a host. In most situations, the parasite benefits from this relationship, often at the expense of the host organism. Traditionally, parasites include protozoans and helminths. However, today, the term *parasite* is sometimes used to describe the multitude of viruses, bacteria, fungi, plants, and animals, including ticks, mites, and lice, that act in a parasitic fashion. Traditional parasites (protozoans and helminths) are responsible for many diseases in animals and humans and are transmitted to their host most often through the ingestion of contaminated food or water or arthropods, which act as intermediate hosts and vectors. Parasites pose health risks and economic costs in livestock and in humans and are often associated with epidemics when a disease occurs at a higher rate than would be expected within a defined area. The high prevalence of parasitic disease in humans provides opportunity for epidemiological studies that examine parasite pathogenicity, hosts, environment, and social conditions that may play a role in the spread of disease.

Traditional Parasites

Research has shown that parasites existed in ancient civilizations as evidenced by written records and the discovery of eggs of parasites in ancient Egyptian mummies. In 1875, Fedor A. Lösch demonstrated that the causative agent of dysentery was the protozoan *Entamoeba histolytica*. Protozoa are single-celled, heterotrophic eukaryotes, most of which are free-living. The discovery of *E. histolytica* as a pathogen led to the identification of other species of pathogenic protozoa. The flagellated protozoa *Trypanosoma rhodesiense* that is transmitted to humans through the bite of infected tsetse flies causes sleeping sickness (African trypanosomiasis). The organisms reproduce rapidly, avoiding recognition by antibodies in the blood and possibly outnumbering red blood cells. They travel through the bloodstream and eventually reach the spinal cord and brain, leading to coma and death. In a healthy human infected with *T. rhodesiense*, the disease may become a chronic condition, with the organism later becoming opportunistic if the immune system is weakened. The protozoa of the *Leishmania* species are transmitted to humans by infected sand flies and infect macrophages that attempt to engulf and digest the foreign pathogen. Eventually, the macrophages and immune defenses become overwhelmed causing leishmaniasis. This is a debilitating and fatal disease and epidemics have occurred in India, China, Africa, and Brazil.

Descriptions of malarial disease have dated back to ancient Chinese and Greek civilizations; however, the actual cause of malaria, protozoans of the genus *Plasmodium*, was not discovered until 1898, when it was found that humans could become infected through the bite of an infected mosquito. Once in the bloodstream, the *Plasmodium* travels to the liver where it infects and replicates within cells. The burden of organisms within a single cell will cause it to burst, releasing the *Plasmodium*, and allowing it to infect red blood cells, where it replicates rapidly, again causing the cell to rupture. The infection cycle into red blood cells may happen several times, resulting in a large quantity of *Plasmodium* and the symptoms of infection, such as intermittent fever.

Helminths include roundworms, also called nematodes, and flatworms, such as flukes and tapeworms. Filarial disease may be caused by one of several species of helminth nematodes. The filarial nematode *Wucheria bancrofti* is transmitted to humans by arthropods and is commonly found in Africa, the Middle East, Mexico, and Brazil. Humans and mosquitoes are the only suitable hosts in which *Wucheria* is able to complete its life cycle. Once injected into the bloodstream, the immature worms make their way into a lymph duct and mature into adults, which may take between 6 months and a year and result in a worm about 3 to 4 inches in length. Multiple adult females will exist in streams of clusters within a lymph duct where they reproduce, shedding thousands of microfilia every day, sometimes remaining in the lymph duct for 5 to 10 years. The accumulation of microfilia in the lymph ducts blocks the flow of lymphatic fluid causing swelling in affected body parts. Microfilia eventually migrate into the bloodstream and are drawn into the proboscis of a mosquito when it bites the host. In general, the immune system is able to defend against and kill the majority of microfilia, resulting only in minor illness associated with the lymphatic system and a low rate of morbidity.

Flatworms, such as the tapeworm, can cause infection and disease in humans. The tapeworm species *Diphyllobothrium latum* or one of several different species in the genus *Taenia*, in addition to several other genera, can be infectious. Tapeworms are highly specialized worms that attach themselves to the lining of the human intestinal wall using hooks that keep them firmly in place, or burrow into tissues such as muscle, the spinal cord, or the brain. Adult tapeworms tend to stay within their host as long as possible, with just one adult tapeworm per host growing and reproducing continuously, shedding eggs that are excreted in the feces. Juvenile tapeworms pose the greatest health risks to humans because of their tendency to burrow through the intestinal wall, migrating to internal organs where they interfere with normal tissue function. Infection with adult tapeworms may be asymptomatic; sometimes abdominal pain or diarrhea occurs but is not immediately known to be the result of a tapeworm infection. Infection with juvenile tapeworms can cause cysticercosis, typified by the formation of cysts under the skin, inflammation, mental disorientation, and seizures.

Parasite Life Cycles

All parasites have a life cycle that involves a period of time spent in a host organism and the phases of which can be divided into growth, reproduction, and transmission. Life cycles of parasites can be divided into two categories: direct (monoxenous) and indirect (heteroxenous). Parasites with direct life cycles spend most of their adult lives in one host, known as the parasitic stage, with their progeny transmitted from one host to another, known as the free-living stage. Direct parasites often lack an intermediate stage and must leave their host. To do this, they must be able to survive in an environment outside their original host and then locate and establish in a new host. Parasites that depend on the host stage are called obligate parasites, whereas parasites that can skip the parasitic stage for several generations are called facultative parasites. Roundworms, trypanosomatids, and *Cryptosporidium* are examples of parasites with direct life cycles. Parasites with indirect life cycles are characterized by two host stages, which require a definitive host and an intermediate host. The definitive host stage is required for reproduction and the adult life phase. Within the intermediate host, parasite development occurs, after which it can be transmitted to a definitive host. Multiple developmental stages may take place in an intermediate host, which plays an important role in facilitating disease transmission in the form of vectors, such as mosquitoes, which pass immature parasites through their proboscis directly into the bloodstream of the definitive host. Filarial nemotodes, *Plasmodium*, and *Leishmania* are examples of parasites with indirect life cycles. Reservoir hosts typically tolerate parasites with no ill effects; however, the introduction of a new host into a population of reservoir hosts will often result in severe disease in the newly introduced host.

Epidemiology

Close to 3 billion people worldwide are infected with parasites. Parasites are often endemic and sometimes epidemic in certain regions of the world. For instance, the pathogenic parasite *Plasmodium* that causes malaria is a constant concern in Africa and often occurs in endemic and epidemic proportions, and sleeping sickness, caused by a species of *Trypanosoma*, has resulted in epidemic disease in Uganda. The emergence of diseases resulting from pathogenic parasites is always an issue of concern in many tropical regions around the world. Studies of infected populations and of pathogenic parasites have provided, and continue to provide, insight into ways to prevent, treat, and control disease. Following simple sanitation procedures, such as washing hands, cooking meat, and keeping human waste separate from humans, food supplies, pets, and livestock can prevent many diseases caused by parasites. However, these sanitary guidelines are not so easy to follow in Third World countries, which may lack monetary support to provide clean water sources or proper medications, or in cultures where humans maintain intimate dwellings with their livestock and their coexisting parasites. A more difficult problem to overcome is the presence of arthropod hosts in numbers sufficient to infect large number of people over a short period of time, especially in tropical climates. These diseases can be maintained indefinitely in human populations that have a lack of access to medical relief to break the parasite infection cycle.

Treatment

Unsanitary conditions are often the underlying cause of parasitic disease, especially in areas that are overpopulated or have poor water quality, or among populations that lack knowledge of parasites. In addition, parasites have evolved in ways that enable them to avoid antibody recognition and elimination by the immune system by entering into the cells of the body. This results in a cell-mediated immune response, including activation of helper and cytotoxic T cells, cytokines, and interleukins. Protozoa such as *Toxoplasma gondii*, *Leishmania*, and *Plasmodium* have each found ways to avoid or use the human immune system to their advantage, facilitating their replication and increasing their pathogenicity. Antiparasitic drugs can be divided into antiprotozoan agents and antihelminthic agents. Antiprotozoans are typically designed to be effective in disrupting a specific stage in a parasite life cycle. Drugs against *Plasmodium* can be taken as prophylactics in the case of oral chloroquine or as treatment for acute attacks in the case of oral chloroquine in combination with sulfadoxine or oral quinine in combination with tetracycline. Other commonly used antiprotozoal drugs include metronidazole, amphotericin B, and suramin.

Antihelminthic drugs cause physical damage to parasitic worms, in most cases targeting adult worms, and inhibit their metabolism, inhibit their ability to lay eggs, or facilitate their excretion from the host. The class of benzimidazole antihelminthics, which includes mebendazole and albendazole, causes degeneration of microtubules that inhibits glucose uptake. These drugs are used as first line therapy for most roundworm and some tapeworm infections. Ivermectin, synthesized from a group of naturally occurring substances, is often used to treat leishmaniasis by causing paralysis of the infecting worms and is effective against *W. bancrofti*. Other antihelminthic agents include diethylcarbamazine and praziquantal.

—*Kara E. Rogers*

See also Epidemiology in Developing Countries; Malaria; Waterborne Diseases

Further Readings

Fernando, R. L., Fernando, S. S. E., & Leong, A. S.-Y. (2001). *Tropical infectious diseases*. Boston: Cambridge University Press.

Hardman, J. G., & Limbird, L. E. (Eds.). (2001). *Goodman and Gilman's the pharmacological basis of therapeutics* (10th ed.). New York: McGraw-Hill.

Mehlhorn, H. (Ed.). (2001). *Encyclopedic reference of parasitology: Biology, structure, function* (2nd ed.). New York: Springer.

PARTICIPATION RATE

See RESPONSE RATE

PARTICIPATORY ACTION RESEARCH

Research oriented toward action and/or change can take three forms: (1) It can apply the professional expert model, in which the researcher makes a study and recommends a course of action to decision makers in the organization studied; (2) it may involve action research controlled by the researcher, in which the researcher aims to be a principal change agent as well as controlling the research process; or (3) it may involve participatory action research (PAR), in which the researcher seeks to involve some members of the organization studied as active participants in all stages of the research or action process.

Investigations in the PAR context indicate a systematic effort to generate knowledge about specific conditions that can influence changes in a given situation. The term *action* in research indicates that the research is meant to contribute to change efforts or accompany action by the part of participants, such as workers and their representative trade unions, or change for employers, through the research learning process. PAR has its roots in social psychology and is a relatively new research technique in epidemiology but can be applied fruitfully in many contexts, for instance, to understand the causes of and reduce the number of worker injuries in an occupational setting or to reduce morbidity and mortality from diabetes in a community. The entry uses the example of PAR in a workplace setting to illustrate the principles of PAR. Workplace PAR is a process of systematic inquiry in which those who are experiencing a work-related problem participate with trained researchers in deciding the focus of knowledge generation, in collecting and analyzing information, and in taking action to improve the conditions or to resolve the problem entirely.

PAR as a Multidisciplinary Methodology

PAR methodology has been used in community development and health-related research, such as with community health workers and nurses, in industrial and other types of organizations, and in research in agriculture. In these settings, researchers using PAR have focused primarily on oppressed groups to empower and generate collective action, where new knowledge based on research led to local level and industrial actions aimed at improvements for workers. PAR has also been used extensively in organizational development in industry and by management's application of human resource theories, particularly those with a systems perspective focusing on the fit, or lack of fit, between technical and social systems. When participatory systems work well, they produce results because they apply a wide range of information and ideas to problems in an organizational context.

Applying PAR as a methodology requires ensuring that those participating in the research feel that the researchers have genuine respect for them and their experiences, that their opinions are valued, and that they are perceived as partners in the process. Research tool choice should depend on what is being studied as well as why a subject is being studied. PAR can be used to extend the principles of education for empowerment, which espouse learning that is participatory, based on real-life experiences. The primary purpose of PAR has, thus, often been to encourage the poor and oppressed, and those who work with them, to generate and control their own knowledge. As a research methodology, PAR assumes that knowledge generates power and that people's knowledge is central to social change.

PAR for Workplace-Based Research

The application of PAR methodology in occupational health research starts from a belief that adults are self-motivated, rich with information that has immediate application to their lives and work. In research where workers' health is in question due to work processes, some degree of change in the organization is likely to be necessary to prevent further work-related injury and illness.

Few problems can be resolved in modern industrial organizations through the use of any single academic discipline; the complex nature of work calls for integrating ideas and methods from a variety of disciplines. The increasingly complex nature of the workplace gives rise to greater need to understand the causes and methods of prevention of work-related accidents, injuries, and illnesses, with the transmission of this information to workers, managers, and others being a critical dimension of preventing these negative outcomes. Important advantages of PAR methods include the qualitative information obtained about workers involved in the study, the potential to obtain a precise picture of work-related risks and the root

causes, and the semiquantitative data on adverse health outcomes. Use of the research process as a means of catalyzing a process of consciousness raising and organization among workers is a further advantage, enabling positive actions for workplace improvements.

The need for a holistic view of occupational disease is a compelling reason for occupational physicians to view workers as a member of an occupational health team and gives rise to the fundamental need for a systems approach to health-related problems, involving workers as an indispensable source of information and valuable agent of change.

In conducting PAR-based occupational health research, both qualitative and quantitative techniques can be applied. Quantitative techniques may include survey-based data collection and systematic analysis by structured questionnaire with closed- and open-ended questions. Qualitative techniques may include structured individual interviews with open-ended questions, participant observation on the job, focus group interviews and discussions, videotaping, and examination of work process, workstation analysis, document and archival review, and broad or well-defined literature review. Engaging in discussion with workers and management at various stages of the research process is an important means of increasing confidence in the research findings by both groups, and it can strengthen the process and outcomes aimed at eventual change.

Comparisons by Laurell, Noriega, Martinez, and Villegas (1992) of workplace-based study results based on PAR methodology made with results from an individual questionnaire have affirmed that PAR-generated results are more revealing than individual questionnaire-generated results. Rosskam (2007) applied PAR methodology in a study of airport check-in workers; the process and findings led to direct improvements in various airports and contributed to policy changes in a number of countries. Hugentobler, Israel, and Schurman (1992) used PAR methods to implement a longitudinal multimethodological research and intervention project investigating occupational stress, psychosocial factors, and health outcomes; their findings were combined with intervention to improve worker health. Israel, Schurman, and Hugentobler (1992) used PAR methodology to better understand and try to reduce the negative effects of work-related stress. Ritchie (1996) described the workplace as a useful venue for research, where social and environmental factors in a work environment can be relatively easily explored, a defined community where one can legitimately explore and help develop improvement-oriented and empowerment-based strategies for action. Schurman (1996) used a PAR approach to study stress in an automobile factory, involving the factory workers in the investigation. The process was designed to improve the system's performance through work organization redesign and to contribute to the body of scientific knowledge at the same time.

Participatory action researchers put into question domination and dominating research structures and relationships, including how actual organizational structures, processes, and practices shape and influence the ways in which those holding decision-making power relate to those not holding decision-making power. This questioning is particularly relevant and important to work-related research given the complex nature of worker-management relationships; indeed, it is the very process of human inquiry that provides the impetus toward action. At its core, PAR in work-related health issues promotes worker participation in decision making in the workplace, which implies an inherent redistribution of power between workers and management. In workplace PAR, this can also be conceived of as sharing and providing information and access to resource mobilization to help others as well as oneself.

PAR methodology incorporates the recognition that research can involve workers as an integral part of the process. The process can be a tool to encourage workers to question and challenge the very systems that may keep them passive and not able to participate in decision making, which in turn adversely affects their well-being. Dialogue and participation in the research process are means for workers to gain a critical understanding of the causes of workplace problems and their role in accepting or challenging these forces. Where workers are consulted and participate in projects likely to affect them, positive outcomes and changes are more likely to be sustainable, and participants can critically analyze the barriers to change in systems of work organization.

PAR in the workplace, like education, is most effective when it includes a holistic view of the context of behaviors, including an analysis of obstacles to safe or healthful work practices, without becoming narrowed to specific behaviors or competencies. Employing a holistic and systems view is concordant with the reality that improvement in working conditions takes place in a wider organizational context of worker and management relations.

PAR Compared With Other Research Methodologies

The professional expert model could be appropriate for examining contributing factors and moderating variables posited to cause a given health outcome. Case studies are not developed as a means of measuring a variety of causal factors. PAR, however, lends itself as a useful method by which multiple factors and outcomes can be examined. The contribution of detailed information from study participants is a key means of learning about factors thought to contribute to, or cause, outcomes, which is not inherent in the professional expert model. The descriptive aspects of a case study model may be useful for detailing a worker population and depicting working conditions. A detailed work analysis is indispensable for understanding how jobs are performed. While observation and questioning can be applied in case study development, the researcher maintains a more distant attitude than that used in a PAR methodology. The difference in researcher attitude between PAR and the professional expert model is significant in determining how a study process unfolds. Where participants feel themselves viewed as the object of scientific research rather than part of a process designed to benefit them, engendering a sense of trust and involvement becomes more difficult.

For a worker health study, where a change process is part of the study design, direct involvement with the participants is essential. Direct involvement with participants is of particular importance to identify problems associated with the job, as these are best known by the person performing the job. The professional expert model does not include the use of focus group discussions as part of the research process, as this could "contaminate," or influence the research process, compromising objectivity. In contrast, focus group discussions are accepted and even encouraged in a PAR methodology as a key means of obtaining rich, qualitative information, and for obtaining support for participation in the study. Focus group discussions can be also very useful for generating hypotheses.

In both the professional expert model and a case study methodology, there is no demarcation between theory and practice. In both these methods, it is the researcher who defines the problem to be studied. There is no feedback mechanism built into these methodologies, no requirement that knowledge gained be shared directly with the study participants. The professional expert model contributes to the body of knowledge shared by only a limited group of "experts." These methods neither include an action component meant to contribute to change on the part of the participants nor are they designed to create a learning process for the participants. In contrast, PAR is designed to create a learning process among participants and to ensure the dissemination and application of knowledge and experience gained. For research on workers' health problems, where entire systems are questioned, one can argue that research needs to be directly relevant to those involved and that the findings are shared, and have the potential to contribute to organizational change, in addition to contributing to the existing body of knowledge.

Limitations of PAR

One of the difficulties in PAR is to ensure that all groups understand the process and feel validated and valued in their contributions to the research design, process, and any outcomes. PAR researchers must be careful not to speak only in academic terms with the various groups and not to presume the same understanding of research terminology and ability to interpret data—but without appearing condescending or technocratic. This entails a delicate balance on the part of PAR researchers, who should see themselves as learners and facilitators in addition to being scientists. Listening to and learning from workers and managers about workplace issues is valuable and enriching, albeit time-consuming. PAR researchers have the additional responsibility to help the various participants learn from the process, which can be time-consuming.

An additional difficulty in applying a PAR approach is arriving at consensus with workers and employers, establishing a relationship with each group, and bringing them into the process. These can be both difficult and lengthy processes for the researcher. The processes are more time-consuming than research based on, for example, the professional expert model, where input from various groups is not involved and where consensus building is not required at any stage. The consultative process in PAR methodology is likely, therefore, to be more costly in terms of researchers' time and in analysis of qualitative data.

As with any research methodology, there exists the potential for bias to be introduced. This can occur in defining the issues to be addressed, or if the participating groups want more emphasis on certain issues of greater importance or concern to them, which may also be areas of political concern. Stronger emphasis on particular issues by any one participating group could skew results. In working with management and unions, researchers must exercise caution to not fall into political traps, based on the agendas of any one group. While the research team must gain the confidence of all groups involved, if they are perceived to lean more toward one group's interest than another's, they may lose the confidence of the other group. Maintaining what can be a delicate balance is necessary, apart from being perceived as neutral with all groups, while ensuring that all concerns are addressed. There is also a risk of researcher bias through personal involvement with the participant community as well as in any change process that may develop. The researcher can influence how the change process unfolds and how the research findings are interpreted and applied within and beyond the participating groups. Care must be exercised to maintain a distance from the process, allowing the stakeholder groups to define how a change process is envisioned and formulated. In the end, it is the workers and managers who will have to live with the effects of any changes they implement, or any changes they do not implement, since nonimplementation of changes, after awareness has been raised, can also have consequences.

Validity and Reliability of Data Collected

A debate exists about the validity and reliability of data, in particular when they are qualitative and obtained through participatory appraisal. In the course of data collection, researchers' interpretation and conclusions can be confirmed or disputed by participants in the research process. Confirmation by the participant community of the accuracy of the study findings and analysis of the data greatly increases the credibility of the research findings. PAR is open to various interpretations that can include the researcher and participant community designing the study together or researchers designing the study and then collecting the data with the help of the participating group. Perhaps this is the best means of ensuring that research contributes to an organizational change process given the complex nature of today's organizations.

PAR is important to epidemiology and to epidemiologists. Some epidemiologists would challenge PAR as being "not objective." Many epidemiologists do not involve themselves in PAR because intervention studies are often more difficult to carry out than strictly quantitative research and can take more time and, thus, may cost more. It can be easier to analyze an existing data set than to talk to groups of people, build consensus, and aim for real change to improve health. Yet it is precisely through intervention-based research and the adequate evaluation of this research that public health and occupational health get improved. For epidemiological research to not remain "ivory tower" in nature, epidemiologists need to be aware of the importance of PAR, perhaps today more than ever before. Epidemiologists stand only to gain from joint research together with working people.

—Ellen Rosskam

See also Environmental and Occupational Epidemiology; Health Disparities; Qualitative Methods in Epidemiology

Further Readings

Abrams, H. (1983). The worker as teacher. *American Journal of Industrial Medicine, 4,* 759–768.

Dash, D. P. (Ed.). (1998). *Problems of action research: As I see it.* Lincoln, UK: Lincoln School of Management.

De Koning, K., & Martin, M. (Eds.). (1996). *Participatory research in health: Issues and experiences.* London: Zed Books.

Deshler, D., & Ewert, M. (1995). *Participatory action research: Traditions and major assumptions.* Ithaca, NY: Cornell University, Department of Education.

Elden, M. (1981). Political efficacy at work: The connection between more autonomous forms of workplace organization and more participatory politics. *American Political Science Review, 75*(1), 43–58.

Elden, M. (1981). Sharing the research work: Participative research and its role demands. In P. Reason & J. Rowan (Eds.), *Human inquiry: A sourcebook of new paradigm research* (pp. 253–266). Chichester, UK: Wiley.

Hugentobler, M., Israel, B. A., & Schurman, S. J. (1992). An action research approach to workplace health: Integrating methods. *Health Education Quarterly, 19*(1), 55–76.

Israel, B., Schurman, S. J., & Hugentobler, M. K. (1992). Conducting action research: Relationships between organization members and researchers. *Journal of Applied Behavioral Science, 28*(1), 74–101.

Khanna, R. (1996). Participatory action research (PAR) in women's health: SARTHI, India. In K. De Koning & M. Martin (Eds.), *Participatory research in health: Issues and experiences* (pp. 62–81). London: Zed Books.

Laurell, A., Noriega, M., Martinez, S., & Villegas, J. (1992). Participatory research on workers' health. *Social Science and Medicine, 34*(6), 603–613.

Mergler, D. (1987). Worker participation in occupational health research: Theory and practice. *International Journal of Health Services, 17*(1), 151–167.

Ritchie, J. (1996). Participatory research in the workplace. In K. De Koning & M. Martin (Eds.), *Participatory research in health: Issues and experiences* (pp. 205–215). London: Zed Books.

Rosskam, E. (2007). *Excess baggage: Leveling the load and changing the workplace.* New York: Baywood.

Schurman, S. (1996). Making the New American workplace safe and healthy: A joint labor-management-researcher approach. *American Journal of Industrial Medicine, 29,* 373–377.

Smith, S., Willms, D., & Johnson, D. (Eds.). (1997). *Nurtured by knowledge: Learning to do participatory action-research.* New York: Apex Press.

Whyte, W. F. (Ed.). (1991). *Participatory action research.* Newbury Park, CA: Sage.

Whyte, W. F. (1991). *Social theory for action: How individuals and organizations learn to change.* Newbury Park, CA: Sage.

PARTNER NOTIFICATION

Partner notification (PN) is a fundamental component of sexually transmitted infection (STI) prevention and control programs in many state jurisdictions and may help prevent the spread of STIs and human immunodeficiency virus (HIV) among individuals who engage in risky sexual behaviors outside the context of a monogamous relationship. Traditional PN uses three different strategies for notifying the sexual partners of patients infected with an STI or HIV: provider referral (notification of sexual partners via a third party, such as an individuals' medical provider), partner referral (notification of sexual partners via the index patient), and contract referral (an agreement between the patient and provider, whereby the patient is given the opportunity to notify their sexual partners on their own, with the understanding that their partners will be notified by a third party if they have not been notified by a predetermined date).

PN was previously referred to as contact tracing, though more recently it includes the comprehensive category of partner services—the process of obtaining from individuals recently diagnosed with an STI information about their sexual partners and facilitating the triage procedure for the examination and treatment of those partners. Conducting PN assumes that the index patient has identifying and locating information for their sexual partners, which is often not the case for individuals with multiple anonymous partners, such as individuals who meet their partners on the Internet sexual Web sites or public and private sex venues. It is also important to note that laws regarding PN for STIs and HIV infection differ from state to state, and that PN is traditionally a voluntary process, and that patient confidentiality is protected by law.

Partner Services for Individuals Diagnosed With STIs

In an attempt to avoid STI reinfection and/or continued transmission and acquisition of infection, it is imperative that examination and treatment of the sexual partner(s) be addressed when medical providers diagnose patients with an STI. The partner services process includes notification of partners in the case of STIs and HIV partner counseling and referral services (PCRS). PCRS programs provide services to HIV-infected persons and their sexual and needle-sharing partners in an attempt to curb infection or, if already infected, to prevent transmission to other individuals. In addition, these programs aid sexual partners of the index patient in gaining earlier access to individualized counseling, HIV testing, medical evaluation, treatment, and other prevention and health services.

Partner Counseling and Referral Services for HIV Infection

In addition to providing partner services for individuals diagnosed with an STI, some state-level PN programs also provide partner services for individuals infected with HIV. PCRS are typically available to individuals with HIV infection as long as contact with program staff is voluntary. Traditionally, the individual does not have to identify himself or herself and may choose whether or not to identify partners after discussion with the PN staff. Program staff do not have access to individuals' medical records related to the HIV infection unless they have the consent of the patient, typically requiring a medical release form.

Discussion about disclosing HIV infection to past and current sexual and injection-drug-using partners should routinely occur for all HIV-infected people and be integrated into the larger system of preventive and clinical care. Whereas the central goal of PCRS for STIs is the eradication of infection through treatment, the success of PCRS for HIV is evidenced by the prevention of new infections. HIV-infected patients should be informed of the benefits and advantages of PCRS, facilitating informed decision making about this service.

Nontraditional, Internet-Based PN

Traditional PN strategies may be appropriate for notification of partners under certain circumstances; however, much of the literature on PN strategies argues for cultural sensitivity and attention to special circumstances in assessing their appropriateness and potential for success as an intervention strategy. In particular, there are numerous considerations when evaluating the success of such strategies for men who have sex with men (MSM), such as the feasibility of notifying anonymous partners.

Internet-based interventions and PN efforts have evolved as a way to counteract the risks associated with seeking sexual partners, particularly anonymous encounters, on the Internet. Online health information on STI and HIV has become more pervasive, and there have been several initiatives to develop online PN systems that permit notification of sexual partners who may not otherwise be identified by the index patient. One such initiative, conducted by Klausner, Wolf, Fischer-Ponce, Zolt, and Katz (2000), found online PN via an Internet chat room for MSM to be moderately successful. These researchers designed a notification system in which the partners of index patients were notified of their possible exposure by an e-mail message sent via their online profile and found that an average of 5.9 partners per index patient sought testing.

In an attempt to assess the acceptability and perceived utility of a PN system for STI exposure among MSM, Mimiaga et al. (2006) recruited 1,848 men using one of the largest MSM sexual Web sites. Participants were recruited via a banner advertisement accessible by U.S. users of the Web site. The vast majority responded favorably to questions about receiving a PN e-mail containing information about being exposed to an STI (80.9%), education about the STI to which the person was exposed (77.8%), where to get tested (82.1%), a contact phone number (75.5%), and a number/e-mail address allowing the recipient to verify e-mail authenticity (78.8%). The majority were "somewhat to very likely" to use the following components of a PN e-mail: a contact phone number (61.0%), a Web site link providing information about where to get tested (82.6%), an educational Web site about the STI (86.2%), and a number/e-mail address allowing the recipient to verify e-mail authenticity (70.5%). Overall, 70.0% of participants indicated they would use a public health specialist in some capacity to inform partners via an online notification e-mail of possible exposure to an STI had they been infected. These findings demonstrate that high-risk MSM reported high levels of willingness to use electronic media in conjunction with public health specialists for PN if they were infected with or exposed to an STI.

The Role of the Health Care Provider

For STIs that are priority cases, such as chlamydia, gonorrhea, and syphilis, it is helpful for the health care provider to inform patients that a state department of public health official will need to get in touch with them to discuss their sexual partners, specific behaviors that they engaged in with them, and when necessary, a mechanism of action for notification. With regard to STIs that are not priority cases, such as human papillomavirus (HPV) or herpes simplex virus (HSV), typically, the state department of public health relies on the health care provider to discuss the importance of examination and treatment of sexual partners. In most of these cases, the patients will inform their sexual partners themselves. It is recommended that patients infected with chlamydia or gonorrhea be informed to contact all sexual partners within 60 days preceding their diagnosis or contact the most recent partner if more than 60 days occurred since their last sexual contact. If a patient provides consent, their health care provider can contact his or her sexual partners to make them aware of their exposure to a given STI; typically, this process is confidential, in that the index patient is not identified. Health care providers are generally required to report priority cases of STIs promptly and directly to the appropriate state department of public health.

PN is an important public health strategy for preventing STIs and HIV among at-risk populations. Traditional and nontraditional PN efforts have yielded success with respect to curbing continued transmission of STIs and HIV, as well as getting asymptomatic patients in for evaluation and treatment. For continued success, evaluation of PN programs should be conducted and documented with various at-risk groups as nontraditional methods, such as the Internet, might need to be employed with populations who engage in sexual behavior with anonymous or otherwise nonnotifiable individuals.

—*Matthew J. Mimiaga and Margie Skeer*

See also Ethics in Health Care; Ethics in Public Health; HIV/AIDS; Sexually Transmitted Diseases

Further Readings

Centers for Disease Control and Prevention. (2002). Sexually transmitted diseases treatment guidelines. *Morbidity and Mortality Weekly Report, 51,* 4–5.

Centers for Disease Control and Prevention. (2003). Using the Internet for partner notification of sexually transmitted diseases: Los Angeles County, California. *Morbidity and Mortality Weekly Report, 53,* 129–131.

Klausner, J. D., Wolf, W., Fischer-Ponce, L., Zolt, I., & Katz, M. H. (2000). Tracing a syphilis outbreak through cyberspace. *Journal of the American Medical Association, 284,* 447–449.

Mathews, C., Coetzee, N., Zwarenstein, M., Lombard, C., Guttmacher, S., Oxman, A., et al. (2002). A systematic review of strategies for partner notification for sexually transmitted diseases, including HIV/AIDS. *International Journal of STD and AIDS, 13,* 285–300.

Mimiaga, M. J., Tetu, A., Novak, D., Adelson, S., VanDerwarker, R., & Mayer, K. H. (2006, August). *Acceptability and utility of a partner notification system for sexually transmitted infection exposure using an Internet-based, partner-seeking Web site for men who have sex with men.* Oral presentation at the XVI International AIDS Conference, Toronto, Ontario, Canada.

PASTEUR, LOUIS
(1822–1895)

Louis Pasteur, a French chemist, is often called the father of modern microbiology. Through the development of vaccines for cholera, anthrax, rabies, staphylococcus, and streptococcus, he discovered much about the nature of infection and laid the groundwork for the microbial theory of disease. Pasteur also contributed greatly to the field of infectious epidemiology by demonstrating how pathogens spread through animal and human populations.

Pasteur examined the role of microorganisms in the transformation of organic matter, which at the time was greatly misunderstood. Instructed by Napoleon to investigate diseases infecting wines, he determined that fermentation results from the action of a specific microorganism. To enable fermentation, the right microorganism must be introduced, and microorganisms that could alter the process must be kept out. With Claude Bernard, Pasteur developed a process, eventually known as "pasteurization," in which wine, beer, vinegar, and milk were heated to kill bacteria and molds present within them.

Pasteur discredited the theory of spontaneous generation by demonstrating that microorganisms in a presterilized medium could be explained by outside germs. His research also showed that juice will not ferment if environmental yeasts are prevented from being deposited on grapes. By analogy, Pasteur believed that infectious diseases are probably caused by germs and that just as grapes can be protected against yeast, it might be possible to protect human beings against germs.

In 1879, Pasteur discovered that fowl cholera is caused by a type of bacteria now known as "Pasteurella." Chickens inoculated with a few drops of these bacteria would die. However, chickens inoculated with an old, weakened culture of Pasteruella did not die and were protected against a later inoculation with a more virulent culture. Through this chance observation, Pasteur discovered the principle of vaccination with attenuated pathogens. Because of Edward Jenner's work on vaccination, scientists knew that a weakened form of a disease could provide immunity to a more virulent version. However, whereas Jenner's vaccines used cowpox, a naturally occurring infection similar to but much less severe than smallpox, Pasteur's cholera and anthrax vaccines used artificially generated, weakened forms of disease organisms.

Pasteur grew the rabies virus in rabbits and then weakened it by drying the affected nerve tissue. He gave these artificially weakened diseases the generic name of "vaccines" to honor Jenner. In 1885, Pasteur conducted the first experimental rabies inoculations on a human. Joseph Meister, a 9-year-old boy who had been bitten multiple times by a rabid dog, was brought to Pasteur by his mother. Since the death of the child appeared inevitable, Pasteur attempted a method of inoculation that had proved consistently successful on dogs. Pasteur was not a licensed physician and could have faced prosecution for this.

Ultimately, Meister's health improved after 12 inoculations, and Pasteur was hailed as a hero.

—Emily E. Anderson

See also Public Health, History of; Vaccination; Zoonotic Disease

Further Readings

Debré, P. (1998). *Louis Pasteur* (E. Forster, Trans.). Baltimore: Johns Hopkins University Press.
Geison, G. L. (1995). *The private science of Louis Pasteur.* Princeton, NJ: Princeton University Press.
Schwartz, M. (2001). The life and works of Louis Pasteur. *Journal of Applied Microbiology, 91,* 597–601.

Pearson Correlation Coefficient

The sample Pearson product-moment correlation coefficient (r) is a measure of the linear association between two independent continuous variables, namely X and Y, measured on the same individuals or units. The values of the Pearson correlation coefficient measures the strength of the linear relationship between X and Y, while the sign of the correlation coefficient indicates the direction of the relationship between X and Y.

Given two continuous variables, X and Y, the Pearson correlation coefficient, r_{XY}, is obtained as the ratio of the covariance between the two variables over the product of the respective standard deviations.

$$r_{XY} = \frac{\text{Degree to which } X \text{ and } Y \text{ vary together}}{\text{Degree to which } X \text{ and } Y \text{ vary separately}}$$

$$= \frac{\text{Cov}(X, Y)}{\sqrt{\text{Var}(X)}\sqrt{\text{Var}(Y)}}$$

$$= \frac{\sum_{i=1}^{n}(x_i - \bar{x})(y_i - \bar{y})}{\sum_{i=1}^{n}(x_i - \bar{x})^2 \sum_{i=1}^{n}(y_i - \bar{y})^2},$$

where $\bar{x}$ and $\bar{y}$ are the sample means for the variables X and Y, respectively.

The correlation coefficient is defined only if both the standard deviations are finite and both of them are nonzero.

Assumptions

To be able to correctly interpret and make valid inferences about the Pearson correlation coefficient, the following assumptions must hold:

- The observation $x_1, x_2, \ldots, x_n$ and $y_1, y_2, \ldots, y_n$ of X and Y are independent and identically distributed.
- The variables X and Y are jointly normally distributed with means μ_X and μ_Y, variances σ_X^2 and σ_Y^2 and correlation ρ_{XY}.

Under these assumptions, the sample Pearson correlation coefficient r_{XY} represents a valid estimate of the correlation ρ_{XY}.

Properties

The Pearson correlation coefficient assumes values within the $(-1; 1)$ range. A correlation coefficient equal to -1 indicates a perfect negative linear relationship between two variables (see Figure 1a), while a correlation coefficient of 1 indicates a perfect positive linear relationship between two variables (Figure 1b). The correlation coefficient is equal to zero when either the two variables are independent (Figure 1c)

or they are associated through a nonlinear relationship (Figure 1d).

Values in the middle of the $(-1; 1)$ range indicate the degree of linear dependence of the X and Y variables. A correlation coefficient >0 is called a positive correlation and indicates that the variables X and Y tend to increase or decrease together. A correlation coefficient <0 is called a negative correlation and indicates that increases in one variable correspond to decreases in the other. There are no rules on what defines a high or a low correlation, and the interpretation of the correlation coefficient depends on the context and the data on which it is calculated.

The Pearson correlation coefficient is not affected by changes in location or scale in either variable.

Although r_{XY} can be used to determine the degree of association between two variables, it is not a measure of the causal relationship between X and Y.

The value of r_{XY} can be affected greatly by the range of the data values, and extreme observations (outliers) can have dramatic effect on r_{XY}. Thus, the full range of scores should always be used when calculating the correlation coefficient. Extreme observations should be treated with caution in the calculation of the correlation coefficient.

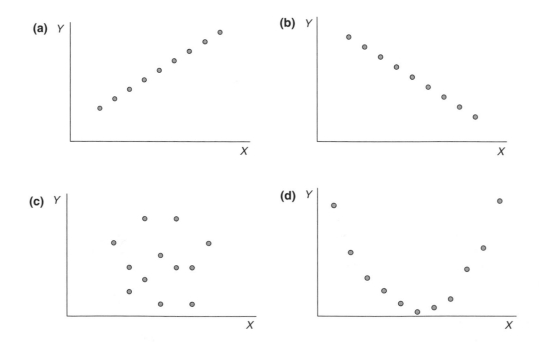

Figure 1   Correlation Coefficient Under Different Scenarios

Applications

The Pearson correlation coefficient can be used in a number of different applications.

- *Prediction.* Knowing that a strong relationship exists between two variables allows one to make an accurate prediction about one of them using the other.
- *Validity.* The Pearson correlation coefficient is often used to validate a new measurement scale. A high correlation between the new scale and an established one would assure that the new instrument is measuring what it is supposed to.
- *Reliability.* The Pearson correlation coefficient may also be used to establish reliability of an instrument. A high correlation between successive measures on the same individuals, for example, would indicate that the instrument is reliable.

Hypothesis Testing About ρ_{XY}

When interest is in testing the null hypothesis that there is no linear association between two continuous variables (H_0: $\rho_{XY} = 0$) against an alternative hypothesis that such association exists (H_A: $\rho_{XY} \neq 0$), then a Student's t approximation can be used to test this hypothesis. Under the assumption that the distribution of X and Y is bivariate normal, the test statistic

$$t^* = \frac{r_{XY}\sqrt{n-2}}{\sqrt{1-r_{XY}^2}}$$

follows a Student t distribution with $(n-2)$ df, under the null hypothesis. Thus, values of this test that exceed the critical value $t_{(n-2),(1-\alpha/2)}$ for a prespecified Type I error α would lead to reject the null hypothesis of no linear association or independence of X and Y.

When interest is in testing a more general null hypothesis that specifies a particular value for ρ_{XY}, H_0: $\rho_{XY} = \rho_0$ against the alternative H_A: $\rho_{XY} \neq \rho_0$, then an inference is carried out using the Fisher's transformation:

$$z = \frac{1}{2}\log_e\left(\frac{1+r_{XY}}{1-r_{XY}}\right).$$

When the sample size n is large, z is approximately normally distributed with mean

$$\varsigma = \frac{1}{2}\log_e\left(\frac{1+\rho_0}{1-\rho_0}\right)$$

and variance $\sigma^2(z) = 1/(n-3)$, under the null hypothesis.

The test statistic $\lambda = (z-z_0)\sqrt{n-3}$ will reject the null hypothesis if its value exceeds the critical value $z_{1-\alpha/2}$ on the standard normal distribution, for a prespecified Type I error α.

Confidence Intervals for ρ_{XY}

The upper and lower bound of a $100(1-\alpha/2)\%$ confidence interval for the Fisher's transformation z are given by $z_L = z - z_{1-\alpha/2}\sqrt{n-3}$ and $z_U = z + z_{1-\alpha/2}\sqrt{n-3}$.

A $100\%(1-\alpha)$ confidence interval for ρ_{XY} is given by

$$\rho_L = \frac{e^{2z_1}-1}{e^{2z_1}+1}; \rho_U = \frac{e^{2z_2}-1}{e^{2z_2}+1}.$$

Relationship Between r_{XY} and Regression Parameters

In a straight line model $r_{Y|X} = \hat{\beta}_1(S_X/S_Y)$, where $\hat{\beta}_1$ is the estimate of the slope, r_{XY} and $\hat{\beta}_1$ have the same sign.

When $r_{Y|X} = \pm 1$, then $\hat{\beta}_1 = \pm(S_Y/S_X)$. Thus, r_{XY} does not indicate the magnitude of the slope of the regression line. But in a straight line model, testing for $\rho_{XY} = 0$ is the same as testing for $\beta_1 = 0$.

When $\rho_{XY} = 0$, then $\beta_1 = 0$. There is no linear relationship between X and Y although a nonlinear relationship may exist.

In a linear model $r_{YX} = \text{sign}(\hat{\beta}_1)\sqrt{R^2}$, where R^2 is the model coefficient of determination. Note that although r_{XY} is related to the coefficient of determination, it should never be interpreted as a proportion (e.g., the proportion of Y predicted by X).

—Emilia Bagiella

See also Coefficient of Determination; Hypothesis Testing; Normal Distribution; Regression

Further Readings

Gravetter, F. J, & Wallnau, L. B. (1992). *Statistics for the behavioral sciences* (3rd ed.). St. Paul, MN: West.

Neter, J., Kutner, H. M., Nachtsheim, C. J., & Wasserman, W. (1996). *Applied linear regression models* (3rd ed.). Chicago: Irwin.

PEER REVIEW PROCESS

Peer review is a process whereby experts help judge the value of a work that they were not part of creating. Editorial peer review involves scientific or academic manuscripts submitted for publication or meeting presentation, while grant peer review involves review of funding applications. This entry focuses on editorial peer review of work submitted to scientific journals, although some of the issues discussed apply to other types of peer review as well. The primary function of editorial peer review is gate-keeping—selecting the best from a pool of submissions. In addition, peer review often involves constructive criticisms intended to improve a submitted work prior to publication. A common misunderstanding is that peer review validates the scientific integrity of a published article. Expecting such validation is unrealistic, as reviewers typically have access only to what the author or authors present in the manuscript. Important logistical and methodological decisions made along the way will be unknown to the reviewers, as will key details that the authors might omit. In essence, we must trust the authors.

Early forms of editorial peer review go back as far as the beginning of the 18th century, most notably within the Royal Societies of London and Edinburgh. The first modern peer review system was developed in the late 19th century by Ernest Hart, editor of the *British Medical Journal*. Yet it was only after World War II, as medical research methods became more sophisticated and journals became more selective, that peer review systems became institutionalized in the scientific and academic journals of the United Kingdom, the United States, and elsewhere.

In this context, the term *peer* is loosely interpreted to include subject-area experts, statisticians and methodologists, journal editors, editorial boards, and sometimes others, such as graduate students or nonexperts. Outside experts are usually sought because of their specialized knowledge in the submitted manuscript's content area or their advanced statistical or methodological skills. Ideally, these reviewers will have more expertise than the authors of the submitted work. But because of the proliferation of scientific journals and the many competing demands on experts' time, this specialized ideal is not always reached. It is therefore not uncommon for less qualified reviewers to assume this role.

A variety of peer review systems are employed across the world's 10,000 or so journals. Systems vary in their relative reliance on external reviewers, such as outside experts, versus in-house reviewers, such as editors and editorial boards. Acceptance rates can differ widely across journals, ranging from around 2% for the most highly selective journals to 90% and above for some electronic journals where publication space is less of an issue, and pay-per-page journals such as those that serve primarily as outlets for routine pharmaceutical studies.

Postpublication peer review is an important, if often neglected, type of review. This can include letters to the editor or full articles critiquing a published work, sometimes going so far as to involve reanalysis of the original data. While the need for postpublication review is now receiving more attention, challenges remain. Authors sometimes choose to ignore a published critique or respond minimally to peripheral issues in place of the specific criticisms made. Even when serious errors are detailed in a critique, retractions or corrections are the exception. Medline and other databases rarely link postpublication critiques to the original article, and literature reviews that cite a criticized work frequently ignore the critique.

Criticisms of Peer Review

Many criticisms of peer review have been raised by authors and reviewers as well as journal editors. A common criticism is that peer review is prone to bias. Bias can take various forms, including ad hominem bias, affiliation bias, ideological bias, and publication bias, among others. Ad hominem bias and affiliation bias are found when a review is influenced, either consciously or unconsciously, by knowledge of the author's identity or affiliation. Mixed evidence has been found on the presence and extent of these two biases. Some have argued that such influences are not necessarily biases but can be valid considerations in reviewing a manuscript. Yet the prevailing opinion remains that these potential influences are inappropriate for editorial peer review. It is for this reason that the norm is blinded review, where the author's name and affiliation are not known to the reviewer. The opposite is true, however, in grant peer review, where authors' names and affiliations, as well as other detailed information about the authors' past experience and accomplishments, are typically an integral part of the reviewed application.

Ideological bias, where a reviewer's antecedent value-based views for or against an author's position unduly influence a review, has been demonstrated in several studies on the peer review process. Closely related is confirmation bias, the more general and well-documented tendency to less critically evaluate evidence that is consistent with one's existing beliefs. Numerous experimental demonstrations of these types of biases have led some to call for use of only the introduction and methods section of a paper in publication decisions, but this strategy has not yet been widely embraced or studied. Also related is publication bias, the selective publication of manuscripts based on the direction and magnitude of their results. It is widely accepted that research reporting statistically significant positive results is more likely to be published than research with null or nonsignificant results, and that this can, among other problems, lead to serious negative consequences for meta-analyses and other types of systematic reviews. Interestingly, studies have failed to support the belief that editorial decisions are biased in this matter. Instead, publication bias appears to result primarily from authors' reduced likelihood of submitting papers with null or negative results.

Other commonly voiced criticisms are that peer review is conservative and stifles innovation; is secretive and without accountability of reviewers to authors; suffers from low interrater reliability (typically found to be .30 or less); produces reviews of low quality; allows too many papers to slip thorough the system; frequently lacks adequate statistical and methodological review; is slow and expensive and delays publication; and is unscientific, with little or no evidence of its effectiveness. It is sometimes said that, like democracy, the peer review system is deeply flawed, yet better than all the alternatives. While no serious candidates for replacement of peer review have emerged, the many challenges to the current system have been increasingly publicized, and many suggestions for improvements in current practice have attracted attention.

Improving the Peer Review Process

One proposal to increase reviewer accountability and to generate more constructive reviews is to employ a signed rather than anonymous review process, in which reviewers' names are provided to the reviewed author. Several major journals, including the *British Medical Journal* (*BMJ*), now use signed review systems, while other journals encourage but do not require signed reviews. Yet most journals—and reviewers—do not yet support such a process, primarily due to reviewers' concerns about retribution, especially in the case of younger researchers who are fearful of criticizing senior colleagues. With reviewer recruitment already a difficult and time-consuming task, additional disincentives to accept review invitations would not be ideal.

Other suggestions for improving overall review and editorial decision quality include providing more training and support to reviewers and employing statistical and methodological review of all manuscripts. Reviewer training can take the form of workshops, tutorials, guides, apprentice models, and other strategies and should be targeted not only to existing reviewers but also to graduate students as future reviewers. Statistical and methodological review can be done concurrently with review by subject-area experts or subsequent to initial reviews by these experts. It can involve either in-house or external methodologists. Some journals, such as the *BMJ* and *Lancet*, already institutionalize separate methodological reviews, yet the majority of medical journals do not. In spite of the challenges in recruiting sufficient numbers of methodologists, this strategy has tremendous potential power, given that it has been found across several different fields that most published articles do contain nontrivial methodological flaws.

It is said that if peer review were not already widely in use and someone were to propose it today, the evidence of its effectiveness would be so lacking that it would not be given serious consideration. But evidence is accumulating as research on the peer review process becomes more widespread and sophisticated. An International Congress on Peer Review in Biomedical Publication is held every 4 years since 1989. These meetings are an attempt to encourage systematic research on the peer review process. And a large-scale collaborative mixed-methods study is currently underway to investigate the peer review processes at three prestigious medical journals: *Lancet*, *Annals of Internal Medicine*, and *BMJ*.

—*Norman A. Constantine*

See also Meta-Analysis; Publication Bias

Further Readings

Altman, D. G. (2002). Poor quality medical research: What can journals do? *Journal of the American Medical Association, 287*, 2765–2767.

Cicchetti, D. V. (1991). The reliability of peer-review for manuscript and grant submissions: A cross-disciplinary investigation. *Behavioral and Brain Sciences, 14*, 119–134.

Cole, S., Cole, J. R., & Simon, G. A. (1981). Chance and consensus in peer-review. *Science, 214*, 881–886.

Fiske, D. W., & Fogg, L. (1990). But the reviewers are making different criticisms of my paper! Diversity and uniqueness in reviewer comments. *American Psychologist, 45*, 591–598.

Giles, J. (2006). Journals submit to scrutiny of their peer-review process. *Nature, 439*, 252.

Godlee, F., & Jefferson, T. (Eds.). (2003). *Peer review in health sciences* (2nd ed.). London: BMJ Books.

Rennie, D. R. (1998). Freedom and responsibility in medical publication: Setting the balance right. *Journal of the American Medical Association, 280*, 300–302.

Rennie, D. R. (2002). Fourth international congress on peer review in biomedical publication. *Journal of the American Medical Association, 287*, 2759–2758.

Schmelkin, L. P. (2003, August). *Peer review: Standard or delusion?* Division 5 Presidential Address delivered at the annual meeting of the American Psychological Association, Toronto, Ontario, Canada.

Shatz, D. (2001). *Peer review: A critical inquiry.* New York: Rowman & Littlefield.

Wagner, E., Godlee, F., & Jefferson, T. (2002). *How to survive peer review.* London: BMJ Books.

Web Sites

Fifth International Congress on Peer Review and Biomedical Publication home page: http://www.ama-assn.org/public/peer/peerhome.htm.

PELLAGRA

See GOLDBERGER, JOSEPH

PERCENTILES

The percentile is a concept often used to summarize data and place the score or measurement taken on an individual into the context of a larger population. For any particular number p between 0 and 100, the pth percentile of a set of n measurements arranged in order of magnitude is the value that has at most $p\%$ of the observations below it and at most $(100 - p)\%$ above it. Roughly speaking, the first percentile is the number that divides the bottom 1% of the data from the top 99%; the second percentile is the number that divides the bottom 2% of the data from the top 98%; and so on. Therefore, if a man has a body mass index score at the 98th percentile for his age, it means roughly 98% of men his age have a body mass index score lower than him, and only 2% have a higher score.

A percentile may be viewed as the division of a data set into 100 equal parts. Smaller groupings are often used; for instance, the median of a data set is also the 50th percentile, which specifies that at least half the observations are equal or smaller than it. Other commonly used percentile groupings include deciles, which divide a data set into tenths (10 equal parts), quintiles, which divide a data set into fifths (5 equal parts), and quartiles, which divide a data set into quarters (4 equal parts). Of these, quartiles are the most commonly used.

Percentiles are often used to describe large data sets; for instance, in the body mass index example above, the percentiles may have been calculated using a sample of thousands of American men. However, researchers sometimes want to calculate percentiles, quartiles, and so on, for a smaller data set, in which case the following procedure may be used to establish cut points.

1. Arrange the observations into increasing order from smallest to largest.

2. Calculate the product of the sample size n and proportion p you wish to include in each division (for quartiles, $p = 0.25$; for deciles, $p = 0.10$; etc.)

3. If np is an integer, say k, calculate the average of the kth and $(k + 1)$th ordered values; if np is not an integer, round it up to the next integer and find the corresponding ordered value.

For example, a study of serum total cholesterol (mg/L) levels recorded the following ordered levels for 20 adult patients (the data were adapted by the author from data presented in Ott and Longnecker (2001, p. 83).

To determine the first quartile, we take $p = 0.25$, and calculate $np = (20)(0.25) = 5$, then the first quartile is the average of the fifth and sixth observations,

Table 1 Serum Total Cholesterol (mg/L) Levels Recorded the Following Ordered Levels for 20 Adult Patients

Ordered Observation	Cholesterol (mg/L)
1	133
2	137
3	148
4	149
5	152
6	167
7	174
8	179
9	189
10	192
11	201
12	209
13	210
14	211
15	218
16	238
17	245
18	248
19	253
20	257

Source: Adapted from data presented in Ott and Longnecker (2001, p. 83).

$$Q_1 = \frac{152 + 167}{2} = 159.5.$$

Therefore, data points falling at or below this cut point are in the first quartile of the data set. To calculate the cut point for the median, we take $p = 0.5$, and $np = (20)(0.5) = 10$, so the median is the average of the 10th and 11th observations, the

$$\text{median} = \frac{192 + 201}{2} = 196.5.$$

Values falling between 159.5 and 196.5 are in the second quartile. For the third quartile, we take $p = 0.75$,

and $np = (20)(0.75) = 15$, so the cut point for the third quartile is the average of the 15th and 16th observations:

$$Q_3 = \frac{218 + 238}{2} = 228.$$

Values falling between 196.5 and 228 are in the third quartile, and values above 228 are in the fourth quartile.

A related concept, the interquartile range (IQR) of a data set is defined to be the difference between the upper and lower quartiles—that is,

$$IQR = Q_3 - Q_1.$$

The IQR measures the distance needed to cover the middle 50% of the data only, so it totally ignores the variability in the lower and upper 25% of data. Thus, the IQR does not provide a lot of useful information about the variability of a single set of measurements but can be quite useful when comparing the variability of two or more data sets. This is especially true when the data sets are skewed or contain outliers. For the above data set, IQR = 228 − 159.5 = 68.5.

If we need to calculate the 87th percentile of this data set, we can take $p = 0.87$ and calculate $np = (20)(0.87) = 17.4$. Because this is not an integer, we take the next largest integer, 18, so that the 18th ordered observation, 248 is at the 87th percentile.

—*Renjin Tu*

See also Box-and-Whisker Plot; Histogram; Measures of Central Tendency; Measures of Variability

Further Readings

Johnson, R. A., & Bhattacharyya, G. K. (2006). *Statistics principles and methods* (5th ed.). Hoboken, NJ: Wiley.
Ott, R. L., & Longnecker, M. (2001). *Statistical methods and data analysis* (5th ed.). Pacific Grove, CA: Duxbury.

PERSON-TIME UNITS

It is common in medicine and epidemiology to express the frequency of occurrence of some event in terms of the number of events per person-time unit; for instance, the number of complications per 100 patient-days or the number of deaths per 100,000 person-years. A good example is the incidence rate, also known as the incidence density or force of morbidity or mortality. The incidence rate is calculated as

$$\frac{\text{No. of new cases of a disease}}{\text{Total person-time of observation}}.$$

The numerator is always the number of new cases of the disease in the time period studied, and the denominator is the sum of the time of observation for all the subjects in the study. This fraction is usually converted to a standard unit such as cases per 100 to facilitate comparisons.

Person-time units are used when the subjects in a study have been observed for different lengths of time and have, therefore, been at risk for the event in question for longer or shorter times. Using a person-time denominator allows each subject to contribute to the denominator in proportion to the length of time they were observed and allows comparison across units (e.g., complication rates in different hospitals or mortality rates in different countries).

Consider the following example. We want to compare the quality of care for a particular condition in a particular year at two hospitals using the mortality rate for that condition. Table 1 presents hypothetical data on eight patients treated for this condition at two hospitals and includes the days observed (i.e., the number of days they were in that hospital and thus eligible for the event of death to occur at that hospital). Assuming this is the total patient population treated at those hospitals for that condition in the year under study, we can see that in Hospital A, two patients died (because they have a "Y" for "yes" in the "Event" column), whereas in Hospital B, only one patient died. We might interpret this as meaning that Hospital A was somehow less safe or had a lower quality of care for this condition because they had two deaths per year versus one death per year for Hospital B, but we would be ignoring the fact that Hospital A had more patients at risk of death from this condition during this time period.

A more sensible comparison would be made using the mortality rate per 100 patient-days. In this case, Hospital A had 2 deaths per 100 patient-days, while Hospital B had 1 event in 20 patient-days or a rate of 5 deaths per 100 patient-days. By the criterion of mortality rate, Hospital A seems to be doing a better job in treating this condition. Of course, this example is

Table 1   Data to Calculate Complication Rate per 100 Patient-Years for Two Hospitals

Hospital	Patient	Days Followed	Event?
A	1	10	Y
A	2	20	Y
A	3	25	N
A	4	30	N
A	5	15	N
Total Person-Days		100	
B	6	10	Y
B	7	5	N
B	8	5	N
Total Person-Days		20	

greatly simplified, and hospital-to-hospital comparisons are generally done after correcting for expected mortality and morbidity, considering factors such as patient mix, but it illustrates why person-time units are commonly used in epidemiology.

—*Sarah Boslaugh*

See also Incidence; Mortality Rates; Public Health Surveillance; Rate

Further Readings

Hennekens, C. H., & Buring, J. E. (1987). Measures of disease frequency. In S. L. Mayrent (Ed.), *Epidemiology in medicine* (ch. 4, pp. 54–98). Boston: Little, Brown.

Rothman, K. J., & Greenland, S. (1998). *Modern epidemiology* (2nd ed.). Philadelphia: Lippincott-Raven.

PHARMACOEPIDEMIOLOGY

Pharmacoepidemiology is the study of the use and effects of medical products (drugs, biological products, and medical devices) in human populations. One of the newer branches of epidemiology, pharmacoepidemiology has emerged as a unique field of study in parallel with the development of large, comprehensive, health care databases. However, it is not the reliance on large databases, but the nature of medical products as exposures that truly differentiates pharmacoepidemiology as a subspecialty of epidemiology. First, medical products are regulated by government entities. They are approved for a particular use or indication with dosing, labeling, and monitoring requirements. Second, exposures to medical products are made consciously for the treatment of a known medical condition or to prevent or delay the occurrence of a disease. The regulatory nature of pharmaceutical products drives the type and timing of studies and often the source of funding and perspective as well. The nonrandom nature of treatment decisions can introduce bias and, as such, drives many research design decisions and ultimately affects interpretation of study results. The entry is organized into the following sections: (1) the drug development and approval process, (2) adverse drug events, (3) postmarketing safety, (4) risk management, and (5) training and careers.

Drug Development and Approval

Approval of a pharmaceutical product for marketing in the United States requires extensive testing and a determination by the Food and Drug Administration (FDA) that its benefits outweigh its risks for the intended use or indication. Before a medicine is tested in humans, it is studied and evaluated extensively in the laboratory and in animal models. The type and extent of testing depends on the nature of the chemical being studied and the indication for use that the sponsor is pursuing. Before clinical testing can begin, the product sponsor submits an investigational new drug application (IND) to the FDA. An IND summarizes the preclinical study results and contains a detailed plan for clinical testing.

Clinical testing is divided into three unique phases. Phase I is the first use of a medication in humans and, as such, is usually limited to a small group of healthy individuals. The primary purpose of this first phase is to determine the safety of the drug in humans. Within Phase I, scientists seek to determine a safe dosing range, how the drug is handled by the body (pharmacokinetics), and its action or effect at various dosages (pharmacodynamics). Phase II studies are generally small clinical trials in which a drug is tested in patients to further characterize its safety profile and determine

which dosages and dosing schedules will be tested for approval. Phase III clinical trials are the randomized studies in the intended patient population. In Phase III trials, the new drug is compared with a placebo, or in cases where it is unethical to deny or delay treatment, an alternative treatment—typically the standard of care. The use of such "active-control" trials relies on historical data for assurance that the alternative treatment is more effective than placebo, while testing for equivalence between the new and control drugs.

From 1,000 to 5,000 patients are typically exposed to a new drug on submission of a New Drug Application (NDA) to the FDA. If the FDA determines that the NDA is complete, a team of reviewers evaluates all the study results and determines whether or not the medication can be marketed in the United States. It takes approximately 15 years and $800 million to take a drug from discovery through approval, according to the Pharmaceutical Research and Manufacturers Association (PhRMA).

Adverse Drug Events

The basis for approval of a new pharmaceutical agent is that it is safe and effective for its intended or labeled use. This does not mean that it is absolutely safe but that relative to its benefits as established in the clinical trials, the risks are acceptable. At the time of approval, the FDA may require additional studies to follow-up on outstanding questions. These postmarketing studies are often called Phase IV studies or commitments. Additionally, all sponsors are required to monitor and report any serious adverse events that may be related to the use of the drug. Pharmacovigilance refers to the process of collecting, monitoring, and evaluating adverse events reports.

Often, adverse effects of a drug are related to its pharmacokinetics (how it is processed by the body) or pharmacodynamics (how it affects the body). A drug may cause adverse events by the same mechanism that provides the intended therapeutic benefit. For example, an agent that effectively prevents blood clotting can be a contributing cause of excessive bleeding and subsequent hemorrhage.

Genetic variation, concomitant drugs, and other medical conditions can contribute individually or in unison to increase the risk of an adverse event. For example, the amount of an active metabolite can be increased to toxic levels by genetic polymorphisms that impede its breakdown, renal or liver impairment (depending on the route of metabolism), and/or the use of a concomitant drug that successfully competes for binding sites. These "Type A" adverse drug events are considered predictable because they are based on known properties of the drug. Less common are Type B adverse events, those that are idiosyncratic or unpredictable such as allergic or immunologic reactions. Type B events include anaphylaxis and Stevens Johnson syndrome.

Extensive preclinical and clinical testing ensures that on marketing approval, the more common adverse events, occurring at rates of 1% or greater, are well characterized. As approval is conditioned on the benefits of therapy outweighing the risks, commonly occurring adverse events are typically nonserious. Pre-approval studies are limited not only in the total number of persons exposed but also on the duration of exposure and the diversity of the patient populations. Therefore, rare adverse events, occurring at rates below 1/10,000 persons, and events associated with extended duration use are often not identified until after a drug is marketed. New safety problems, for example drug-drug or drug-gene interactions, may also emerge on use within a larger and more diverse patient population.

Postmarketing Safety

Once a product is marketed, manufacturers are required to monitor, evaluate, and submit reports of serious adverse events potentially caused by their products to the FDA. Health care professionals and the general public may voluntarily report problems to the manufacturer or directly to the FDA through their MedWatch® program. The FDA maintains databases of these reports: the Adverse Event Reporting System (AERS) for drugs and biologics, the Vaccine Adverse Event Reporting System (VAERS) for vaccines, and the Manufacturer and User Facility Device Experience Database (MAUDE) for devices.

The initial evaluation of a potential product safety problem has many similarities to outbreak investigations, beginning with the development of a case series of adverse event reports. Once a case definition is created, ineligible reports are excluded and the remaining reports evaluated in terms of person, place, and time. A crude reporting rate may be estimated and a causal assessment conducted. Case series investigations guide the decision to conduct further research, either observational or experimental, and provide information about exposures, latency period, and potential risk factors.

There is no magic number of case reports that identify a real problem. The volume of adverse event reports varies over time and is typically highest during the first several years of marketing. Labeling changes, marketing programs, and publicity have all been shown to affect reporting levels. Also, the uniqueness and severity of the adverse event may also affect reporting. For example, an abnormal laboratory test for liver enzymes is less likely to be reported as an adverse event than a case of acute liver failure. Similarly a unique syndrome of birth defects is more likely to be associated with an exposure and reported because of its uniqueness, than a more common pregnancy outcome such as a spontaneous abortion. A clinical expert evaluates each new report of an adverse drug event within the context of previous reports. The application of data mining techniques, which use statistical algorithms to aid in the identification of new and otherwise unexpected adverse events, shows promise as an additional screening tool. Data mining algorithms identify drug-event or drug-drug-events that occur in excess of expected rates.

Once a hypothesis is formulated, the feasibility for conducting an epidemiological study must be determined. In rare situations, one or more cases can be so definitive that no further information is needed to prove a causal link between exposure and adverse outcome. Pharmacoepidemiological investigations use the methods and study designs of epidemiology. The field relies heavily on the use of databases such as health care service utilization data, automated medical records, and health care and pharmaceutical claims. Databases have a distinct advantage over original data collection in the speed it takes to complete a study as well as the size of the underlying population. The terms *historic cohort*, *nonconcurrent prospective cohort*, and *retrospective cohort studies* are used synonymously to describe research studies that rely on data from health care or claims databases to identify their study cohort and create variables to characterize subjects by exposure, outcome, demographics, and so on.

Each database has distinct characteristics that can affect internal and external validity. For example, claims databases are established to provide reimbursement for a covered service. As such, services that are not covered or are charged to another insurer (e.g., patients who are covered by both Medicaid and Medicare) may not be captured. Medical practice and changes in coding practices may also influence the validity of diagnostic codes. The likelihood that a patient was exposed to a medication also varies across and within databases. An assumption of an exposure is based on a record in a database though there is no proof that the patient ever took the medication. A claim for reimbursement by the pharmacy for a filled prescription is a step closer to a potential exposure than a record of a prescription having been written by the physician. Two filled prescriptions, one following the other at an interval equivalent to the allotted days supply, further increases the likelihood of an exposure compared with a single filled prescription. Knowledge of database characteristics, local medical practice, and the covered population, and how these unique database characteristics influence the potential to be prescribed a particular drug and the likelihood of diagnosing the study outcome, are critical to designing a valid epidemiological study.

Physicians make a variety of treatment choices, first whether or not to prescribe a medication, and if so, which medication and dosage schedule to use. These decisions are not random. Thus, therapeutic decision making can introduce a number of potential biases that, if not accounted for in the study design, can obscure a true association between exposure and outcome. "Confounding by indication" refers to a bias introduced into a study when the choice of treatments is in some way (noncausally) related to the outcome being studied. Consider an observational study comparing rates of oral cancer among men with and without heavy use of mouthwash. Because heavy mouthwash users (exposed) were predominantly smokers and the unexposed predominantly nonsmokers, the statistical association with mouthwash use and oral cancer is confounded by the "indication" for the study exposure. Confounding by indication is best accounted for in the design of a study. In the mouthwash example, the study population could be limited to heavy smokers. Protopathic bias occurs when a particular treatment is used to treat a symptom or other factor that is directly associated with the risk of the outcome under study. For example, an antidiabetic agent may be associated with an increased risk of birth defects because gestational diabetes itself increases the risk of adverse fetal outcome.

Risk Management

In March 2005, the U.S. FDA released an industry guidance document on the Development and Use of Risk Management Action Plans (RiskMAP) simultaneously with guidances on premarketing risk assessment and postmarketing pharmacovigilance practices. These guidance documents articulated the need to articulate and assess known and potential risks of a product at the earliest stages of preclinical development. They outline a framework to identify, evaluate, and monitor safety throughout a product's life cycle. This life cycle approach, particularly the anticipation and evaluation of the risk to cause serious adverse events, such as blood dyscrasias, liver toxicity, and Q-T prolongation, is designed to save lives by identifying and characterizing safety issues earlier in the process. Potentially, this may allow important therapies, which would have previously been withdrawn for safety reasons, to be available to patients for whom the benefits do outweigh the risks.

At the time of approval for marketing, the FDA may require the sponsor to conduct further studies, often called Phase IV studies or Phase IV commitments, as they come after the definitive Phase III clinical trials conducted for approval. Phase IV studies are done to answer questions that arise during clinical development but are outside the scope of the Phase III trials. This might include questions on the impact of an extended duration of use or the safety of use in special populations, such as patients with common chronic conditions or pregnant women.

The ultimate risk management decision is the FDA's approval (or withdrawing of approval) to market a medication in the United States. Product labeling is the next line of risk management describing approved indications as well as contraindications, dosing and prescribing considerations, and known safety issues. There are additional levels of regulation that can be used to improve the benefit-risk ratio for products with unique risks that may be avoided or managed with appropriate knowledge and/or action. In escalating levels of intervention, this includes education and outreach, informed consent or prescribing checklists, and performance-based access. The most stringent level of regulation, performance-based access, requires certain conditions for medication access such as laboratory assessment to rule out pregnancy before a prescription for a teratogen such as isotretinoin or thalidomide can be filled. There is a great need to evaluate ongoing risk management programs as well as develop and assess new methods to communicate product risk and risk management to patients and providers.

Training and Careers

The practice of pharmacoepidemiology requires sound knowledge of epidemiology, including both its methods and limitations. Clinical expertise in medicine and pharmacy is important as is an understanding of pharmacology. Practitioners have come to pharmacoepidemiology from many disciplines, clinical and nonclinical. This same diversity is also seen in training programs, which are based within schools of public heath, medicine, pharmacy, or in multidisciplinary programs. Training is almost exclusively at the graduate and postgraduate levels.

Pharmacoepidemiologists apply epidemiological methods to study the risks, benefits, and utilization of drugs, vaccines, biologics, and/or devices. They are employed in three principal areas: industry, regulatory agencies, and academia. An industry pharmacoepidemiologist may work for a pharmaceutical company or a company that provides consulting, pharmacovigilance support, research, or some combination of these services. Within a regulatory agency, a pharmacoepidemiologist might evaluate adverse drug events, conduct independent research, evaluate industry studies, oversee external research, and develop standards. Academic researchers typically teach, train graduate and postgraduate students, conduct research, and consult. There are a number of professional societies that provide forums for the exchange of new knowledge, professional development, and training in pharmacoepidemiology. The International Society for Pharmacoepidemiology (ISPE) is the most specific professional organization within the field. Through the society, ISPE members develop and promulgate standards for pharmacoepidemiology research, provide training programs, provide forums for scientific exchange, advertise jobs and training programs, and recognize expertise through their Fellow program. There are a number of more broad-based professional societies that include Pharmacoepidemiology—for example, the Society for Epidemiologic Research (SER), Drug Information Association (DIA), International Society for Pharmacovigilance (IsoP), and the International Society of Pharmacoeconomics and Outcomes Research (ISPOR). ISPE maintains a list of hyperlinks to these and other professional associations, as well as Pharmacoepidemiology-related resources, including training programs, government agencies, research centers, professional journals, and tools.

—*Sheila Weiss Smith*

See also Case Reports and Case Series; Clinical Trials; Confounding; Food and Drug Administration; Secondary Data

Further Readings

Begaud, B. (2000). *Dictionary of pharmacoepidemiology.* New York: McGraw-Hill.

Center for Drug Evaluation and Research and Center for Biologics Evaluation and Research. (2005). *Guidance for industry development and use of risk minimization action plans.* Rockville, MD: U.S. Department of Health and Human Services, Food and Drug Administration. Retrieved July 24, 2007, from http://www.fda.gov/cber/gdlns/riskminim.pdf.

Center for Drug Evaluation and Research and Center for Biologics Evaluation and Research. (2005). *Guidance for industry good pharmacovigilance practices and pharmacoepidemiologic assessment.* Rockville, MD: U.S. Department of Health and Human Services, Food and Drug Administration. Retrieved July 24, 2007, from http://www.fda.gov/cder/guidance/6359OCC.htm.

Center for Drug Evaluation and Research and Center for Biologics Evaluation and Research. (2005). *Guidance for industry premarketing risk assessment.* Rockville, MD: U.S. Department of Health and Human Services, Food and Drug Administration. Retrieved July 24, 2007, from http://www.fda.gov/cder/guidance/6357fnl.htm.

Goldman, S. A. (2004). Communication of medical product risk: How effective is effective enough? *Drug Safety, 27,* 519–534.

Goldman, S. A., Kennedy, D. L., & Lieberman, R. (2005). *Clinical therapeutics and the recognition of drug-induced disease.* MedWatch continuing education article. Rockville, MD: Staff College, Center for Drug Evaluation and Research, Food and Drug Administration. Retrieved July 24, 2007, from http://www.fda.gov/medwatch/articles/dig/ceart.pdf.

Hartzema, A. G., Porta, M. S., & Tilson, H. H. (Eds.). (1998). *Pharmacoepidemiology: An introduction* (3rd ed.). Cincinnati, OH: Harvey Whitney.

International Society for Pharmacoepidemiology. (2003). *Hyperlinks of interest.* Retrieved September 8, 2006, from http://www.pharmacoepi.org/resources/links.cfm.

Nelson, R. C., Palsulich, B., & Goglak, V. (2002). Good pharmacovigilance practices technology enabled. *Drug Safety, 25,* 407–414.

Pharmaceutical Research and Manufacturers Association. (n.d.) *Drug development in the United States.* Retrieved September 28, 2006, from http://www.phrma.org/innovation.

Strom, B. (Ed.). (2005). *Pharmacoepidemiology* (4th ed.). West Sussex, UK: Wiley.

Waning, B., & Montagne, M. (2000). *Pharmacoepidemiology: Principles & practice.* New York: McGraw-Hill.

Wysowski, D. K., & Swartz, L. (2005). Adverse drug event surveillance and drug withdrawals in the United States, 1969–2002: The importance of reporting suspected reactions. *Archives of Internal Medicine*, *165*, 1363–1369.

PHENOTYPE

The *phenotype*, a term used extensively in the field of genetics since its development in the early 1900s, comprises the characteristics, traits, values, or abnormalities that we observe, measure, test, or evaluate in an individual. As such, the phenotype may include behavioral, biochemical, clinical, molecular, morphological, physical, and physiological characteristics, as well as the presence or absence of disease. In genetics, we think of the phenotype as the outcomes and results that are determined by the interplay between the genotype and environmental factors. It is important to consider that the environment can also include the so-called genetic environment—that is, the genes at other genetic loci whose products might interact with a specified gene or its product during development or during processes later in life.

With respect to genetic disease, the phenotype includes the clinical signs and symptoms of the disease, clinical features that are observed or measured on an individual as the disease progresses, and various disease outcomes such as impairments, disabilities, and quality of life measures. Clinical diagnosis of a genetic disease usually occurs following the initial recognition of the phenotypic manifestations of the disease, which then spurs the physician to request genetic testing for confirmation and specification of the genetic mutation. For example, the muscular dystrophies comprise a group of hereditary diseases characterized by the progressive wasting of skeletal and sometimes cardiac and smooth muscles. The Muscular Dystrophy Association recognizes 9 different muscular dystrophies among 34 other various types of diseases affecting neuromuscular function. The presence of progressive muscle wasting and weakness often suggests the diagnosis of a form of muscular dystrophy. The presence of these symptoms in early childhood further narrows the diagnostic consideration to (1) Duchenne muscular dystrophy (DMD), (2) Becker muscular dystrophy (BMD), (3) one of the various limb-girdle muscular dystrophy (LGMD), or (4) several other less common dystrophies. The presence of progressive weakness with a predominantly limb and trunk distribution with weakness occurring more in the lower versus upper limbs suggests the possibility of either DMD, BMD, or one of the LGMD, at which point genetic testing for mutations in the appropriate genes underlying these disorders may be ordered based on the phenotypic manifestations.

In DMD, genetic mutations in the dystrophin gene lead to incorrect coding for the protein dystrophin with varying degrees of severity. The decreased expression of the fully functioning form of dystrophin leads to a loss of internal muscle structure, leading to slowly progressive muscle weakness and wasting, the clinical phenotype of DMD. The phenotypic expression of a disease may also correlate with the severity of the genetic mutation. This information may enhance or even redefine what we know about disease. DMD and BMD were originally considered to be two separate genetic diseases because of the variation in clinical disease symptom severity and prognosis of death between them. It is now known that DMD and BMD represent a spectrum of the phenotypic expression of differing mutations in the dystrophin gene. DMD (clinically severe, leading to death in the third decade of life) and BMD (milder clinical disease than DMD with significantly improved survival) are now classic examples of how minor variations in genotype may cause major variations in phenotype.

Much current research focuses on the relationship of the genotypes in individuals affected with a genetic disorder to the resultant phenotypic outcomes. Different genotypes of a genetic disorder could be predictive of the severity of the disease among affected individuals or even the phenotypic manifestations of the disease. For example, if we could predict the resultant phenotype of individuals with mutations in the dystrophin gene, specifically whether and when common secondary complications, such as cardiomyopathy, scoliosis, and pulmonary disease, will manifest, then it is possible that physicians may provide more effective prevention and treatment. It has been well documented that improved clinical management of these complications does prolong the life and improve the quality of that life in patients with DMD. Understanding the relationship between the genotype and resultant phenotype will likely prove to enhance our understanding of these disorders and our abilities to care for those affected.

New methods for detecting mutations in specific disease-causing genes have enabled the identification of mutant genotypes heretofore not possible in many genetic disorders. The hope has been that this would allow us to predict phenotypic variance that in turn would improve prognosis and treatment of genetic diseases. However, as with most diseases, the phenotypic outcomes that are observed in the clinical evaluation are the result of a complex and lengthy series of biological events, both genetically and environmentally influenced. These events occur during development and well into adult life, adding to the complexity of the situation. By and large, what has followed is the realization of the complexity of the phenotypic expression in genetic diseases. It is this realization that has caused many geneticists to question the common ways that we have classified some of the genetic disorders, and there is currently a trend to view even single gene (monogenic) traits as complex and multifactorial. Contributing to this changing perspective is the realization that if we examine the multitude of phenotypic outcomes in any genetic disorder, we find a variety of factors that can contribute to the widely different phenotypic expressions among affected individuals. What accounts for differences in phenotypic outcomes include, but are not limited to, variation among the alleles for a single gene, the effects of interaction between the disease gene and other genes (modifier genes), and the effects of environmental exposures on the products of disease genes during development. Even for simple monogenic disorders, the biology remains complicated and multifaceted.

—*F. John Meaney, Jennifer Andrews, and Timothy Miller*

See also Association, Genetic; Gene; Gene-Environment Interactions; Genotype; Mutation

Further Readings

Nussbaum, R. J., McInnes, R. R., & Willard, H. F. (2001). *Thompson and Thompson genetics in medicine* (6th ed.). Philadelphia: W. B. Saunders.

Scriver, C. R., & Waters, P. J. (1999). Monogenic traits are not so simple: Lessons from phenylketonuria. *Trends in Genetics, 15*, 267–272.

Strachan, T., & Read, A. P. (2004). *Human molecular genetics 3* (3rd ed.). New York: Garland Science.

PHYSICAL ACTIVITY AND HEALTH

Prior to 1900, virtually every aspect of life, including transportation, work, food preparation, and caring for one's property required physical exertion or movement. However, beginning with the Industrial Revolution, an immense number of inventions have provided convenience and relief from physical effort. This has created an environment in which people can be almost completely sedentary on any given day. This changed environment has unintended consequences as we are now beginning to fully understand the negative impact a sedentary lifestyle can have on health.

The benefits of physical activity (PA) have been extolled throughout Western history, but it was not until the latter half of the 20th century that scientific evidence supporting these beliefs began to accumulate. A significant amount of this evidence has come from prospective epidemiology studies involving large numbers of people followed for several years in which the relationship between PA and various health outcomes have been documented.

This entry summarizes the evidence from such studies to provide an understanding of the association between PA and different health benefits and risks. Where sufficient evidence exists, answers to the question, "How much physical activity is enough?" are provided. However, since the vast majority of the epidemiology studies have involved participants above 18 years of age, only evidence on adults is considered. Research with adults shows that regular PA independently confers significant health benefits as indicated by marked reductions in the risk of developing several chronic diseases that are today's leading causes of death and disability. In some cases, the optimal dose of PA is unclear. However, current data suggest that at least 30 min/day of moderate intensity PA is very beneficial and, in some cases, more is better. The resultant health benefits are available to all persons across the adult life span and, therefore, a lifetime of PA should be a priority.

Terminology

Physical activity is defined as bodily movement produced by skeletal muscle that increases energy expenditure above the resting level. As such, PA involves all movement associated with occupational, household, leisure time, recreational, sport, or transportation activities. *Exercise* is a subcategory of PA and is planned, structured, repetitive, and for the purpose of improving or maintaining one or more components of physical fitness. Both PA and exercise can be categorized by type, duration, frequency, and intensity.

Physical fitness is the ability to carry out daily tasks with vigor and alertness, without undue fatigue. Health-related fitness includes cardiorespiratory (aerobic) endurance, muscle endurance, muscle strength, flexibility, and body composition. *Health* is a human condition with physical, social, and psychological dimensions. Positive health is associated with a capacity to enjoy life and withstand challenges, not just the absence of disease. Negative health is associated with morbidity and, sometimes, premature mortality.

The intensity of PA is known to influence the health benefits derived. Thus, a correct knowledge of this component is helpful. *Moderate intensity* PA requires 3 to 6 times as much energy as rest. This is equivalent to brisk walking. *Vigorous intensity* PA requires 7 times as much energy as rest, or greater. This is equivalent to jogging. *Energy expenditure* is a product of the frequency, intensity, and duration of PA and is commonly reported as kilocalories per week (kcal/week).

Physical Activity and Mortality

Does PA add years to life? The resounding answer is yes. A number of studies indicate that physically active men and women live longer than sedentary people, meaning that the health benefits of PA outweigh the risks.

The cumulative evidence indicates a linear reduction in mortality risk with an increased level of PA. On average, a threshold of about 1,000 kcal/week (4,200 kJ/week) of energy expenditure from PA is associated with a 20% to 30% reduction in mortality from all causes. This amount of energy expenditure is attainable by walking briskly for 30 min/day. Further risk reduction may be observed with energy expenditure greater than 1,000 kcal/week.

The protective effect of cardiorespiratory fitness has also been reported with the most fit men and women having 70% to 80% lower death rates than the least fit men and women. Interestingly, adults in the next to lowest fitness group have exhibited 48% to 60% lower rates of all-cause death than the least fit group, indicating that even modest increases in aerobic fitness promote longevity. The amount of PA required for achieving even minor improvements in aerobic fitness and significant risk reductions in premature death equates to 130 to 140 min/week of walking, 100 to 130 min/week of aerobics, or 90 min/week of jogging.

Of special note is that the research indicates that higher-activity and higher-fitness groups had lower risk of death whether or not they smoked, had high cholesterol, had high blood pressure, had high blood glucose, had a family history of heart disease, had a healthy baseline examination, or were overweight. Thus, PA and fitness can improve health for men and women, regardless of their health and risk factor status.

One limitation to most of the epidemiology studies is that PA is only measured once. However, it can change over time. Stronger evidence that PA and fitness *cause* health improvements comes from studies illustrating that changes in PA predict changes in risk of mortality. In the Harvard Alumni Study, more than 10,000 men aged 45 to 84 years reported their PA at two time periods with subsequent deaths monitored. Compared with those who remained inactive at both times, those who became active decreased their risk of dying by 15%. Those who were active the first time but became inactive by the second assessment increased their risk of death by 10%. This cause and effect relationship has been confirmed with research linking changes in aerobic fitness to changes in mortality. Another important finding is that gains in longevity are noted for persons across a large age range demonstrating that changes in PA or fitness at any age are beneficial.

The evidence is irrefutable for regular PA significantly reducing the risk of premature death. To put this in perspective, one can determine the number of deaths for which sedentary lifestyle is responsible. Considering the most common causes of death, more than 250,000 deaths in the United States could be prevented *each year* if sedentary lifestyle was eliminated. This figure accounts for approximately 23% of all deaths as compared with those caused by smoking (33%), obesity (24%), and high cholesterol (23%). As such, sedentary lifestyle is one of the most important public health challenges facing us today.

Physical Activity and Cardiovascular Disease (CVD)

Physical activity reduces the risk of premature death by primarily decreasing the risk of cardiovascular diseases, which are the leading causes of death in the United States and other industrialized countries. Many associate CVD with men, but heart disease is also the leading cause of death in women, resulting in approximately 500,000 deaths in U.S. women each year.

Coronary Heart Disease

Coronary heart disease (CHD) resulting from plaque accumulating in the coronary arteries is the most deadly form of CVD, and there is overwhelming evidence that PA and aerobic fitness are protective factors. Results show that the least active or fit persons had an 80% higher risk of dying from CHD than the most active or fit groups. In addition, the largest risk reduction typically occurs between persons in the least active or fit group and persons in the next highest activity or fitness group, once again indicating that even slight increases in activity or fitness confers significant benefits. For example, women have experienced 20% to 50% reductions in risk of CHD death with as little as 1 hr/week of walking. As with all-cause mortality, the association between PA or aerobic fitness and CHD risk is significant for both men and women across different races, levels of body fatness, preexisting medical conditions, and age groups. These results signify the capacity to use PA as an effective intervention for both primary and secondary prevention of CHD.

Similar to findings for premature death from all causes, *changes* in PA and fitness have been shown to affect CHD risk. Men who were unfit or inactive at baseline but increased in fitness or activity level over time reduced their risk of CHD by 52% and 45%, respectively, compared with men who remained unfit or inactive at both assessments.

There appears to be a window of protection from CHD death by expending 750 to 2,000 kcal/week through *moderate* intensity, dynamic, endurance PA (such as walking or jogging 7.5–20 miles/week). In the absence of other activity, at least 1 hr/week of intermittent hard physical labor also significantly reduces the risk of CHD. Most evidence shows that the largest reductions occur with moderate levels of activity or fitness as compared with those who are least active or fit. Therefore, something is better than nothing, but exactly how much is enough remains unclear. Regardless, in very inactive or unfit persons, brisk walking daily for at least 30 min should stimulate fitness gains and energy expenditure associated with CHD benefits.

Stroke

Recent reviews on PA and stroke risk found that moderately or highly active individuals had lower risk of stroke occurrence or mortality than did low active persons. Being moderately or highly active during leisure time was associated with a 15% to 20% and 20% to 27% lower risk of total stroke occurrence and mortality, respectively, compared with being inactive. Although there were relatively few studies available, results showed that being moderately and highly active at work was associated with a 36% and 43% lower risk of stroke, respectively, compared with being sedentary. It has also been demonstrated that daily commuting PA on foot or by bicycle was modestly associated with a decreased risk of stroke in both men and women. The risk of having a stroke was decreased by 8% and 11% in persons accumulating 1 to 29 min/day and >30 min/day of active commuting, respectively, compared with those who did not actively commute to work. Overall, the results indicate that moderate PA achieved through a variety of daily activities is protective against stroke and additional benefits may be realized with greater than moderate amounts of PA. However, more information is needed to develop specific recommendations with regard to the intensity, duration, and frequency of PA associated with a meaningful reduction in stroke risk.

Hypertension

Hypertension (HTN) is a significant risk factor for all-cause and CVD death, stroke, CHD, heart failure, kidney malfunction, and peripheral vascular disease. Fortunately, PA can serve as a low cost intervention in the prevention and management of HTN.

Epidemiology studies reveal that regular PA has potential for reducing or preventing mild hypertension. Participation in vigorous sports was associated with a 19% to 30% reduction in risk of developing HTN in U.S. men. Investigations with Japanese and Finnish men have also demonstrated significant inverse associations between baseline levels of commuting and leisure-time PA and future HTN. High levels of aerobic fitness have also been reported to reduce risk of HTN by 50% to 90% as compared with the lowest levels of fitness. None of the studies in women have observed significant relationships between PA and future HTN, although one did report a 30% lower risk for developing HTN in active versus sedentary women. In the only study to date including black men, PA was not associated with HTN risk; however, more studies are needed before definitive conclusions can be made.

Clinical studies indicate that regular exercise is effective for reducing systolic blood pressure by about 6 to 11 mmHg and diastolic blood pressure by about 6 to 8 mmHg in men and women with mild HTN. The recommendation to achieve such benefits is to accumulate at least 30 min of moderate intensity endurance type PA on most (at least 5) days of the week. For now, it doesn't appear that PA of a higher intensity confers any further benefits above those attained with moderate intensity activity.

Physical Activity and Cancer

Cancer is the second leading cause of death in many industrialized nations with the most common cancers being lung, colon, breast, and prostate. Because each cancer is likely to have somewhat different causal factors, the protective effects for PA have been examined for specific types of cancer.

Colon Cancer

The cumulative evidence from more than 50 studies clearly shows that physically active men and women have about a 30% to 40% reduction in risk of developing colon cancer, compared with inactive persons. It appears that 30 to 60 min/day of moderate to vigorous intensity PA is required to decrease risk. The optimal amount, intensity, duration, and frequency of PA associated with a reduced risk of colon cancer remains uncertain. However, the findings do indicate that total energy expenditure, whether from a job or leisure-time activities, is associated with colon cancer risk reduction.

Breast Cancer

Substantial evidence documents that physically active women have a 20% to 30% reduction in risk of breast cancer, compared with sedentary women. As with colon cancer, 30 to 60 min/day of moderate to vigorous intensity PA is needed to decrease breast cancer risk with risk declining further at the higher levels of PA. Although the biological mechanisms explaining how PA affects breast cancer risk remain unknown, lifetime moderate intensity PA appears to be a protective measure against breast cancer for all women.

Other Cancers

The available data reveal that PA is not associated with the risk of future rectal cancer. Data do suggest that physically active persons have a lower risk of lung cancer, but separating the effects of smoking is difficult. There is scant information on the role of PA in preventing other cancers.

Physical Activity and Diabetes

A substantial reduction in the occurrence of type 2 diabetes is consistently found among physically active persons compared with their sedentary peers. The magnitude of the reduced risk is 30% to 50% for active individuals with the benefit related to favorable effects of PA on body weight, insulin sensitivity, blood glucose control, blood pressure, and blood lipids. Most of these studies have observed significant benefits with daily walking for 30 min or more with additional benefits exhibited through participation in regular vigorous intensity PA. Some studies indicate that persons with an elevated risk of diabetes at baseline (such as higher body weight and fasting blood glucose) also demonstrate marked reductions in type 2 diabetes risk via regular PA or attainment of high aerobic fitness.

Physical activity combined with modest weight loss may exert optimal reduction in type 2 diabetes risk. In the U.S. Diabetes Prevention Program, combining 150 min/week of PA and a low-fat diet resulted in a 5% weight loss and 60% reduced risk of future type 2 diabetes. This benefit was superior to the nearly 30% risk reduction after treatment with an oral drug. This lifestyle intervention was found to be effective in men and women of all ethnic groups, including persons aged 60 years and older.

Regardless of the underlying biological mechanisms involved, regular PA is strongly related to a reduced risk of type 2 diabetes. The general recommendation is 30 min/day of moderate intensity endurance PA. Even further benefits may be attained with higher intensity aerobic activity, and performing strength-training exercises 2 to 3 days/week has also resulted in positive changes in biological markers of type 2 diabetes. However, further research is needed to uncover the ideal methods and intensities of PA, and more studies with women and minority groups need to be conducted.

Physical Activity and Obesity

Obesity is a problem of epidemic proportions with nearly two thirds of American adults suffering from overweight or obesity. The prevalence of overweight and obesity continues to increase among all age groups and ethnicities, but PA plays a vital role in reversing this trend. The research shows an inverse relationship between levels of PA and body fatness, and men and women who are minimally active are 3 to 4 times more likely than their more active counterparts to experience weight gain.

Thirty minutes of moderate intensity PA, preferably all days of the week, is adequate to minimize health risks for chronic diseases, yet it may be insufficient for prevention of weight gain, stimulation of weight loss, or prevention of weight regain. The International Association for the Study of Obesity recommends 45 to 60 min/day of moderate intensity PA to prevent unhealthy weight gain and 60 to 90 min/day of moderate intensity PA or lesser amounts of vigorous PA to prevent weight regain in formerly overweight and obese individuals. There is no conclusive evidence regarding the amount of PA needed to incur significant weight loss; however, most studies indicate that exercise combined with modest caloric restriction is most effective in promoting weight loss.

Regular PA, independent of substantial weight loss, can provide improvements in health. Those who are overweight, yet engage in regular PA, have been termed the *fit fat*. Research shows that unfit lean adults have twice the risk of all-cause mortality as fit lean and fit obese adults. Although there is a direct relationship between body fatness and all-cause and CVD mortality, being active or fit decreases high mortality risk in obese persons.

—Steven P. Hooker and Anna E. Price

See also Cancer; Cardiovascular Disease; Obesity

Further Readings

Bassuk, S. S., & Manson, J. E. (2005). Epidemiological evidence for the role of physical activity in reducing risk of type 2 diabetes and cardiovascular disease. *Journal of Applied Physiology*, *99*, 1193–1204.

Dishman, R. K., Washburn, R. A., & Heath, G. W. (2004). *Physical activity epidemiology*. Champaign, IL: Human Kinetics.

Lee, I. (2003). Physical activity and cancer prevention: Data from epidemiologic studies. *Medicine and Science in Sports and Exercise*, *35*, 1823–1827.

Pescatello, L. S., Franklin, B. A., Fagard, R., Farquhar, W. B., Kelley, G. A., & Ray, C. A. (2004). American College of Sports Medicine position stand. Exercise and hypertension. *Medicine and Science in Sports and Exercise*, *36*, 533–553.

Sallis, J. F., & Owen, N. (1999). *Physical activity and behavioral medicine*. Thousand Oaks, CA: Sage.

Saris, W. H. M., Blair, S. N., van Baak, M. A., Eaton, S. B., Davies, P. S. W., Di Pietro, L., et al. (2003). How much physical activity is enough to prevent unhealthy weight gain? Outcome of the IASO 1st stock conference and consensus statement. *Obesity Reviews*, *4*, 101–114.

U.S. Department of Health and Human Services, Centers for Disease Control and Prevention. (1996). *Physical activity and health: A report of the surgeon general*. Atlanta, GA: Author.

PHYSICIANS' HEALTH STUDY

The Physicians' Health Study (PHS) is a randomized, double-blind, placebo-controlled trial that was initially designed as a cohort study to test the effect of two medications: (1) the effect of aspirin on mortality due to cardiovascular disease and (2) the effect of beta-carotene on reducing the incidence of cancer. The initial planning for the PHS began in 1978, with Phase One (PHS-I) beginning in 1982 and ending in 1995. Phase Two of the cohort study (PHS-II) began in 1997 and is expected to conclude in 2007. This entry provides a general overview of the two phases of PHS and briefly discusses the major findings from PHS-I.

Physicians' Health Study Phase I

Study Population

The first phase of the Physicians' Health Study began in 1982, with funding from the National Cancer Institute and the National Heart, Lung, and Blood Institute. The study had two arms. One group of study participants were used to test whether aspirin prevented cardiovascular events such as a heart attack (myocardial infarction). A second group of participants were used to determine whether beta-carotene was useful in preventing cancer. Physicians aged 40 to 84 years were recruited between 1980 and 1982 as the study participants, and the study was conducted by mail-in survey between 1984 and 1995. A total of 22,071 physicians were eventually randomized into the trial. Principal investigators used physicians as the study population to obtain more accurate medical history and other pertinent health information.

Study Design

PHS-I was constructed to assign study participants to one of four possible treatment scenarios. Study participants received one of the following: two active medications (aspirin and beta-carotene), one active drug and one placebo (active aspirin and a beta-carotene placebo, or an aspirin placebo and active beta-carotene), or two placebos (neither pill was an active medication). Using blood samples and follow-up questionnaires, information was obtained regarding each participant's ability to adhere to the medication regimen, their use of other medications, significant health outcomes, and whether a participant had any illness or disease during the course of the study.

Major Findings

The aspirin arm of the study was stopped in 1988 after a finding that aspirin reduced the risk of myocardial infarction by 44%. This was a highly significant result when compared with the experience of those participants taking the aspirin placebo. Partly as a result of this finding, low-dose (325 mg) aspirin is now recommended as standard care for patients with cardiovascular disease.

The beta-carotene arm of PHS-I concluded in 1995. Although the medical literature had suggested that individuals consuming fruits and vegetables high in beta-carotene had lower rates of cancer, the results of PHS-I failed to demonstrate any positive or negative effect of beta-carotene supplementation on the incidence of cancer.

Physicians' Health Study Phase II

The second phase of the Physician's Health Study was initiated in 1997 and is expected to conclude in 2007. Funding is provided by the National Institutes of Health and additional private sponsors. This particular study is designed to determine whether certain dietary supplements have any effect on reducing the incidence of certain chronic diseases. Specifically, PHS-II investigates whether vitamin C, vitamin E, multivitamins, and beta-carotene serve to prevent colon cancer, prostate cancer, diseases of the eye, memory loss, and cardiovascular disease.

Participants in this study are physicians aged 50 years or older and who did not participate in the first Physician's Health Study. Similar to the design of PHS-I, physicians are assigned to one of 16 treatment scenarios. These include supplementation with one of the following: active forms of vitamins C and E, beta-carotene and a multivitamin, a set of four placebos, or a combination of both active supplements and placebos. A total of 14,642 physicians are randomized into the trial. The collection of information from each participant is also similar to the design of PHS-I: Blood samples and annual follow-up questionnaires are being used to obtain information about individual adherence to the supplement regimen, use of other medications, significant health outcomes, and incidence of major illness or disease during the course of the study.

Results from PHS-II are yet to be published, although information about the design and rationale for the trial is available in the medical literature. Findings regarding the long-term use of vitamin supplementation and the impact of supplements on the prevention of chronic disease are expected to follow the conclusion of the study, which is expected in December of 2007.

—*Ashby Wolfe*

See also Cancer; Cardiovascular Disease; Chronic Disease Epidemiology; Nutritional Epidemiology

Further Readings

Christen, W. G., Gaziano, J. M., & Hennekens, C. H. (2000). Design of Physicians' Health Study II: A randomized trial of beta-carotene, vitamins E and C, and multivitamins, in prevention of cancer, cardiovascular disease, and eye disease, and review of results of completed trials. *Annals of Epidemiology, 10*(2), 125–134.

Hennekens, C. H., Buring, J. E., Manson, J. E., Stampfer, M., Rosner, B., Cook, N. R., et al. (1996). Lack of effect of long-term supplementation with beta carotene on the incidence of malignant neoplasms and cardiovascular disease. *New England Journal of Medicine, 334*(18), 1145–1149.

Steering Committee of the Physicians' Health Study Research Group. (1989). Final report on the aspirin component of the ongoing Physicians' Health Study. *New England Journal of Medicine, 321*(3), 129–135.

Web Sites

Physicians' Health Study: http://phs.bwh.harvard.edu.

PIE CHART

A *pie chart* is a graphical representation of data as a disk divided into wedge-shaped "pieces" or "slices" whose sizes are proportional to the relative frequencies of the categories they represent. Because pie charts are most useful when they include only a small number of categories, they are most often used to display the relative frequencies of a categorical data set. Pie charts are a logical choice for graphical presentation when the focus of interest is on the relative frequencies of the data—that is, how much of the whole each category represents, rather than the absolute frequency of each category (in the latter case, a bar chart would be more appropriate).

Florence Nightingale, a founder of modern nursing, was also well versed in statistics. She invented a type of pie chart to show that in the Crimean War, far more soldiers died of illness and infection than those who died of battle wounds. Her campaign succeeded in improving hospital conditions and nursing so that many lives were saved.

Pie charts are most often created using statistical software but may also be created by hand: to obtain the angle for any category—that is, the size of the "slice," we multiply the relative frequency by 360°, because there are 360° in a complete circle.

For example, there were 863 kidney transplant patients who had their transplant performed at the Ohio State University Transplant Center during the period 1982 to 1992. There were 432 white males, 92 black males, 280 white females, and 59 black females.

Table 1   Race and Sex of Kidney Transplant Patients: Demographics of Kidney Transplant Recipients at the Ohio State University Transplant Center (1982–1992)

Race and Sex	Frequency	Relative Frequency
White male	432	0.501
Black male	92	0.107
White female	280	0.324
Black female	59	0.068
Total	863	1.000

Source: Adapted from data presented in Klein and Moeschberger (2003, p. 262).

Table 1 gives the race and sex information and calculates the relative frequencies for the four response categories.

To make a pie chart for this data set, we need to divide a disk into four wedge-shaped pieces that comprise 50.1%, 10.7%, 32.4%, and 6.8% of the disk. We do so by using a protractor and the fact that there are 360° in a circle. Thus, four pieces of the disk are obtained by marking off 180.36°, 38.52°, 116.64°, and 24.48°, which are 50.1% of 360°, 10.7% of 360°, 32.4% of 360°, and 6.8% of 360°, respectively. The pie chart for the relative frequency distribution for the above table is shown in Figure 1.

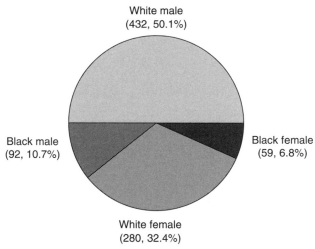

Kidney Transplant Patients

White male (432, 50.1%)

Black male (92, 10.7%)

Black female (59, 6.8%)

White female (280, 32.4%)

Figure 1   Race and Sex of Kidney Transplant Patients: Demographics of Kidney Transplant Recipients at the Ohio State University Transplant Center (1982–1992)

—*Renjin Tu*

See also Bar Chart; Graphical Presentation of Data; Nightingale, Florence; Proportion

Further Readings

De Veaux, R. D., Velleman, P. F., & Bock, D. E. (2005). *Stats data and models.* Boston: Addison-Wesley.

Klein, J. P., & Moeschberger, M. L. (2003). *Survival analysis: Techniques for censored and truncated data* (2nd ed.). New York: Springer.

Nightingale, F. (1958). *Polar-area diagram: Biographies of women mathematicians.* Retrieved November 10, 2006, from http://www.scottlan.edu/lriddle/women/ nightpiechart.htm.

PLACEBO EFFECT

The placebo effect is an improvement in an individual's medical condition or an alleviation of adverse symptoms that occurs when the person receives an inert treatment. It may result from the person's expectation of improvement or from the increased motivation to make improvements in general health that may result. The placebo effect was first described in 1955 by Henry K. Beecher, an American physician, who described it in his frequently cited article, "The Powerful Placebo." The placebo effect has been explained as a result of the Pavlovian conditioning theory, the expectancy-value theory, and increased motivation on the part of the participant.

A placebo may be contact with a physician, cognitive or behavioral intervention, lifestyle changes in diet or level of physical activity, or a sugar pill. Regardless of the form, the aim of a placebo is to have no biologic effect at all. Placebos are typically used in placebo-controlled clinical trials where a treatment group receives the medical intervention being tested and the control group receives a placebo. The aim of this experimental design is to ensure that the study participants do not know whether they are receiving the treatment or the placebo. When the experimenter knows who is receiving the treatment and who is receiving the placebo, the study is single blind; if neither the participants nor the researcher knows, the study is double blind. Such studies minimize potential bias that may distort the true relationship between the exposure to the treatment and the outcome.

Although the aim of a placebo is primarily related to improving the methodology of a trial by blinding the participants to the status of the received treatments, one of the results of offering a placebo is that some individuals actually feel better and experience a beneficial effect despite the fact that the placebo has no known mechanism of action that may induce this effect. It seems that for illnesses such as depression, headache, stomach ailments, and pain, about a third of patients taking a placebo actually start to feel better because they believe they are receiving medical treatment, when in fact they are receiving an inert treatment.

The biologic mechanism by which a placebo can create this effect is unclear. However, it has been suggested that it is primarily a psychological effect that results from the individual's expectation that the treatment will work. Another theory of the mechanism of the placebo effect is that it is a conditioned response reflecting people's experience of treatment followed by symptom relief.

There are several ethical issues in the use of a placebo. Some bioethicists suggest that patients participating in trials cannot truly give informed consent if they do not know which treatment they will be receiving. Another criticism is that single-blind studies introduce an element of deception into health care and practice, because patients are told or allowed to believe that they are receiving a drug when the researchers know otherwise. Furthermore, in some cases, the placebo effect may actually result in adverse side effects, rather than only beneficial ones; this phenomenon is often called the nocebo effect. This may occur when individuals expect to experience negative side effects from the treatment.

—*Kate Bassil*

See also Ethics in Human Subjects Research; Hawthorne Effect; Randomization

Further Readings

Beecher, H. K. (1955). The powerful placebo. *Journal of the American Medical Association, 159,* 1602–1606.
Turner, J. A., Deyo, R. A., Loeser, J. D., Von Korff, M., & Fordyce, W. E. (1994). The importance of placebo effects in pain treatment and research. *Journal of the American Medical Association, 271*(20), 1609–1614.
Walsh, B. T., Seidman, S. N., Sysko, R., & Gould, M. (2002). Placebo response in studies of major depression: Variable, substantial, and growing. *Journal of the American Medical Association, 287,* 1840–1847.

PLAGUE

Yersinia pestis is the causative organism of plague, an enzootic vector-borne disease usually infecting rodents (e.g., rats) and fleas. Over the past 2,000 years, three devastating pandemics have occurred. Plague pandemics have caused social and economic devastations on a scale unmatched by any other infectious disease except for smallpox. Although at the present time the organism is not considered a major health concern, approximately 2,500 cases annually are reported worldwide, and recently the World Health Organization categorized plague as a reemerging infectious disease. Despite major advances in diagnosis and treatment that were made since the discovery of the causative organism, the disease persists in several parts of the world, causing significant recurrent outbreaks in rodents and humans.

History

Reports of plague date back to ancient times, but the first undoubted account of bubonic plague is the *Great Plague of Justinian*. This first plague pandemic originated around AD 532 in Egypt and quickly spread to the Middle East and around the Mediterranean basin. In the following years, the disease spread as far north as into the territories of France and Germany. The estimated population losses in North Africa, Europe, and central/southern Asia were between 50% and 60% of the population. In contrast, the second pandemic—also known as the great medieval plague, Black Death, or Great Pestilence—is well described by many authors and many documents. It originated around the year 1334 in China and spread westward along the trade routes in Tauris on the Black Sea and eventually reached Constantinople (today's Istanbul) and the Crimea in 1347. From the Crimea, the disease was imported into Venice, Genoa, and Sicily by Italian merchant ships. The disease spread slowly but inevitably from village to village and eventually extended all over Europe, killing more than one third of its population. Despite the high mortality rate of the Black Death pandemic, the most devastating effects resulted from smaller, recurrent outbreaks that continued well into the 18th century. The third pandemic originated in China around 1855, rapidly spreading to its southern coast. The disease reached the city of Hong Kong in the 1890s. At this time, larger epidemics occurred all over China, marking the beginning of the next pandemic. Plague rapidly spread throughout the world to all inhabited continents, except for Australia.

Since then, smaller outbreaks have occurred around the world, with most recent outbreaks in Africa and Madagascar. In 1900, plague was introduced into North America (San Francisco), and between 1900 and 1924 most plague cases in the United States occurred in port cities along the Pacific and Gulf coasts. The disease spread slowly eastward with sporadic cases now being reported mainly in Arizona, New Mexico, Colorado, Utah, and Texas.

The causative organism of plague was discovered in 1894 during the early years of the third pandemic. Independent from each other, the Japanese microbiologist Shibasaburo Kitasato and the French microbiologist Alexandre Yersin conducted the experiments that led to the identification of the causative organism. Yersin's descriptions and explanations were published only a few days after Kitasato's; however, they seemed to be somewhat more accurate. Over the past decades, the literature has been quite inconsistent in crediting Yersin or Kitasato with the discovery of the plague bacillus. Finally, in 1970, the organism was officially named *Yersinia pestis*. In 1898, Paul-Louis Simond discovered that plague is transmitted by fleas. In 1927, Ricardo Jorge found an explanation for the occurrence of sporadic cases of plague.

Epidemiology and Clinical Manifestations

Plague occurs worldwide, with most cases reported in rural underdeveloped areas of Third World countries. In developed countries, advances in living conditions, public health, and antibiotic treatment made outbreaks of urban rat-borne plague less likely to occur in the decades after the third pandemic. However, the disease continues to be a problem in rural areas in the Americas, Africa, and Asia. This form of plague, termed the *sylvatic plague*, is maintained in wild rodents. Most recently, plague has resurged in sub-Saharan Africa and particularly in East Africa and Madagascar. In addition to its occurrence in nature, plague has been extensively researched for its role in biowarfare during the times of World War II and the Cold War. The possibility of plague being used as a biological weapon in the hands of military or terrorists remains as an important national security threat requiring special measures for medical and public health preparedness.

The organism is a gram negative, nonmotile bacillus and belongs to the family of Enterobacteriaceae. Based on historical data and bacteriological characteristics of strains isolated from remnant foci, Devignat described the three biovars Antiqua, Medievalis, and

Orientalis, which caused the first, second, and third pandemic, respectively. In nature, plague is primarily an infection of wild rodents and is transmitted by fleas. Worldwide, the domestic rats *Rattus rattus* and *Rattus norvegicus* are the most important reservoirs. The most common vector for transmission is the oriental rat flea.

Infection of *Y. pestis* in humans occurs in one of three clinical forms: *bubonic plague* is characterized by regional lymphadenopathy resulting from cutaneous or mucous membrane exposure to the organism; *primary septicemic plague* is an overwhelming plague bacteremia usually following cutaneous exposure; *primary pulmonary plague* follows the inhalation of aerosolized droplets containing *Y. pestis* organisms. Most cases of naturally occurring human plague represent the classic form of bubonic plague when victims are bitten by infected fleas. Plague can effectively be treated using antibiotics such as gentamicin, doxycycline, or tetracycline.

—Stefan Riedel

See also Bioterrorism; Epidemic; Insect-Borne Disease; Zoonotic Disease

Further Readings

Mandell, G. L., Bennett, J. E., & Dolin, R. (Eds.). (2005). *Principles of infectious diseases* (6th ed.). Philadelphia: Churchill Livingstone.

Murray, P. R., Baron, E. J., Jorgensen, J. H., Pfaller, M. A., & Yolken, R. H. (Eds.). (2003). *ASM manual of clinical microbiology* (8th ed.). Washington, DC: ASM Press.

POINT ESTIMATE

Most statistical analysis is done with the desire to reach a conclusion or decision about one or more parameters associated with a population of interest (statistical inference). Two types of estimators are used to assist in reaching a conclusion: point estimators and interval estimators. The goal of estimation is to provide a "best guess" at the true value of an unknown population parameter. To this end, a point estimator is a rule or function for computing a single quantity from a sample that will be used to approximate most closely a population parameter. Statistically, the point estimate is the value itself that is obtained when the rule is applied to sample data. Often the term point estimate is used to refer to any value computed from the data that is used to estimate a population parameter, even if it is not the "best" estimator.

The point estimate is the most common way that an estimate is expressed. Table 1 contains a list of the names or symbols for commonly used estimators along with the population parameters they estimate. Note that often point estimators are descriptive statistics.

Point estimates are quick and easy to calculate. They allow for a first look at the population based on sample data. Researchers hope that the single value obtained for a point estimator will be close to the parameter it is estimating. Since a point estimate is a random variable, it is in some way distributed about the true value of the population parameter. However, since the point estimate consists of a single number or a single point on the real number scale, there is room for questions. For example, a point estimate does not tell us how large the sample was on which it is based. Nor does it tell anything about the possible size of the error.

Since a researcher will infer that the population parameter is equal to the value of the point estimator, a little more knowledge of statistical inference is necessary. Statistical inference differs from ordinary inference in that not only is an inference made, but typically a measure is provided of how good the inference is. The error of estimation for a particular point estimate is defined to be the absolute value of the difference between the point estimate and the true population value. For example, the error of estimation for the mean is $|\bar{x} - \mu|$. However, the magnitude of the error of estimation is unknown since the true population parameter value is unknown. If a probability sample was taken, then statistical reliability may be calculated for the estimate by either using a confidence interval or by using the bound on the error of estimation.

Table 1   Common Parameters and Their Point Estimators

Parameter	Population	Point Estimator
Mean	μ	$\overline{X}$
Variance	σ^2	s^2
Proportion	p or π	$\hat{p}$
Relative risk	RR	$\widehat{RR}$

Sometimes a point estimate is referred to as the "realized value" since it is the actual numerical value of a random variable. Also, the phrase "point estimate" is sometimes used as an infinitive verb, as in the following: To point estimate is to compute a value from a sample and accept that value as an estimate of the unknown parameter.

Estimation of the Mean

Most often, researchers are interested in the value of the population mean for some variable. There are two points about estimating the mean. First, each of the measures of central tendency is a valid estimator for the population mean. However, the "best" or most robust estimator of the population mean is the sample mean. Thus, it is the estimator used in this article. Second, if the sampling distribution is approximately normal (i.e., the data have a bell-shaped curve or a mound-shaped histogram), then the Empirical Rule applies. By the Empirical Rule, the error of estimation will be less than $2(\sigma_{\bar{X}}) = 2(\sigma/\sqrt{n})$ approximately 95% of the time. The quantity $2(\sigma/\sqrt{n})$ is called the bound on the error of estimation. This quantity is a measure of how good our inference is. The smaller the bound on the error of estimation, the better the inference is. Since σ is unknown, we estimate it with the sample standard deviation (s) and obtain an approximate bound on the error. Point estimation with a bound on the error of estimation is used when no more than a crude statement of precision is required. If more precision is needed, confidence intervals are used.

—*Stacie Ezelle Taylor*

See also Confidence Interval; Histogram; Inferential and Descriptive Statistics; Measures of Central Tendency; Probability Sample; Random Variable; Robust Statistics; Sampling Distribution

Further Readings

Freund, J. E., & Smith, R. M. (1986). *Statistics: A first course* (4th ed.). Englewood Cliffs, NJ: Prentice Hall.
Hurlburt, R. T. (2006). *Comprehending behavioral statistics* (4th ed.). Belmont, CA: Thomson/Wadsworth.
Ott, R. L., & Longnecker, M. (2001). *An introduction to statistical methods and data analysis* (5th ed.). Pacific Grove, CA: Duxbury.

POISSON REGRESSION

See REGRESSION

POLIO

Polio is a viral disease that has caused considerable suffering for much of human history. The oldest clearly identifiable reference to paralytic poliomyelitis is an Egyptian stone engraving from 14th century BCE. Prior to the introduction of effective vaccines in the 1950s, polio was a common infection of childhood, with a small proportion of infections resulting in death or lifelong paralysis. Control began in 1955 after the first inactivated poliovirus vaccine (IPV) and subsequently several years later an oral polio vaccine (OPV) was also introduced. In most developed countries, a good level of control was achieved by the mid 1960s. In 1985, the Pan American Health Organization (PAHO) launched an initiative to eradicate polio in the Americas by 1990. Based on the success of the PAHO program, in May 1988, the 41st World Health Assembly committed the Member States of the World Health Organization (WHO) to the global eradication of poliomyelitis by the year 2000 (resolution WHA41.28). Despite great progress, by the end of 2006, there were still four countries in which polio was endemic (Nigeria, India, Pakistan, and Afghanistan), with another eight countries experiencing importations (Angola, Cameroon, Ethiopia, Indonesia, Nepal, Niger, Somalia, and Yemen).

Infectious Agent and Transmission

The poliovirus is an enterovirus with man as the only reservoir. There are three antigenic types: 1, 2, and 3. Type 1 most commonly causes paralysis, Type 3 less frequently, and Type 2 uncommonly. Most epidemics historically are due to Type 1. The risk of vaccine-associated poliomyelitis per million persons vaccinated ranged from .05 to .99 (Type 1), 0 to .65 (Type 2), and 1.18 to 8.91 (Type 3).

Infection is spread from person-to-person with fecal-oral transmission most common in developing countries where sanitation is poor, while oral-pharyngeal transmission is more common in industrialized countries and during outbreaks. The mouth is the usual site of entry, and the virus first multiplies at the site of implantation in the lymph nodes in the pharynx and gastrointestinal tract. Incubation is usually from 7 to 10 days and may range from 4 to 40 days. The virus is usually present in the pharynx and in the stool before the onset of paralytic illness. One week after onset, there is low virus concentration in the throat, but the virus continues to be excreted in the stool for several weeks. Cases are most infectious during the first few days before and after onset of symptoms. For poliomyelitis, the ratio of inapparent (either subclinical or mild) infections to paralytic cases is very high, somewhere between 100 and 1,000 to 1. Long-term carriers are not known to occur.

Immunity

Susceptibility to poliomyelitis is universal. Epidemiologic evidence indicates that infants born to mothers with antibodies are naturally protected against paralytic disease for a few weeks. Immunity is obtained from infection with the wild virus or from immunization. Immunity following natural (including inapparent and mild) infections, or a completed series of immunizations with live OPV, results in both humoral (related to antibody production) and local intestinal cellular responses (a more localized response). Such immunity is thought to be lifelong and can serve as a block to infection with subsequent wild viruses and, therefore, helps in breaking chains of transmission. Vaccination with the IPV confers humoral immunity, but relatively less intestinal immunity; thus, vaccination with IPV does not provide resistance to carriage and spread of wild virus in the community. There is thought to be little, if any, cross-immunity between poliovirus types.

Clinical Features

Many infected with the wild poliovirus exhibit minor illnesses, but these cannot be distinguished clinically from illnesses caused by a number of other etiologies. Symptoms associated with minor illnesses include mild fever, muscle pains, headache, nausea, vomiting, stiffness of neck and back, and less frequently, signs of aseptic (nonbacterial) meningitis. Other conditions that may present similar to paralytic poliomyelitis include traumatic neuritis and tumors, followed less frequently by meningitis/encephalitis and illnesses produced by a variety of toxins. The most prominent

difference between poliomyelitis and other causes of acute flaccid paralysis (AFP) is that for polio, the paralytic sequelae is generally severe and permanent, while for many other causes of AFP, paralysis tends to resolve or improve by 60 days after onset.

Susceptible older children and adults, if infected, are at greatest risk of paralytic illness. For persons with paralytic disease, the case-fatality rate varies between 2% and 20%; however, with either bulbar or respiratory involvement, case-fatality rates may reach as high as 40%. The majority of the deaths occur within the first week following onset of paralysis.

Epidemiology

Polio epidemics in both developed and developing countries were common during the first half of the 20th century. For example, in the United States more than 20,000 cases of paralytic disease were reported in 1952. Dramatic reductions in polio incidence was achieved in countries incorporating either IPV or OPV into their routine schedule. For example, in the United States cases dropped to < 100 in 1965 and < 10 in 1973. The last cases of indigenously transmitted wild-type poliovirus in the United States were in 1979.

The molecular epidemiology of wild poliovirus has recently proved to be useful in helping identify whether different virus isolates originate from a common ancestral source of infection. With this information, geographic foci or reservoirs of transmission can be defined and help trace sources of outbreaks throughout large geographical areas, such as have been seen in Africa during 2006.

Vaccines

There are currently two effective polio vaccines available: IPV, which first became available in 1955, and live attenuated OPV, first used in mass campaigns in 1959. In 1987, an enhanced inactivated poliovirus vaccine (eIPV) was introduced. In developing countries, OPV has been the vaccine of choice due to ease of administration, since it simulates natural infection and induces both circulating antibody and intestinal resistance, and by secondary spread protects susceptible contacts. In the Americas, using OPV mass campaigns interrupted transmission in areas where routine delivery had failed. Under ideal conditions in temperate countries, a primary series of three doses of OPV produces seroconversion to all three virus types in more than 95% of vaccine recipients and is thought to have a clinical efficacy of nearly 100%. Three properly spaced doses of OPV should confer lifelong immunity. In developing tropical countries, the serologic response to OPV may be only 85%. This may be due to breaks in the cold chain, interference with intestinal infection by other enteroviruses, presence of diarrhea that causes excretion of the virus before it can attach to the mucosal cell, and other factors. Schedules may vary; WHO recommends that children receive four doses of OPV before 1 year of age. In endemic countries, a dose should be given at birth or as close to birth as possible. This is called the "birth dose," or "zero dose." The other three doses should be given at least 4 weeks apart and usually at the same time as DPT. For IPV, the current schedule is for four doses of the vaccine (2, 4, 6 to 18 months, and at 4 to 6 years) although the duration of immunity is not known with certainty.

OPV Versus IPV

In countries where polio is no longer endemic or there is little or no threat for reimportation, and cost is not a major consideration, increased use of IPV has been recommended since 1996. This has successfully reduced the risk of vaccine-associated paralytic polio. The overall risk in the United States for OPV vaccine-associated paralytic polio in vaccine recipients was one case per 5.2 million doses distributed. The risk of vaccine-associated paralytic polio in vaccine recipients for first dose was one case per 1.3 million doses. On the other hand, there are a number of advantages that favor OPV over IPV for use in an eradication programs. The rationale to use OPV includes the following: the development of intestinal immunity and ability to reduce intestinal spread of wild virus, duration of immunity, ease of administration in both routine and mass campaigns, and cost. Probably, the most critical issue relates to the effect of the vaccine on wild poliovirus transmission. It has been well documented that the use of OPV can successfully interrupt wild poliovirus transmission in both developed and developing countries. IPV protects against clinical disease and suppresses pharyngeal excretion of the virus but has little effect on intestinal excretion. Vaccinating children with IPV would reduce the number of paralytic cases due to the vaccine but, comparatively, would have little effect on the transmission of the wild poliovirus, which in developing countries is primarily by the fecal-oral route.

Vaccination Strategies

High immunization coverage is a key factor in the success of maintaining a polio-free environment or for eradication. Vaccination coverage of 90% or higher at 1 year of age with three or more doses of OPV or IPV must be maintained, not only at the national level but also at local levels. Immunization activities at the local level should be evaluated as to (1) the availability of routine immunizations, including the reduction of missed opportunities (e.g., false contraindications are one of the major causes of missed opportunities), (2) the extent of infant and preschool immunization programs, and (3) the availability of vaccination coverage data. If vaccination coverage is low, it is necessary to improve routine and outreach immunization activities and to determine whether mass immunization campaigns are needed to substantially raise low levels of coverage.

Mass Vaccination Campaigns

Conducting vaccination days (a selected time period in which a large number of people are vaccinated en masse) is an integral part of the polio eradication strategy, and without such campaigns polio is unlikely to be eradicated. Widespread vaccination produces extensive dissemination of the vaccine virus that competes with circulation of the wild virus and can abruptly interrupt virus transmission. Such activities are intended to supplement the routine immunization programs and can be held at the local or national levels. During the organization of these vaccination days, special attention needs to be paid to those locations in which coverage is below the national average. This is particularly true in areas with deficient health services. Not all endemic countries can successfully reach all high-risk populations with routine delivery and national vaccination days; therefore, it is necessary to mount special efforts to reach pockets of children in areas of potential wild poliovirus foci or in those areas not being served by existing health resources, a process known as mop-up.

Control and Eradication

Surveillance

Surveillance is the key to controlling and ultimately eliminating any disease threat. For polio, the reporting system must cover key hospitals and clinics with at least one reporting source for each geopolitical unit. A concept of weekly reporting of all AFP cases rather than only poliomyelitis cases is critical to this effort. A concept of negative reporting of AFP (i.e., reporting even when no cases occur) must be integrated in the reporting system. Surveillance systems need to be continually monitored and feedback issued. Immediate response to reports in the surveillance system by trained epidemiologists must occur with every suspected case within 48 hr. Cooperation from the private medical community is essential for all surveillance efforts, and of course the public needs to be informed about reporting AFP.

Environmental Monitoring

In the latter stages of eradication when no cases are being reported, community monitoring may be considered. However, countries planning to start environmental surveillance should consult the WHO regional office at an early stage.

Methods of collection, concentration, and identification of viruses in the environment differ depending on the type of system that is being sampled, as well as the type of virus. Different methods for each of these steps have advantages and disadvantages, although the best chance of finding poliovirus is in stools of the cases and their contacts.

Global Eradication

In 1962, just 1 year after the introduction of Sabin's OPV in most industrialized countries, Cuba began using the oral vaccine in a series of nationwide polio campaigns. The success of these efforts demonstrated that polioviruses could be successfully eliminated from a developing country. In 1985, PAHO, under the leadership of Dr. Ciro de Quadros, launched an initiative to eradicate polio in the Americas by 1990.

On September 7, 1993, PAHO announced that 2 years had elapsed since the occurrence of the last case of poliomyelitis associated with wild poliovirus isolation in the Americas (Peru, August 1991). Although in 2000 and 2001, outbreaks occurred in the Dominican Republic and Haiti, respectively, these outbreaks were caused by a virus derived from the Sabin vaccine (a reversion of the vaccine virus to neurovirulence), and the same strategies that had eliminated polio previously were successful in bringing these outbreaks under control. The overall achievement in the Americas presented a new milestone in efforts to eradicate a disease.

An initiative to eradicate polio globally was launched in 1988. This has become one of the largest public health initiatives in history. In 1988, polio existed in more than 125 countries on five continents, and there were more than 35,251 reported cases of children paralyzed that year. By the end of 2006, there were 1,902 cases reported (provisional), with two countries, India and Nigeria, reporting more than 90% of the cases. The dominant type reported is Type 1 although some cases of Type 3 are still being reported.

Poliomyelitis transmission has been interrupted in the American, European, and Western Pacific Regions, and by end 2002, more than 180 countries and territories were polio free. With the eradication of polio and the eventual cessation of polio immunization, it is estimated that the world will save U.S.$ 1.5 billion (2006) dollars per year. The only other infectious disease eradicated previously was smallpox, the last case of which was reported during August 1977 in Somalia, and now it is hoped that polio will soon join this short list.

—Marc Strassburg

Acknowledgment: The author worked as a consultant for the PAHO polio eradication program, and in that capacity he assisted in writing a number of earlier versions of the polio eradication field guide. Sections from both previous and current field guides were adapted for this entry.

See also Disease Eradication; Pan American Health Organization; Public Health Surveillance; Vaccination

Further Readings

Andrus, J. A., de Quadros, C. A., Olivé J.-M., & Hull, H. F. (1992). Screening of cases of acute flaccid paralysis for poliomyelitis eradication: Ways to improve specificity. Bulletin of the World Health Organization, 70(5), 591–596.

Cáceres, V. M., & Sutter, R. W. (2001). Sabin monovalent oral polio vaccines: Review of past experiences and their potential use after polio eradication. Clinical Infectious Diseases, 33, 531–541.

Centers for Disease Control and Prevention. (2005). Poliomyelitis. In W. Atkinson, J. Hamborsky, L. McIntyre, & S. Wolfe (Eds.), Epidemiology and prevention of vaccine-preventable diseases (8th ed., pp. 89–100). Washington, DC: Public Health Foundation.

Cherry, J. D. (2004). Enteroviruses and parechoviruses. In R. D. Feigin, J. Cherry, G. J. Demmler, & S. Kaplan (Eds.), *Textbook of pediatric infectious diseases* (5th ed., pp. 1984–2041). Philadelphia: W. B. Saunders.

Halsey, N. A., & de Quadros, C. A. (Eds.). (1983). *Recent advances in immunization: A bibliographic review.* Scientific and Technical Publication No. 451. Washington, DC: Pan American Health Organization.

Heymann, D. (Ed.). (2004). *Control of communicable diseases in man* (18th ed.). Washington, DC: American Public Health Association.

Kew, O. M., Sutter, R. W., de Gourville, E. M., Dowdle, W. R., & Pallansch, M. A. (2005). Vaccine-derived polioviruses and the endgame strategy for global polio eradication. *Annual Review of Microbiology, 59,* 587–635.

Pan American Health Organization. (2006). *Poliomyelitis eradication field guide* (3rd ed.). Washington, DC: Author.

de Quadros, C. A., Andrus, J. A., Olivé, J.-M., Da Silveira, C. M., Eikhof, R. M., Carrasco, P., et al. (1991). Eradication of poliomyelitis: Progress in the Americas. *Pediatric Infectious Disease Journal, 10,* 222–229.

de Quadros, C. A., Andrus, J. A., Olivé, J.-M., de Macedo, C. G., Henderson, D. A. (1992). Polio eradication from the Western hemisphere. *Annual Review of Public Health, 12,* 239–252.

World Health Organization, Department of Vaccines and Biologicals. (2003). *Guidelines for environmental surveillance of poliovirus circulation.* Geneva, Switzerland: Author. Retrieved July 24, 2007, from http://www.who.int/vaccines-document.

POLLUTION

Pollution can be defined as the presence of a substance or agent in the environment that is potentially harmful to health, safety, or comfort. In addition to affecting the health of humans or the ecosystem, pollution may have adverse effects on agricultural products or infrastructure such as buildings or monuments. Pollutants include naturally occurring and industrial chemicals, biological pathogens, and forms of energy such as noise.

The primary significance of pollution to epidemiology lies in its relation to human health. In some cases, this has been well studied, but for thousands of chemicals, it has not. The potential for a pollutant to cause adverse health outcomes is related not only to its toxicity but also on the extent of exposure. Briggs (2003) has estimated that 8% to 9% of the total global burden of disease is attributable to environmental or occupational pollution. Children and people in developing countries are disproportionately affected, and the most important routes of exposure are water and indoor air. Although this is only one estimate, it serves to underscore the impact of pollution on human health. This entry describes characteristics, sources and health effects of key pollutants, focusing on those affecting air and water.

Air Pollution

Human use of fire was perhaps the first anthropogenic source of air pollution, but it was the beginning of industrialization that really initiated a rapid escalation of the phenomenon. Several early-20th-century events brought with them recognition that circumstances of extreme air pollution could be threatening to health and even deadly. In 1930, in the Meuse River valley of Belgium, an atmospheric inversion during a period of cold, damp weather trapped pollutants of industrial origin close to the ground, resulting in 60 deaths, mostly among older persons with preexisting heart or lung disease. A similar event occurred in Donora, Pennsylvania, in 1948, and the infamous London smog of 1952 also involved similar meteorological conditions with pollutants created by burning of coal. In this case, thousands of deaths resulted. Following these incidents, efforts were made to reduce air pollution levels in the United States and Western Europe. However, air pollution remains a serious problem for humankind, as health effects of pollutants are discovered at even lower concentrations, formerly less developed nations undergo rapid industrialization, and greenhouse gas concentrations increase on an unprecedented scale.

Ambient Air Pollutants

Pollutants are released to the ambient air from an array of stationary or point sources (e.g., power plants, industrial sites), area sources (e.g., forest fires), and mobile sources (e.g., motor vehicles, boats, lawn mowers). Indoor sources are discussed separately below. Human exposure generally involves complex mixtures rather than individual pollutants.

The U.S. Environmental Protection Agency (EPA) is required by the Clean Air Act to set national ambient air quality standards for the protection of public health and welfare. The six major pollutants for which these standards are set, known as "criteria" pollutants, are carbon monoxide (CO), sulfur dioxide

(SO_2), nitrogen dioxide (NO_2), ozone, airborne particulates, and lead.

• *CO* is formed by incomplete combustion of carbon-based fuels such as gasoline or natural gas. The primary outdoor source is motor vehicles, while indoor sources include gas appliances and environmental tobacco smoke. CO has a high affinity for hemoglobin and interferes with oxygen transport. It causes acute poisoning at high levels; for typical environmental levels, associations with cardiovascular endpoints have been observed.

• *SO_2* is formed by the combustion of fossil fuels containing sulfur (primarily coal). Levels were very high in urban areas of the United States and Europe in the early to mid-20th century and have declined since the 1970s. However, high levels are now observed in other regions such as China, where coal use is currently high. SO_2 is associated with decreased lung function and respiratory symptoms, especially in asthmatics, and contributes to the formation of acid rain.

• Primary sources of *NO_2* include motor vehicle and power plant emissions and burning of fossil fuels. Local levels vary with the density of traffic. NO_2 is associated with lung irritation and lowered resistance to respiratory infection. In the presence of sunlight, NO_2 contributes to the formation of ozone.

• *Ozone* is a secondary pollutant formed by solar radiation and other pollutants such as nitrogen oxides and volatile organic chemicals (VOCs) from sources such as gasoline vapors, solvents, and consumer products. Due to the role of solar radiation in its formation, ozone levels are higher in summertime and in sunnier areas. Concentrations are higher downwind of urban centers than in cities themselves because of the time needed for these photochemical reactions to occur. Ozone in our ground-level air is considered a pollutant that contributes to formation of urban smog and is associated with reduced lung function and sensitization to other irritants; however, depletion of stratospheric ozone is associated with global warming and decreased protection from UV exposure.

• *Particulate matter* (PM) is a heterogeneous mixture of small particles and liquid droplets. Components include acids, organic chemicals, metals, soil, and dust particles from sources, including fuel combustion, high temperature industrial processes, atmospheric reactions of other pollutants, and mechanical processes such as demolition or road wear. PM is classified according to the diameter of the particles, which affects how far they can penetrate into the respiratory system: coarse PM (PM10) is <10 μm, fine (PM2.5) is <2.5 μm, and ultrafine particles are <0.1 μm. Respiratory and cardiovascular outcomes and visibility impairment have been associated with PM.

• *Lead* is a naturally occurring metal. For much of the last century, motor vehicles were the principal source of lead in air, and ambient concentrations have decreased markedly in the United States since the phase-out of lead from gasoline. Current sources for lead pollution in air include metal processing and waste incinerators. Lead exposure can have adverse effects on many of the body's organs and systems. It is considered of particular concern for infants and young children as one of the primary targets is the nervous system and exposure can lead to impaired neurodevelopment and reduced IQ.

Numerous air pollutants in addition to these six are known or suspected to pose health threats. The Clean Air Act amendments of 1990 designated 188 of these as "hazardous air pollutants." Chemicals in this category have been associated with cancer or other adverse health effects, including neurological, reproductive, developmental, immune, and respiratory outcomes. Examples include benzene, formaldehyde, perchloroethylene (used in dry cleaning), polycyclic organic matter (produced as combustion byproducts), and compounds of metals such as mercury and cadmium. The World Health Organization (WHO) and European Union (EU) also set air quality guidelines.

Indoor Air Pollutants

Because many people spend a large portion of time indoors, indoor air pollution may be as important as that of outdoor air in determining potential exposures. The quality of indoor air is influenced by that of the ambient outdoor air, but there are additional concerns arising from the built environment or indoor activities.

According to the WHO, more than half of the world's population uses solid biomass fuels (i.e., dung, wood, crop waste) or coal for cooking and heating. Burning these materials in open fires or simple, nonvented stoves produces indoor smoke, with specific components, including CO, particulate matter, and VOCs. Depending on the composition of coal, its combustion can also produce SO_2 and toxins such as fluorine and arsenic. Exposure to smoke from these solid fuels is a risk factor for pneumonia and other lower respiratory infections, especially in young children, chronic obstructive pulmonary disease (COPD), and lung cancer. It may also be associated with other adverse outcomes, including cataracts, tuberculosis, asthma, and low birth weight.

Modern buildings raise air quality concerns related to building, furnishing, and consumer products contained within. They are often composed of synthetic materials and contained within airtight structures. Asbestos insulation and lead-based paints are instances in which products that were once widely used were subsequently recognized as posing serious threats to health. Other chemicals have been associated with sensory irritation, nervous system symptoms, and cancer. Common concerns include formaldehyde occurring in pressed-wood building materials, organic chemicals in paints or cleaning products, and pesticides. Microorganisms and allergens arising from sources, including humidifiers, air-cooling equipment, household pets, insects, and mold have been associated with allergies, asthma, and infections such as Legionnaires' disease. The phenomenon of *sick building syndrome*, a term used to describe various types of medically unexplained symptoms reported by people living or working in the same building, has drawn attention to possible health effects of indoor air exposures.

Environmental tobacco smoke (ETS), like smoking itself, is a concern worldwide. ETS consists of exhaled smoke plus secondary smoke produced by burning tobacco, and it is associated with lower respiratory infections, asthma, lung cancer, and adverse perinatal outcomes.

Radon is a naturally occurring, odorless, and colorless gas formed during the decay of uranium in the earth's crust. Higher levels tend to occur in homes on sandy or gravelly soil. Radon and its decay products result in radiation exposure in persons who breathe the affected air. The primary concern related to radon exposure is lung cancer; this association has been demonstrated in uranium miners. Because of a synergistic effect, risks are greater for smokers than for nonsmokers.

Water Pollution

The importance of clean drinking water for human life has been accepted for thousands of years. However, direct consumption accounts for only a minute fraction of human water use. Other uses include cooking, bathing, washing laundry, personal and industrial waste disposal, recreation, and irrigation. While some of these activities provide additional occasions for human exposure to pollutants in water, they may also be mechanisms of water contamination in and of themselves. Recognition of the idea that water can transmit disease is typically attributed to John Snow, who mapped cholera cases and traced them to a common water source during an 1854 cholera outbreak in London.

Sources of Water Pollution

There are numerous ways in which pollutants can enter water supplies. Point sources are those such as industrial or sewage treatment facilities, where discharges occur at an explicit location and are more easily identified and controlled than nonpoint or diffuse sources. These include agricultural and urban runoff. Deliberate discharges of pollutants may occur legally or illegally, and other sources include leakage or spills, seepage from landfills, and atmospheric deposition. Naturally occurring contaminants, such as arsenic, can leach into groundwater from geological formations. Water distribution systems are another source where water may pick up contaminants—for example, iron, lead, or copper due to leaching or corrosion from pipes. Finally, disinfectants added to water to treat microbial contamination may react with organic matter to form halogenated chemicals known as disinfection by-products.

Health Effects of Water Pollutants

In developing countries, many cities lack infrastructure for waste treatment and discharge the majority of sewage directly into water sources such as rivers and streams. Hence, in many areas of the world, human feces is the most important contaminant, and waterborne diseases (such as diarrheal illness, cholera, typhoid, and amebic dysentery) are the greatest human health risks associated with water contamination. Waterborne disease outbreaks still occur in developed countries as well. For example, a 1993 cryptosporidium outbreak in Milwaukee, Wisconsin, caused more than 400,000 cases of illness.

Contamination from naturally occurring substances such as arsenic and fluoride can be a concern in both developed and developing countries, although they are associated with greater morbidity for the latter, where water testing and treatment facilities are often not in place. Arsenic exposure is associated with skin, lung, and bladder cancer; keratosis; and peripheral vascular damage and is particularly prevalent in Bangladesh. Areas with high levels of fluoride in drinking water include India, Africa, China; this can cause fluorosis, which involves dental discoloration, decay, and skeletal deformity.

Chemical contaminants of water supplies include agricultural products such as nitrates, pesticides, and fertilizers; chemicals from urban or industrial sources, especially heavy metals and solvents; pharmaceuticals or their breakdown products; and disinfection by-products such as trihalomethanes. Some of these pollutants are volatile so that exposure may occur via absorption through the skin or inhalation, for example, during showering. Epidemiological studies on possible health effects of these contaminants have tended to focus on cancer and reproductive/developmental effects such as miscarriage or low birth weight; however, the overall evidence for association is generally inconclusive.

Other Types of Pollution

Pollution affecting air and water are highlighted here as two categories of major import for the health of populations worldwide. However, there are other media affected by pollution and other possible ways of classifying pollutants. Some of these are mentioned below.

Food in its various manifestations is at once life sustaining and a potential source of exposure to a variety of pollutants. Plant products are vulnerable to sources, including pesticides that are applied intentionally, deposition from traffic or industry, sludge application, and waste disposal or spills. Pollutants may directly deposit on plants, as in a sprayed pesticide, or be taken up from soil in which they are contained. For example, cadmium concentrates in leafy vegetables. Contaminated soil itself may be a source of exposure by ingestion, especially for young children playing near the ground with abundant hand-to-mouth behavior. Animals can also ingest contaminated soil, water, plants, or feed, and then become a source of exposure for humans who consume their milk, eggs, or meat. Bioaccumulation is a process whereby concentration of a chemical within organs or tissues of an organism exposed to it increases over the

concentration of the chemical in the surrounding environment. This can lead to increasing concentrations up the food chain, the potentially detrimental consequences of which were illustrated in Minamata Bay, Japan, in the 1950s. Wastes containing mercury were discharged by a chemical company and concentrated in fish and shellfish living in the contaminated waters. People who then ate large quantities of fish caught from the bay were affected by methyl mercury poisoning, resulting in neurological impairment and in some cases, death. A congenital form affecting infants exposed in utero showed cerebral-palsy-like symptoms.

Persistent organic pollutants (POPs) are chemicals that persist in the environment, accumulate in fat tissue of animals, circulate globally achieving a wide geographic distribution, and have health effects on humans and animals, most notably disruption of endocrine systems and reproduction. POPs include DDT and other pesticides, polychlorinated biphenyls (PCBs), dioxins, and furans. Of relatively recent concern are the polybrominated diphenyl ethers (PBDE), which are used as flame retardants. POPs may be present in the food supply, air, and water; infants can also be exposed through breast milk.

Greenhouse gases are gases, especially carbon dioxide, methane, and nitrous oxide that trap and retain heat from the sun. The primary anthropogenic source is carbon dioxide from the burning of fossil fuels. Evidence indicates that rising atmospheric levels of these gases are contributing to an observed increase in global temperatures over the last century. Global warming and associated climate change may eventually have a variety of effects with direct impact on human health, including illness or injury from extreme weather events, changes in geographic distribution of disease vector organisms, impaired crop or livestock production, and displacement of populations.

Physical agents may also be considered as pollutants. For example, noise pollution can be described simply as unwanted noise, coming from sources such as airports and traffic. Radiation and heat are other examples that fall into this category.

—Keely Cheslack-Postava

See also Environmental and Occupational Epidemiology; Harvard Six Cities Study; Lead; Love Canal; Mercury; Sick Building Syndrome; Urban Health Issues; Waterborne Diseases

Further Readings

Briggs, D. (2003). Environmental pollution and the global burden of disease. *British Medical Bulletin, 68*, 1–24.

Gordon, B., Mackay, R., & Rehfuess, E. (2004). *Inheriting the world: The atlas of children's health and the environment.* Geneva, Switzerland: World Health Organization. Also available online at http://www.who.int/ceh/publications/atlas/en.

Moeller, D. W. (2005). *Environmental health* (3rd. ed.). Cambridge, MA: Harvard University Press.

Patz, J. A., & Balbus, J. M. (2001). Global climate change and air pollution. In J. L. Aron & J. A. Patz (Eds.), *Ecosystem change and public health: A global perspective* (pp. 379–408). Baltimore: Johns Hopkins University Press.

Tibbetts, J. (2000). Water world 2000. *Environmental Health Perspectives, 108*, A69–A73.

World Health Organization. (2005). *Indoor air pollution and health* (Fact sheet no. 292). Retrieved December 20, 2006, from http://www.who.int/mediacentre/factsheets/fs292/en/print.html.

Web Sites

U.S. Environmental Protection Agency. Office of Air and Radiation: http://www.epa.gov/air.

POPULATION PYRAMID

The population pyramid is a graphical representation of the age and gender composition of a specific population. The shape of the graph depends on the age and gender structure of the population. The representation may take the form of a pyramid, but it may have a columnar shape, with vertical sides rather than sloped sides, or it may have an irregular profile.

Population pyramids provide a summary view of the overall age-gender structure of a specific population. The size of the population is depicted on the horizontal axis, and age is aligned on the vertical axis. The depiction actually contains two graphs, in mirror image format, on either side of a central vertical axis; the female population is represented on the right side of the axis, and the male population is shown on the left side.

The population pyramid is made up of bars stacked on top of one another, each representing an age category, typically in 5-year age groups, with the youngest age group represented by the bottom bar, and the oldest age group by the uppermost bar. The length of each bar, on either side of the central vertical axis,

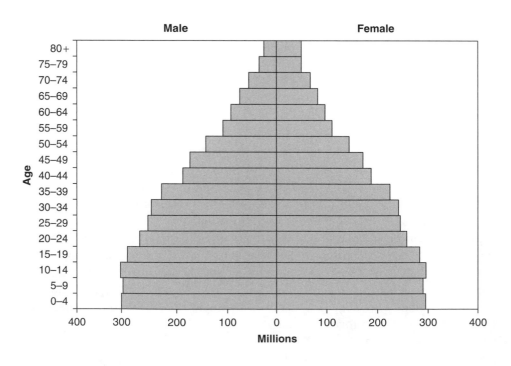

Figure 1   Age-Sex Structure of Global Population: 2002

Source: U.S. Census Bureau (2004a).

represents the number of males (left side) and females (right side) in the specific age group, in the population depicted. The age groups are displayed along the central axis or along one side, and often the years of birth for each age category are also displayed on the graph. To maintain proportionality, the age groups are all of the same size (typically in 1-year, 5-year, or 10-year age groups), and the bars are all of equal height. However, the age axis is often truncated at the age group 80 to 84, depending on the data available for the population depicted. For some populations, the data for the older age groups are incomplete or inaccurate, or there are few people in the older age categories.

The population pyramid can depict the proportion of the total population in each age-gender group rather than the actual count. In this case, for example, the length of the bar for females in the 5- to 9-year-old group would represent the proportion that group consists of within the total population. When calculating the proportions, the denominator used is always the number in the entire population, and the numerator is the number in the specific age-gender group. The sum of all the groups represented by the bars should add up to 100% of the population depicted.

When comparing population pyramids, it is important to note whether proportions or counts are represented and whether the scale of the bars and the age categories are the same. Population pyramids intended for comparison should be drawn to the same scale, and should depict the same age categories. The population pyramid can be used to represent additional characteristics of the population, such as marital status, race, or geographic location. In this case, the bar for each age-gender group is further subdivided and formatted to represent the additional categories. The formatting system used to depict the additional categories should be applied consistently throughout the graph. The same sequence should be used on either side of the vertical axis, in mirror image form. For example, if race is depicted, and the categories are white, black, and other, the categories would be arranged in the same sequence for males and for females, working outward from each side of the central axis.

The shape of the population pyramid efficiently communicates considerable information about the age-gender structure of a specific population. A broad-based pyramid indicates people in the younger age categories make up a relatively large proportion of the population, and a narrow or pointed top indicates older people make up a relatively small proportion of the population. In the older age groups in many populations, the number of females is much greater than the number of males, and this is reflected in the shape of the pyramid; the bars on the right side of the central axis (the female side) are longer than those on the left (male) side. The median age of the population would be the age group (bar) represented by the point on the vertical axis that equally divides the area within the pyramid, that is, about equal areas within the pyramid fall above and below the age represented by this bar. The fertility and mortality of the population are also reflected in the shape of the population pyramid. A broad base and sharply tapering sides (a true pyramid shape) reflects a high fertility rate and high mortality rates in younger age groups. Irregularities in the profile of the population pyramid convey information about changes in the population or aberrations. A bulge or an indentation in the profile of the population pyramid may indicate unusually high fertility or mortality, or changes in the population due to in-migration or out-migration. For example, the bulge in the age groups of 35 to 54 years in the pyramid representing the 2000 U.S. population reflects a period of high fertility, the post–World War II baby boom (Figure 2).

Demographers who have studied the historical changes in the age and gender composition, fertility, and mortality of the world's populations have articulated

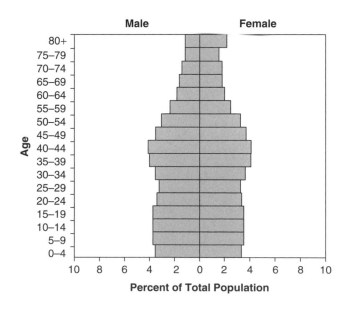

Figure 2   Bulge in a Population Pyramid Due to a Baby Boom (United States, 2000)

Source: U.S. Census Bureau (2004a).

Population at Stage 1 of the Demographic Transition

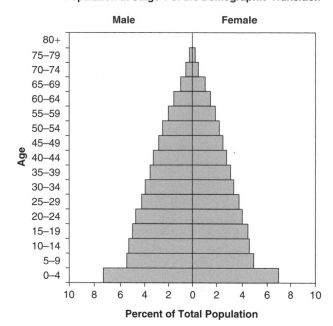

Population in Stage 2 of the Demographic Transition

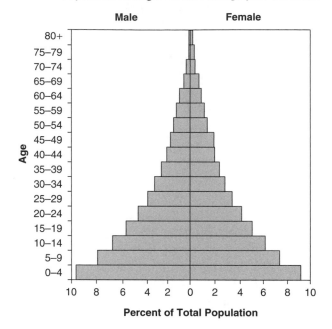

Population at the End of Stage 3 of the Demographic Transition

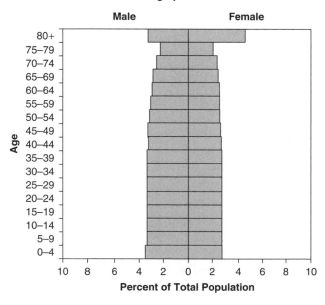

Figure 3   Stages in the Demographic Transition

Source: U.S. Census Bureau (2004a).

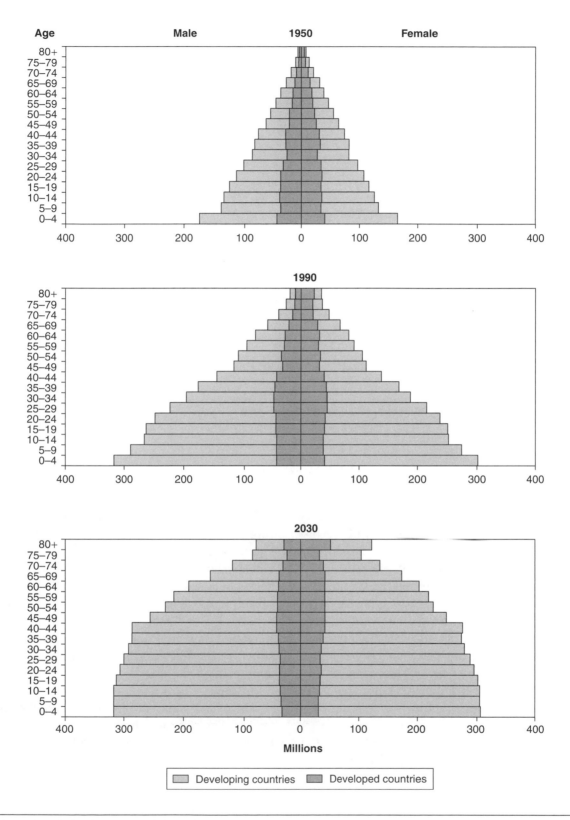

Figure 4   Population by Age and Sex: 1950, 1990, and 2030

Source: Kinsella and Velkoff (2001).

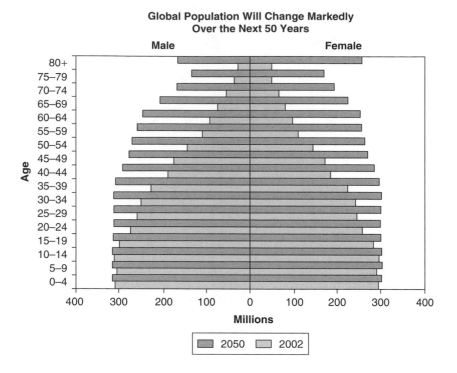

Global Population Will Change Markedly Over the Next 50 Years

Figure 5   Age-Sex Structure of World Population: 2002 and 2050

Source: U.S. Census Bureau (2004b)

a theory of "demographic transition." This theory seems to provide a useful approximation of the historical changes that have taken place in the populations in many different regions of the world. The stages of this transition are represented by dramatically different population pyramids (Figure 3).

Stage 1 is represented by a tapering pyramid sitting on a broad base, reflecting high fertility, but also a high mortality rate among the younger age groups, so the population increases slowly, and remains relatively small. The shape of the population pyramid for Stage 2 of the demographic transition reflects lower mortality, especially among the youngest age groups, coupled with high fertility; the population increases rapidly but remains relatively young. The population pyramid that represents Stage 3 in the demographic transition is roughly rectangular, reflecting lower fertility, lower childhood mortality, and longer survival; the older age categories make up a larger proportion of the population than in earlier stages, and the size of the population stabilizes.

The world's population does appear to be progressing through the stages of the demographic transition. Figure 4 shows changes in the age structure of the global population over time and shows the contrast between developed countries and developing countries. It is apparent from this figure that the developed countries are further ahead in the demographic transition than are the developing countries, but the structure of the world's population as a whole is approaching the third stage of the demographic transition.

The overall aging of the world's population can be seen in Figure 5, which shows the dramatic changes that are expected to occur by 2050.

The variety in the age and gender structure of the population in different regions of the world is graphically depicted in Figure 6, which superimposes regional population pyramids on the global population pyramid.

—Judith Marie Bezy

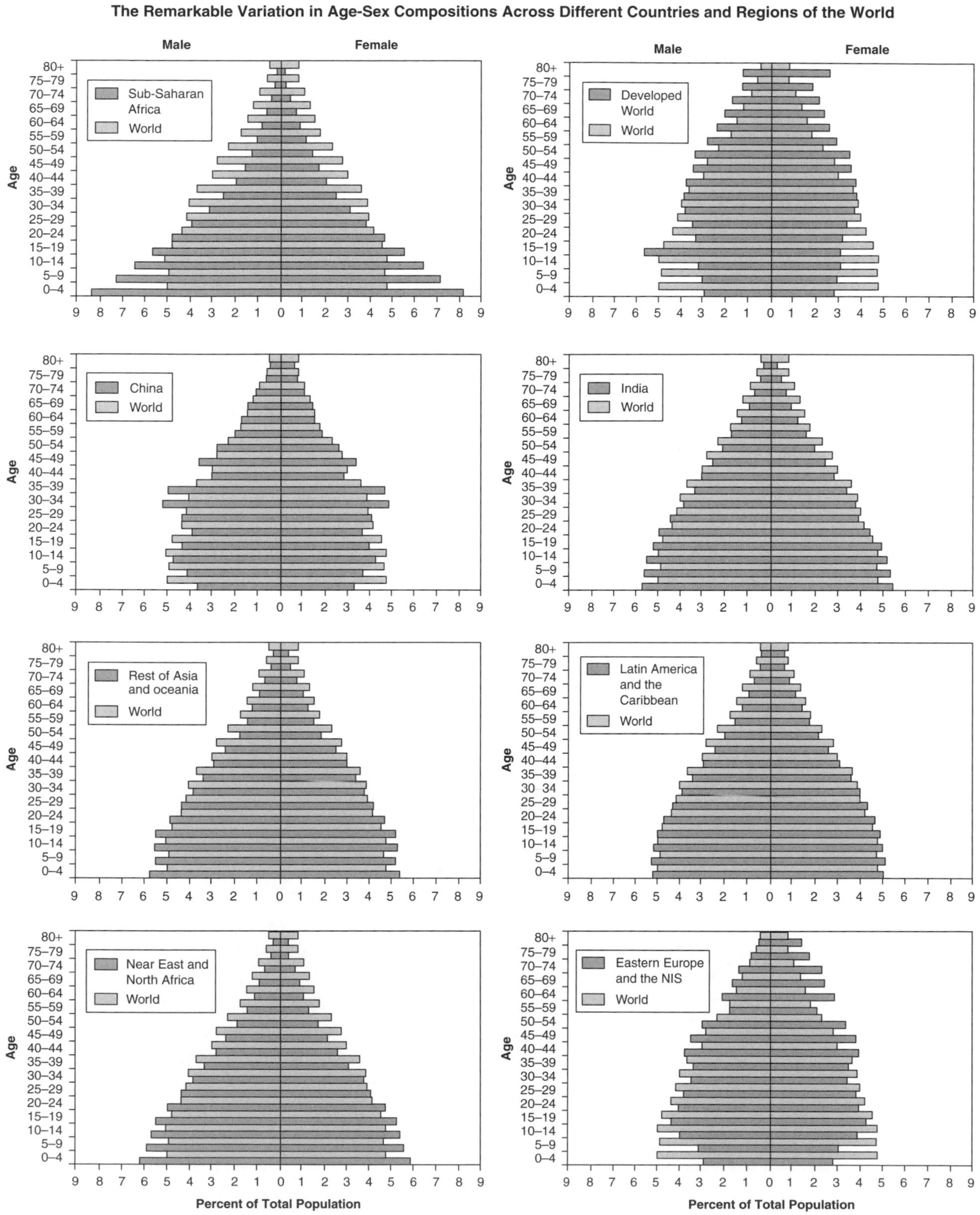

The Remarkable Variation in Age-Sex Compositions Across Different Countries and Regions of the World

Figure 6   Population Pyramids by Region and Selected Countries: 2002

Source: U.S. Census Bureau (2004a).

See also Demography; Graphical Presentation of Data; Proportion

Further Readings

Kinsella, K., & Velkoff, V. A. (2001). *An aging world: 2001* (U.S. Census Bureau, Series P95/01-1). Washington, DC: Government Printing Office.

Siegel, J. S., & Swanson, D. A. (Eds.). (2004). *The methods and materials of demography* (2nd ed.). San Diego, CA: Elsevier Academic Press.

U.S. Census Bureau. (2004a). *Global population profile: 2002* (International Population Reports, WP/02). Washington, DC: Government Printing Office.

U.S. Census Bureau. (2004b). *Global population at a glance: 2002 and beyond* (International Brief, WP/02-1).Washington, DC: Government Printing Office.

POSITIVE PREDICTIVE VALUE

See CLINICAL EPIDEMIOLOGY

POST-TRAUMATIC STRESS DISORDER

Post-traumatic stress disorder (PTSD) was adopted by the American Psychiatric Association (APA) as part of the official classification of psychiatric disorders in the third edition of the *Diagnostic and Statistical Manual of Mental Disorder* (*DSM-III*), published in 1980. The adoption of PTSD in *DSM-III* was motivated by pressures from advocates on behalf of Vietnam War veterans. The definition of PTSD in the *DSM-III* and subsequent *DSM* editions, *DSM-III-R* and *DSM-IV*, is based on the concept that traumatic events, in contrast with other stressful events, are linked etiologically to a specific syndrome. The PTSD syndrome is defined by three symptom groups: (1) reexperiencing the traumatic event, (2) avoidance of stimuli that resemble the event and numbing of emotional responsiveness, and (3) increased arousal. These features are defined in terms of their connection with the traumatic event that caused them. Temporal ordering is also required: These disturbances must not have been present before the trauma occurred.

Since 1980, research on PTSD has focused chiefly on Vietnam War veterans and to a lesser degree on victims of specific types of traumas, such as natural disasters or rape. With the growth of the field of psychiatric epidemiology, PTSD has been studied in samples of the general population in the United States and other countries. From the time of its introduction into the official psychiatric nosology, PTSD has been a controversial diagnosis. Some critics question its validity as a distinct disorder. Others contest the trend toward a broader, more inclusive definition of what constitutes a traumatic event. Concerns have been expressed about the proliferation of PTSD-related disturbances other than *DSM-IV* PTSD (e.g., subthreshold PTSD) and about potential distortion in recalling traumatic experiences, especially when the diagnosis of PTSD entitles victims to compensation. Despite extensive efforts, neurobiological research has not yielded laboratory tests that can be used diagnostically.

Exposure to *DSM-IV* Traumatic Events and PTSD

In the latest edition of the *DSM*, the *DSM-IV* (APA, 1994), the definition of traumatic events that can potentially cause PTSD has been enlarged to include a wider range of stressors than the typical stressors of the initial definition (combat, concentration camp confinement, natural disaster, rape, or assault). The stressor definition in *DSM-IV* requires that "the person experienced, witnessed or was confronted with an event(s) that involved actual or threatened death or serious injury or a threat to the physical integrity of self and others," and which evoked "intense fear, helplessness, or horror." Thus, learning that someone else was threatened with harm qualifies as a traumatic event. The defining features of the PTSD syndrome have remained unchanged, although the specific configuration of symptoms was revised somewhat. *DSM-IV* introduced a new condition—that the disturbance causes clinically significant distress or impairment— in recognition that distress in itself or in commonly experienced symptoms, such as sleep problems, is not equivalent to a mental disorder. Survey data from the United States, where results based on earlier definitions are available for comparison, show that the broader definition of stressors has resulted in a considerably higher proportion of the population having experienced traumatic events that qualify for PTSD. However, prevalence estimates of *DSM-IV* PTSD have not increased. In the United States, the vast majority of the population (approximately 80%) has experienced one or more traumatic events. A similarly high figure has been reported in a Canadian study. Much lower figures have been reported in surveys in Germany and Switzerland (from 20% to 28%).

Although most of the U.S. population has been exposed to one or more traumatic events, only a minority of victims has succumbed to PTSD (< 10%). The lifetime cumulative incidence of *DSM-IV* PTSD in a national sample of the U.S. population, circa 2000, was 6.8%. Table 1 presents published estimates of lifetime cumulative incidence and 12-month prevalence of PTSD from surveys in the United States, Canada, Germany, the Netherlands, Switzerland,

Lebanon, and Australia. Both lifetime and 12-month estimates are higher in the United States than in other countries.

A consistent finding across epidemiologic studies is the higher PTSD prevalence in women compared with men. Although men are more likely to experience trauma, the likelihood of developing PTSD following exposure to traumatic events is higher in women. Rape and sexual assault occur more frequently in women, and victims of either sex are more likely to succumb to PTSD than victims of other traumatic events. However, the sex difference in PTSD is not accounted for by women's greater risk of experiencing rape and sexual assault.

Table 1   Cumulative Incidence in Lifetime and 12-Months Prevalence of *DSM-IV* Post-Traumatic Stress Disorder (PTSD)

Study	Sample	Interview	Total Lifetime	Total 12-Months
Breslau et al. (1998)	Detroit PMSA, United States Age 18–45 ($n = 2,181$)	WHO-CIDI (telephone interview)	12.2% (8.3%)	—
Breslau, Wilcox, Storr, Lucia, and Anthony (2004)	Mid-Atlantic City, United States Age 19–22 ($n = 1,698$)	WHO-CIDI (personal interview)	7.1%	—
Kessler et al. (2005a, 2005b)	U.S. national Age ≥ 18 ($n = 9,282$)	WMH-CIDI (personal interview)	6.8%	3.5%
Stein, Walker, Hazen, and Forde (1997)	Winnipeg, Canada Age >18 ($n = 1,002$)	PTSD Symptom Scale (telephone interview)	—	2.0%
Hapke et al. (2005)	Luebeck, Germany Age 18–64 ($n = 4,075$)	M-CIDI	1.4%	—
Perkonigg, Kessler, Storz, and Wittchen (2000)	Munich, Germany Age 14–24 ($n = 3021$)	WHO-CIDI (personal interview)	1.3%	0.7%
Van Zelst, de Beurs, Beekman, Deeq, and van Dyck (2003)	The Netherlands Age 55–85 ($n = 422$)	WHO-CIDI (personal interview)	—	0.9%
Hepp et al. (2006)	Zurich, Switzerland Age 34–35 and 40–41	Zurich Cohort Study (personal interview)	—	0.0%
Karam et al. (2006)	Lebanon national Age ≥ 18 ($n = 308$)	WHO-CIDI (personal interviews)	—	2.0%
Creamer, Burgess, and McFarlane (2001)	Australian national Age 18 ($n = 10,641$)	WHO-CIDI modified (personal interview)	—	1.3%

Sources: Breslau et al. (1998), Breslau, Wilcox, Storr, Lucia, and Anthony (2004), Creamer, Burgess, and McFarlane (2001), Hapke et al. (2005), Hepp et al. (2006), Karam et al. (2006), Kessler et al. (2005a, 2005b), Perkonigg, Kessler, Storz, and Wittchen (2000), Stein, Walker, Hazen, and Forde (1997), and Van Zelst, de Beurs, Beekman, Deeq, and van Dyck (2003).

Note: Dash represents not published. CIDI, Composite International Diagnostic Interview; WMH, World Mental Health; *DSM-IV*, *Diagnostic and Statistical Manual of Mental Disorders*, 4th edition (1994).

Suspected Risk Factors, Course, and Co-Occurring Disorders

Because traumatic events cause PTSD in only a small fraction of victims, researchers have sought to identify risk factors that predict who succumbs to the disorder among those who have experienced trauma. Suspected risk factors include personality traits (neuroticisms), preexisting psychiatric disorders, family history of psychiatric disorders, and prior exposure to traumatic events. High intelligence (more than 1 *SD* above the population mean) has been found to protect individuals against PTSD effects after exposure to traumatic events. PTSD is more likely to occur following events involving assaultive violence than other types of traumatic events, such as natural disasters or severe accidents. Recently, there has been a growing interest in the relationship between PTSD and terrorist attacks on civilian populations. Surveys following the September 11, 2001, terrorist attacks on the World Trade Center indicate that, with the exception of persons directly involved, any increase in the prevalence of PTSD among New York City residents was transient.

The onset of PTSD symptoms among victims with the disorder occurs within days of the traumatic experience. Cross-sectional surveys of the general population shows recovery over time, although the disorder is generally chronic, lasting longer than 6 months in the majority of cases. Victims who develop PTSD are at an increased risk for the first occurrence of other psychiatric disorders, chiefly major depression, anxiety disorders, drug use disorders, and nicotine dependence. Trauma victims who do not succumb to PTSD (i.e., most victims) are not at a markedly increased risk for subsequent onset of other psychiatric disorders, compared with community residents who have not experienced traumatic events.

Treatment

Both psychological and pharmacological approaches have been developed for patients with PTSD. Of the psychological treatments, specialized versions of cognitive behavior therapies (CBT) that help patients confront fear and avoidance in a structured format have been found in randomized clinical trials to be efficacious in improving PTSD symptoms. With respect to medication, to date, two serotonin reuptake inhibitors, sertraline and paroxetine, have been approved by the Food and Drug Administration (FDA) for the treatment of PTSD. Debriefing, a popular technique involving immediate post-trauma intervention that encourages victims to recount their experiences, has been found to be ineffective and at times damaging.

—*Naomi Breslau*

See also Psychiatric Epidemiology; Stress; Violence as a Public Health Issue; War

Further Readings

Breslau, N., Kessler, R. C., Chilcoat, H. D., Schultz, L. R., Davis, G. C., & Andreski, P. (1998). Trauma and posttraumatic stress disorder in the community: The 1996 Detroit area survey of trauma. *Archives of General Psychiatry, 55*, 626–632.

Breslau, N., Wilcox, H. C., Storr, C. L., Lucia, V. C., & Anthony, J. C. (2004). Trauma exposure and posttraumatic stress disorder: A study of youths in urban America. *Journal of Urban Health, 81*, 530–544.

Brewin, C. R., Andrews, B., & Valentine, J. D. (2000). Meta-analysis of risk factors for posttraumatic stress disorder in trauma-exposed adults. *Journal of Consulting and Clinical Psychology, 68*, 748–766.

Creamer, M., Burgess, P., & McFarlane, A. C. (2001). Post-traumatic stress disorder: Findings from the Australian National Survey of Mental Health and Well-being. *Psychological Medicine, 31*, 1237–1247.

Foa, E. B., Keane, T. M., Friedman, M. J., & International Society for Traumatic Stress Studies. (2000). *Effective treatments for PTSD: Practice guidelines from the International Society for Traumatic Stress Studies.* New York: Guilford Press.

Hapke, U., Schumann, A., Rumpf, H. J., John, U., Konerding, U., & Meyer, C. (2005). Association of smoking and nicotine dependence with trauma and posttraumatic stress disorder in a general population sample. *Journal of Nervous and Mental Disease, 193*, 843–846.

Hepp, U., Gamma, A., Milos, G., Eich, D., Ajdacic-Gross, V., Rossler, W., et al. (2006). Prevalence of exposure to potentially traumatic events and PTSD: The Zurich Cohort Study. *European Archives of Psychiatry and Clinical Neuroscience, 256*, 151–158.

Karam, E. G., Mneimneh, Z. N., Karam, A. N., Fayyad, J. A., Nasser, S. C., Chatterji, S., et al. (2006). Prevalence and treatment of mental disorders in Lebanon: A national epidemiological survey. *Lancet, 367*, 1000–1006.

Kessler, R. C., Berglund, P., Demler, O., Jin, R., Merikangas, K. R., & Walters, E. E. (2005). Lifetime prevalence and age-of-onset distributions of DSM-IV disorders in the National Comorbidity Survey Replication. *Archives of General Psychiatry, 62*, 593–602.

Kessler, R. C., Chiu, W. T., Demler, O., Merikangas, K. R., & Walters, E. E. (2005). Prevalence, severity, and comorbidity of 12-month DSM-IV disorders in the National Comorbidity Survey Replication. *Archives of General Psychiatry*, *62*, 617–627.

Perkonigg, A., Kessler, R. C., Storz, S., & Wittchen, H. U. (2000). Traumatic events and post-traumatic stress disorder in the community: Prevalence, risk factors and comorbidity. *Acta Psychiatrica Scandinavica*, *101*, 46–59.

Rose, S., Bisson, J., Churchill, R., & Wessely, S. (2002). Psychological debriefing for preventing post traumatic stress disorder (PTSD). *Cochrane Database of Systematic Reviews*, Article No. CD000560.

Stein, M. B., Walker, J. R., Hazen, A. L., & Forde, D. R. (1997). Full and partial posttraumatic stress disorder: Findings from a community survey. *American Journal of Psychiatry*, *154*, 1114–1119.

Van Zelst W. H., de Beurs, E., Beekman, A. T., Deeq, D. J., & van Dyck, R. (2003). Prevalence and risk factors of posttraumatic stress disorder in older adults. *Psychotherapy and Psychosomatics*, *72*(6), 333–342.

POVERTY AND HEALTH

The adverse effects of poverty on health are well documented and continue to be a major public health concern all over the world. Much of the early pioneering work in public health has its roots in the study of the health consequences of poverty. And, although poverty has long been known to cause numerous public health problems, billions of people globally continue to be affected by poverty. This entry examines the extent of poverty, its impact on health, methods for measuring poverty, and strategies for alleviating poverty and addressing the health needs of the poor.

Demographics

The World Bank estimated that in 2001, 2.7 billion people worldwide lived on less than $2 per day and more than a billion subsisted on less than $1 per day. Some regions, such as eastern and southern Asia, have seen reductions in extreme poverty (from a rate of 33% in 1990 to 14% in 2002 in eastern Asia and from 39% in 1990 to 31% in 2002 in southern Asia). Yet the percentage of persons living in extreme poverty has increased in some of the transition economies of southeastern Europe and many of the countries of the former Soviet Union (from 0.4% in both regions in 1990 to 1.8% and 2.5% in 2002, respectively). While Latin America and the Caribbean have seen marginal reductions in poverty rates, more than 47 million people continue to live in poverty in those regions. With more than 300 million people living in extreme poverty, sub-Saharan Africa continues to have the largest regional proportion of extreme poverty in the world.

While poverty is often a great concern for developing nations, poverty continues to affect developed nations as well. In the United States, the Census Bureau reported that in 2005, more than 12% of Americans were living in poverty (37.0 million people). Furthermore, poverty rates in the United States are higher for some racial/ethnic groups than for non-Hispanic whites. Nearly 25% of blacks, 25% of American Indian and Alaska Natives, and nearly 22% of Hispanics lived in poverty in 2005 in the United States, compared with 8.3% of non-Hispanic whites and 10.9% of Asians. Poverty rates vary widely by geographic areas within the country as well. For example, the proportion of persons in poverty for some areas of the United States is in excess of 40%, whereas other areas have poverty rates of less than 5%.

Poverty and Health Outcomes

Poverty has been shown to influence many health outcomes, including all-cause mortality, infectious diseases, chronic diseases, and health behaviors. Millions of people die from poverty-related diseases each year. Many of the diseases associated with poverty are infectious, such as tuberculosis, diarrheal illnesses, and malaria. Lack of appropriate health care, malnourishment, and disease are likely responsible for more than half a million childbirth-related deaths in women each year. However, with increased industrialization and globalization in developing nations, social and behavioral changes that lead to chronic diseases such as diabetes, hypertension, circulatory diseases, respiratory diseases, and cancer are being observed at higher rates. While these diseases affect persons of all socioeconomic strata, socioeconomic gradients in disease incidence, prevalence, treatment, and survival have been shown, most often revealing that poorer individuals have poorer health outcomes. Also, many risk factors for poor health outcomes are poverty-related, such as substandard housing, environmental pollution, and lack of health insurance. While poverty contributes to the development of disease, there is likely a two-way relationship whereby illness also directly influences poverty due to lost wages and productivity, plus prohibitive health care costs for those without health insurance. Furthermore, people living in extreme poverty tend to have more frequent and severe disease complications and make greater demands on the health care system.

Childhood Poverty

Children often disproportionately suffer the effects of poverty. Many children die each year from communicable, maternal, perinatal, or nutritional causes, largely due to the effects of poverty. Countries with high rates of child mortality have been shown to have higher rates of extreme poverty. Diseases such as pneumonia, diarrhea, malaria, measles, and HIV/AIDS have been estimated to account for more than half of global under-5 deaths, much of which is associated with preventable malnutrition. In the United States, the poverty rate for children below 18 years was 17.6%, which is higher than any other age group. Nearly 53% of related children below 6 years living in families with a female householder with no husband present were in poverty, compared with 9.9% of children below 6 living in married-couple families. Moreover, the consequences of childhood poverty have been shown to extend into adulthood and effect health throughout the life course, whereby poor and uninsured children are at greater risk of experiencing health problems such as obesity, heart disease, and asthma.

How Poverty Influences Health

One primary way that poverty influences health is through material deprivation and inability to meet basic human needs. Factors such as low income, lack of education and employment opportunities, poor and/or crowded housing conditions, substandard working conditions, insufficient nutrition, unsafe water and inadequate sanitation, environmental pollution, and limited access to health care all contribute to poor health outcomes. Furthermore, poor countries often have limited or weakened health care systems in the context of inadequate governmental infrastructure, along with shortages in health care workers, to adequately respond to the health needs of the poor.

Additional ways that poverty may influence health is through its influence on social relationships, caring for children, psychological health, and lifestyle factors such as smoking, alcohol, exercise, and diet. Poverty may influence the degree of control that people feel

they have over their lives. Experiencing such economic and psychosocial strains can lead to unhealthy lifestyle behaviors. Moreover, the cumulative effects of poverty experienced over the life course have been observed. Socioeconomic deprivation experienced in early life has been linked to increased risk of chronic conditions such as cardiovascular disease, respiratory disease, and some cancers in adulthood.

Measuring Poverty

There has been considerable debate over the best way to measure poverty. Poverty is most often considered economic deprivation, with income or consumption as the primary components of the measurement. A poverty line is classified as an income level falling below some minimum level necessary to meet basic needs. Poverty can be conceptualized in absolute or relative terms that vary across time and societies. For example, the World Bank's poverty definitions of $1 or $2 per day are absolute definitions that adjust for the country-specific prices needed to "buy" one or two dollar's worth of goods. Conversely, an example of a commonly used relative definition of poverty is the use of a threshold set at 50% of a country's median income. This particular measurement will constrain the poverty rate to 50% and may not be rooted in a meaningful threshold for unmet basic needs. Relative poverty measures vary from country to country making it difficult to compare rates across countries.

It has been argued that conventional poverty calculations inadequately define poverty and that estimates should include additional items such as indicators of well-being, education, health, access to services, infrastructure, social exclusion and social capital taxes, job-related expenses, and the value of noncash benefits.

Measuring Poverty in the United States

The U.S. Census Bureau releases poverty statistics for the U.S. population every fall. These statistics are based on thresholds that represent the annual amount of income required to support families of various sizes. Despite some criticism, these thresholds remain the official benchmarks for defining economic deprivation for children and adults in the Unites States. Census-based poverty statistics are used in a variety of ways in epidemiologic research. With an increased interest in multilevel modeling and capturing the effects of neighborhood poverty, aggregated regional poverty measures within various census-defined geographic boundaries (i.e., county, tract, block group, etc.) have been used to determine how area-level poverty influences health outcomes.

Addressing Poverty and the Health Needs of the Poor

Many strategies have been developed to address the health needs of the poor. Although there are thousands of articles addressing poverty in the health literature, relatively few evidence-based interventions have been targeted to serve the poor. There are several distinct but related approaches to bringing attention to the specific health problems faced by the poor. Some approaches target the alleviation of poverty, some target inequality reduction, and some focus on equity enhancement. While these schools of thought differ in some ways, many have argued for moving beyond the epidemiologic understanding of poverty and health into intervention development and policy making. As such, there has been an increase in intercountry research projects that address poverty and health supported by many entities and with the participation of more than 100 countries. Some specific strategies have included the following: preventative and curative interventions for infectious and nutritional-related diseases in children and adults; improved quality and access to education, particularly among women; improved access to necessary drugs, vaccinations, and health care services; microcredit programs, innovative sustainable health care financing alternatives, social and behavioral interventions; family planning services; prevention and rehabilitation of disability; health education programs; and increased access to clean water and sanitation.

The issues surrounding poverty and health have received global attention. Strategies aimed at reducing extreme poverty and hunger were a focus of the Millennium Development Goals (MDGs) developed during the United Nations Millennium Summit of 2000. In addition to poverty and hunger reduction, the MDGs provide a framework for other poverty-related issues such as increasing education; promoting gender equality; reducing child mortality; improving maternal health; combating HIV/AIDS, tuberculosis, and malaria; ensuring environmental sustainability; and developing a global partnership for development.

—*Amy B. Dailey*

See also Epidemiology in Developing Countries; Health Disparities; Health Economics; Malnutrition, Measurement of; Socioeconomic Classification

Further Readings

Betson, D. M., & Warlick, J. L. (2006). Measuring poverty. In J. M. Oakes & J. S. Kaufman (Eds.), *Methods in social epidemiology* (pp. 112–133). San Francisco: Jossey-Bass.

Chuhan, P. (2006). Poverty and inequality. In V. Bhargava (Ed.), *Global issues for global citizens: An introduction to key development challenges.* Washington, DC: World Bank. Retrieved January 31, 2007, from http://siteresources.worldbank.org/EXTABOUTUS/Resources/Chapter2.pdf.

DeNavas-Walt, C., Proctor, B. D., & Hill, L. C. (2006). *Income, poverty, and health insurance coverage in the United States: 2005* (U.S. Census Bureau, Current Population Reports, P60-231). Washington, DC: Government Printing Office.

Gwatkin, D. R. (2000). Health inequalities and the health of the poor: What do we know? What can we do? *Bulletin of the World Health Organization, 78,* 3–18.

Shaw, M., Dorling, D., & Davey Smith, G. (1999). Poverty, social exclusion, and minorities. In M. Marmot & R. G. Wilkinson (Eds.), *Social determinants of health* (pp. 211–239). New York: Oxford University Press.

United Nations. (2006). *The millennium development goals report.* Retrieved January 31, 2007, from http://unstats.un.org/unsd/mdg/Resources/Static/Products/Progress2006/MDGReport2006.pdf.

Wagstaff, A. (2002). Poverty and health sector inequalities. *Bulletin of the World Health Organization, 80,* 97–105.

PRECLINICAL PHASE OF DISEASE

The preclinical phase of a disease is the period of time during the natural course of a disease where symptoms are not yet apparent, but the disease is biologically present. The concept of a preclinical phase of a disease is most widely referred to in the topic of screening.

Every disease has a natural history that represents the process of the disease in the absence of an intervention. The preclinical phase is one component of this natural history. It begins at the biologic onset of disease and ends when an individual begins experiencing disease-related symptoms. Thus, this phase is when the disease is present but the individual is asymptomatic. When symptoms appear, the preclinical phase ends, and the clinical phase of the disease begins. The length of the preclinical phase varies for different diseases and between individuals and depends on how quickly the disease progresses. For example, the preclinical phase of many cancers may be quite long, sometimes several years. Many neurodegenerative diseases such as Alzheimer's disease and Creutzfeldt-Jakob disease also have a long preclinical phase.

The preclinical phase of disease can be divided into the nondetectable component and the detectable preclinical phase (DPCP). The former represents the phase that is not yet detectable by screening methods, whereas the latter represents the time window when screening methods can detect the presence of asymptomatic disease. Diseases must have a DPCP to be a candidate for screening.

One of the aims of screening is to detect disease at an early stage so that an intervention can be implemented early and prevent future morbidity and mortality. However, for this to be achieved, the disease in question must have a DPCP. Although there are several criteria for screening, this is a key one of several criteria that indicate whether a screening program could be useful in combating a particular disease. For a screening test to be successful, the disease in question should have a relatively long DPCP with a relatively high prevalence in the population. If it does not, the individuals will pass through to the clinical phase of disease so quickly that the presence of disease will already have been detected by the presence of symptoms, and a screening test will no longer be of use. For example, colorectal cancer has a relatively long DPCP and thus is an ideal candidate for screening by colonoscopy. This is in contrast to other more aggressive tumors that have a very short DPCP, and this screening is not as effective.

For screening to be effective, the DPCP must contain a critical point where intervention is more effective if started at this earlier point than after clinical symptoms appear. Without this early critical point of intervention during the DPCP, screening is not of benefit as early intervention will not make a difference in the progression of disease.

—*Kate Bassil*

See also Alzheimer's Disease; Cancer; Screening

Further Readings

Hennekens, C. H., & Buring, J. E. (1987). Screening. In S. L. Mayrent (Ed.), *Epidemiology in medicine* (chap. 13). Boston: Little, Brown.

PREDICTIVE AND ASSOCIATIVE MODELS

See REGRESSION

PREGNANCY RISK ASSESSMENT AND MONITORING SYSTEM

The Pregnancy Risk Assessment and Monitoring System (PRAMS) is a surveillance project conducted cooperatively by the Centers for Disease Control and Prevention (CDC) and state health departments, with the goal of reducing adverse birth outcomes and improving the health of mothers and infants. PRAMS collects data about pregnancy and the first few months after birth which supplement that available on birth certificates, including maternal experiences and attitudes during pregnancy, while giving birth, and shortly after giving birth. PRAMS was initiated in 1987, and the first participants were the District of Columbia, Indiana, Maine, Michigan, Oklahoma, and West Virginia. Twenty-nine states plus New York City participated in PRAMS in 2006, and six other states have participated at some point in the past.

Two factors led to the establishment of PRAMS: research that indicated that maternal behaviors during pregnancy could influence infant mortality rates and birth weight and the fact that by the mid-1980s birth outcomes were not improving as expected. In particular, the incidence of low-birth-weight babies had changed little over the past 20 years, and infant mortality rates were not declining as rapidly as they had in previous years. PRAMS provides state-specific data for planning and assessing maternal and infant health because responsibility to develop, implement, and evaluate programs to improve birth outcomes rests primarily with individual state health departments. For this reason, some degree of customization is allowed, including differing sample plans so a state may target groups of women who are perceived to be at high risk for poor birth outcomes in a particular state, and some customization of the types of information collected (although there is a common core of information collected in all states).

Each month, PRAMS data are collected from a stratified sample of women in each participating state who recently gave birth to a live infant. Sample size for each participating state varies between 1,300 and 3,400 women per year and may include oversampling among populations of particular interest to state health officials. Examples of populations include women who gave birth to low-birth-weight children and specific racial and ethnic groups who are perceived by state officials as being at high risk for poor birth outcomes. PRAMS data collection procedures are standardized to allow comparison of data collected in different states. Most data are collected by a questionnaire mailed to selected women 2 to 4 months after delivery; telephone interviews are used if the women selected do not respond after three attempts to contact them by mail.

The PRAMS questionnaire consists of two parts: *core* questions asked in all states and *standard questions* that are chosen from a list of pretested questions supplied by the CDC or developed by the individual state. Topics covered by the Phase 5 Questionnaire, which will be used in the years 2004 to 2008, include attitudes and feelings about the pregnancy, content and source of prenatal care, use of alcohol and tobacco, physical abuse, pregnancy-related illness, infant health care, contraceptive use, and knowledge of pregnancy-related health issues such as the benefits of folic acid and risks of HIV. Topics included in the Phase 5 standard questionnaire cover a broad range of topics, including fertility treatments, child care, HIV testing, breast-feeding, living arrangements, and physical activity. PRAMS questionnaires for Phase 3 (in use 1996–1999), Phase 4 (2000–2003), and Phase 5 (2004–2008) are currently available in English and Spanish for download from the PRAMS Web site.

The PRAMS data sets also include data drawn from birth certificates, including maternal demographics and pregnancy outcomes. To preserve confidentiality, PRAMS files omit information that could identify a particular birth, such as the birth certificate number and the dates of birth of the infant and its mother.

Researchers must apply for permission to use PRAMS data. Those who wish to use data from multiple states must submit a proposal to the CDC; guidelines for developing such a proposal are available on the PRAMS Web site. Those who wish to use PRAMS data from only one state should contact that state's PRAMS coordinator for permission: Contact information for these individuals is available on the PRAMS Web site.

—*Sarah Boslaugh*

See also Maternal and Child Health Epidemiology; Preterm Birth; Reproductive Epidemiology

Further Readings

Suellentrop, K., Morrow, B., Williams, L., D'Angelo, D., & Centers for Disease Control and Prevention. (2006). Monitoring progress toward achieving maternal and infant healthy people 2010 objectives: 19 states. Pregnancy Risk Assessment Monitoring System (PRAMS), 2000–2003. *MMWR Surveillance Summaries, 55*(9), 1–11.

Web Sites

Pregnancy Risk Assessment Monitoring (PRAMS): http://www.cdc.gov/prams.

PRETERM BIRTH

Preterm birth is an adverse outcome of pregnancy in which delivery of a live-born infant occurs before the completion of 37 gestational weeks. Infants born between 32 and 36 gestational weeks are considered moderate preterm births, while those delivered earlier than 32 gestational weeks are classified as very preterm births. This entry reviews the occurrence and public health impact of preterm birth and describes the mechanisms and risk factors associated with preterm birth. It also describes approaches used for the detection and prevention of preterm delivery as well as measurement issues encountered in epidemiological studies.

Public Health Impact

Preterm birth is associated with increased infant and childhood morbidity such as neurodevelopmental deficits and behavioral problems. Several adult diseases, such as diabetes, hypertension, and cardiovascular disease, are more likely to occur among preterm infants. Preterm birth is also associated with increased mortality with two thirds of perinatal deaths occurring among preterm infants. Although preterm delivery is associated with birth defects and other causes of mortality, one third of these deaths have been shown to be directly attributable to preterm delivery.

Preterm births can exact a considerable toll on health care systems since most premature babies require extensive neonatal and postneonatal medical care. In the United States, the disease burden associated with preterm deliveries was estimated at $26 billion a year. The annual cost of neonatal care alone was estimated at $1 billion for preterm births occurring in Canada (excluding costs associated with long-term medical care).

Mechanisms

Preterm birth can occur via at least four major pathophysiologic pathways that may work independently or simultaneously. These include the following:

1. inflammation and infection associated with maternal and fetal cytokine response ($\sim 40\%$ of preterm births);

2. maternal/fetal stress and the production of placental and fetal-membrane derived corticotropin-releasing hormone, which in turn enhances placental estrogen and stimulates fetal cortisol production ($\sim 25\%$ of preterm births);

3. abruption or decidual hemorrhage with thrombin-induced protease expression and disturbances in uterine tone ($\sim 25\%$ of preterm births); and

4. mechanical stretch due to multifetal pregnancy or polyhydramnios-induced uterine or cervical distention ($\sim 10\%$ of preterm births).

These pathways result in activation of the uterine myometrium which can initiate a preterm delivery through uterine contractions, cervical dilation, and premature rupture of the membranes.

Risk Factors

Preterm delivery is a multifactorial outcome in which the cause is unknown in nearly half of preterm births (i.e., idiopathic). Nonidiopathic preterm births can be classified by clinical subtypes, including spontaneous preterm labor, premature membrane rupture, and induction of labor or cesarean section triggered by maternal or fetal indications (e.g., hypertensive disorders of pregnancy, cervical incompetence). Risk factors for preterm birth identified in epidemiological studies include young and old maternal age, African American race, smoking, alcohol use, drug use, nutritional deficiency, poverty/neighborhood factors, stress/anxiety, inadequate prenatal care, inadequate weight gain during pregnancy, hypertension, uterine bleeding, short interconceptual interval, and previous preterm delivery. Systemic maternal infections such as pneumonia and periodontal disease have been associated with preterm delivery in epidemiological studies. Genital tract infections such as bacterial vaginosis have also been linked with an increased risk of preterm delivery. Associations have also been reported in epidemiological studies between risk of preterm birth and various environmental and occupational exposures, including pesticides, organochlorinated compounds (e.g., 1,1-dichloro-2, 2-bis(p-chlorophenyl)ethylene) and air pollutants (e.g., sulfur dioxide and particulate matter $< 10 \, \mu m$).

Heredity may play a role in the onset of preterm birth, since certain genetic polymorphisms may increase the risk of preterm delivery. Gene-environment interactions are becoming increasingly important considerations for reproductive and developmental epidemiological studies since genetic factors may also modify associations between risk of preterm birth and environmental pollution or other lifestyle/behavioral factors. Molecular epidemiological studies may also be used to determine the contribution of social deprivation, biological differences, and other factors to the racial disparities observed in preterm birth prevalence.

Occurrence

The prevalence of preterm birth ranges from 5% to 15% and is 5% to 10% in most Western societies. The prevalence of preterm delivery was 7.6% in Canada in 2000 and 12.5% in the United States in 2004. Notable disparities by ethnicity exist in the United States for preterm delivery. In 2004, the prevalence of preterm birth was 17.8% for African Americans compared with 11.5% for non-Hispanic Caucasians.

Temporal trends indicate an increase in preterm births over the past few decades in many countries. Most of the increase in preterm prevalence in the United States has occurred among moderate preterm births, since the prevalence of very preterm birth has remained about 2%. This temporal increase may be a reflection of obstetrical intervention in which many more high-risk fetuses are surviving than in previous years due to medical advances. The increased frequency of multiple gestations due to assisted reproductive technologies (i.e., fertility treatment) in many developed countries may also account for some of these trends.

Estimation Techniques

Preterm birth is a common health endpoint examined in epidemiological studies. The validity of preterm birth as an epidemiological endpoint depends on the accuracy of the gestational age estimation technique, since these estimates are not as precise as other clinical measures of fetal development (e.g., birthweight). Common methods for estimating gestational age include ultrasonography, menstrual dating, and clinician estimate. Ultrasound dating based on various measures (e.g., biparietal diameter, crown-rump length, fetal length, abdominal circumference) is considered the most accurate gestational age estimate technique. Gestational age estimates based on last menstrual dating and clinician estimate are commonly recorded on birth certificate data and used to derive preterm birth endpoints in epidemiological studies. Menstrual dating of gestational age depends on maternal recall of the last menstrual period, which can be subject to considerable measurement error. Clinical estimate of gestational age is another method used to gauge the developmental status of the infant but is also subject to measurement error. Random and systematic errors in estimating gestation can result in under- and overestimation of gestational duration and misclassification of the health endpoint being examined. This has potential clinical implications and may also lead to biased relative risk estimates due to false-positive and false-negative cases in the classification of preterm, term, and post-term births.

Detection and Prevention

Early detection and treatment of preterm labor symptoms and maternal infections are keys to reducing the risk for preterm delivery. Biomarkers and other diagnostic tools such as fetal fibronectin, endovaginal ultrasound, and salivary estriol can be used to predict risk of preterm delivery. Avoidance of drugs, alcohol, cigarettes, and other modifiable risk factors are important preventative measures. Adequate weight gain and proper nutrition are essential to the health of a fetus and should be discussed with health care practitioners during prenatal care visits early in pregnancy. As the use of fertility treatment increases the incidence of preterm birth, there will be an increasing need to expand management and treatment alternatives for early deliveries. Promising new hormone treatments, such as 17-alpha-hydroxprogesterone caproate, may decrease the risk of preterm delivery by preventing shortening of the cervix among high-risk pregnant women.

—*J. Michael Wright*

See also African American Health Issues; Child and Adolescent Health; Gestational Age; Prevalence; Reproductive Epidemiology

Further Readings

Behrman, R. E., & Stith Butler, A. (Eds.). (2006). *Preterm birth: Causes, consequences and prevention.* Washington, DC: National Academies Press.

Callaghan, W. M., MacDorman, M. F., Rasmussen, S. A., Qin, C., & Lackritz, E. M. (2006). The contribution of preterm birth to infant mortality rates in the United States. *Pediatrics, 118*(4), 1566–1573.

Crider, K. S., Whitehead, N., & Buss, R. M. (2005). Genetic variation associated with preterm birth: A HuGE review. *Genetics in Medicine, 7*(9), 593–604.

Green, N. S., Damus, K., Simpson, J. L., Iams, J., Reece, E. A., Hobel, C. J., et al. (2005). Research agenda for preterm birth: Recommendations from the March of Dimes. *American Journal of Obstetrics and Gynecology, 193*(3), 626–635.

Hanke, W., & Jurewicz, J. (2004). The risk of adverse reproductive and developmental disorders due to occupational pesticide exposure: An overview of current epidemiological evidence. *International Journal of Occupational Medicine and Environmental Health, 17*(2), 223–243.

Savitz, D. A., Terry, J. W., Jr., Dole, N., Thorp, J. M., Jr., Siega-Riz, A. M., & Herring, A. H. (2002). Comparison of pregnancy dating by last menstrual period, ultrasound scanning, and their combination. *American Journal of Obstetrics and Gynecology, 187*(6), 1660–1666.

Sram, R. J., Binkova, B., Dejmek, J., & Bobak, M. (2005). Ambient air pollution and pregnancy outcomes: A review of the literature. *Environmental Health Perspectives, 113*(4), 378–382.

PREVALENCE

In epidemiology, the term *prevalence* quantifies the proportion of a population with disease or a particular condition at a specific point in time (sometimes called point prevalence). Prevalence is used widely in the media and by government agencies, insurance companies, epidemiologists, and health care providers. Often confused with prevalence, *incidence* (described in detail elsewhere) quantifies *new* cases while prevalence describes *existing* cases.

While the term *prevalence rate* is often used synonymously with *prevalence*, the strict definition restricts prevalence to a proportion, not a rate. The difference is in the denominator: Rates describe risk of disease during a given time *interval* among a *population at risk*, while proportions describe the likelihood of disease at a specific *point* in time among the *population*. The point in time may be a specific calendar date or a time that varies from person to person, such as the onset of menopause or puberty, or discharge from the hospital.

For prevalence, the numerator is the number of existing cases or conditions, and the denominator is the total population or group. For example, the prevalence of type 2 diabetes among children aged 2 to 12 years equals the number of children aged 2 to 12 years with type 2 diabetes divided by the total number of children aged 2 to 12 years.

While incidence helps investigators understand the etiology (or cause) of disease, prevalence is especially useful to health system planners and public health professionals. Knowledge of the disease burden in a population, whether global or local, is essential to securing the resources required to fund special services or health promotion programs. For instance, the director of a nursing home must be able to measure the proportion of seniors with Alzheimer's to plan the appropriate level of services for the residents. Legislators and public health professionals need good population statistics to prioritize funding for health promotion programs, such as obesity and smoking cessation. On a community level, understanding the prevalence of English as a second language would be helpful to school administrators. National- and state-level prevalence of behaviors and diseases are usually calculated using data collected systematically from the population through major health surveys, such as the CDC's Behavioral Risk Factor Surveillance Survey (BRFSS), the National Health Interview Survey (NHIS), and National Health and Nutrition Examination Survey (NHANES).

Understanding the difference between prevalence and incidence allows the epidemiologist to apply the terms correctly, define denominators for measures, and conceptualize the study design best suited to a specific research question. In addition, these terms are related mathematically, a property that can prove useful when moving from a measure of incidence to prevalence or vice versa. When the incidence of disease is stable over time, such as in the absence of epidemics or changes in treatment effectiveness, prevalence is the product of the incidence and the average duration of disease or condition ($P = I \times D$). More complex mathematical relationships exist between incidence and prevalence when these assumptions cannot be met.

—Allison Krug and Louise-Anne McNutt

See also Incidence; Proportion; Rate

Further Readings

Hennekens, D. H., & Buring, J. E. (1987). *Epidemiology in medicine.* Boston: Little, Brown.

Last, J. M. (2001). *A dictionary of epidemiology* (Handbooks sponsored by the IEA and WHO). New York: Oxford University Press.

PREVENTION: PRIMARY, SECONDARY, AND TERTIARY

The term *prevention* refers to planning for and taking action to avoid the occurrence of an undesirable event. As it relates to health, prevention aims to hinder the development of diseases or illnesses or avoid injuries. Prevention can be divided into three levels: primary, secondary, and tertiary. The entry discusses each of these levels of prevention and presents examples applied to both communicable and noncommunicable diseases as they relate to individual as well as community efforts.

The importance of prevention in improving health cannot be overlooked. Though the death rates have been decreasing in the United States, preventive actions could further lower these rates. Approximately one third of Americans live with a chronic disease, and almost 70% of the deaths that occur each year are the result of chronic diseases. Furthermore, approximately one third of all U.S. deaths are related to three modifiable health-damaging behaviors—tobacco use, lack of physical activity, and poor eating habits. Establishing healthy habits and making lifestyle changes, which are critical prevention efforts, can significantly decrease the morbidity and mortality rates of Americans.

Levels of Prevention

The first level of prevention, *primary prevention*, sometimes just referred to as *prevention*, is aimed at stopping any occurrence of disease or illness before the disease process begins or taking measures to avoid injury. Thus, many primary prevention activities focus on health education and health promotion programs that are aimed at changing individuals' health behavior and lifestyle.

Injury and illness cannot always be avoided. Some chronic diseases, such as cancer or heart disease, can develop and cause damage before being detected and treated. In such situations, the sooner medical intervention can occur, the greater the chance of preventing death or limiting disability. *Secondary prevention*, sometimes referred to as *intervention*, is aimed at health screening and detection activities that lead to early diagnosis and prompt treatment of a disease or an injury before the disease becomes advanced or the disability becomes severe.

Tertiary prevention, often referred to as *treatment*, is aimed at retraining, reeducating, and rehabilitating the individual who has already incurred a disability. Tertiary prevention measures are applied after the disease, disability, impairment, or dependency has already occurred.

Application of Prevention Principles

The principles of the various levels of prevention can be applied to both communicable and noncommunicable diseases. Furthermore, these principles can be applied to the actions undertaken by single individuals or entire communities.

Prevention of Communicable Diseases

Stopping the spread of communicable diseases in a population is based on stopping the transmission of the pathogens causing the diseases. Successful application of primary, secondary, and tertiary strategies to communicable diseases, particularly primary prevention, resulted in unprecedented declines in both morbidity and mortality during the 20th century. Examples of primary prevention activities undertaken by individuals to stop the spread of communicable diseases include hand washing, proper cooking of foods, and getting immunized against specific diseases. To these can be added community primary prevention measures, including laws dealing with food handling and safety, chlorination of the water supply, the proper collection and disposal of solid waste, and the control of vectors and rodents.

Secondary preventive actions against communicable diseases for individuals can include the self-diagnosis or diagnosis by a physician and treatment of the disease with either over-the-counter medications or those prescribed by a physician. Secondary prevention measures that communities can use are usually aimed at the spread of the disease once it is present in a group of people. Such activities may include case findings and treatment and the reporting of notifiable diseases (those that physicians, clinics, and hospitals are legally required to report to their local health department). Less commonly, communities may isolate or quarantine those infected or exposed, respectively.

The tertiary preventive measures for control of communicable disease in individuals usually include convalescence from infection, recovery to health, and return to normal activities. Tertiary prevention measures at the community level are aimed at the recurrence of the disease. An example would be the removal, embalming, and burial of the dead.

Prevention of Noncommunicable Diseases

Unlike communicable diseases that are caused by pathogens, the strategies used to prevent noncommunicable diseases focus on the risk factors associated with a particular disease. Thus, the prevention principles are applied a bit differently to noncommunicable diseases, but as with communicable diseases, they can be applied to both individual and community activities. Primary prevention measures for noncommunicable diseases at the individual level begin with a solid education about health and health practices. With such knowledge, individuals can take the necessary steps to prevent noncommunicable disease such as getting enough exercise, maintaining a healthy body weight, eating properly, wearing safety belts, and avoiding excess exposure to the sun by wearing sunscreen. Community primary prevention measures include providing a safe and healthful environment. Examples may include smoke-free environments, exercise trails, and appropriate lighting in parking lots and on sidewalks to reduce injury and crime.

Secondary prevention measures for individuals for noncommunicable diseases include actions, for example, personal screenings such as self-examination for cancer of the testes or breasts, or participating in screenings provided by the medical community such as mammograms, Pap tests, or PSA (prostate-specific antigen) tests for cancer. The goal of such screenings is early detection, referral, and prompt treatment to either cure the disease or slow the progress of disease, disability, disorder, or death. Behavior change programs are another example of individual secondary prevention efforts. Smoking cessation, weight loss, stress reduction, or early admission in to a drug prevention program are examples of such behavior change programs.

Community secondary prevention measures include the provisions of mass screenings and case finding for chronic disease and the provision of adequate health care personnel and facilities to conduct such screenings. Examples may include blood pressure screenings provided by the paramedics at the local fire house or a local voluntary health agency partnering with a cancer center offering the various array of cancer screenings.

Tertiary prevention measures for noncommunicable diseases by individuals often require significant lifestyle changes. For a person with diabetes, it may include testing oneself regularly for blood sugar levels, taking prescribed medications or injections of insulin, and faithfully watching one's diet and getting enough exercise. Patient education, after care, support groups, and health counseling are some important community health promotion components of tertiary prevention efforts.

It has been commonly reported that in the United States, 95% of all health care dollars is used for medical care services, while only 5% is used for preventive activities. If the health of the American people is going to improve and health care costs are going to be controlled, a greater emphasis needs to be placed on prevention.

—*James F. McKenzie*
and Denise M. Seabert

See also Community Health; Health Behavior; Notifiable Disease; Quarantine and Isolation; Screening

Further Readings

Centers for Disease Control and Prevention. (2003). *The power of prevention: Reducing the health and economic burden of chronic disease.* Atlanta, GA: U.S. Department of Health and Human Services. Retrieved July 24, 2007, from http://www.cdc.gov/nccdphp/publications/ PowerOfPrevention.

McGinnis, J. M., Williams-Russo, P., & Knickman, J. R. (2002). The case for more active attention to health promotion. *Health Affairs, 21*(2), 78–93.
McKenzie, J. F., Neiger, B. L., & Smeltzer, J. L. (2005). *Planning, implementing, and evaluating health promotion programs: A primer* (4th ed.). San Francisco: Benjamin Cummings.
McKenzie, J. F., Pinger, R. R., & Kotecki, J. E. (2005). *An introduction to community health* (5th ed.). Sudbury, MA: Jones & Bartlett.
Timmreck, T. C. (1998). *An introduction to epidemiology* (2nd ed.). Sudbury, MA: Jones & Bartlett.

PROBABILITY SAMPLE

A probability sample is one in which members are chosen from a target population using methods that rely on chance such as random number tables. In probability sampling, all members of the target population have a nonzero probability of being chosen; the probability of selection for each can be calculated. Probability samples are superior to nonprobability samples in that the extent to which the sample varies from the target population can be calculated, and in the absence of other biases, study results may be generalizable to the target populations.

Probability Versus Nonprobability Sampling

Due to limits on resources and time, researchers are rarely able to observe every member of a target population, or the group for which a researcher wishes to generalize the results of a study. Instead, a subset must be chosen. Members may be selected for study using either nonprobability or probability sampling methods. In nonprobability sampling, selection occurs in a nonrandom fashion usually based on availability. Two examples of nonprobability sampling methods are convenience and snow-ball sampling. Because all members of a population chosen via nonprobability sampling methods do not have a nonzero chance of being selected for the study, it is not possible to determine how closely a nonprobability sample resembles the target population and, therefore, results from these studies are not generalizable to the entire target population. However, probability sampling, which involves selection of members from the target population using random selection techniques, produces results that, in the absence of other biases, are generalizable. In probability sampling, all members of the target population have a nonzero opportunity of being chosen to be in the sample and the probability that any given one will be chosen can be calculated.

Types of Probability Sampling

Simple random sampling, systematic sampling, and stratified or cluster sampling are types of probability sampling. In simple random sampling, members are randomly and independently chosen from a list of all target population members; every member of the target population has an equal chance of being chosen for participation in a study. In systematic sampling, a sample is chosen by selecting the first member from a list at random and then by taking every kth member from the population list thereafter. In stratified or cluster sampling, a population is first subdivided into groups that share at least one common characteristic, then a sample is chosen from each stratum using simple random or systematic selection.

Probability Sampling and Sampling Error

The degree to which a sample obtained through probability sampling varies from the target population is measured by estimating the sampling error. Sampling error arises when only part of a population is observed; for any given target population, many alternative sample realizations, or sets of members or individuals selected for a sample, can be obtained by employing a given sampling method, and each may lead to a different summary statistic, such as mean, for the parameter being studied. Theoretically, sampling error is derived from the amount of variation that exists between the summary statistics for all possible realizations. In practice, the standard error of the study sample is used to construct a confidence interval for which with a certain level of confidence the true parameter of interest lies.

Probability Sampling and Bias

The use of probability sampling methods does not guarantee that a sample accurately represents the target population; various biases may affect the results of a study despite the use of probability sampling techniques. For example, sample bias may occur in studies that have low response rates as study participants who choose to respond to a survey may differ significantly from those who choose not to, therefore causing the study summary statistic to vary from that of the target population. Sample size, which is inversely correlated with sampling error, is also important in obtaining precise measures.

—*Michelle Kirian*

See also Bias; Convenience Sample; Sampling Techniques; Stratified Methods

Further Readings

Groves, R. M., Fowler, F. J., Couper, M. P., Lepkowski, J. M., Singer, E., & Tourangeau, R. (2004). Sample design and standard error. In *Survey methodology* (pp. 93–136). Hoboken, NJ: Wiley.

Scientists and Engineers Statistical Data System. (2001, September). *Sampling errors for SESTAT.* Retrieved March 1, 2007, from http://sestat.nsf.gov/docs/stderr00.html.

Statistics Canada. (2006, August). *Sampling methods.* Retrieved March 1, 2007, from http://www.statcan.ca/english/edu/power/ch13/first13.htm.

PROGRAM EVALUATION

Evaluation has at its root the word *value*. Program evaluation is the part of the evaluation field that determines the merit or worth of a program. A program is a set of planned activities designed to reach a predetermined goal—for instance, to encourage employees in a company to begin and maintain an exercise program or to discourage teenagers from beginning to smoke. Program evaluation consists of the activities that determine the value, merit, or worth of the program—whether the program activities are making a difference and accomplishing the program's goal (outcomes). The question may be asked, "Why evaluate?" Evaluation is the process that allows decision makers to determine whether programs are making a difference and to identify changes that may be necessary for success. It provides program planners, policymakers, legislators, and other decision-making stakeholders with information on which to base decisions concerning program continuation or closure. Since epidemiologists are often in the roles of determining needs and influencing policy, understanding policy is important. An example of these activities would be the input of epidemiologists in determining government policy surrounding immunization of school-age children. Program evaluation provided evidence that immunizations make a difference. Epidemiologists used that information to advocate for a policy requiring school-age children to be immunized prior to attending public schools.

Program evaluation is considered a *transdiscipline.* That is, it is an area of inquiry that provides services to many disciplines, using methodologies drawn from social and applied sciences and applied broadly across various disciplines such as social services, industry and business, health care, education, and mental health care, among others. The application of a transdiscipline is not uniform across all contexts; some methods are more useful and applicable in some contexts or situations than in others. Michael Scriven describes transdisciplines as disciplines such as logic and statistics that provide tools for other disciplines such as sociology and psychology. Transdisciplines apply across a broad range of inquiry and creative endeavors, yet maintain disciplinary autonomy.

Another way to view program evaluation is through the concept of *appreciative* inquiry (AI). Hallie Preskill and Anne Coghlan describe appreciative inquiry as a method of inquiry that is participatory, collaborative, and systematic in determining an organization's capacity to develop a positive potential in planning its preferred future. In evaluation, appreciative inquiry is a process that promotes positive change, especially in organizations, to build the capacities of the organization.

In the past 10 to 15 years, program evaluation as a discipline has come into its own. This has been one of the concrete long-term outcomes of the federal mandate for accountability through the Government Performance Results Act (GPRA) of 1993 and, more recently, the Program Assessment Rating Tool (PART) developed by the Office of Management and Budget and released in 2002. PART is a questionnaire used to evaluate federally funded programs in terms of their purpose, design, planning, management, results, and accountability to determine its overall effectiveness. The PART established another layer of accountability at the federal level and ensured that evaluation activities are systematically included in program implementation. Yet to truly understand program evaluation as a field, one needs an understanding of its history,

knowledge of the key concepts, and its applications in epidemiology and public health.

History of Program Evaluation

Program evaluation as it is known today evolved over several hundred years. Michael Quinn Patton subscribes to the view that program evaluation was used by Daniel when in the lion's den. However, program evaluation as a systematic form of inquiry has its origins in the 19th century. During the 1800s, the British government appointed commissions that reviewed (i.e., evaluated) educational institutions of the time. These commissions established external boards to inspect schools. In the United States in the mid 1800s, Massachusetts assessed student achievement and used those assessments for school comparisons. The accreditation movement for schools and institutions of higher learning (secondary and postsecondary schools) began in the late 1800s.

The early 1900s brought the review of social service and health programs that addressed problems such as slum conditions and infectious diseases. Development of the educational testing movement also began in the early 1900s, due in large part to the psychometric work of E. L. Thorndike and the intelligence testing work of Alfred Binet and Louis Terman. The use of norm-referenced and then criterion-referenced tests moved evaluation of educational programs forward significantly. Egon Guba and Yvonna Lincoln call this first generation of evaluation the measurement generation.

Simultaneously, social service fields were establishing methods for assessing efficiency of their social programs. The management movement of Fredrick Taylor was of notable significance. Yet these efforts were neither widespread, nor did they have government support. The Great Depression changed all that as there was a proliferation of government-supported entitlement and social services programs such as welfare, health, and urban development. These field-based programs served as living laboratories for the applied social scientists who were attempting to determine the effects of these programs.

During World War II, social scientists established mechanisms by which governmental programs were developed to assist the military and, later, the programs for returning veterans. The results of psychological and personality testing for job placement received much attention. It was also during this time that skill-based teaching and testing were initiated. This objective-based teaching guided curriculum development, and the extent to which students achieved those objectives was then described by developers. This largely descriptive process identified strengths and weaknesses of the curriculum, rather than the abilities of the students. Ralph Tyler did much to advance the use of objectives expressed in measurable terms. Guba and Lincoln refer to this period as the second generation of evaluation.

The second half of the 20th century nurtured the advancements that led to evaluation as it is known today. The concepts of judgment, merit, and worth became the keystone for evaluation. Many scholars developed various models that employed criteria against which programs were judged (e.g., Robert Stake's countenance model; Daniel Stufflebeam's CIPP (context, input, process, product) model; Malcolm Provus's discrepancy evaluation model; Michael Scriven's goal-free model; and Elliot Eisner's connoisseurship model. Guba and Lincoln describe this as the third generation of evaluation. They developed yet another model, the responsive constructivist evaluation model, which they labeled fourth generation.

Government policies in the latter half of the 20th century supported and even demanded evaluation. The Elementary and Secondary Education Act (ESEA) of 1965 was probably the single piece of legislation most responsible for moving program evaluation forward. This legislation funneled massive amounts of governmental funds to local, state, and regional educational institutions and at the same time required the recipients of the funds to provide the funding agency with an evaluation report detailing the program results supported by federal funds.

By the late 1900s, evaluation had come into its own as a profession. The American Evaluation Association was formed in 1986 through a merger of the Evaluation Research Society and the Evaluation Network. Universities had developed graduate programs for preparing evaluation specialists, professional development institutes provided continuing education for practicing evaluators, standards of practice were developed and approved, and scholars were developing theories of program evaluation.

To ensure effective use of scarce fiscal resources, the federal government passed the GPRA and implemented PART mandating evaluations of programs both funded by and housed within the federal government. Evaluation societies proliferated internationally, with more than 20 societies existing around the world. The International Organization for Cooperation in Evaluation (IOCE) ratified its constitution in 2003. As an organization of various national and international professional evaluation societies, the IOCE mission is promoting cooperation and partnership in evaluation worldwide through the exchange of information, ideas, and resources and promoting a high level of professional standards.

Key Evaluation Concepts

Any discussion about program evaluation will typically involve some, if not all, of the following terms: informal evaluation, formal evaluation, formative evaluation, summative evaluation, needs assessment, process evaluation, internal evaluation, external evaluation, logic modeling, outcome evaluation, qualitative evaluation, and quantitative evaluation. Understanding how these terms form the framework of program evaluation provides the reader with a foundation to understand program evaluation.

Informal and Formal Evaluation

Informal evaluation is the process used by individuals in daily activities to make judgments and to make choices based on those judgments. Consumers use informal evaluation in choosing a brand of cereal or canned vegetables. Teachers make observations of students and form judgments of the student's ability. Typically informal evaluations are unsystematic, based on incomplete evidence. For example, in choosing a cereal, it is unlikely that an individual will have tasted every type of cereal available in the store. In addition, other stores may have different brands. Consequently, informal evaluation typically provides incomplete data on which to base the decision of value or worth. Personal and situational biases also contribute to this inadequacy of informal evaluation. Nevertheless, even though informal evaluations may provide incomplete data, they may be the only evaluation possible in many situations.

Formal evaluation is systematic, planned, and context specific. Typically, specific methods are applied to determining the value or merit of a program. One can consider program evaluation, or evaluation of any object, a continuum from informal to formal. Finding the balance providing between unstructured evaluation and rigorous but excessive formal evaluation is the challenge facing evaluators.

Formative and Summative Evaluation

Formative and *summative evaluation* are terms that Michael Scriven coined in 1967 to distinguish between evaluations that were conducted for program improvement only (formative) and evaluations that were typically conducted for decision making only (summative). Formative evaluation is the evaluation typically occurring during the program's implementation and often evaluates only a part of a program. Formative evaluation allows for midcourse corrections in program implementation. Summative evaluation is the evaluation typically occurring after the program implementation is completed. It provides information to decision makers for a "go-no go" decision on program continuation.

The audiences for the reports of formative and summative evaluation are typically different. The audiences for formative evaluation reports are the program planners or program staff. The audiences for summative evaluation reports are consumers, funding sources, policymakers, and other decision-making stakeholders.

Needs Assessment

Programs are typically planned to answer questions about a condition currently existing. To garner clear and unambiguous information about the nature of the condition, evaluators typically conduct a "needs assessment." The information gathered helps establish the extent to which a need or problem exists and provides information for making recommendations to address that problem.

Process Evaluation

A process evaluation determines the "how" of a program. It details the delivery, the administrative structure, and the successes encountered as the program is implemented. One way to look at process evaluation is to structure the process evaluation around the following questions: (1) What challenges were encountered? (2) What was done to overcome those challenges? and (3) What lessons were learned from this approach? Challenges may be both positive and negative. Answering these questions helps program planners and decision makers when similar programs are being planned.

Outcome Evaluation

An outcome evaluation documents what changes have occurred as a result of implementing a program. Changes can occur in program participants, in those who interact with the program participants, and in the communities in which program participants live. Changes may occur in knowledge, behavior, or practice or in social, environmental, or economic conditions. Outcome evaluations are often conducted as a part of a comprehensive evaluation that includes a needs assessment, a process evaluation, and an output evaluation.

One often hears the term *outcome evaluation* being used synonymously with *summative evaluation.* Outcome evaluations may be summative, and summative evaluations may not describe outcomes. Huey-Tsyh Chen proposed a typology showing the relationship between formative and summative evaluations and among needs assessment, process, and outcome evaluations. It is clear that needs assessments, process, and outcome evaluations can be either formative or summative, depending on the questions being answered by the evaluation.

Internal Evaluation and External Evaluation

When an evaluation is conducted by an employee of the program, the evaluation is typically considered an internal evaluation. When an evaluation is conducted by an individual who is outside the organization conducting the program, the evaluation is typically considered an external evaluation. Although the use of these terms seems reasonably clear, there may be variations whereby an employee of an organization (internal) is not part of the program being conducted (external) (e.g., when there is a multisite program and an evaluation team unfamiliar with the program being evaluated is sent from corporate headquarters).

It is important to consider the advantages and disadvantages of each position when designing evaluations. The external evaluator typically brings greater credibility and perhaps objectivity to the task as well as greater specialized evaluation knowledge. The internal evaluator typically understands the corporate and programmatic culture. The external evaluator will not know the corporate culture, while the internal evaluator may be burdened by personal and situational biases related to the corporate/programmatic culture.

Blaine Worthen, James Sanders, and Jody Fitzpatrick (2003) propose a 2 × 2 matrix for the combinations of formative and summative evaluations and internal and external evaluation. They are formative-internal, formative-external, summative-internal, and summative-external. Most commonly, individual evaluators are either formative-internal (because of their knowledge of the program) or summative-external (because of the perceived objectivity).

Logic Modeling

Logic modeling is simply a map of the program executed in a series of if-then statements. Logic modeling is employed during the program planning stages to detail the long-term expectations (often called impacts) of the program. Program planners describe what conditions will change if the program is successful. They attempt to outline what difference the program will make. Program planners then look at medium-term outcomes (often called intermediate outcomes) and short-term outcomes (often called immediate outcomes). One will also see the term *proximal outcome* used to describe short-term and medium-term outcomes and *distal outcomes* to describe long-term outcomes.

Once these outcomes are identified in a time frame, the question is posed by program planners as to what must be done to reach these outcomes. Specifically, what activities will need to be conducted to which audience with what resources? The activities and audience are typically called outputs, while the resources are typically called inputs.

Outputs consist of the number of sessions, encounters, publications, and so on that the specified number of targeted audience will receive in the time frame specified. Inputs are the budgets, personnel, time, equipment, materials, facilities, and so on that are required to perform the activities to the targeted audiences.

Logic models are often linear, although not necessarily so. As with formative evaluations, midcourse corrections can be made in models, implying that the models are more accurately an iterative rather than a linear activity.

Quantitative Evaluation and Qualitative Evaluation

Evaluation traditionally employed methods from the social and applied sciences, such as the quasi-experimental designs, objective measurement techniques,

and statistical analyses. These quantitative methods were employed in the comparisons, providing the evaluator with indicators of validity and reliability for making judgments. Quantitative evaluation drawing from applied social science research provides information about two important criteria found in social science research: *internal validity*, or causality, and *external validity*, or generalizability to other settings and times. It is difficult to secure measures for these criteria using the rich narrative found in qualitative evaluation.

Qualitative evaluation, on the other hand, employs qualitative, or nonnumerical, data. Sources of these data are verbal descriptions of observations, interviews, and individual collective perceptions (such as data gathered from focus groups). One could not reasonably use the same criteria one used with quantitative data to determine the value of the program evaluated using a qualitative evaluation. Instead, one would employ *accuracy*, or the extent obtained data are reflective of the real situation; *utility*, or the extent results serve practical needs; *feasibility*, or the degree of prudence, diplomacy, and reality employed; and *propriety*, or the legal and ethical parameters of an evaluation.

The value of each form is clear. Numeric data are typically more precise, while narrative data are typically more descriptively rich. Using both, called *mixed methods*, is the approach more often used by today's evaluators. In using mixed methods, evaluators draw from across disciplinary boundaries and employ methodologies from such varying disciplines as agronomy, anthropology, sociology, psychology, philosophy, mathematics, history, and economics. Policy analysis often draws from legal frameworks.

These methodological approaches are classified into five evaluation approaches relating to the models employed. These approaches are objective-oriented, management-oriented, consumer-oriented, expertise-oriented, and participant-oriented. Qualitative and quantitative methods are used in varying degrees in each of these, so that these approaches form a continuum from utilitarian evaluation to intuitionist-pluralist evaluation, and quantitative to qualitative evaluation.

Application of Program Evaluation

Often, the incidence and prevalence of an event change as a result of a program or intervention. Program evaluation is the discipline that will aid in determining what change has occurred and assist in identifying the attribution of that change to a specific intervention. Although program evaluation does not explicitly identify causality, it is the discipline that will provide information for decision making by determining the merit or worth of a program and often provides the tools for determining causality later.

—*Molly Engle*

See also Economic Evaluation; Qualitative Methods in Epidemiology; Quantitative Methods in Epidemiology; Study Design

Further Readings

Chelimski, E., & Shaddish, W. R. (Eds.). (1997). *Evaluation for the 21st century: A handbook.* Thousand Oaks, CA: Sage.

Chen, H.-T. (1990). *Theory-driven evaluations.* Newbury Park, CA: Sage.

Guba, E. G., & Lincoln, Y. S. (1989). *Fourth generation evaluation.* Newbury Park, CA: Sage.

Mark, M. M., Henry, G. T., & Julnes, G. (2000). *Evaluation: An integrated framework for understanding, guiding and improving policies and programs.* San Francisco: Jossey-Bass.

Patton, M. Q. (1996). *Utilization-focused evaluation* (3rd ed.). Thousand Oaks, CA: Sage.

Preskill, H., & Coghan, A. T. (Eds.). (2003). *Using appreciative inquiry in evaluation.* New Directions for Evaluation, no. 100. San Francisco: Jossey-Bass.

Rossi, P. H., Lipsey, M. W., & Freeman, H. E. (2004). *Evaluation: A systematic approach* (7th ed.). Thousand Oaks, CA: Sage.

Scriven, M. (1967). The methodology of evaluation. In R. E. Stake (Ed.), *Curriculum evaluation* (American Educational Research Association Monograph Series on Evaluation, No. 1, pp. 39–83). Chicago: Rand McNally.

Scriven, M. (1991). *Evaluation thesaurus* (4th ed.). Newbury Park, CA: Sage.

Shaddish, W. R., Cook, T. D., & Leviton, L. (1991). *Foundations of program evaluation.* Newbury Park, CA: Sage.

Stufflebeam, D. L. (2001). Evaluation models. In G. T. Gary & J. C. Greene (Eds.), *New directions for evaluation* (Vol. 89, pp. 7–99). San Francisco: Jossey-Bass.

Wholey, J. S., Hatry, H. P., & Newcomer, K. E. (2004). *Handbook of practical program evaluation* (2nd ed.). San Francisco: Jossey-Bass.

Worthen, B. R., Sanders, J. R., & Fitzpatrick, J. L. (2003). *Program evaluation: Alternative approaches and practical guidelines* (3rd ed.). New York: Allyn & Bacon.

Web Sites

Government Performance and Results Act (1993): http://www.whitehouse.gov/omb/mgmt-gpra/gplaw2m.html.

International Organization for Cooperation in Evaluation: http://ioce.net/index.shtml.

Program Assessment Rating Tool: http://www.whitehouse.gov/omb/part.

PROPENSITY SCORE

Propensity score adjustment is a method of adjusting for all covariates in an observational case-control study, using scalar matching. In case-control studies, the goal is typically to determine if one group (cases) of subjects has a different outcome than another group (controls). These groups might be defined by which treatment they received or which factor they were exposed to, and the purpose of the study is to determine if the treatments or factors result in different outcomes in the cases than in the controls. For example, we can observe people who smoke (cases) and people who don't smoke (controls) and compare the rates of cancer between the two groups. Because people cannot ethically be assigned to one or the other condition (smoking or nonsmoking) we have to accept the groupings that exist. However, because random assignment to condition was not used, the two groups very likely differ on other factors, which can introduce bias into the study. Historically epidemiologists have dealt with this issue by matching subjects in the case group with subjects in control group based on observed covariates, for example, age category and gender, to attempt to remove the influence of these factors on the outcome by equalizing their distribution in the two groups. However, matching can be performed on only a limited number of covariates before the sample size within each matching group becomes too small for statistical analysis. For instance, if we divided age into four categories (e.g., < 30, $31–50$, $51–70$, ≥ 71), then matching on age and gender would divide the sample into eight separate subgroups. In addition, by dividing a continuous variable (age) into categories, we are losing some of the information contained in the variable.

Propensity score adjustment overcomes this limitation using scalar matching as follows. Let the data measured on subjects be classified into three sets of variables: X is the set of all covariates to be adjusted for, Y is the group membership (case or control, smoker or nonsmoker in this example), and Z is the outcome (cancer or no cancer in this example). Each subject observed has the set of variables (X, Y, Z) measured on them. Note that the covariates X may be continuous, categorical, or both, and the outcome variable Z may also be either categorical (e.g., develop cancer or not) or continuous (e.g., number of pounds lost).

In the simplest propensity-score-matching approach, a logistic regression model is fit using all the covariates in X to predict the group membership Y. Note that this analysis excludes the use of the outcome Z in the model fitting. The logistic regression model assigns each subject a predicted log-odds value for belonging to the smoking group (case), whether they smoked or not. Matching cases with controls can then be done based on the log-odds of smoking number (the scalar) calculated for each subject. Matching cases with controls who have a similar log-odds of smoking value results in an adjustment for all the covariates in X.

After matching cases with controls, a comparison of the outcome Z in the matched sets is done using standard statistical methods. If matching is done on a one-to-one basis, with a categorical outcome, as in the smoking example, a paired test of proportion (McNemar's test) can be used to determine if death is more likely to occur in the smokers than in the nonsmokers). Stratified matching can also be done by grouping subjects according to the distribution of the log-odds scalar. For instance, to form five strata in the smoking study, the first group would be the cases and controls whose log-odds of smoking are in the lowest 20th percentile, the next group in the 21st to 40th percentile, and so on. The analysis of the outcome can then be performed on each subgroup separately, using Fisher's exact test, or over all the subgroups, using the Mantel-Haenzel test.

—*William D. Shannon*

See also Bias; Logistic Regression; Observational Studies; Study Design

Further Readings

Connors, A., Speroff, T., Dawson, N., Thomas, C., Harrell, F. E., Jr., Wagner, D., et al. (1996). The effectiveness of right heart catheterization in the initial care of critically ill patients. *Journal of the American Medical Association, 276,* 889–897.

Juang, P., Skledar, S. J., Zgheib, N. K., Paterson, D. L., Vergis, E. N., Shannon W. D., et al. (2007). Clinical outcomes of intravenous immune globulin in severe *Clostridium difficile*-induced diarrhea. *American Journal of Infection Control, 35*(2), 131–137.

Rosenbaum, P. (2002). *Observational studies* (2nd ed.). New York: Springer-Verlag.

Rosenbaum, P., & Rubin, D. (1984). Reducing bias in observational studies using subclassification on the propensity score. *Journal of the American Statistical Association, 79,* 516–524.

PROPORTION

The proportion is a statistic that is used to describe how much of a population has a particular characteristic or attribute and is usually expressed as a fraction or decimal. The defining characteristic of the proportion, as distinct from the ratio, is that every individual in the numerator of a proportion is also included in the denominator. Consider a population in which each member either has or does not have a specified attribute. The population proportion is the percentage (or rate) of the entire population that has the specified attribute. For examples, we might be interested in the proportion of U.S. adults who have health insurance or in comparing the proportions of prevalence of CF antibody to Para influenza I virus among boys and girls in the age group 5 to 9 years. In the first case, the population consists of all U.S. adults and the specified attribute is "has health insurance." For the second case, the population consists of all boys and girls in the age group of 5 to 9 years.

Frequently, the population under consideration is large, and determining the population proportion by taking a census is therefore usually impractical and often impossible; for instance, imagine trying to interview every U.S. adult for the purpose of ascertaining the proportion that have health insurance. Thus, in practice, we mostly rely on sampling and use the sample data to make inferences about the population proportion.

The sample proportion is the percentage of a sample from the population that has the specified attribute. The sample proportion $\hat{p}$ can be computed by the formula

$$\hat{p} = \frac{x}{n},$$

where x denotes the number of members in the sample that have the specified attribute and n denotes the sample size. For example, a study is undertaken to compare the rates of prevalence of CF antibody to Para influenza I virus among boys and girls in the age group of 5 to 9 years. Among 113 boys tested, 34 are found to have the antibody; among 139 girls tested, 54 have the antibody. Let p_1 denote the population proportion of boys who have the CF antibody and p_2 the population of girls who have the CF antibody. Then sample proportions are

$$\hat{p}_1 = \frac{34}{113} = 0.301 \text{ and } \hat{p}_2 = \frac{54}{139} = 0.388.$$

We may use these sample proportions, in accordance with statistical theory, to make inferences about the difference of these two population proportions.

—Renjin Tu

See also Confidence Interval; Hypothesis Testing; Inferential and Descriptive Statistics; Ratio

Further Readings

Johnson, R. A., & Bhattachayya, G. K. (2006). *Statistics principles and methods* (5th ed). Hoboken, NJ: Wiley.

Weiss, N. A. (2005). *Introductory statistics* (7th ed.). Boston: Addison-Wesley.

PSYCHIATRIC EPIDEMIOLOGY

Psychiatric epidemiology is the study of distribution, determinants, and causes of psychiatric conditions or mental health in human populations. The term *psychiatric epidemiology* was first coined at the 1949 Annual Conference of the Milbank Memorial Fund and was later documented in a Milbank Memorial Fund publication in 1950. Long before then, however, studies of mental health in populations had been conducted. Edward Jarvis, a mid-19th-century physician, described the distribution of "insanity" and "idiocy" and health care utilization in a wide range of facilities in Massachusetts from 1850 through 1855. This period marks the beginning of descriptive epidemiology where focused efforts were being made to describe disease distribution in the population. Not long after, psychiatric research began to use analytical epidemiology techniques as well. With methods still in use today, researchers examined hypotheses using various study designs, such as case-control and cohort studies, aimed to understand the nature, etiology, and prognosis of mental disorders.

Diagnosis

Psychiatric disorders include disturbances of thinking, such as schizophrenia, dementia, and mental retardation; disturbances of feeling, such as bipolar disorder, anxiety, and depression; and disturbances of acting, such as alcohol and drug disorders and antisocial disorders. Important childhood psychiatric disorders include autism, depression, and attention deficit disorders. Psychiatric disorders always involve biological or neurological adaptation of some sort and often include disruption of social life as well. These disorders are among the most disabling in the world, accounting for higher percentages of disability-adjusted life years than most other categories of disorder.

The diagnosis of psychiatric disorder is made almost totally on the basis of observed symptoms and behaviors because, to date, no biomarkers or laboratory tests are conclusive in diagnosis. The most commonly used diagnostic systems in psychiatry are the *Diagnostic and Statistical Manual of Mental Disorders* (*DSM*) and the International Classification of Diseases (ICD). Since its birth in 1952, DSM has been revised a number of times, with the most recent version being *DSM-IV*. *DSM-V* is expected in the near future. The number of psychiatric disorders listed increased from 159 in *DSM-II*, to 227 in *DSM-III*, to 357 in *DSM-IV*, and more are expected in *DSM-V*. The number of disorders has increased with revisions of the ICD also. As a result of the increasing numbers of diagnoses, as expected, the number of comorbid diagnoses also increased. This makes it more challenging to determine independent etiologies or measure an impact from a single disorder.

The use of standard criteria to define a mental disorder allows measurement of prevalence, related impairments, financial burden, and resulting mortality, and also makes it possible to compare these features across different regions, sex, and ethnic groups, as well as groups defined by other characteristics. But despite the many advances that have been accomplished in classifying mental disorders since the 1950s, case definitions are still controversial. Since the birth of the DSM and ICD, categorical diagnoses have been used for psychiatric disorders. However, many argue that mental disorders are best conceptualized as dimensional and that diagnostic thresholds may not be meaningful for etiologic determination. A categorical diagnostic decision is made depending on whether a patient meets or fails to meet a series of criteria, whereas a dimensional system acknowledges the continuum of symptom severity that may fall above or below a categorical diagnostic threshold. Most researchers suggest that for nosology (the systematic classification of diseases), the need for retaining categorical distinctions is compelling but that dimensional models may be more useful for clinical treatment, epidemiologic research, and policy development.

Psychiatric screening instruments have served the purpose of measuring symptoms and behaviors dimensionally. Historically, screening instruments were developed before diagnostic schedules/systems were established. Screening instruments are shorter and simpler and can be either filled out by participants themselves or by research staff with minimal training. On the other hand, structured or semistructured diagnostic schedules are more comprehensive in coverage of disorders, but more time-consuming, and require psychiatric professionals or trained interviewers to administer. For example, the Center for Epidemiologic Studies Depression Scale (CES-D), the most commonly used short screener for depression in the U.S. epidemiologic studies, consists of 20 items describing behaviors and feelings such as "I felt fearful" and "I talked less than usual" and takes about 5 to 10 min for most people to complete. A cutoff score of 16 was suggested by epidemiologic studies, meaning that a person whose score is greater than or equal to 16 is considered likely to be clinically depressed. In contrast, a diagnosis of major depressive disorder (MDD) using *DSM-IV* criteria requires a clinical evaluation and at least five of nine symptoms for 2 weeks or more, such as "A significantly reduced level of interest or pleasure in most or all activities" and "Behavior that is agitated or slowed down." Because prevalence of a psychiatric disorder (in this example, depression) is highly influenced by its definition, it is not surprising to see differences in CES-D-determined prevalence and *DSM-IV*-diagnosed prevalence.

Study Designs

Epidemiologic study designs developed to study infectious diseases and chronic diseases are frequently used in psychiatric epidemiologic studies. There are also hybrid studies that modify traditional designs and can be tailored to meet a specific study's needs. We describe below some common epidemiologic study designs frequently used in psychiatric epidemiologic studies, with particular focus on unique challenges in studying mental health using each design.

Incidence and Prevalence

Incidence and prevalence are measures of the extent of disorder in the population. Incidence is a measure of the occurrence of new cases per unit of time, and prevalence is the proportion of cases in the population at a defined time point. When depression is defined as a positive score on the CES-D, its prevalence will probably be higher for the same population than if depression were defined according to *DSM-IV* criteria for an MDD. This is because the CES-D taps a wider range of less severe symptoms. Comparisons of the incidence and prevalence of psychiatric disorders in different populations or geographic regions, require that studies use a consistent definition of depression. Other factors may also reflect the measured incidence and prevalence of depression, including, but not limited to, the awareness of the condition in a population, relative access to the health care system, and cultural acceptance of depressive symptoms.

Many persons with psychiatric disorders do not enter into treatment, and thus, population-based incidence and prevalence studies are preferred to clinic-based studies whenever feasible. In addition, population-based studies are more likely to detect a psychiatric condition (e.g., depressed mood) that has a wide spectrum and is common in a population. Individuals with such a condition might not be seen in clinical settings because the condition is so common and people might not be aware of the need for medical treatment, or the condition might be overshadowed by other more severe disorders.

Although measures of incidence are generally preferred over measures of prevalence in risk factor epidemiology, incidence can be difficult to measure for some psychiatric disorders, because many have an insidious onset. Therefore, it is often difficult to determine the precise time of onset and, consequently, what constitutes a new occurrence of disease. This is particularly true for disorders that begin as early as in utero (before birth). In such cases, prevalence rather than incidence is more commonly used as a measure of psychiatric disorders.

Cohort Studies

Cohort studies provide great potential to study the sequence of exposure and event/outcome, which is essential to determine causality, and allow researchers to investigate psychiatric comorbidities (e.g., MDD, anxiety symptoms, post-traumatic stress disorders) after an exposure of interest (e.g., traumatic stress). A *prospective cohort study* is most successful when the duration between exposure and detectable outcome is not exceedingly lengthy and the outcome is not a rare event (e.g., depression). Because cohort studies follow participants for a defined time period, an accurate exposure measure can be more easily obtained and is less likely to suffer from recall bias. However, the cost of a prospective study can be substantial because a large cohort and long-term follow-up may be necessary to observe sufficient cases of the disease. A *retrospective cohort design* is often used to study conditions that occur less frequently (e.g., schizophrenia) or when there is a lengthy lag between exposure and the event/outcome (e.g., early childhood exposure and dementia). Although the disorder can be determined at the current time point, making follow-up unnecessary, the accuracy of retrospective exposure measures can be problematic for reasons such as recall bias or missing information on exposure. Psychiatric disorders often have slow onset, over years and decades, which lead many psychiatric epidemiologists to favor the life course paradigm in epidemiology.

Case-Control Studies

Case-control studies are more efficient in terms of cost and time as compared with cohort studies, especially prospective cohort studies. The case-control design is frequently used in psychiatric epidemiologic research because many psychiatric disorders are uncommon in the population. A major challenge in implementing this study design is to select controls who come from the same source population as cases. Controls can come from a variety of sources, such as hospitals or the community. Often in psychiatric epidemiologic research, studies that use cases from a psychiatric clinic use controls from a primary care clinic. However, regardless of whether the source of controls is the clinic or community, it can be difficult to know whether controls come from the same source population as cases. Selection bias is an important threat to validity in case-control studies and can obscure the relationship between exposure and disease by introducing extraneous factors that influence this relationship.

There are ways in which selection bias can be reduced. One way is to use the same eligibility criteria for both groups and to treat both groups similarly. For example, cases should not be probed more than controls for exposure information. Another way is to adopt a nested case-control study strategy using an already existing cohort study. This way, cases and controls come from the same source population. However, a parent cohort study is not always available for a nested case-control study. A third example is to use more than one control group. Making comparisons with control groups that may have different sources of bias can aid in the interpretation of results and/or evaluate the extent of bias. If the results are similar for both groups, the investigator is more confident that the results are not affected by selection bias. If, however, they are different, the reasoning for the difference, potentially selection bias, should be explored. Recall bias is another important source of bias that can frequently occur when conducting case-control studies in psychiatric epidemiology. This is because many putative exposures have to be assessed by recall of the individual, or a relative of the individual, with the disorder. It is possible that such persons search their memories and work harder to "explain" a possible cause of their condition than do comparable controls who have no need of an explanation.

Cross-Sectional Studies

A study with a cross-sectional design collects outcome and exposure data at the same time point. Cross-sectional studies are relatively inexpensive and may often use a survey approach in which large numbers of people fill out questionnaires or answer simple questions regarding their mental health and other factors. A study with a cross-sectional design provides an opportunity to have a relatively large number of cases to better detect statistical differences. A major drawback to this approach is that the temporal relationship between exposure and outcome cannot be confidently determined because both measures are collected at the same time point. Another limitation is that survey approaches that depend on self-report measures of psychiatric disorders may be subject to many biases. For instance, persons with low income or low educational levels may be more likely to have an undiagnosed psychiatric condition, resulting in inaccurate reporting of psychiatric disorders, and thus introduce a confounding factor that may obscure the relationship between psychiatric disorders and the factors of interest to the researcher.

Randomized Controlled Trials (RCTs)

An RCT is an experimental study design in which study participants are randomly assigned to either a treatment or comparison group. An RCT is often used to evaluate treatment or intervention effect rather than to study disease etiology; however, its results can complement etiology studies and lend further credence to a hypothesis. Although the RCT is often considered the gold standard study design, there are drawbacks. One of these is that the eligibility criteria to participate in an RCT may be stringent, allowing only a select group of people into the study. For example, this may occur in treatment studies that exclude sicker people for potential safety reasons. Limiting study participation to select individuals does not, in itself, lead to invalid results but it can make them nongeneralizable to other populations. Similarly, results from an RCT study may not be generalizable to real-life situations because an RCT operates under ideal conditions, which will be unlikely to be repeated outside the trial, so that a treatment or intervention shown to be efficacious under ideal conditions may not prove to be effective when used in a community setting.

Multilevel Studies

Results from many psychiatric epidemiologic research studies have indicated that most psychiatric conditions have complicated causal pathways with risk factors from multiple levels. For environmental determinants, this multilevel hierarchy may include factors measured on many levels, including cellular, neurological, physiological, psychological, family, neighborhood, county, state, and national. Depression is a disorder that has risk factors at multiple levels. Risk factors at the individual level include genes, gender, age, neurotic temperament, and life event stressors; at the family level, risk factors include family history and family cohesion; while at the neighborhood level, risk factors may include community disorganization and economic deprivation. Evaluation of the contribution of factors at different levels requires use of multilevel modeling.

Multisite and Multinational Studies

There is a growing demand for studies involving multiple sites and multiple nations in psychiatric epidemiology because of the low incidence of many psychiatric conditions and the large sample size needed to provide sufficient statistical power for multilevel and multifactorial analyses. An example of a cross-national study is the World Mental Health 2000 Surveys recently conducted in 29 countries. Findings from this study provided important insights into the similarities and differences between psychiatric disorders across the world. However, studies implemented at this scale pose a number of challenges due to differences in administrative systems, cultures, and languages across nations.

Environmental and Genetic Factors

Most psychiatric disorders involve an inherited predisposition interacting with environmental exposures in complex ways. Autism, schizophrenia, and bipolar disorder have the strongest degrees of inheritance, while depression, anxiety disorders, and conduct disorders have moderate or small inherited factors. Environmental factors include prenatal complications, psychological experiences, physical conditions, neighborhood risk, life event stresses, social supports, or toxicant exposure. Although gene-environment interaction is a highly popular topic in psychiatric epidemiological research, only a few substantive findings have been reported. These include the interaction of perinatal risk factors with genetic risk exemplifying the neurodevelopmental model of schizophrenia, and genetic risk and the serotonin transport gene interacting with life stressors of one sort or another, exemplifying the diathesis-stress model for depression. This research is still in its infancy. No evident candidate genes have been identified for most psychiatric conditions, and measures for environmental exposures are still problematic. Furthermore, it can be challenging to define and distinguish whether an effect is genetically or environmentally based. For example, psychosocial events seem to have an influence on the prevalence of depression in a population. Although a psychosocial event, at face value, is an environmental risk factor, the means by which life events have an impact on depression may not be independent from genetically determined vulnerability. In fact, it may be that individuals "choose" and "create" their own environmental exposures due to their inherited genotype.

Age, Gender, and Culture

Age

Mental health should be studied with a life course approach that incorporates elements such as genetic risk, parental psychopathology, prenatal exposure or complications, socioeconomic status, and environmental and contextual factors. These elements consist of a causal pathway over the life span, with critical periods for disease susceptibility in some instances. These elements may also interact with early exposure and later risk/outcome on top of an individual's genetic predisposition. This can be seen in some childhood conditions and adult-onset disorders where subtle deviances are observed in early brain development, although the full adverse consequences are not manifest until later developmental stages. An example is autism spectrum disorders (ASD). Some young children with ASD do not show "full blown" symptoms until 3 or 4 years of age, but abnormalities in brain development and behaviors may have been present from infancy. Likewise, research has uncovered evidence that childhood motor, language, cognitive, emotional, and behavioral problems are precursors to adult-onset schizophrenia.

Gender

Epidemiologic research in the field of psychiatry has shown that gender is a crucial determinant of some mental disorders. Women have a higher prevalence of mood disorders, anxiety disorders, somatoform disorders, and nonaffective psychosis, while men have higher rates of substance use disorders and antisocial personality disorder. Evidence also suggests that women have higher prevalence of three or more comorbid psychiatric disorders than men. Gender differences in mental disorders are not only observed in adults, they are also seen in some childhood diagnoses. The male-to-female ratio is, approximately, 1.5:1 in mental retardation, 3:1 to 10:1 in ADHD (attention deficit/hyperactivity disorder), and 4:1 in autism spectrum disorders. Reasons suggested for the disparity between males and females include gender differences in exposure to risk factors, symptom reporting, symptom expression and severity, natural history of a disease, service utilization, comorbidity and disability, socioeconomic control and position, and gender stereotypes. Inclusion of gender-related perspectives into psychiatric epidemiological research has important implications for clinical practice and policy making.

Culture

Much effort has been put into developing universal diagnostic systems that set criteria for each psychiatric disorder; however, many culture-specific syndromes and conditions remain and are not classified in either *DSM* or ICD. There are more than two dozen culture-specific syndromes acknowledged and listed in *DSM-IV*, and these syndromes remain closely allied with culture and resist universal classification. For example, *locura* is a severe form of chronic psychosis seen in Latinos; *boufee delirante* is a brief delusional syndrome observed in West Africa and Haiti; and *Latah* is a startle-match-obey syndrome found in Southeast Asia. These culture-specific conditions presumably reflect basic human physiologic processes, constrained or precipitated by cultural contexts, and investigations on the effect of culture will improve our understanding of how environmental factors modify disease symptomatology.

Future Directions and Prospects

Through the application of epidemiologic methods, studies of psychiatric disorders have greatly contributed to informed mental health policies and improved prevention and treatment efforts. With advances in methodology and technology, the field of psychiatric epidemiology will continue to have a great impact on improving the quality of life for many people. One important aspect of more advanced research in future psychiatric epidemiology lies in the replacement of simple case-control comparison of groups with and without specified environmental exposures with more complex designs in which multilevel environmental exposures and genotypic variants may be ascertained and interactions between genetic and environmental risk factors may be investigated. A major challenge faced by today's psychiatric epidemiologists is to keep pace with advances in techniques available for measuring environmental risk factors, especially those that occur as early as before birth (e.g., preconception, prenatal). These challenges are amplified because new causal models need to address variables from various levels and perspectives in order to understand the complex nature of most forms of psychiatric disorders. Another challenge is that gene-environment interaction research is struggling to find well-established candidate genes for most psychiatric conditions, and there is a lack of firm conceptual frameworks for environmental exposures. Although knowledge on both genetic and environmental causal factors is still fragmentary, some progress has been made for a few psychiatric disorders. Most of the challenges described above can be overcome only if studies are not narrowed by disciplinary orientation. Epidemiology is essentially a collective science; therefore, a multidisciplinary research team that integrates expertise is essential in psychiatric epidemiologic research.

Successfully fighting mental diseases will require research in many disciplines, intervention on every level, and involvement across nations. Research needs to incorporate environmental factors, socioeconomic conditions, gender, culture, individual behaviors, biologic components, and molecular genetics. Interventions need to include social changes, individual behavior changes, and effective treatments and should have political support. Because psychiatric disorders impose a heavy burden on population health in many countries, the World Health Organization (WHO) has initiated collaborative work to lay the foundation to extend the use of instruments across diverse cultures and in different languages. One of the clearest messages is that the application of question and answer techniques can no longer be limited to North America and Europe; the perspective must be global, and the techniques need to be adapted for studies in all parts of the world.

—Li-Ching Lee, Rebecca Harrington,
and William W. Eaton

Note: Dr. William Eaton's effort on this work was supported by NIMH grant MH 47447.

See also Alzheimer's Disease; Anxiety Disorders; Autism; Bipolar Disorder; Gene-Environment Interaction; Life Course Approach; Multilevel Modeling; Post-Traumatic Stress Disorder; Schizophrenia; Study Design

Further Readings

American Psychiatric Association. (1994). *Diagnostic and statistical manual of mental disorders* (4th ed.). Washington, DC: Author.

Cannon, T. D., Mednick, S. A., & Parnas, J. (1989). Genetic and perinatal determinants of structural brain deficits in schizophrenia. *Archives of General Psychiatry, 46*(10), 883–889.

Caspi, A., Sugden, K., Moffitt, T. E., Taylor, A., Craig, I. W., Harrington, H., et al. (2003). Influence of life stress on depression: Moderation by a polymorphism in the 5-HTT gene. *Science, 301*(5631), 386–389.

Demyttenaere, K., Bruffaerts, R., Posada-Villa, J., Gasquet, I., Kovess, V., Lepine, J. P., et al. (for the WHO, World Mental Health Survey Consortium). (2004). Prevalence, severity, and unmet need for treatment of mental disorders in the World Health Organization World Mental Health Surveys. *Journal of the American Medical Association, 291*(21), 2581–2590.

Jarvis, E. (1971). *Insanity and idiocy in Massachusetts: Report of the commission on lunacy, 1855.* Cambridge, MA: Harvard University Press.

Kendler, K. S., Thornton, L. M., & Gardner, C. O. (2001). Genetic risk, number of previous depressive episodes, and stressful life events in predicting onset of major depression. *American Journal of Psychiatry, 158*(4), 582–586.

Kessler, R. C., Haro, J. M., Heeringa, S. G., Pennell, B. E., & Ustun, T. B. (2006). The World Health Organization World Mental Health Survey initiative. *Epidemiologia e Psichiatria Sociale, 15*(3), 161–166.

Susser, E., Schwartz, S., Morabia, A., & Bromet, E. J. (2006). *Psychiatric epidemiology: Searching for the causes of mental disorders.* New York: Oxford University Press.

Tsuang, M. T., & Tohen, M. (Eds.). (2002). *Textbook in psychiatric epidemiology* (2nd ed.). New York: Wiley.

World Health Organization. (1993). *The ICD-10 classification of mental and behavioural disorders: Diagnostic criteria for research.* Geneva, Switzerland: Author.

World Health Organization. (2001). *World health reports: Mental health new understanding, new hope.* Geneva, Switzerland: Author.

PUBLICATION BIAS

Publication bias can result from the selective publication of manuscripts based on the direction and magnitude of results, multiple publication of results, and selective reporting of results within a published study. In particular, research with statistically significant positive results is more likely to be submitted for publication, to be published, and to be published more quickly than research with negative or nonsignificant results. Consequently, published studies on a particular topic might not be representative of all valid studies conducted on the topic, leading to distortion of the scientific record.

Publication bias tends to be greater in clinical research than in public health research, and in observational studies as opposed to randomized studies. Nevertheless, it has been demonstrated across all these types of research. One area where a variety of publication biases have been documented is pharmaceutical industry studies of new drug applications.

The primary sources of publication bias are commonly assumed to be editorial decision making, together with authors' reluctance to submit research with null or negative results—sometimes referred to as the file drawer problem. While research has supported the latter explanation, studies of publication bias in editorial decision making have yielded mixed findings. Less well-recognized sources of publication bias include multiple publication of results and within-study selective reporting among multiple outcomes, exposures, subgroup analyses, and other multiplicities. Although these types of publication bias have until recently received little attention, they are likely to cause even greater bias in the literature than does selective publication.

Publication bias presents a serious threat to the validity of systematic reviews and meta-analyses. Undetected publication bias not only can lead to misleading conclusions but at the same time can also give the impression of unfounded precision of results. A screening method for selective-publication bias in meta-analysis involves correlating observed effect sizes with study design features that are potential risk factors for publication bias, such as sample size. A funnel plot provides an informal graphical method where effect sizes are plotted against sample sizes, while the null hypothesis of no publication bias can be tested using rank correlation approaches such as Kendall's tau or Spearman's rho. Detecting within-study selective reporting presents a greater challenge, unless access is available to a study's original protocol and complete results of all analyses performed.

Several strategies exist for reducing or adjusting for publication bias. *Sampling methods* involve tracking down unpublished manuscripts, sometimes referred to as the grey literature, as well as broader systemic solutions such as requiring prospective registration of clinical trials. *Analytic methods* include the file drawer adjustment strategy, where the number of zero-effect studies needed to eliminate significant findings in a meta-analysis is estimated. More complex analytic approaches involving weighted distribution theory are also available. All analytic methods involve important assumptions, which in many situations can be questionable. Perhaps most important, consumers of meta-analyses and systematic reviews are cautioned to be constructively skeptical in interpreting results.

—*Norman A. Constantine*

See also Evidence-Based Medicine; Meta-Analysis; Peer Review Process

Further Readings

Chan, A. W., Hrobjartsson, A., Haahr, M. T., Gotzsche, P. C., & Altman, D. G. (2004). Empirical evidence for selective reporting of outcomes in randomized trials: Comparison of protocols to published articles. *Journal of the American Medical Association, 291,* 2457–2465.

Easterbrook, P. J., Berlin, J. A., Gopalan, R., & Matthews, D. R. (1991). Publication bias in clinical research. *Lancet, 337,* 867–872.

Melander, H., Ahlqvist-Rastad, J., Meijer, G., & Beermann, B. (2003). Evidence b(i)ased medicine: Selective reporting from studies sponsored by pharmaceutical industry. *British Medical Journal, 326,* 1171–1173.

Phillips, C. V. (2004). Publication bias in situ. *BMC Medical Research Methodology, 4*(20).

Thornton, A., & Lee, P. (2000). Publication bias in meta-analysis: Its causes and consequences. *Journal of Clinical Epidemiology, 53,* 207–216.

PUBLIC HEALTH, HISTORY OF

Human concern with health dates back to the earliest writings and civilizations. Excavations of Mohenjo Daro and Harappa in the Indian subcontinent reveal bathrooms and drainage systems more than 4,000 years old. Hygiene is a vital component of many religions, governing the cultural and culinary traditions of numerous societies. In addition, people throughout history have considered illness, especially plagues, a judgment or punishment from god(s).

The great writers, philosophers, and physicians of ancient Greece tell us of the beginnings of public health. Hippocrates in "Airs, Waters and Places" distinguished between endemic and epidemic diseases and the factors affecting them, including climate, soil, water, mode of life, and nutrition. He also discussed the link between health and the environment, suggesting conditions to avoid and others to seek out in the interest of health.

The Romans continued the medical inquest of the Greeks and added to the administration of public health. Not only did they construct impressive baths and sewer systems, but aqueducts and water supply systems were carefully erected and monitored as well. There was a government position dedicated to the maintenance of the water supply and the supervision of public use and another office for oversight of the drainage system. Eventually, individuals also would be charged with assessment of the food supply.

Despite the impressive gains in sanitation made by both the Greeks and the Romans, many of the poorest citizens of both societies, including slaves, lived in deplorable conditions. City water and sewage systems typically did not extend into the poorer neighborhoods, leading to filthy living conditions and higher disease incidence. There is little in Greek literature relating to occupational health, but the Romans recognized increased disease frequency among slaves as well as workers in specific trades, such as miners, blacksmiths, and sulfur workers.

Greek physicians often treated the destitute and wealthy alike, and eventually Rome followed suit, implementing a publicly funded medical service in the second century BCE. In Greece, doctors had offices, but it seems hospitals—and certainly charity hospitals—originated in fourth century Rome.

The Middle Ages, bookended by the Plague of Justinian in 543 and the Black Death in 1348, was a time of frequent and profound epidemics. During these years, citizens lived rural lives within the narrow confines of a city, which often lacked reliable municipal water supplies and sewage disposal systems. Overcrowding was common, and livestock in addition to humans contributed to the waste. These cities generally lacked paved roads and drainage systems. Hygiene and health remained connected to religion, though medical care reverted to more pagan traditions and spiritual cleansings. Around 1200, cities throughout Europe began drafting laws to improve public health. Slaughterhouses were established and the possession of animals was regulated. Dumping waste into rivers was prohibited, roads were paved, and covered drainage systems were constructed. The market, the center of city life, became the impetus for food regulation as it was recognized as a common site for the origination of disease outbreaks. Isolation of patients with communicable diseases developed early in the Middle Ages in response to leprosy. In addition, laws required citizens to report others exhibiting symptoms of disease. The isolation premise extended to plague, and from it the segregation of ships coming into Venice's ports led to the term *quarantine* from the Italian *quarantenaria*, meaning 40 days.

The Renaissance brought great strides in scientific discovery, laying the groundwork for advances in public health. During the Renaissance, two theories on the origin of epidemics prevailed. The first, taken from Hippocrates, held that environmental factors dictated the potential for outbreaks and an individual's susceptibility determined whether he would fall ill. The opposing theory of contagion, championed by Giolamo Fracastoro (1478–1533), gave us our present understanding of infection. Fracastoro believed that microscopic agents were responsible for disease and these agents could be transmitted by direct contact, through the air, or by intermediate fomites (inanimate objects that transmit contagious disease). He and his contemporaries, however, did not imagine these infectious agents to be alive. It was not until Anton von Leeuwenhock (1632–1723) observed the first microscopic organisms that people believed this to be possible. And despite earlier conjecture by some leading scientists, the germ theory of disease did not truly take hold until the late 19th century.

As mercantilism and the conquest for wealth and power swept Europe from the 16th to the 18th centuries, public health was encapsulated in the national interest. The necessity to quantify people and their health became clear. William Petty (1623–1687) coined the term *political arithmetic* and advocated the collection of data on income, education, and health conditions. Gottfried Achenwall introduced the term *statistics* in 1749 to replace "political arithmetic." It was John Graunt (1620–1674), however, who published the first statistical analyses of a population's health, noting associations of a variety of demographic variables with disease. He recognized the imperfections in his data but worked to determine the reliability and errors in it. Graunt produced the first calculations of life expectancy. It was during this time that people began to recognize the need for state-supported programs to prevent early death and societal loss, yet it was not until the 19th century that government was able to enact a true national health plan, and even then, most public health measures continued to be administered locally.

As France led the world into the Enlightenment, public health began in earnest. A humanitarian spirit and the desire for equality led to a social understanding of health. Infant mortality was high on the list of concerns and disparities. The public health movement involved concerned citizens lobbying their government to regulate alcohol and to provide for the safe conditions and fair treatment of all infants and children, whether illegitimate, poor, or disabled. Simultaneously, health education became popular, in line with the Enlightenment tenets of universal education and information dissemination. Despite earlier interest in the relationship of environment, social factors, and disease, health surveys were first employed during this era. Occupational health received additional attention as well. John Howard (1726–1790) exposed the deplorable conditions in English prisons, rousing public sentiment that led to improved conditions. Mental illness, which carried a severe stigma and was generally treated by confining the affected individual, began to be viewed as a public health problem, especially after physicians demonstrated that kind treatment and a stable, nurturing environment produced better results in the insane than restraints and physical punishment.

Variolation (deliberate infection with smallpox), a common practice originating in China and spreading through the East over the centuries, became popular in the West in the 1700s. Although somewhat effective, the practice could induce severe forms of disease and contributed to epidemics. In 1798, Edward Jenner (1749–1823) used naturally acquired cowpox to inoculate others against smallpox. Within 3 years, more than 100,000 people had been vaccinated in England alone. As early as 1800, publications heralded the impending eradication of smallpox, an event that would be officially achieved in 1980.

As the Industrial Revolution spread, first in England then throughout Europe and eventually in the United States, the health of workers quickly deteriorated and calls for improved public health measures followed. The industrialization process widened gaps in income, causing the number of poor supported by local governments to increase beyond capacity. In 1834, Edwin Chadwick (1800–1890) led the development of England's Poor Law Amendment Act, which withdrew government support from the able-bodied poor in an effort to encourage self-sufficiency. The only assistance offered was placement in workhouses. The administration of this system occurred at the national level, with a hierarchy of regional and local boards below. This market system ideology mobilized the workforce, leading to a significant social change. Factories appeared and the population moved toward industrial centers, creating crowded urban areas and work conditions ripe for the spread of disease. Little, if any, city planning occurred as builders rushed to provide enough housing for the influx of workers. Meanwhile, the wealthy, who could afford transportation into the city, moved to suburban or rural areas vacated by the masses. Sanitation systems and public parks were not planned in most cities. Few toilets were available to city-dwellers, and there was no infrastructure for garbage or sewage removal. In 1833, the passage of the Factory Act dealt with working conditions, as well as the poor living conditions of those workers it sought to protect. Throughout the 1830s and 1840s, legislation regulating mines, factories, and child labor were passed in England and Europe.

Disease outbreaks certainly were associated with the poorest, dirtiest parts of cities, but quickly began to affect all social classes. Chadwick understood the poverty-disease cycle and sought statistics to quantify the relationship. Surveys on sanitary conditions resulted in the *Report ... on and Inquiry into the Sanitary Condition of the Laboring Population of Great Britain* in 1842. The *Report* became a standard for epidemiologic investigation and community health action, and it formed the basis for sanitary reform. Chadwick clearly linked disease and environment and called for city engineers rather than physicians to wage the war on disease outbreaks. The General Board of Health, created by the Public Health Act of 1848, was an attempt at organized government responsibility for the health of its citizens. Though disbanded after a few years, the Board laid the groundwork for public health as we know it. In the United States, Lemuel Shattuck (1793–1859) produced his own *Report on the Sanitary Condition of Massachusetts* in 1850, calling for the establishment of state and local boards of health, increased attention to vital statistics collection, improved health education, and other regulations not standard in his day but now considered part of the basic public health services.

The explosion of vital statistics and survey data collection prompted the publication of several volumes during the mid-1850s. Few, however, employed the same methods, citing the inapplicability of mathematics to health. Adolphe Quetelet (1796–1874) began the work necessary to remedy the perceived incompatibility with his compendium of practical applications of mathematics.

During a cholera outbreak in London in 1848, John Snow (1813–1858), often deemed the Father of Epidemiology, identified a particular water pump as the likely source of the epidemic. Again in 1854, he mapped the reported cholera deaths and associated the clusters with a water supply company that drew its supply downstream of London on the Thames River. Snow hypothesized that cholera transmission was possible through water. In addition, he is generally credited with ending the 1848 outbreak by breaking the handle off the Broad Street Pump, although some historians believed that the epidemic had already begun to recede by this point. It would be several decades, however, before his hypothesis was proven correct.

In 1866, the New York Metropolitan Health Bill created the Metropolitan Board of Health, reorganized 4 years later into what is today the New York City Health Department. This Board was the foundation for the U.S. public health system. In 1869, Massachusetts used Shattuck's recommendations to create the first effective state health department. Around the same time, efforts to create a National Board of Health failed. In 1878, the authority for port quarantine was bestowed on the Surgeon General of Marine Hospital Services. Eventually, this led to the creation of the U.S. Public Health Service (USPHS).

During the 19th century, two theories relating to communicable disease prevailed. The first was the miasma theory, which held that disease was due to a particular state of the air or environment. The second theory was that a specific contagion was responsible for each disease. In fact, many people believed that some combination of the two was the real explanation: that some contagious agent, whether disease-specific or not, produced disease in combination with social or environmental factors. By the end of the century, the germ theory of disease had been firmly established by Robert Koch, Louis Pasteur, and many others. From 1880 to 1898, the causative agents for a multitude of diseases, from malaria to tuberculosis, plague to typhoid, were identified. Antiseptics became popular in medical care, decreasing morbidity and mortality. Active and passive immunity were established late in the 19th century, and the development of vaccines proceeded nearly as rapidly as the discovery of pathogenic organisms. The U.S. Marine Hospital established one of the first bacteriologic laboratories in the world in 1887. Although the United States was not the site of most scientific discovery in the era, it was the leader in public health application of new knowledge.

Armed with increasingly more effective weapons against disease, public health's mission throughout most of the 20th century continued to be preventing and controlling communicable disease. Public health remained largely a local enterprise until the social change following the Depression, when people needed, and thus allowed, government intervention and subsidy. Throughout the 1900s public health achievements such as water fluoridation, mass immunizations, motor vehicle safety, occupational safety, food supply safety and fortification, improved maternal and child health, family planning, antismoking campaigns, prevention of heart disease and stroke, and of course, control of infectious diseases have led to substantially reduced morbidity and mortality. Public health has been credited with a 25-year increase in life span over the course of the 20th century. The establishment of agencies such as the Centers for Disease Control and Prevention in 1946 (born out of the Office of Malaria Control as the Communicable Disease Center—part of the USPHS) and the World Health Organization in 1948 (the United Nations' dedicated health agency) have allowed for the advancement of public health by establishing centralized agencies to which people can turn for information and assistance.

The definition of public health was also largely established during the 20th century by individuals such as C. E. A. Winslow and through groundbreaking works such as the series of reports by the Institute of Medicine (IOM) dedicated to the field. IOM's 1988 report *The Future of Public Health* clearly defined public health as "assuring conditions in which people can be healthy." It also delineated steps needed to improve a fractured public health infrastructure, and unequivocally determined the three core functions of public health: assessment, policy development, and assurance. In 2002, *Who Will Keep the Public Healthy* established requirements for the training of the public health workforce, and *The Future of the Public's Health in the 21st Century* translated the 1988 recommendations into practice while embracing the Healthy People 2010 initiative of "healthy people in healthy communities."

Public health continues to evolve, although some of the ancient concerns remain. At the dawn of the 21st century, when the industrialized world seemed to be close to conquering major infectious diseases, HIV/AIDS emerged as a deadly contagious disease with no known cure. It makes the infected person vulnerable to diseases not generally of concern to the uninfected population, such as pneumocystis pneumonia (pneumocystis carinii or PCP). Antibiotic resistance has also made the apparent victory over common infections less certain. High rates of nosocomial infections are disconcerting, and as in the field, the prevalence of antibiotic resistant organisms in hospitals is growing. Medical care and insurance in the United States continue to cost more than most people can afford, and as the population ages, the federal government will face increasing fiscal demands. Bioterrorism and natural disasters have required planning for mass immunization, prophylaxis, evacuation, and treatment.

The future of public health will be busy indeed, but the number of trained workers is increasing to meet the need. New schools of public health are being established, and undergraduates at some institutions can take coursework and complete degrees in public health. Strong partnerships between government, private, and nonprofit agencies exist, and public health on an international scale is becoming more integrated. Laboratory science continues to make discoveries that allow public health improvements in disease treatment and prevention, and as we continue to build our understanding of the human genome, the public health implications will continue to expand. Public health comes from a varied and tumultuous past, and its future lies in continuing to form interdisciplinary alliances while focusing on its core disciplines and functions to assure a continuity of practice in a world of change.

—*Erin L. DeFries*

See also Emerging Infections; Epidemiology, History of; Graunt, John; Snow, John

Further Readings

Rosen, G. (1993). *A history of public health.* Baltimore: Johns Hopkins University Press.
Turnock, B. J. (2004). *Public health: What it is and how it works* (3rd ed.). Sudbury, MA: Jones & Bartlett.

Web Sites

Centers for Disease Control, information and history: http://www.cdc.gov/od/oc/media/timeline.htm and http://www.cdc.gov/od/oc/media/tengpha.htm.
Institute of Medicine reports: http://www.iom.edu.
World Health Organization, information and history: http://www.who.int/about/en.

PUBLIC HEALTH AGENCY OF CANADA

The Public Health Agency of Canada (PHAC) was created in September 2004, after the SARS outbreak of 2003, due to concerns about the capacity of the Canadian public health system to anticipate and respond effectively to public health threats. The agency's role is to help build an effective public health system in Canada, which allows Canadians to achieve better health and well-being, while protecting them from threats to their health security. The PHAC has three main areas of responsibility: preventing and responding to outbreaks of infectious disease and other public health emergencies, preventing chronic disease and injury, and promoting good health.

The agency is directed by the Chief Public Health Officer, who reports to the Minister of Health. The Chief Public Health Officer fills a dual role of overseeing the daily operations of the PHAC and advising the Minister on public health matters. The agency is headquartered in Winnipeg and also has an office in Ottawa, as well as regional offices across Canada. Related organizations in the Canadian government's Health Portfolio include Health Canada, the Canadian Institutes of Health Research, and the Hazardous Materials Information Review Commission.

Due to the inherent difficulties in eliciting the requisite level of collaboration among federal, territorial, provincial, and local governments, the agency was specifically designed to encourage collaboration between these entities. All relevant stakeholders were included in the development of a national public health strategy, to serve as a framework for the agency's efforts. A new Pan-Canadian Public Health Network was established in 2005 to formalize communication links between public health experts and officials from all jurisdictions and to facilitate a nationwide approach to public health policy, planning, and implementation.

The PHAC has a mandate to lead federal efforts and mobilize action throughout Canada to prevent disease and injury, and to promote and protect national and international public health, through the following activities:

1. Anticipate, prepare for, respond to, and recover from threats to public health.

2. Carry out surveillance; monitor, research, investigate, and report on diseases, injuries, other preventable health risks and their determinants, and the general state of public health in Canada and internationally.

3. Use the best available evidence and tools to advise and support public health stakeholders nationally and internationally in their work to enhance the health of their communities.

4. Provide public health information, advice, and leadership.

5. Build and sustain a public health network with stakeholders.

The Public Health Agency of Canada publishes annual performance reports, and annual reports on plans and priorities; these are available on the Web site.

Organizational Structure

The PHAC has four main branches; each of the branches includes several agencies and centers. The branches are organized as follows.

Infectious Disease and Emergency Preparedness (IDEP) Branch

1. The Centre for Infectious Disease Prevention and Control is responsible for decreasing the transmission of infectious diseases and improving the health status of those infected via programs in surveillance and risk assessment. Program areas include the following: foodborne, zoonotic, and environmentally acquired infections; immunization; respiratory infections; community acquired infections (hepatitis C, sexually transmitted infections, and tuberculosis); blood safety surveillance and health care acquired infections; HIV/AIDS.

2. The Centre for Emergency Preparedness and Response (CEPR) is Canada's central coordinating point for public health security. Its responsibilities include developing and maintaining national emergency response plans for the Agency, monitoring outbreaks and global disease events, assessing public health risks during emergencies, laboratory safety and security, quarantine issues and travel health advisories, and bioterrorism and emergency health services.

3. The National Microbiology Laboratory (NML) consists of four programs, supported by a Division of Core Services, which includes DNA sequencing, Animal Resources, and a Central Laboratory for Decontamination and Wash-up Services. The four programs are as follows:

- Bacteriology and Enterics, focusing on bacterial diseases such as tuberculosis and meningitis, food- and waterborne pathogens, and infections affecting the nervous system
- Host Genetics and Prion Disease, dealing with transmissible spongiform encephalopathies

- Viral Diagnostics, for a range of viral diseases
- Zoonotic Diseases and Special Pathogens, dealing with viral, bacterial, and rickettsial diseases transmitted to humans from other species

4. The Laboratory for Foodborne Zoonoses (LFZ) provides scientific evidence and advice on human illnesses that arise from the interface between humans, animals, and the environment, with emphasis on intestinal-disease-causing agents.

5. The Pandemic Preparedness Secretariat (PPS) was established in March 2006 to coordinate and facilitate pandemic preparedness and response activities nationwide and internationally, such as those related to avian and pandemic influenza.

Health Promotion and Chronic Disease Prevention (HPCDP) Branch

1. The Centre for Chronic Disease Prevention and Control (CCDPC). The activities of CCDPC focus on facilitating the development of prevention, screening, and early detection programs for chronic diseases; providing project funding to community and support groups; developing national strategies for the management and control of chronic diseases; maintaining an integrated surveillance system to assist in developing chronic disease policy; providing a stimulus for international links in the area of chronic disease prevention and control.

2. The Centre for Health Promotion (CHP) is responsible for implementing policies and programs that enhance the conditions within which healthy development occurs. Programs include healthy child development, active living, families, aging, lifestyles, public information, education, and issues related to rural health.

3. The Transfer Payment Services and Accountability Division promotes excellence in management practices via initiatives on performance measurement and evaluation and the management of grants and contributions. It manages the Population Health Fund and provides administrative services for several grants and funding programs.

Public Health Practice and Regional Operations (PHPRO) Branch

The Office of Public Health Practice (OPHP) was created to support and improve the public health infrastructure necessary for effective public health practice. Its priority issues are information and knowledge systems, the public health workforce, and public health law and information policy. Regional offices throughout Canada carry out the Agency's mandate by engaging in program delivery, research, policy analysis, community capacity building, and public and professional education.

Strategic Policy, Communications, and Corporate Services (SPCCS) Branch

The Strategic Policy Directorate gathers and synthesizes key policy information, cultivates partnerships, and provides evidence-based policy advice. The branch also includes the Communications Directorate, the Finance and Administration Directorate, the Human Resources Directorate, the Information Management and Information Technology Directorate, and the Audit Services Division.

—*Judith Marie Bezy*

See also Bioterrorism; Centers for Disease Control and Prevention; Governmental Role in Public Health; Public Health Surveillance; U.S. Public Health Service

Further Readings

Public Health Agency of Canada. (2005). *Performance report for the period ending March 31, 2005* (BT31-4/98-2005). Ottawa, Ontario, Canada: Canadian Government Publishing.

Public Health Agency of Canada. (2006, September 26). *Report on plans and priorities 2006–2007*. Retrieved July 24, 2007, from http://www.tbs-sct.gc.ca/rpp/0607/phac-aspc/phac-aspc_e.asp.

Wilson, K. (2004). A Canadian agency for public health: Could it work? *Canadian Medical Association Journal, 170*(2), 222–223.

Web Sites

Public Health Agency of Canada: http://www.phac-aspc.gc.ca.

PUBLIC HEALTH NURSING

Public health nursing is a specialty within nursing whose primary focus is on the health care of communities and populations rather than individuals, families, or groups. The goal of public health nursing is to prevent disease and preserve, promote, and protect health for the community, a focus that allies it closely with the concerns of epidemiology and public health in general. This entry reviews the history of public health nursing and describes the varied settings and functions of work by public health nurses.

The primary emphasis in public health nursing is on populations that live in the community, as opposed to individuals or families. In public health nursing, problems are defined (assessments/diagnoses) and solutions (interventions) implemented for or within a defined population or subpopulation as opposed to diagnoses, interventions, and treatments carried out at the individual level.

In contrast, community-based nursing is setting specific, whereby care is provided for "sick" individuals and families where they live, work, and attend school. Emphasis is on acute and chronic care and the provision of comprehensive, coordinated, and continuous care. Nurses who work in the community may be generalists or specialists in adult, geriatric, pediatric, maternal-child, or psychiatric mental health nursing. Community health nursing practice focuses on the health of individuals, families, and groups and how their health status affects the community.

History

Public health nursing evolved in the United States in the late 19th and early 20th centuries. Lillian Wald emerged as a leader in the field because of her pioneering work in public health nursing in New York City. Growing up in Rochester, New York, Wald worked as a nurse tending to immigrant families on the Lower East Side of New York. Her experiences provided evidence that many injustices existed in society with differences in health care for those individuals who were able to pay for care versus those who were poor and unable to pay. Wald could not tolerate situations where poor people had no access to health care. With the support of others, Wald moved to the Lower East Side of New York and began campaigning for health-promoting social policies to improve environmental and social conditions affecting health. As author of *The House on Henry Street*, Wald described her work as a public health nurse as well as the development of payment by life insurance companies for nursing services. The Henry Street Settlement, established in New York City, is an example of a settlement house or neighborhood center that serves as a center for health care and social welfare programs. At Henry Street Settlement, nurses took care of the sick in their homes and tended to the overall population of low-income people in the community. Wald believed that the beginning efforts at Henry Street Settlement needed to be associated with an official health agency. The establishment of rural health nursing services through the American Red Cross was led by Wald, and it addressed public health issues such as tuberculosis, pneumonia, and typhoid fever in areas outside large cities.

Public health nursing was recognized as a legitimate specialty within public health early in the development of the profession and remains an important part of public health practice today. In 1872, the American Public Health Association (APHA) was established to facilitate interdisciplinary efforts and promote the practice of public hygiene. In 1923, the Public Health Nursing Section was formed within APHA to provide a national forum for discussion of strategies for public health nurses within the context of the larger public health organization. By 1981, APHA affirmed the importance of public health nursing and defined it as a specialty that brings together knowledge from the public health sciences and nursing to improve the health of the community.

The Work of Public Health Nurses

A variety of settings and a diversity of perspectives are available to nurses interested in working in public health. Nurses employed at local, state, and federal agencies integrate community involvement and knowledge about populations with a clinical understanding of the health and illness experiences of individuals and families in the population. Nurses work in partnership with other public health staff that include physicians, nutritionists, health educators, epidemiologists, and outreach workers.

The work of public health nursing includes population-based assessment, policy development, and assurance processes that are systematic and comprehensive. Regardless of setting, the role of the public health nurse focuses on the prevention of illness, injury, or disability, and on the promotion and maintenance of the health of populations. Examples of what public health nurses can accomplish include providing preventive services to high-risk populations; establishing programs and services to meet

special needs; recommending clinical care and other services to individuals and their families in clinics, homes, and the community; providing referrals through community links; participating in community provider coalitions and meetings to educate others and identify service center for community populations; and providing clinical surveillance and identification of communicable disease.

—*James A. Fain*

See also American Public Health Association; Community Health; Health Care Delivery; Health Disparities; Public Health, History of

Further Readings

American Public Health Association. (1981). *The definition and role of public health nursing in the delivery of health care: A statement of the public health nursing section.* Washington, DC: Author.
Backer, B. A. (1993). Lillian Wald: Connecting caring with action. *Nursing & Health Care, 14,* 122–128.
Stanhope, M., & Lancaster, J. (2006). *Foundations of nursing in the community: Community-oriented practice.* St. Louis, MO: Mosby Elsevier.

PUBLIC HEALTH SURVEILLANCE

Effective public health practice relies on current, relevant information on which to base actions. The information base that serves this core function is called public health surveillance—it is often called information for action. This entry describes the development of public health surveillance as well as information about some surveillance systems themselves.

History

Although the use of information in health decision making can be found as early as Hippocrates, the modern origins of public health surveillance are usually dated to the late 18th century by which time there were organized health authorities and an accepted classification system of diseases. William Farr's analysis of death certificates in England and Wales in the mid-19th century is recognized as one of the first functional surveillance systems. In the United States, as elsewhere, there was growing application of surveillance tools to infectious disease. In colonial times,

Rhode Island required innkeepers to report what we now know to be infectious diseases, and shortly thereafter reporting of cholera, yellow fever, and smallpox was codified. It was only in 1850 that national reporting of deaths was required in the United States, and it was not until 1874 that Massachusetts created a voluntary communicable disease reporting system using postcards submitted by physicians. Michigan initiated compulsory reporting in 1881. Voluntary national reporting of communicable diseases followed, but it was only after the influenza pandemic of 1918 to 1919 that all states began reporting. It is worth noting that to this day, with the exception of conditions required by international treaty (cholera, smallpox, plague, and yellow fever), reporting by states remains voluntary since the Constitution does not delegate authority over health to the federal government. Since 1961, these data have been published weekly by the Centers for Disease Control and Prevention, a federal agency, in the *Morbidity and Mortality Weekly Report* (MMWR).

Early surveillance systems monitored illness in individuals. A major conceptual shift occurred in the context of the first widespread vaccination campaign for polio (poliomyelitis). States reported small number of cases of polio among patients who received the new vaccine. Very rapidly a system for daily reporting of cases was established with rapid follow-up of cases. This led to identification of a single lot of vaccine contaminated with live virus as the source of the cases. This lot was removed from the market, and the vaccination program was able to continue. A potentially devastating disaster had been averted. Here was a clear demonstration of the value of surveillance. Alexander Langmuir led the movement to evolve the concept from monitoring disease in individuals to monitoring the health of populations and established the current definition of surveillance as the ongoing collection, analysis, and dissemination of those who need the information to take action.

In response to public health's attention to a broader range of health conditions and determinants, contemporary public health surveillance systems now embrace a broad array of health conditions, including behavioral risk factors, chronic disease, intentional and unintentional injuries, worksite diseases and injuries, birth defects, medical safety, adverse effect of drugs and vaccines, and quality of health care.

Uses of Surveillance Systems

Surveillance systems are intrinsically action oriented. Although they may capitalize on a variety of data systems, they differ from those data systems in having specific purposes that warrant their ongoing use. Surveillance systems measure health outcomes, such as cases of influenza, or important markers of health outcomes that drive programmatic action, such as obesity or tobacco smoking. This information can be used to detect outbreaks of disease or epidemics; understand the burden of disease; facilitate planning and resource allocation; understand the natural history of diseases and injuries and who in the population is affected; evaluate the impact of public health programs; and monitor changes in infectious organisms, such as antibiotic resistance.

Characteristics of Surveillance Systems

Public health resources are always limited, so surveillance systems are targeted at public health issues based on a number of factors. The public health burden of the condition or the potential public health burden should be substantial based on mortality, frequency, severity, and economic impact. In addition, the condition should be preventable or controllable.

Case definitions are specific criteria used to report and count cases. Case definitions may be straightforward, such as death from diabetes as reported on a death certificate, or based on a set of symptoms as used in syndromic surveillance, or combinations of clinical signs, symptoms, and laboratory data as is often the case for infectious diseases. Case definitions may not accurately capture all cases, but the sensitivity (the degree to which cases are identified) and specificity (the degree to which noncases are not included) need to be known so that the reliability of the data is fully understood. For example, although deaths among people with diabetes may be counted based on death certificates, it is important to realize that approximately half of the people with diabetes who die do not have diabetes recorded on their death certificates. By the same token, using symptoms of influenza will capture many cases that are actually due to other diseases. Thus, laboratory confirmation of at least a subset of cases is important to establish the type of influenza as well as the proportion of influenza-like illness actually due to influenza.

The timeliness required may vary widely. For many infectious diseases, interventions are needed rapidly because of the need to identify outbreaks and prevent further spread. For influenza, several different strategies have emerged to meet the varying surveillance needs. Thus, absence from school is a good measure of the scope of disease, since it is by far the most common reason for large-scale absenteeism during the influenza season. Sentinel physicians are used to identify early cases and to provide specimens for identification of the specific virus. A system that reports pneumonia and influenza deaths weekly from most large cities provides a measure of severity and is also used to assess when influenza exceeds expected rates. All these provide information very rapidly. For many conditions, however, daily, weekly, or even monthly surveillance would be excessive, since rates do not change rapidly. Thus, for many chronic diseases or risk factors, surveillance is conducted at less frequent intervals, often annually.

The data for surveillance may come from case reports provided directly to health departments, from surveys (e.g., the Behavioral Risk Factor Surveillance System), vital records (birth and death certificates), administrative data (e.g., medical claims data), or other sources. Data need to be collected at a sufficient level of detail to meet the public health need, but since there is usually a trade-off between feasibility and detail, efforts are made to keep the data requirements to a minimum. In addition to the condition, basic descriptors of person (age, race, sex) and place are usually collected. Additional information is often needed to provide understanding of risk characteristics to facilitate public health action. Active surveillance systems involve solicited, direct collection of data, whereas passive systems rely on spontaneous reporting. Surveillance of infectious diseases is typically achieved through passive reporting.

Tabulation and analysis of the data need to be completed in a regular and timely fashion, usually with a core set of basic descriptive analyses. More detailed analyses are conducted as needed. Descriptive analyses usually include counts of cases or events based on person (age, race, and sex of cases), location (e.g., by state or county), and time (e.g., by date or trends in number of cases over time).

The results are provided to those who need to act on the results. To facilitate this process, interpretation is often provided along with the analyses themselves. Users of surveillance information are diverse. National, state, and local health departments are the traditional users, but there are many others. For example, infectious disease practitioners rely on antimicrobial resistance patterns in their hospitals in making antibiotic choices; the Food and Drug Administration monitors safety of drugs, biologics, and devices; employers may use surveillance of the quality of managed care organizations, for example, HEDIS (Healthcare Effectiveness Data and Information Set), in making decisions about selection of health insurance plans to offer employees; and cancer researchers may use information about cancer survival trends to generate research hypotheses.

Public health surveillance serves as the nervous system for public health, providing the information to guide action. It is a dynamic process, responding to the changing needs of society and public health. Unlike most research-generated data, surveillance systems must be highly efficient and the strengths and limitations of the data must be well understood so that users can respond appropriately. Modern information systems should enhance the capacity of public health surveillance to meet future demands.

—Steven Teutsch

See also Behavioral Risk Factor Surveillance System; Birth Certificate; Centers for Disease Control and Prevention; Death Certificate; Governmental Role in Public Health

Further Readings

Centers for Disease Control and Prevention. (2001). Updated guidelines for evaluating surveillance systems: Recommendations from the guidelines working group. *Morbidity and Mortality Weekly Report, 50*(RR13), 1–35.

Teutsch, S. M., & Churchill, R. E. (Eds.). (2000). *Principles and practice of public health surveillance* (2nd ed.). New York: Oxford University Press.

p VALUE

A *p* value expresses the probability that a given statistical result is due to chance. *p* Values are automatically produced for many statistical procedures by analysis packages such as SAS, SPSS, and Stata, and they are commonly cited in epidemiological and medical research as evidence that results should be considered significant. For instance, a clinical trial concerning the effect of two different drugs on a medical outcome would almost certainly cite one or more *p* values as evidence of the influence, or lack thereof, of the drugs on the outcome. In the example above, perhaps we would expect that if the two drugs are no different in their effect, we would expect the outcome to be the same in each group. Therefore, we would expect the difference between the two groups to be zero, and would be interested in determining whether the actual difference we found could be attributed to chance or whether it is likely to indicate true difference between the groups.

Generally speaking, the greater the difference between the expected and observed results, the smaller the *p* value and, therefore, the less likely it is that the difference is due to chance (random variation). As the likelihood of chance explaining the difference diminishes, so does its plausibility—giving way to an alternative explanation: that the difference is not due to chance, the difference is due to the expected value being wrong.

We will illustrate the concept of *p* value using the simple example of 10 tosses of a coin. Without saying more, it is reasonable to believe the coin is fair: There is an equal chance of either heads or tails on each toss. Following this line of reasoning, it is logical to expect 5 heads from 10 tosses, so the *expected value* of heads is 5. On 10 tosses, however, a variety of outcomes are not at all remarkable. For example, 6 heads (H) and 4 tails (T); 5H and 5T; 4H and 6T do not surprise or call into question the reasonable presumption of a fair coin. Further departures from the 5H and 5T, however, credibly cause doubt, increasing doubt with increasing departure.

Consider the result 8H and 2T. Such an outcome is not expected and causes doubt about the fairness of the coin (or process). Certainly, chance could have produced the outcome, but it is unlikely. The *p* value is the measure of that chance. The probability that such a result is due to chance is derived from the binomial distribution and is .0439. This calculation assumes that the coin is fair, that is, that the probability of heads on each toss is .5. Therefore, the *p* value calculation is a conditional probability with the condition being that the expected value is true. Such an assumption is important since we are determining the probability of the observed difference (departure) from the expected value if the expected value was correct in the first place.

In statistics, we are usually concerned with the probability not of achieving a particular result but of obtaining results at least as extreme as our result. In our example, the expected result is 5H and 5T, so we consider deviations from that expectation to be more extreme as they are less likely. So 9H and 1T is even less likely than 8H and 2T (the probability of 9H and 1T, given a fair coin, is .0098), and 10H and 0T is yet more extreme (with a probability of .0010). To calculate the probability of a result at least as extreme as 8T and 2H, we add together these probabilities: .0439 + .0098 + .0010 + .0547.

A final comment to this illustration: The calculation of .0547 is based on a one-sided *p* value. In other words, it only considers the probability of getting 8 or more heads in 10 tosses of a fair coin and ignores the probability of getting 8 or more tails, which would be equally as extreme. If we would consider a deviation toward either more heads or more tails to be a significant result, then the *p* value should be a two-sided calculation incorporating all the outcomes consistent with observation. In our illustration, the set of outcomes would number six: 10H and 0T; 9H and 1T; 8H and 2T; 2H and 8T; 1H and 9T; 0H and 10T. The probability would be the sum of these six independent outcomes: .0010 + .0098 + .0439 + .0439 + .0098 + .0010 = .1094. (The fact that this is exactly two times the one-sided *p* value is because the binomial distribution is symmetrical when the probability of a success is .5, the expected probability of an H when assuming a fair coin.) Thus, there is approximately 11% chance (.1094) that 10 fair tosses of a fair coin would produce any one of the six "extreme" values: 10H and 0T; 9H and 1T; 8H and 2T; 2H and 8T; 1H and 9T; 0H and 10T.

The *p* value can be calculated for any difference between an observed and an expected value provided that the probability distribution is known. Modern statistical analysis software calculates *p* values automatically for many different types of statistical tests, and *p* values are typically reported in epidemiological literature.

p Values are excellent metrics if properly used, because they incorporate information about sample size, sampling variation, and differences from expectation into one convenient number yielding a measure of chance for observations differing from expectations.

For example, if an epidemiologist is studying whether a suspected risk factor is associated with a disease, he or she may derive an odds ratio (for a case-control study) or a relative risk or risk ratio (*RR*, for a cohort study) for the risk factor. Until sufficient evidence indicates otherwise, the epidemiologist will assume an expected value of 1.00: that there is no increased (or decreased) risk of the disease with exposure to the risk factor. After collecting data from his cohort study, however, he discovers a *RR* of 1.25, which indicates a slightly elevated risk of the disease for those exposed to the risk factor. This of course could simply be chance. Let us assume that the correct *p* value calculation based on the probability distribution of a *RR* produces a value of .04. This result is a one-sided *p* value consistent with the epidemiologist's suspicion that the risk factor was harmful (antagonistic) rather than protective. Had he suspected an effect, but with no expectation toward a protective or antagonistic effect, he may advocate the use of a two-sided *p* value.

The value .04 takes into account the sample size, the probability distribution of *RR*, and the variability of the observations recorded from the cohort study. Taken together, this evidence suggests that if there is no effect from the risk factor in truth, then there is only a 4% ($p = .04$) chance of obtaining a *RR* of 1.25 or higher for a randomly selected data set of the same size from this cohort.

In practice, this simply means that it is unlikely that the $RR = 1.25$ is due to chance. Therefore, a more plausible explanation for the departure from $RR = 1.00$ is that the risk factor is actually associated with the disease. Typically, when a *p* value is less than .05, an epidemiologist will set aside chance as the explanation in favor of a real association. The value of .05 is based on a long history of scientific precedent memorialized in the concept of Type I error and its presumptive measure, $\alpha = .05$. As a formal rule, when the *p* value is less than α, then reject the null hypothesis (usually the expected value). Otherwise, the null hypothesis is tenable.

Because the *p* value is a practical metric summarizing much of the evidence and avoids the formal language of hypothesis testing, it is a popular way to report results. Unfortunately, the *p* value is taken to be more than what it actually is. One problem is that the *p* value may be heavily influenced by sample size: It is a truism in epidemiology that if you have a large enough sample you will likely find significant results. For this reason, a distinction is often made between statistical and clinical significance—that is, between a difference that is merely improbable in a statistical sense versus one that is large enough to make a difference in a person's health. For the same reason, some journals require the presentation of confidence intervals, which give an indication of the magnitude of differences found. Second, a *p* value is purely a statistical calculation, and its usefulness is limited to reliability and has no bearing on validity.

—*Mark Gerard Haug*

See also Confidence Interval; Significance Testing; Type I and Type II Errors

Further Readings

Gigerenzer, G., Krauss, S., & Vitouch, O. (2004). The null ritual: What you always wanted to know about significance testing but were afraid to ask. In D. Kaplan (Ed.), *The Sage handbook of quantitative methodology for the social sciences* (pp. 391–408). Thousand Oaks, CA: Sage.

Poole, C. (2001). Low *p*-values or narrow confidence intervals: Which are more durable? *Epidemiology, 12*, 291–294.

Sheskin, D. J. (1997). *Handbook of parametric and nonparametric statistical procedures*. Boca Raton, FL: CRC Press.

Tietjen, G. L. (1986). *A topical dictionary of statistics*. London: Chapman & Hall.

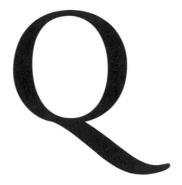

QUALITATIVE METHODS IN EPIDEMIOLOGY

Qualitative methods (QM) are used to explore a wide range of experiences in epidemiology and public health. These methods examine the depths of experience to identify why or how complex events happen, and they are particularly useful for exploring new and complicated topics. Characteristics of QM studies generally include field contact and are intended to provide a holistic perspective. If an estimate of the magnitude of a problem is needed, QM will not be useful. Generalizability from the purposive sample (which samples the topic of interest) to the general population is not a goal of QM research.

The goals of QM are usually exploratory and descriptive, with the aim of understanding and describing a phenomenon and focusing on perceptions of the "lived experience" from the perspective of the research respondent. For example, after determining whether or how well a prevention program works using quantitative methods, a researcher may turn to QM to examine how the program works and what aspects of the program the research participants and the staff believe are and are not working. A QM approach is particularly necessary in participatory research, where giving voice to vulnerable populations is often a particular concern.

QM approaches are derived from various philosophies that inform each of the steps in the research process: framing the research purpose, collecting data, analyzing, and interpreting. Data are generally collected using interviews, focus groups, existing documents, and observation. The most common methods of QM are grounded theory, phenomenology, ethnography, and case study, with the latter two using quantitative data in addition to qualitative data.

Grounded theory examines a process, usually a psychosocial process of change such as adapting to a new diagnosis of a health problem. A first sample of data is collected using "purposive sampling," which refers to sampling to cover the topic of interest. Next, an initial analysis is done, and it then informs the further collection of data, which is followed by analysis of the new data. This process is called "constant comparison." When new data yield no additional information, "data saturation" has been reached, and data collection stops. Analysis involves coding the meaning for each segment of the document, aggregating the codes into themes and then, usually, formulating a core category. The context, conditions, covariances, and consequences are explored in formulating how the core category relates all the themes together. Symbolic interaction theory informs this approach.

Phenomenology focuses on the essential core meaning of a phenomenon, with primary importance given to the social meanings people ascribe to the phenomenon. Recognizing that interpretation is an intermediate step between recognition and behavior, the researcher uses reflective description and meditation to identify the essence. Models or theories are not the goal of this approach. This approach arose from the philosophical traditions of Edmund Husserl and Martin Heidegger.

Ethnography aims to describe a group or a culture, focusing on the routines and usual lives of the people as observed in behaviors and information from records. As with the other QM, ethnography emphasizes a holistic perspective, the multiple realities of the different respondents, and the embeddedness of data in the specific context. Structure and function, symbol and ritual, and micro- and macrolevels of data are concepts that guide this approach. Analysis often involves identification of patterns of thoughts and actions, making flowcharts of major concepts, and the use of simple nonparametric statistics and scales.

Case study is an approach that first establishes bounds for a unit such as a school or a health system. A thorough description is produced of the activities in the actual setting(s) using multiple sources of information rich in social, historical, and economical context. A single case would be of interest because it belongs to a set of cases or is exceptional in some way that is of interest. Issues are selected to help focus the data collection. Patterns and conclusions are developed.

Recently, more attention has been given to the advantages of combining QM with quantitative methods, sometimes called "mixed methods" or "integrated methods." The techniques need to be planned to support each other, either sequentially or concurrently. For a new area of study, a common process is to use focus groups or interviews to identify the domains and the natural vocabulary needed in questionnaire development. QM can be used along with questionnaires to expand, explain, or reinforce the quantitative results.

To be useful, research must be credible and be perceived as appropriately rigorous, whether it is descriptive or posits a causal model. The concepts of reliability and validity are not applied in QM as they usually are in quantitative studies. Rigor of the results has been examined in terms of credibility, transferability, dependability, and confirmability. More recently, some attention has been focused on the research process to ensure rigor. Verification involves checking data, confirming the data links to theory or themes, inclusion of a clear audit trail, and the logic connection between purpose (goal), process (sampling and analysis), and product (knowledge).

Ethical issues are of primary concern in QM, which often involve close contact with research participants. It is important to plan for "leaving the field"; respondents may have considered the researcher a confidant,

and they will need closure. In focus groups, the researcher cannot guarantee that the group members will maintain the conversation in confidence. Also, in a group setting, a member may disclose more than he or she intended to; the group leader needs to carefully monitor to prevent this occurrence.

Computer programs can assist with the organization of data files and can reduce some burden for the researcher. For medium to large projects, any of the several available are worth becoming familiar with. Quantitative data, such as demographics and videos, can also be linked to the qualitative data for analysis.

—*Martha Ann Carey*

See also Community-Based Participatory Research; Ethics in Human Subjects Research; Interview Techniques; Measurement; Survey Research Methods

Further Readings

Glaser, B., & Strauss, A. (1967). *The discovery of grounded theory: Strategies for qualitatve research.* Chicago: Aldine.

Miles, M., & Huberman, M. (1994). *Qualitative data analysis: An expanded handbook* (2nd ed.). Thousand Oaks, CA: Sage.

Morse, J., & Field, P. (1995). *Qualitative research methods for health professionals* (2nd ed.). Thousand Oaks, CA: Sage.

QUALITY OF LIFE, QUANTIFICATION OF

The term *quality of life*, as used in health research and policy, refers primarily to the quantification of the cost of being in a less-than-perfect health state. Such quantification is motivated largely by economic analyses, which require comparison of all costs and benefits of a policy or situation, including not only mortality and resource costs but also morbidity. Without such quantification, it is impossible to assess the net benefits of policies that affect health or to make formal analyses comparing the costs and benefits of different treatments. Various methods exist for eliciting quality of life quantifications and calculating quality-adjusted life years (QALYs). However, all of them have major drawbacks, and thus while it is always possible to generate the needed numbers, it is difficult to defend them as accurate in most contexts.

Quality of life is a concept that permeates modern and ancient philosophy. It invokes two interrelated but fundamentally different meanings, creating some practical confusion. One sense of the term captures concepts related to happiness, satisfaction, and freedom from pain, while another refers to the worthiness of people's lives. In modern health science, researchers are interested in the former concerns, and particularly with assigning cardinal values to different states of well-being. However, subtle influences of the latter interpretation sometimes confuse measures and understanding.

In the post-Enlightenment world, where everyone's life is considered to have worth and everyone's well-being is considered a legitimate concern, there is near universal agreement that improving people's quality of life is a worthwhile endeavor. Making people happy (comfortable, functional), and not just long-lived, is seen as a goal of health care, health policy, and health research.

The motivation for quantifying quality of life in health science is largely driven by the limits of the ordinal concept—increased longevity or health or happiness is better—in economic analysis (which is the study and assessment of trade-offs) of health care. While it is straightforward to quantify the number of lives (or life years) saved for a given expenditure on mortality-reducing interventions, it is more difficult to quantify the trade-off when the benefits are a reduction in morbidity rather than mortality. Comparison of the value of interventions that reduce morbidity to those that reduce mortality, and analysis of interventions that substantially affect both, is impossible without a common metric. That metric is also useful for descriptive epidemiology and other research, apart from economic analysis.

A naive and inappropriate measure of the cost of morbidity is the loss of productivity (often measured in terms of lost wages). This implicitly invokes the "worthiness" sense of *quality*, equating the value of someone's life to what they produce. Lost wages are often the basis of payouts from insurance contracts or policies designed to mimic insurance (e.g., the settlements paid to survivors of victims of the 9/11 attacks). Such measures have a legitimate economic basis (roughly speaking, rational insurance contracts should replace what can be replaced with money, but not pay for those things which cannot be replaced).

But they should not be mistaken for the appropriate value to incorporate into decision making. Individual productivity is a reasonable approximation for the value of someone's life in some sociopolitical systems (e.g., primitive cultures where survival of the community is in question, or modern highly communitarian systems such as fascism or communism), but in modern Western traditions, there is general agreement that someone suffering poor health causes much greater cost than merely the wages lost, as does dying prematurely.

QALYs and Related Measures

In response to these challenges, the concept of *quality-adjusted life years* (QALYs) based on quality of life (QoL) scores was developed. QoL is a score on a scale where perfect health is assigned the value of 1.0 and being dead is assigned the value of 0.0 for a particular (actual or hypothetical) state of health. In this scale, 1 is the maximum possible value, though it is possible to suffer misery that would be valued at less than 0. QALYs are derived from this score by multiplying by the number of person-years spent in a particular state of health. The premise is that loss of a given number of QALYs is equally bad, whether it is, for example, premature death by 10 years of one person who had been in perfect health, or 50 people who suffer a QoL drop from 1.0 to 0.8 for 1 year.

With QALYs, it is possible to compare the cost-effectiveness of an intervention that prevents mortality with one that increases quality of life without changing life expectancy. It is also possible to add or subtract health benefits and mortality effects, such as subtracting the morbidity cost of an unpleasant intervention (e.g., chemotherapy or giving up smoking) from the mortality benefit. The cost-effectiveness measure, dollars (or another common metric) per life-years saved, can be easily reconfigured as the (presumptively equivalent) cost in dollars per QALY gained.

Technically, the QALY measure has these computational properties only if QoL is properly measured as *von Neumann-Morgenstern utility* (typically referred to as simply *utility*). The fundamental property is that if there is a good state with utility h, and a bad state with utility d, then by definition an intermediate state has utility x if the individual is indifferent between the intermediate state, or facing a gamble in which he has a $(h - x)/(h - d)$ probability of being in the good state and a $(x - d)/(h - d)$ chance of being in the bad state. That definition is fairly nonproblematic when applied to monetary wealth: Someone might be just indifferent between getting $50,000 for sure versus a .5 chance of getting $150,000 with a .5 chance of nothing, in which case the utility of having an additional $50,000 is exactly halfway between his current utility and the utility he would have with an additional $150,000. But applying this concept to health states (thus, gaining the mathematical conveniences it allows) requires asking the question, "given a choice between living in a particular poor-health state, or a gamble, with an $x\%$ chance of dropping dead and a $(1 - x)\%$ chance of being perfectly healthy what value of x would make you just indifferent between the prospects?"

Direct Measures of Individual Quality of Life

In the above question, the answer given for x is, by definition, that person's QoL score for the health state in question. (To put this in terms of the previous probabilities, recall that death is typically assigned the score $d = 0$, while perfect health is assigned $h = 1$.) This can be directly assessed by asking some variation of the above question, an approach known as the *standard gamble method.* Not surprisingly, people find it difficult to answer such questions.

In response to that difficulty, a more popular measurement method is the rating scale, in which subjects are simply asked to state a QoL number (or, equivalently, to mark a point on a line segment, a method called a *visual analog scale*) representing a particular health state. While study subjects generally find this much easier, it is not clear what the measure really represents, since there are no real units (such as the probability in the gamble). Another alternative is the *time trade-off* method, wherein subjects state how much time lived in perfect health would be equivalent to a longer given time lived in a diminished health state. This has the advantage of being clearly defined but is complicated by subjects introducing an unknown level of discounting and valuing living at different ages differently.

For methods that do not produce true utility scores, there is no mathematical justification for treating the resulting QALYs as equivalent to healthy life years, though this is often done in practice. This practice continues despite empirically demonstrated problems, such as respondents spreading their scores across

a substantial part of the range $(0, 1)$ for even minor morbidities. When such results are converted to QALYs, they imply that many morbidities count as a much greater fraction of dying than we would generally believe is plausible.

Standard gamble surveys typically produce QoL scores that are very close to 1.0, even for major morbidities such as blindness or loss of a limb. Taken at face value, these measures suggest that the quantified quality of life loss from diseases is usually very small compared with the loss from dying. (The exceptions tend to be depression and other major mental illness, morbidities that severely impair communication and social interaction, and unrelenting physical pain.) These results are rather more plausible than many of those generated by non-gamble-based measures. However, eliciting responses, already difficult for lifelong ailments, becomes prohibitively difficult when measuring a temporary condition. It is nearly impossible to make sense of a question such as, "If you had the choice of a gamble where you might be dead for 5 days and then alive again, or having the flu for 5 days," let alone the answer. But the alternative of using a normal standard gamble question and assuming that temporary and permanent conditions produce the same welfare loss per unit time (e.g., that having the flu for 5 days is 1/1,000th as bad as having it for 5,000 days) cannot be justified.

Further complicating the problem is that the answer to a QoL question depends a great deal on who is asked. While there should be genuine heterogeneity among people (an athlete is more bothered by tendonitis, a guitarist is likely to value loss of his left little finger more than most people, etc.), there are problematic systematic patterns. Most people assess the quality of life loss from losing their eyesight or hearing as very large, perhaps a QoL of 0.5, while blind or deaf people often assess their QoL as better than 0.9. There is no clear basis for choosing one of these over the other when we want to calculate, say, the QALYs lost due to carotene-deficiency-induced blindness in India, which would be a useful number for prioritizing interventions.

Whatever question is used to elicit QoL, a fundamental problem remains: Results cannot be validated other than by asking another hypothetical question. It is very rare for someone to be offered an actual gamble (e.g., the choice about health improving but possibly fatal surgery), and no equivalent exists for other elicitation methods. Despite the very different answers that result from different questions and populations, if QoL quantification is to be used, it is necessary to just assume one measure is right without being able to justify that assumption.

Partial Solutions to the Measurement Challenge

Asking hypothetical questions about potentially fatal rolls of the dice, or even rating scales or time trade-offs, is far beyond the experience and comfort zone of most people, so it is seldom clear what the answers mean. People are more comfortable thinking about hypothetical *willingness to pay* (WTP): How much money they would be willing to part with to get a particular benefit. While such contemplations usually involve simple consumer goods, it is not a major cognitive leap to substitute relief from a minor morbidity. Economists have substantial experience measuring hypothetical WTP and have refined the study methodology, though unless there is actually a real market, such surveys still suffer from the lack of external validation of the hypothetical question.

Most people can assess how much they would pay to get rid of their tendonitis or avoid a case of the flu, while they cannot easily answer questions that measure how many QALYs the condition costs them. Validation studies that compare QoL survey results with WTP results find substantial divergence (which cannot show that either result is correct, but suggests that the QoL responses do not correspond to a measure that appears more robust). WTP measures of morbidity can be entered into a cost-benefit comparison to calculate net benefits. It is not, however, possible to use WTP in cost-effectiveness calculations based on dollars per QALY (an approach that offers no real advantage over cost-benefit comparisons, but is more popular in the medical literature).

For major morbidities, the WTP is less useful. It is difficult to interpret an asserted willingness to pay $5 million to avoid becoming paralyzed when it comes from someone whose lifetime earnings will only be $2 million. But capping the cost of morbidity at the subject's available wealth would clearly be inappropriate. Thus, WTP may be a more promising measure for minor morbidities and benefits that are akin to those from consumer goods, while QoL remains necessary for quantifying major morbidity.

An alternative solution to the measurement problem is to focus on the major motivation for calculating

QALYs—their use in economic policy analyses—and simply declare what QoLs will be used to make economic decisions without actually assuming they are genuine utility scores. This is effectively what is done when an expert group is asked to assess QoLs on behalf of others (often clinicians on behalf of their patients). While those doing such studies perhaps do not realize it, they are declaring answers to questions such as, "How many cases of major cerebral palsy should be considered to be as bad an outcome as one neonatal death?" If the subjects are aware of the role they are playing, this is a valid way of generating QALY measures, not because it is based on individual utility, but because it is based on a studied decision about society's trade-offs.

Health in the Context of Overall Well-Being

Capturing the effects of different QoL scores in policy analysis is a major improvement over measuring only mortality. Inclusion of mental health effects on QoL is particularly important (some studies have found that total QALY loss from mental health problems exceeds that from any physical disease). But diagnosable conditions capture only a small part of psychological well-being.

Analyses that consider only mortality, morbidity, and expenditures—which is to say, most studies of costs and benefits of health care or public health interventions, especially those coming from the "health promotion" tradition—ignore many factors that affect quality of life. This is suggestive again of defining quality as someone's worthiness or contribution to society, since medically defined morbidity is typically related to losses of productivity, but less so general happiness. The bias toward treating quality of life as reflecting only morbidity or productivity is reflected in the condemnation of some unhealthy exposures (e.g., recreational drugs and junk food) that make people happy but may decrease their productivity, and the relative silence on other exposures (e.g., driving and overwork) that are just as dangerous to physical health but may increase productivity.

Negative responses to public health interventions (e.g., "If I do everything they say, I will live to 100, but I won't want to") reflect the popular view that increasing longevity, or diagnosable-morbidity-adjusted QoL, may conflict with other preferences. Failure to consider all sources of individual well-being leads to such cruel absurdities as limiting access to pain-relief medication or forcing psychiatric patients to give up cigarettes (which they relish, and often get substantial symptomatic relief from) so that they can live a longer but less enjoyable or more troubled life.

Quantified quality of life presents the advantages and pitfalls for analysis that any quantification does. It allows a formal measure, for whatever purpose, of an otherwise vague construct, in particular allowing it to be used in economic analysis. However, quantified values tend to overshadow everything that is left unquantified, including uncertainty about the quantification and other values, and thus inaccurate or incomplete quantification can lead to incorrect analyses that are imbued with a false impression of precision.

—Carl V. Phillips

See also Disability Epidemiology; Economic Evaluation; Ethics in Health Care; EuroQoL EQ-5D Questionnaire; Quality of Well-Being Scale (QWB)

Further Readings

Addington-Hall, J., & Kalra, L. (2002). Measuring quality of life: Who should measure quality of life? *British Medical Journal, 32,* 1417–1420.

Bala, M., Wood, L., Zarkin, G., Norton, E., Gafni, A., & O'Brien, B. (1998). Valuing outcomes in health care: A comparison of willingness to pay and quality-adjusted life-years. *Journal of Clinical Epidemiology, 51,* 667–676.

Drummond, M., O'Brien, B., Stoddart, G., & Torrence, G. (1997). *Methods for the economic evaluation of health care programmes.* Oxford, UK: Oxford University Press.

Phillips, C., & Thompson, G. (2001). What is a QALY? *Hayward Medical Communications, 1,* 6.

QUALITY OF WELL-BEING SCALE

The Quality of Well-Being Scale (QWB) is a generic, preference-based measure of health-related quality of life (HRQOL). It has been extensively validated, and its psychometric properties are well established. A self-administered version of the QWB (QWB-SA) has been developed and validated in response to limitations of the QWB, and it is easier to administer in most research and clinical assessment protocols. The questionnaire assesses the presence or absence of symptoms and functioning on specific days prior to administration. The measure produces a single score that ranges from 0 (death) to 1.0 (optimal HRQOL). The score can be integrated with time and mortality to calculate quality-adjusted life years (QALYs) and conduct cost-effectiveness analysis. To place each case on the continuum between death and optimum functioning, the measure uses mean preference weights from a community sample. QWB scores are most commonly used to describe the HRQOL of larger groups or samples and to inform epidemiological research and public health policy. They may be of less value for assessing individual health status.

Health-Related Quality of Life

HRQOL describes a comprehensive picture of health and overall well-being. HRQOL measures differ from one another along several dimensions, including generic versus disease-specific measures and psychometrically based versus preference-based measures. The QWB is a generic measure in that it was designed to be used with any adult population and any health condition, including healthy individuals. The QWB is a preference based measure and was not developed to assess statistically independent domains of HRQOL. It is preference based, meaning that it is scored on the basis of mean health consumer preferences or utilities for the health states. These preferences or utilities are the ratings of observable health states using a continuum anchored by death and optimum health.

Quality of Well-Being

The QWB was developed in the 1970s using theory from the general health policy model. This model includes several components, including mortality (death) and morbidity (HRQOL). The theory proposes that symptoms and disabilities are important for two reasons: First, illness may cause life expectancy to be shortened and, second, illness may make life less desirable at times prior to death. In assessing the impact of a health intervention, the model requires data on both a possible change in mortality as well as a change in HRQOL. In addition to mortality and morbidity, the general health policy model incorporates preference for observed health states (utility) and duration of stay in health states. Preferences or utility for health states are typically measured using economic principles that ask individuals to prioritize or place values on a wide variety of health states involving both symptoms and functioning. The health preferences or utilities are placed on a preference continuum for the desirability of various health states, giving a "quality" rating on an interval scale ranging from $0 = death$ to $1.0 = completely\ well$.

Calculation

Once a value is obtained that describes the level of morbidity or wellness in a sample using a measure such as the QWB, the score can be multiplied by the amount of time at that level of wellness to calculate QALYs. A QALY is defined as the equivalent of a completely well year of life, or a year of life with optimal functioning and no health problems or symptoms. Consider, for example, a person who has a set of symptoms and is in a state of functioning that is rated by community peers as 0.5 on a 0.0 to 1.0 scale. If the person remains in that state for 1 year, he or she would have lost the equivalent of 1/2 of 1 year of life. Thus, a person limited in activities who requires a cane or walker to get around the community would be hypothetically rated at 0.50. If he or she remained in that state for an entire year, the individual would lose the equivalent of one-half year of life. However, a person who has the flu may also be rated as 0.50. In this case, the illness might only last 3 days and the total loss in QALYs might be $3/365 \times 0.50$, which is equal to 0.004 QALYs. This may not appear as significant an outcome as noted for the disabled person. But suppose that 5,000 people in a community get the flu. The well years lost would then be $5,000 \times 0.004$, which is equal to 20 years of perfect health in one person. An important feature of the system is that it is completely generic. It can be used to compare small health consequences that affect a large number of people with large health consequences that affect a small number of people. The quality-adjusted life expectancy is the current life expectancy adjusted for diminished quality of life associated with dysfunctional states and the duration of stay in each state.

The calculation of QALYs is required for conducting cost-utility analysis, which is simply a cost-effectiveness analysis that uses QALYs as its unit measure of health benefit. The QWB was the first assessment instrument developed for the primary purpose of calculating QALYs and conducting cost-effectiveness analysis. Prior to the existence of generic, preference-based measures, many different outcomes were used to represent the effectiveness side of cost-effectiveness analyses. Generic,

preference-based measures and QALYs have become the recommended standard for cost-effectiveness analyses because they provide a common metric for comparing results across studies and populations.

In the original QWB, respondents report whether or not each of 27 groups of symptoms were experienced on each of the 6 days prior to the assessment. Functioning was assessed by questions about the presence of functional limitations over the previous 6 days, within three separate domains (mobility, physical activity, and social activity). Unlike measures that ask about general time frames such as "the past 4 weeks" or "the previous month," the QWB asks whether specific symptoms or functional limitations did or did not occur on a given day. Each symptom complex and functional limitation is weighted using preferences obtained from the ratings of 856 people randomly sampled from the general population. The four domain scores (three functioning, one symptom) are subtracted from 1.0 to create a total score that provides an expression of well-being that ranges from $0 = death$ to $1.0 = asymptomatic\ optimal\ functioning$. References on the validation of the instrument are available from the University of California San Diego Health Outcomes Assessment Program (UCSD-HOAP). The questionnaire must be administered by a trained interviewer because it employs a somewhat complex branching system of questions and probes. The original questionnaire takes an average of about 15 min to complete. The authors believe that the administration time and complexity of the original measure, which require a trained interviewer, have resulted in its underutilization.

Self-Administered Quality of Well-Being

In 1996, a self-administered version of the questionnaire was developed to address some of the limitations of the original version. The QWB-SA improves on the original version in a number of ways. First, the administration of the questionnaire no longer requires a trained interviewer and can be completed in less than 10 min. Second, the assessment of symptoms follows a clinically useful review of systems model rather than clustering symptoms based on preference weights. Third, a wider variety of symptoms are included in the QWB-SA, making it more comprehensive and improving the assessment of mental health.

Preference weights for the QWB-SA were obtained with a new sample, and studies were conducted and published comparing the new and old versions. The QWB-SA and QWB were highly correlated and the test-retest reliability is high. The measure is not designed to be internally consistent because the factors it measures (symptoms and functioning) are interdependent. QWB-SA scores tend to be slightly lower than QWB scores, primarily because mental health symptoms are assessed in much greater detail and are more likely to contribute to decreased scores.

The format for the QWB-SA includes five sections. The first part assesses the presence/absence of 19 chronic symptoms or problems (e.g., blindness, speech problems). The question format does not assess each of the previous 3 days (as in the rest of the questionnaire) with the expectation that these chronic conditions do not vary much over the 3-day assessment period. These chronic symptoms are followed by 25 acute (or more transient) physical symptoms (e.g., headache, coughing, pain), and 14 mental health symptoms and behaviors (e.g., sadness, anxiety, irritation). The remaining sections of the QWB-SA are similar to the QWB and include assessment of mobility (including use of transportation), physical activity (e.g., walking and bending over), and social activity, including completion of role expectations (e.g., work, school, or home).

The period assessed by the QWB-SA is shorter than in the QWB. The QWB asked patients about symptoms and function "over the past 6 days" prior to the day of administration, whereas the QWB-SA questions refer to the 3 days prior to the day of administration. This change was designed to reduce respondents' recall bias without decreasing the instrument's ability to assess over a period of time and resulted in a more rapid administration. The impact on the overall quality of life score of using only the last 3 days was examined by dropping information from Days 4, 5, and 6 and recalculating QWB scores based only on the past 3 days. No significant differences in scores were found.

When compared with other generic, preference-based measures of HRQOL, the QWB-SA remains longer and slightly more time-consuming because its assessment of symptoms and functioning is more comprehensive. However, the more detailed assessment of symptoms and functioning may result in greater sensitivity to change in some populations. The QWB-SA asks about the presence or absence of specific complaints on specific days to reduce the influence of memory, or severity ratings such as pain intensity, that require personal interpretation. In addition, the distribution of QWB-SA scores in most studies is close to normal, suggesting that ceiling or floor effects are less common than with other HRQOL measures.

Both the QWB and QWB-SA are available free of charge to users from nonprofit organizations. A small fee is charged to for-profit users. Information on copyright agreements and user manuals are available at www.medicine.ucsd.edu/fpm/hoap.

—*Erik J. Groessl and Robert M. Kaplan*

See also Confounding; Ecological Fallacy

Further Readings

Groessl, E. J., & Cronan, T. A. (2000). A cost analysis of self-management programs for people with chronic illness. *American Journal of Community Psychology*, 28(4), 455–480.

Groessl, E. J., Kaplan, R. M., Barrett-Connor, E., & Ganiats, T. G. (2004). Body mass index and quality of well-being in a community of older adults. *American Journal of Preventive Medicine*, 26(2), 126–129.

Groessl, E. J., Kaplan, R. M., & Cronan, T. A. (2003). Quality of well-being in older people with osteoarthritis. *Arthritis and Rheumatism*, 49(1), 23–28.

Kaplan, R. M., & Anderson, J. (1996). The general health policy model: An integrated approach. In B. Spilker (Ed.), *Quality of life and pharmacoeconomics in clinical trials* (2nd ed., pp. 309–322). Philadelphia: Lippincott-Raven.

Kaplan, R. M., Sieber, W. J., & Ganiats, T. G. (1997). The quality of well-being scale: Comparison of the interviewer-administered version with a self-administered questionnaire. *Psychology & Health*, 12, 783–791.

Web Sites

University of California San Diego Health Outcomes Assessment Program Web site: http://www.medicine.ucsd.edu/fpm/hoap/index.html.

QUANTITATIVE METHODS IN EPIDEMIOLOGY

See CATEGORICAL DATA, ANALYSIS OF

QUARANTINE AND ISOLATION

Quarantine and isolation are two different ways to limit the spread of certain infectious diseases by reducing contact between individuals at risk of spreading infectious disease and the rest of the population. The types of diseases for which quarantine and isolation are useful public health measures are those that involve direct transmission of infection by close contact (e.g., aerosol or droplet transmission). There must also be detectable symptoms that allow individuals who have been infected to be distinguished from those who have not. The aims of quarantine and isolation can vary and include stopping local spread of disease, global eradication of a disease, or simply slowing down the progress of an epidemic to gain time in which to vaccinate or administer drugs.

Fundamentally, the difference between quarantine and isolation depends on whether the individual has a confirmed infected/infectious status (depending on the specific disease, determining infection may be easier than determining infectiousness, which is the ability to transmit the disease). If an individual's infected/infectious status is confirmed, they are *isolated*, which means removed to an environment designed to prevent them from spreading the infection to other individuals. These environments can range from an individual's own home to a highly secure medical facility. Individuals can also receive treatment while in isolation, with the health workers taking precautions against compromising the isolation (e.g., physical barriers or vaccination). Isolated individuals remain in isolation until they are no longer considered to be at risk of spreading infection (established, e.g., by a serology test or a clinical assessment). Occasionally, isolation is enforced by law, as was done with tuberculosis (TB) in New York City during the 1990s. In this case, the aims included the prevention of rapid emergence of drug-resistant forms of TB, caused in part by patients not completing their drug treatment. At around the same time (1986–1993), Cuban residents who were HIV-positive were isolated in sanitariums, though this controversial policy evolved so that patients had a choice of how and where to be treated.

Individuals may be *quarantined* if they are considered at risk of having been exposed to an infectious disease (from an infected individual or another source) but do not display symptoms of the disease. The "at risk" assessment can be made by the individual who may have been exposed or by a third party (e.g., doctor, public health official), and it can be based on contact tracing (determining an individual's recent close contacts by interview or questionnaire),

or on the individual's having been to a certain region where the infectious disease is endemic or epidemic. The quarantine conditions can be as strict as those for isolation, but they are often based more on clinical observation and can be as simple as self-reporting and staying at home. If an individual develops symptoms, then he or she meets the criteria for isolation. The length of time that an individual is quarantined for is related to the specific infectious disease; in fact, the origin of the word *quarantine* comes from the 40 days that people arriving by ship had to remain on their ships before coming to land in case they had been exposed to the plague but had not yet become symptomatic. Time required to be spent in quarantine should relate to the incubation period of a particular disease, that is, the time between infection and the onset of detectable symptoms. Mathematical modeling has shown how this quarantine period can best be set and modified based on updated information about the incubation period, which is especially useful for emerging infectious diseases where little epidemiological data is known.

Theoretical work has demonstrated that the success of quarantine and isolation in controlling infectious diseases is strongly linked to both the proportion of presymptomatic transmission and the inherent transmissibility of the etiological agent. Although isolation is probably always a desirable public health measure, quarantine is more controversial. Mass quarantine can inflict significant social, psychological, and economic costs without resulting in the detection of many infected individuals. However, quarantine can be enforced by law, and indeed, during the 2003 severe acute respiratory syndrome (SARS) epidemic, governments added this syndrome to the list of diseases for which individuals can be quarantined. Probabilistic models have been developed to determine the conditions under which quarantine is expected to be useful. Results demonstrate that the number of infections averted (per initially infected individual) through the use of quarantine is expected to be very low provided that isolation is effective, but it increases abruptly and at an accelerating rate as the effectiveness of isolation diminishes. When isolation is ineffective, the use of quarantine will be most beneficial when there is significant asymptomatic transmission and if the asymptomatic period is neither very long nor very short. In these cases, quarantine and isolation can be effectively combined to halt the spread of infection, where each on its own would be insufficient. Both quarantine and isolation become effective when contact tracing is efficient (i.e., accurate and speedy). Quarantine and isolation can be used in conjunction with other public health measures such as vaccination and antiviral drugs, as has been recommended by the World Health Organization (WHO) when faced by an influenza pandemic.

—Andrew Park and Troy Day

See also Influenza; Outbreak Investigation; Severe Acute Respiratory Syndrome (SARS); Tuberculosis

Further Readings

Day, T. (2004). Predicting quarantine failure rates. *Emerging Infectious Diseases, 10*, 487–488.

Day, T., Park, A., Madras, N., Gumel, A., & Wu, J. (2006). When is quarantine a useful control strategy for emerging infectious diseases? *American Journal of Epidemiology, 163*, 479–485.

Fraser, C., Riley, S., Anderson, R. M., Ferguson, & N. M. (2004). Factors that make an infectious disease outbreak controllable. *Proceedings of the National Academy of Sciences of the United States of America, 101*, 6146–6151.

James, L., Shindo, N., Cutter, J., Ma, S., & Chew, S. K. (2006). Public health measures implemented during the SARS outbreak in Singapore, 2003. *Public Health, 120*, 20–26.

QUASI EXPERIMENTS

Quasi experiments, like all experiments, manipulate treatments to discover causal effects (quasi experiments are sometimes referred to as nonrandomized experiments or observational studies). However, these experiments differ from randomized experiments in that units are not randomly assigned to conditions. Quasi experiments are often used when it is not possible to randomize ethically or feasibly. Therefore, units may be assigned to conditions using a variety of nonrandomized techniques, such as permitting units to self-select into conditions or assigning them based on need or some other criterion. Unfortunately, quasi experiments may not yield the unbiased estimates that randomized experiments yield because quasi experiments can neither reliably rule out alternative explanations for the effects nor create error terms that are orthogonal to treatment. To improve causal inferences in quasi experiments, however, researchers can use

a combination of design features, practical logic, and statistical analysis. Although researchers had been using quasi-experimental designs long before 1963, it was then that Donald Campbell and Julian Stanley coined the term *quasi experiment.* The theories, practices, and assumptions about these designs were further developed over the next 40 years by Campbell and his colleagues.

Validity and Threats to Validity

In 1963, Campbell and Stanley created a validity typology, including *threats to validity*, to provide a logical and objective way to evaluate the quality of causal inferences made using quasi-experimental designs. The threats are common reasons why researchers may be incorrect about the causal inferences they draw from any cause-probing study, including randomized and quasi experiments. Originally, Campbell and Stanley described only two types of validity: internal validity and external validity. Thomas Cook and Campbell later added statistical conclusion validity and construct validity. We define the validity types shortly. Of the four types of validity, internal validity is the most crucial to the ability to make causal claims from quasi experiments. *Internal validity* concerns the validity of inferences that the relationship between two variables *A* and *B* is causal from *A* to *B*. The act of randomization helps reduce the plausibility of many threats to internal validity. Lacking randomization, quasi experiments have to pay particular attention to these threats:

- *Ambiguous temporal precedence:* the inability to determine which variable occurred first, thereby preventing the researcher from knowing which variable is the cause and which is the effect.
- *Selection:* systematic differences between unit characteristics in each condition that could affect the outcome.
- *History:* events that occur simultaneously with the treatment that could affect the outcome.
- *Maturation:* a natural development over time that could affect the outcome.
- *Regression:* when units are selected for their extreme scores, they may have less extreme scores on other measures, including later posttests, making it appear as if an effect occurred.
- *Attrition:* when units who drop out of the one condition are systematically different in their responses than those who drop out of other conditions.

- *Testing:* repeatedly exposing units to a test may affect their performance on subsequent tests, appearing as if a treatment effect occurred.
- *Instrumentation:* changes over time or conditions in the instrument used to measure responses may make it appear as if an effect occurred.
- *Additive and interactive threats to internal validity:* the impact of a threat can be compounded by, or may depend on the level of, another threat.

The other three types of validity also affect causal conclusions about the treatment and outcome, but they do not necessarily affect quasi experiments more than any other type of experiment. *Statistical conclusion validity* addresses inferences about whether and how much the presumed cause and effect covary. Examples of threats to statistical conclusion validity are low statistical power and violation of statistical assumptions. *Construct validity* addresses inferences about higher-order constructs that research operations represent. Examples of threats to construct validity include reactivity to the experimental situation (units respond as they want to be perceived rather than to the intended treatment) and treatment diffusion (the control group learns about and uses the treatment); note that in both these cases, a question is raised about whether the researchers are actually measuring or manipulating what they intended or claimed. *External validity* addresses inferences about whether a causal relationship holds over variation in persons, settings, treatment variables, and measurement variables. Examples of threats to external validity include interactions of the causal treatment with units or setting, so that the observed causal relationship might not hold in new units or settings.

Basic Types of Quasi Experiments

While there are many variations of quasi-experimental designs, basic designs include, but are not limited to, (a) *one-group posttest only designs*, in which only one group is given a treatment and is then observed for effects using one posttest observation; (b) *nonequivalent control group designs*, in which the outcomes of two or more treatment or control conditions are studied, but the experimenter does not control assignment to conditions; (c) *regression discontinuity designs*, in which the experimenter uses a cutoff score from a continuous variable to determine assignment to treatment and comparison conditions, and an effect is observed if the regression line of the assignment

variable on outcome for the treatment group is discontinuous from that of the comparison group at the point of the cutoff; and (d) *interrupted time-series designs*, in which many (ideally, 100 or more) consecutive observations over time are available on an outcome, and treatment is introduced in the midst of those observations to determine its impact on the outcome as evidenced by a disruption in the time series after treatment; and (e) *single-group or single-case designs*, in which one group or unit is repeatedly observed over time (more than twice, but fewer than in a time series) while the scheduling and dose of treatment are manipulated to demonstrate that treatment affects outcome.

The causal logic of threats to validity can also be applied to two other classes of designs that are not quasi experiments because the cause is not manipulated, as it is in the previous five designs. These are (f) *case-control designs*, in which a group with an outcome of interest is compared with a group without that outcome to see how they differ retrospectively in exposure to possible causes; and (g) *correlational designs*, in which observations on possible treatments and outcomes are observed simultaneously to see if they are related. These designs often cannot ensure that the cause precedes the effect, making it more difficult to make causal inferences than in quasi experiments.

Design Features

To prevent a threat from occurring or to diagnose its presence and impact on study results, researchers can manipulate certain features within a design, thereby improving the validity of casual inferences made using quasi experiments. These design features include (a) adding observations over time before (pretests) or after (posttests) treatment to examine trends over time; (b) adding more than one treatment or comparison group to serve as a source of inference about the counterfactual (what would have occurred to the treatment group if they had not received the treatment); (c) varying the type of treatment, such as removing or varying a treatment; and (d) using nonrandomized assignment methods that the researcher can control or adjust, such as using a regression discontinuity design or matching. All quasi experiments are combinations of these design features, chosen to diagnose or minimize the plausibility of threats to validity in a particular context.

New designs are added to the basic repertoire of designs using these elements. For example, by adding pretest observations to a posttest-only nonequivalent control group design, existing pretest differences between the treatment and control groups can better be measured and accounted for, which helps reduce effects of selection. Likewise, adding a comparison group to a time-series analysis can assess threats such as history. If the outcome for the comparison group varies over time in the same pattern as the treatment outcome, history is a likely threat.

Examples

Martin Atherton examined the effectiveness of a Web-based, interactive intervention aimed to improve self-management of asthma, called MyAsthma™, on the quality of life for asthma suffers. High volume users of the intervention (those visiting the Web site 17 or more times) reported a better quality of life than low volume users over a 6-month period of time. The researcher compared quality of life for users before (pretest) and after (posttest) the intervention. Using a pretest was critical for this study, since the low volume users had higher pretest scores on all measures of quality of life than the high volume users. Without accounting for the pretest scores, it would have been more difficult to assess the effectiveness of the treatment between the high and low volume users. This study might be thought of as a nonequivalent comparison group design with pretests and posttests.

In 1999, as part of the Complying with the Minimum Drinking Age project (CMDA), law enforcement agencies from several communities across the midwestern United States began periodic enforcement checks in which minors attempted to purchase alcoholic beverages from local establishments. A total of 116 observations were collected once every 2 weeks over 4.5 years from both on-premise (i.e., restaurant and bars) and off-premise (i.e., grocery and liquor stores) sites. Alexander Wagenaar, Traci Toomey, and Darin Erickson found a 17% decrease in alcohol sales to minors immediately after the law enforcement checks among both sites, although long-term effects of these checks varied. The off-premise venues eventually returned to their previous rates of illegal sales. However, the on-premise venues were better at reducing alcohol sales to minors, demonstrating a long-term decrease of 8.2% in illegal sales. Although several of the establishments in the control group were threatened by treatment diffusion (law enforcement agencies began checks in these establishments beyond the researchers' control), those establishments in which law enforcement agencies did not check for illegal sales did not decrease their alcohol sales to minors over time. This study was an interrupted time-series quasi experiment using a nonequivalent control group.

Statistical Adjustments

While Campbell emphasized the importance of good design in quasi experiments, many other researchers sought to resolve problems in making causal inferences from quasi experiments through statistical adjustments. One such method uses *propensity scores*, the conditional probability that a unit will be in a treatment condition given a set of observed covariates. These scores can then be used to balance treatment and control units on predictor variables through matching, stratifying, covariate adjustment, or weighting. Another method, *selection bias modeling*, attempts to remove hidden bias that occurs when unobserved covariates influence treatment effects by modeling the selection process. A third method uses structural equation modeling to study causal relationships in quasi experiments by modeling latent variables to reduce bias caused by unreliable measures. While these statistical adjustments have been shown to reduce some of the bias present in quasi experiments, each of these methods has its limitations that prevents it from accounting for all the sources of biased estimates. Therefore, it is often more effective to obtain less biased estimates through good designs than elaborate statistics; and these statistics always perform better when the study was better designed at its start.

Conclusions

Quasi experiments may never rule out threats to internal validity as well as randomized experiments; however, improving the designs can reduce or control for these threats, making causal conclusions more valid for quasi experiments than they would be otherwise. The strategy is to begin with a basic design that is most appropriate for the research question and most feasible given the practical constraints on the study. Then add design features to address particular plausible threats to validity that may exist.

While certain conditions within field studies may hinder the feasibility of using more sophisticated quasi-experimental designs, it is important to recognize the limitations of designs that are used. In some cases, statistical adjustments can be used to improve treatment estimates; however, even then, causal inferences from quasi experiments should be made with caution.

—*Margaret H. Clark and William R. Shadish*

See also Bias; Causation and Causal Inference; Randomization; Study Design

Further Readings

Atherton, M. (2000). Outcome measures of efficacy associated with a web-enabled asthma self-management programme: Findings from a quasi-experiment. *Disease Management and Health Outcomes, 8*(4), 233–242.

Bollen, K. A. (1989). *Structural equations with latent variables.* New York: Wiley.

Campbell, D. T., & Stanley, J. C. (1963). *Experimental and quasi-experimental designs for research.* Chicago: Rand-McNally.

Cook, T. D., & Campbell, D. T. (1979). *Quasi-experimentation: Design and analysis issues for field settings.* Chicago: Rand-McNally.

Heckman, J. J. (1979). Sample selection bias as a specification error. *Econometrica, 47,* 153–161.

Rosenbaum, P. R., & Rubin, D. B. (1983). The central role of the propensity score in observational studies for causal effects. *Biometrika, 70,* 41–55.

Shadish, W. R., Cook, T. D., & Campbell, D. T. (2002). *Experimental and quasi-experimental designs for generalized causal inference.* Boston: Houghton-Mifflin.

Wagenaar, A. C., Toomey, T. L., & Erickson, D. J. (2005). *Addiction, 100,* 335–345.

QUESTIONNAIRE DESIGN

Questionnaires are one of many ways to elicit information. Researchers who design their own questionnaires need to take steps to ensure that they are validly measuring whatever it is they seek to measure. A strong, well-designed questionnaire starts with the conceptualization of the problem and ends with the visual clarity of the presentation. Poor questionnaire design not only leaves a researcher with incomplete and/or inaccurate information but also wastes the time of the individuals who complete the questionnaire.

Conceptualizing the Problem: What Questions Need to Be Asked?

Before specific questions are developed, it is imperative that a researcher identify what problem he or she is trying to understand as well as consider potential explanations for that problem. This process of conceptualization may use established theoretical frameworks typically based on prior research or, if no known framework exists to the researchers knowledge, a generative process of exploring all possible explanations should be pursued. Because this process is often difficult and time-consuming, it is sometimes omitted. However, failure to conceptualize all the possible "whys" that may explain a problem will result in the probable exclusion of important questions in the final questionnaire. It is often not until the conclusion of the study that these omissions become apparent, and it is then too late to remedy them.

To illustrate the process of conceptualizing a problem, consider the researcher interested in understanding smoking behavior by female adolescents. In the medical, biological, and social science literature, there are a number of possible explanations for why a young girl begins to smoke. For example, there are arguments identifying biological, familial, emotional, and social exposures influencing smoking initiation. While a particular researcher may be interested in understanding the impact of parental smoking on an adolescent girl's decision to smoke, going through the generative process of conceptualizing and examining other explanations alerts the researcher to consider including questions about age, psychological well-being, and the environment in which the girl lives. Even if they are not the focus of the study, including these factors will further refine the researcher's ability to understand how parental smoking operates as a risk factor.

Operationalizing the Measures

Once a researcher has identified the concepts to be measured, the next step is to determine the specific ways to measure them. This is referred to as operationalization. To measure a concept accurately, a researcher must ask questions whose answers will provide useful information about the concepts of interest. The questions must be phrased in such a way that the respondent understands what is being asked and can provide a reasonable reply. To ensure clarity in questions, certain types of questions should be avoided, such as "doubled-barreled" questions (which ask more than one question at a time), long questions, and questions that use language that may confuse the respondent. For example, using the problem of female adolescent smoking, a question such as, "When you are feeling overwhelmed, do you tend to want a cigarette?" is doubled-barreled—a "No" could mean that the respondent does not smoke when overwhelmed or that the respondent does not get overwhelmed. Additionally, the word "overwhelmed" may not be understood by all adolescent respondents.

Another important consideration when designing a question is sensitivity. If the researcher asks a question that a person would feel uncomfortable answering, then the researcher risks not only missing responses but also potentially alienating the respondent so that he or she is reluctant to honestly answer any further questions. While some of this can be avoided by considering how the questionnaire is delivered (e.g., face-to-face vs. telephone), it can also be avoided by learning how others have asked these questions in the past and by considering factors such as the culture, age, and religion of the respondent. For example, to ask a question such as, "Do you think smoking after sexual intercourse is common?" may not bother some respondents, whereas it may be very uncomfortable for others.

It is also important to consider recall when asking questions. The ability of respondents to remember whatever is being asked may be a universal problem, that is, one that all respondents would have difficulty with. Or, it may be a problem unique to one set of respondents but not for another. For example, few individuals who smoke could probably recall what their relationship was like with their parents when they bought their first pack of cigarettes. Furthermore, and possibly more problematic, individuals who always have an easy or always have a strained relationship with their parents may have an easier guess at this question, while for those whose parental relationship are sometimes easy and sometimes strained, remembering the specific condition at a given moment in the past could be difficult. This introduces an element of bias into the subjects' responses.

Two other considerations when designing a question relate less to the wording of the question itself but are also important to consider. First, for closed-ended questions (those with delineated response options), the response options must be clear and mutually exclusive. For example, a question about marital status should include not the categories "single" and "divorced" (because they could both apply to the same person), but the categories "single," "never married" and "currently divorced." Second, often a concept cannot be fully measured using only one question. For example, to understand if an adolescent female were a smoker, it would be important to find out not only if she currently smoked but also how much and for how long.

Formatting the Questionnaire

Once the specific questions are determined, it is important that a researcher consider the format of the questionnaire carefully. A common accepted practice is to begin and end a questionnaire with easy to answer questions such as demographics (gender, age, number of siblings). On a similar note, if more sensitive questions are to be asked, these questions are usually placed later in the survey, so that the respondent is comfortable with the survey process by the time he or she reaches those questions, thus increasing the likelihood that the respondent will answer them honestly.

Each new section of questions should be clearly distinguished and, when needed, specific instructions should be provided for each section. This is particularly so if the responses to the questions are in a new format (e.g., "for the next set of questions, please circle all that apply") or if they require reference to a particular time period (e.g., "for the next set of questions, think back to when you started ninth grade").

It is a useful tool to present a series of questions to measure one concept or a similar set of ideas in a similar format (e.g., "for the next 10 questions, please read each scenario and circle True or Untrue as it applies to you"). These series questions are comfortable for respondents to answer and allow for more questions to be asked efficiently. However, depending on the topic, the length of the questionnaire, and characteristics of the respondents, grouped questions can be problematic, as some will disregard the specifics of each question and answer all questions in a set with the same response, for instance, by always choosing the first or last category. Often, reverse-ordered questions are included in these series to encourage more careful reading of each question. For example, rather than asking, "I think kids should be allowed to smoke outside school grounds" and "I think kids should be allowed to smoke if given permission by their parent/guardian," this second question could be reversed to read "Kids should not be able to get permission from a parent/guardian to smoke."

Skip patterns provide the opportunity to ask only certain people certain questions, potentially providing improved efficiency in a questionnaire. For example, following a question that asks, "Do you currently smoke" respondents who answer "Yes" can then be referred to one set of follow-up questions while respondents who answer "No" could be referred to another set. While this saves time and improves cooperation by not subjecting respondents to a number of irrelevant questions, it can potentially be confusing for respondents if directions are not completely clear. Skip patterns are easily implemented in computer-assisted interviewing and are commonly used in that context.

Implementation Options

Questionnaires can be administered in a number of formats each with its own strengths and limitations. Telephone interviews may provide a sense of anonymity and make it easy to reach people who are geographically spread out, and the presence of the interviewer allows for clarification or elaboration of questions when needed. However, many households do not have telephones and this fact is related to other factors such as age, race, income, and disability status, thus introducing an element of bias into phone surveys. In addition, many phone numbers are not accessible (e.g., unlisted or disconnected), and cell phone numbers are often not included in lists of potential respondent households, introducing another element of bias as many households now have only cell phone service. When potential respondents are reached by telephone, response rate is moderate.

Mailed questionnaires can provide a strong sense of anonymity (if a return envelope only contains a return address) and can reach individuals who are geographically spread out. Mailed surveys are potentially less expensive in that less "interviewer time" is needed. However, mailed surveys provide no opportunity to clarify or elaborate on responses, and the response rate (return of completed questionnaires) is typically lower than that of telephone or personal interviews.

Face-to-face interviews can create a sense of comfort that may assist in improving response rate and comfort when answering questions. Ambiguities can be clarified, and elaboration of responses can be obtained. However, it can be costly to do face-to-face interviews with a large sample, particularly if they are geographically spread out.

Computers have been engaged to assist in questionnaire implementation in a variety of ways. Computers have been used to assist during telephone interviews in order to allow the researcher to work through skip patterns with ease and to directly enter responses in order to reduce data entry mistakes. Computers using voice-activated response have also been engaged to conduct the interview over the telephone, saving person-time due to unanswered calls. Computers have also been engaged as a means of questioning respondents directly through Web-based surveys and free-standing touch screen computer kiosks. Computers have also been used in face-to-face interviews to allow subjects to answer particularly sensitive questions, such as those regarding sexual behavior, by entering their responses directly into the computer rather than by responding to the interviewer.

A final implementation option that is crucial to developing a thoughtful questionnaire is pilot testing, preferably on a sample of individuals similar to those who are the target population for the survey. Pilot testing a questionnaire is the best way to determine if questions are clear and written in such a way as to elicit appropriate responses, not misleading or offensive, and to determine if the questionnaire is easy to follow. Any difficulties encountered during pilot testing should be remedied by revisions in the instrument, interviewer training, and so on, before the full survey is implemented. By looking at responses and discussing issues with a pilot sample, questionnaires can be further refined to increase their ability to ultimately measure what the researcher hopes to understand.

—*Eve Waltermaurer*

See also Psychometrics; Reliability; Survey Research Methods

Further Readings

McNutt, L. A., Waltermaurer, E., McCauley, J., Campbell, J., & Ford, D. (2005). Rationale for and development of the computerized intimate partner screen for primary care. *Family Violence Prevention and Health Practice, 3,* 1–12. Retrieved June 18, 2007, from http://endabuse.org/health/ejournal/archive/1-3/McNutt.pdf.

Mitchell, A. A., Cottler, L. B., & Shapiro, S. (1986). Effect of questionnaire design on recall of drug exposure in pregnancy. *American Journal of Epidemiology, 123,* 670–676.

Wacholder, S., Carroll, R. J., Pee, D., & Gail, M. H. (1994). The partial questionnaire design for case-control studies. *Statistics in Medicine, 13,* 623–634.

R

RACE AND ETHNICITY, MEASUREMENT ISSUES WITH

Race and ethnicity are controversial variables in epidemiological studies. Most of the controversy comes from the misuse of these variables as risk factors and from issues concerning validity and consistency of data over time and territory. Substantial inconsistencies in the categorization of race and ethnicity can be found in the literature. For these reasons, some journals have written policies and published glossaries to better define these variables. However, revisions of criteria are often required due to the dynamics of social and demographic change, such as migrations, globalization, and other cultural movements that may change the perception of group identity.

Epidemiological studies may use race and ethnicity variables in several situations. In the sampling process, these variables may be used to determine whether the true diversity of the total population is being represented by the sample and to audit the randomization process. For example, National Institutes of Health (NIH) requires the assessment of these variables to ensure that the traditionally understudied minorities are sufficiently represented. However, the validity of using race and ethnicity as causal explanatory variables or risk factors is very questionable. The detection of statistical differences between racial or ethnic groups should be considered as a starting point to better understand the true underlying genetic, environmental, or socioeconomic risk factors.

Once the relevance of the use of race and ethnicity is established, the measurement of these variables needs to be planned, validated, and analyzed with caution. The main issues are the difficulty in separating the concept of race from the concept of ethnicity, the nonequivalence of data collection methods, and the mutability of use and meaning of terminology.

Race Versus Ethnicity

In the simplest terms, ethnicity can be defined as a socially constructed method of categorization of human beings, while race can be defined as a biologically constructed method. Race takes into account the physical characteristics of the population, such as skin color, that are marked by traces transmissible by descendant. In contrast, ethnicity emphasizes cultural characteristics that lead to a sense of group membership, such as language, religion, traditions, and/or territorial identity.

One of the main problems in accurately measuring race and ethnicity is the fact that these concepts are not always distinguishable. The reason for this is the lack of a clear boundary between perceptions of race and perceptions of ethnicity. For example, while all races can be found within the group Hispanic/Latino, this group is included as a racial category in some questionnaires. Nevertheless, when race and ethnicity are collected in a single question in the questionnaire, and depending on how the question is stated, inconsistency over time may be observed due to ambiguous membership. The Office of Management and Budget

(OMB) sets standards for classification of race and ethnicity in federal data. In 1997, the standard revision provided two options—collecting race/ethnicity in one combined question or in two separate questions, one for race and one for ethnicity—but stated that to allow flexibility and to ensure data quality, separate questions are preferred.

Nonequivalence of Data Collection Methods

Analyses of epidemiological studies may require the combination of data from multiple sources. It is important to make sure that the methods used to collect the information and the categories used are compatible. Special attention should be given to who provided the information (self-reported or by an observer), how the question was stated (allowing multiple answers or not), and what categories were available.

Who Provided the Information?

While self-identification of race and ethnicity is fairly common, many studies also use information on race/ethnicity provided by an observer such as a health care provider or a direct interviewer. The complexity of the concepts of race and ethnicity and the conflicts between the social perceptions of these variables and the individual's self-identity generate differences in the data collected based on who is giving the information. Self-reported race/ethnicity is considered superior by many organizations. According to the OMB standards, self-reporting or self-identification is the preferred method for collecting data on these variables. The Centers for Disease Control and Prevention, in *Use of Race and Ethnicity in Public Health Surveillance*, discontinued the use of the observer-reported method. Independently of who provided the information, the variation in individual self-perception and social perception caused by different backgrounds, beliefs, and countries of origin contributes to limiting the quality of these variables.

How Was the Question Stated?

A second issue concerns the way the question was stated; for example, did it allow for multiple answers? Ideally, each variable—race and ethnicity—should be exclusive and exhaustive, meaning that within the

variable, each subject belongs to exactly one category. That is not always an easy task because of the overlap of races and the heterogeneity of some ethnic groups. Because respondents may identify themselves as multiracial, much inconsistency in answers will be generated. In practice, the researchers may find some of these respondents still choosing more than one category. Because of these possibilities, questions that allow multiple answers are preferred.

What Categories Were Available?

Ideally, the categories should reflect the respondents' self-perception. For example, the terms *Latino* and *Hispanic* are not exchangeable. The reason for this is the variation in respondent preferences for one term or another, depending, for example, on their country of origin. For this reason, the *American Medical Association Manual of Style* recommends that whenever possible, a more specific term (such as Mexican American, Latin American, etc.) be used. Another example is the definition of race for native Hawaiians. The descendants of the original native inhabitants of the State of Hawaii were considered by OBM as Asian or Pacific Islander. However, that was not their self-perception. They perceived themselves as belonging to the category American Indians and Alaska Natives. As a result, the OBM reviewed the racial categories, and Asian or Pacific Islander category was divided into two categories: Asian and Native Hawaiian or Other Pacific Islander. The standards now have five categories of races: American Indian or Alaska Native, Asian, Black or African American, Native Hawaiian or Other Pacific Islander, and White.

A study by Ulrike Boehmer and colleagues compared information on race/ethnicity from clinical files of a large sample of outpatients with their respective surveyed race/ethnicity. These data sets differed in who provided the information (self-reported vs. nonself-reported), how the question was stated (multiple answers vs. single answer), and what categories were available ("American Indian" vs. "American Indian or Alaska Native"; "Asian" vs. "Asian, Native Hawaiian or Pacific Islander"; "Black" vs. "Black or African American"; "Hispanic" vs. "Spanish, Hispanic, or Latino," and the availability of "Unknown"). Results from this study showed that self-reported whites had the fewest "unknown" in their files and the fewest misclassifications. In contrast, self-reported Asians had the most "unknown" and self-reported American Indians the most occurrences of misclassifications in their files. These results demonstrate how different methods can generate differences in the classification of race/ethnicity.

Terminology Changes Over Time and Territory

Classifications of race have changed over time. For example, the terms *mulatto*, *quadroon*, and *octoroon* were used during the 19th century to describe individuals with one half, one quarter, and one eighth of black ancestry, respectively. Later, this terminology was abandoned and the term *black* was used to refer to persons with any black ancestry. Interesting enough, currently the term *mulatto* (or *mulato* in Spanish or Portuguese) is commonly used by several countries in Latin America. This illustrates why translation of race and ethnicity descriptions from the original language used in a questionnaire can lead to additional measurement error.

Recommendations

The appropriate study design to measure race and ethnicity will depend on the research question under investigation. Independently of how terms are defined officially, the respondent may have a different perception of what category of race or ethnicity he or she belongs to. Pretests of the questionnaires/forms and audits for quality assurance are important to verify if the perception of the respondent is captured by the correct category. Different ethnic groups may have different compositions, though sometimes with one race predominating. However, given the underlying complexity of each variable, the combination of race and ethnicity in one question is not always a good idea.

—*Ana W. Capuano*

See also African American Health Issues; Asian American/ Pacific Islander Health Issues; Health Disparities; Latino Health Issues; Race Bridging

Further Readings

Bhopal, R. (2004). Glossary of terms relating to ethnicity and race: For reflection and debate. *Journal of Epidemiology and Community Health, 58*(6), 441–445.

Boehmer, U., Kressin, N. R., Berlowitz, D. R., Christiansen, C. L., Kazis, L. E., & Jones, J. A. (2002). Self-reported vs. administrative race/ethnicity data and study results. *American Journal of Public Health, 92*(9), 1471–1472.
Centers for Disease Control and Prevention. (1993, June). *Use of race and ethnicity in public health surveillance summary of the CDC/ATSDR workshop.* Retrieved March 2, 2007, from http://www.cdc.gov/mmwr/PDF/rr/ rr4210.pdf.
Kaplan, J. B., & Bennett, T. (2003). Use of race and ethnicity in biomedical publication. *Journal of American Medical Association, 289*(20), 2709–2716.
Lin, S. S., & Kelsey, J. L. (2000). Use of race and ethnicity in epidemiologic research: Concepts, methodological issues, and suggestions for research. *Epidemiologic Reviews, 22*(2), 187–202.
Office of Management and Budget. (1997). *Revisions to the standards for the classification of federal data on race and ethnicity.* Retrieved March 2, 2007, from http:// www.whitehouse.gov/omb/fedreg/1997standards.html.
Winker, M. A. (2006). Race and ethnicity in medical research: Requirements meet reality. *Journal of Law Medical Ethics, 34*(3), 520–525.

RACE BRIDGING

Race bridging refers to making data collected using one set of race categories consistent with data collected using a different set of race categories, to permit estimation and comparison of race-specific statistics at a point in time or over time. More specifically, race bridging is a method used to make multiple-race and single-race data collection systems sufficiently comparable with permit estimation and analysis of race-specific statistics such as birth and death rates. This entry provides an overview of the origins of race bridging and race-bridging methods and focuses on race bridging to estimate single-race population counts, as this has been the primary use of race bridging to date.

Background

The need for race bridging arose when the Office of Management and Budget (OMB) issued revised standards in 1997 for the collection, tabulation, and presentation of data on race and Hispanic origin within the federal statistical system. These standards replaced the 1977 OMB standards. The revised standards increased the minimum set of race categories from four (American Indian or Alaska Native [AIAN], Asian or Pacific Islander [AIP], Black, and White) to five (American Indian or Alaska Native, Asian, Black or African American, Native Hawaiian or Other Pacific Islander, and White). In addition, the revised standards require federal data collection programs to allow respondents to select more than one race category when responding to a query on their racial identity. This means that under the revised standards, there are potentially 31 race groups (five single-race and 26 multiple-race groups), depending on whether a respondent selects one, two, three, four, or all five of the race categories. Because of the addition of the multiple-race groups, race data collected under the revised standards are not comparable with race data collected under the 1977 standards.

The question on race on the 2000 census was based on the revised OMB standards and so allowed respondents to select more than one race category. As a result, the race data on the 2000 census are not comparable with historical race data (e.g., previous censuses, administrative records, surveys, population estimates) or with data on other data systems that have not yet transitioned to the 1997 standards. As many data systems use population estimates to create rates, this left many data users unable to compute current statistics and to track changes over time. One such example is the problem faced by the National Center for Health Statistics (NCHS) in computing birth and death rates for 2000 and beyond and measuring and tracking changes in these vital events. As of 2004, most states had not revised the race question on their birth or death certificates and were still collecting race data using the 1977 race categories. Thus, the calculation of post-2000 race-specific birth and death rates (which use birth and death counts in the numerator and population estimates in the denominator) requires population estimates with the 1977 race categories.

OMB-Proposed Bridging Methods

Recognizing the need to make race data collected under the 1997 standards comparable with race data collected under the 1977 standards, the OMB proposed a number of bridging methods. The proposed methods fall into two broad categories, whole allocation methods and fractional allocation methods. Whole allocation methods assign each multiple-race respondent to only one of the possible single-race categories. Fractional allocation methods divide each multiple-race respondent into parts and assign a part to each possible single-race category. The proposed methods include the following:

- *Smallest Group.* Assigns responses with two or more racial categories to the category, other than white, with the smallest single-race count.
- *Largest Group Other Than White.* Assigns responses with two or more racial categories to the category, other than white, with the largest single-race count.
- *Largest Group.* Assigns responses with two or more racial categories to the category with the largest single-race count.
- *Plurality.* Assigns responses based on data from the National Health Interview Survey (NHIS). Since 1982, the NHIS has permitted respondents to select more than one race and has asked them to indicate with which race they identify most closely (primary race). For each multiple-race group, the proportion selecting each race category as the primary race is calculated. Plurality assigns all responses in a particular multiple-race group to the category with the highest proportion.
- *Equal Fractions.* Assigns multiple-race responses in equal fractions to each single-race category identified.
- *NHIS Fractions.* Assigns responses by fractions to each racial category identified, where the fractions equal the NHIS proportions described in the plurality method above.

Regression Bridging Method

NCHS's National Health Interview Survey (NHIS) provides a unique bridging data source as discussed above. NCHS, in collaboration with the Census Bureau, developed a regression bridging methodology that used information about NHIS multiple-race respondents to obtain single-race population estimates. Schenker and Parker (2003) demonstrated that the regression bridging approach can provide better-bridged estimates than the other proposed bridging methods.

The regression bridging methodology used NHIS data for 1997 to 2000 and involved fitting individual logistic and multilogit models for the larger multiple race groups and a composite multilogit model for the smaller multiple race groups. The models included demographic covariates such as age, sex, and Hispanic origin and county-level contextual variables such as region, urbanization level, percentage in single-race categories, and percent multiple-race population.

Each model estimated the probability that members of the multiple-race group would select each possible single-race category. The probabilities obtained from the bridging models were specific for sex, Hispanic origin, single year of age, and county of residence.

The bridging probabilities derived by NCHS from the regression models have been applied by the Census Bureau to county population estimates beginning in 2000 for 31 races to produce county population estimates for four races. The resulting bridged-race population estimates are available for public use. During the transition period, before all or most birth and death data are available in the multiple-race format, NCHS is also using the bridging probabilities to bridge multiple-race responses on birth and death certificates to single-race responses.

Variance of Bridged-Race Population Estimates

Population estimates generally are assumed to be fixed and do not contribute to the variance of rates. However, this is not true for bridged-race population estimates. Nathaniel Schenker (2003) has developed a methodology to compute variances for bridged-race population estimates.

Race Bridging and the Census Quality Survey

The Census Quality Survey (CQS) was conducted by the Census Bureau in 2001 to produce a data file that could be used to bridge between multiple- and single-race distributions. The sample consisted largely of households that reported at least one multiple-race person in Census 2000 (90% of the initial sample). The CQS respondents were asked at one point in time to "mark one race" and at another point in time to "mark one or more races."

NCHS has used the CQS to develop new bridging models that incorporate additional county-level variables from Census 2000. The outcome of this research will inform decisions concerning selection of bridging probabilities (NHIS or CQS) for future bridging of multiple-race data.

Impact of Bridging

Bridging has the greatest impact on estimates for the AIAN and API populations because a large proportion of each of these populations reports multiple races. Bridging has a small impact on estimates for the black population and negligible impact on estimates for the white population.

—*Deborah D. Ingram*

See also Birth Certificate; Death Certificate; Logistic Regression; Mortality Rates; National Health Interview Survey

Further Readings

Bentley, M., Mattingly, T., Hough, C., & Bennett, C. (2005). *Census Quality Survey to evaluate responses to the Census 2000 question on race: An introduction to the data.* Retrieved June 6, 2006, from http://www2.census .gov/census_2000/datasets/CQS/B.3.pdf.

Ingram, D. D., Parker, J. D., Schenker, N., Weed, J. A., Hamilton, B., Arias, E., et al. (2003). United States Census 2000 population with bridged race categories. National Center for Health Statistics [Electronic version]. *Vital Health Statistics 2*(135). Retrieved June 6, 2006, from http://www.cdc.gov/nchs/about/major/dvs/ popbridge/popbridge.htm.

National Center for Health Statistics. (2005). *U.S. Census populations with bridged race categories.* Retrieved June 6, 2006, from http://www.cdc.gov/nchs/about/major/dvs/ popbridge/popbridge.htm.

Office of Management and Budget. (1997). *Revisions to the standards for the classification of Federal data on race and ethnicity* (Federal Register 62FR58781–58790). Retrieved June 6, 2006, from http://www.whitehouse.gov/ omb/inforeg/r&e_app-a-update.pdf.

Office of Management and Budget. (2000). *Provisional guidance on the implementation of the 1997 standards for the collection of Federal data on race and ethnicity.* Retrieved June 6, 2006, from http://www.Whitehouse .gov/omb/inforeg/r&e_guidance2000update.pdf.

Parker, J. D., Schenker, N., Ingram, D. D, Weed, J. A., Heck, K. E., & Madans, J. H. (2004). Bridging between two standards for collecting information on race and ethnicity and application to Census 2000 and vital rates. *Public Health Reports, 119*, 192–205.

Schenker, N. (2003). Assessing variability due to race bridging: Application to Census counts and vital rates for the Year 2000. *Journal of the American Statistical Association, 98*, 818–828.

Schenker, N., & Parker, J. D. (2003). From single-race reporting to multiple-race reporting: Using imputation methods to bridge the transition. *Statistics in Medicine, 22*, 1571–1587.

Symons-Smith, A., & Ingram, D. D. (2006, March 30 to April 1). *Bridging the gap between the old and new race categories: Comparing population estimates prepared using two different sets of bridging factors.* Population Association of America meetings, Los Angeles, CA.

Radiation

In the context of epidemiology, it is useful to divide radiation into two types: ionizing and nonionizing. Ionizing radiation contains sufficient energy to remove electrons from atoms or molecules, leaving positively charged particles known as ions. X rays, neutrons, alpha particles, beta particles, and gamma rays are forms of ionizing radiation. Nonionizing radiation does not contain sufficient energy to remove electrons from their atoms: types of nonionizing radiation include radiowaves and microwaves. Ionizing radiation is known to be harmful to human tissue in some dosages and can cause damage to DNA. Although some people believe that human health can be harmed by nonionizing radiation emitted by electronic products, such as the radiofrequency radiation used by cell phones, this has not been established scientifically.

Everyone is exposed to small amounts of ionizing radiation, often referred to as "background radiation," from the sun, rocks, water, soil, and so on. For this reason, it is critical to calculate the amount of exposure to radiation when evaluating whether radiation poses a threat to health, because while low levels may be apparently harmless, high levels of exposure can cause serious health effects, including skin burns, hair loss, nausea, birth defects, and death. Exposure to high levels of radiation is also associated with increased risk of certain types of cancer. Apart from accidents such as the Chernobyl nuclear power plant explosion, most radiation exposure results from occupational exposures or from medical applications such as X rays and radiopharmaceuticals.

History

Wilhelm Roentgen discovered artificial radioactivity in 1895 with his observation that emissions from a Crookes tube (a glass vacuum tube with a high-voltage electric current flowing through it) caused a paper coated with fluorescent material to glow. He put this discovery to use by taking an "X ray" of his wife's hand by placing the hand on a photographic plate and exposing it using the Crookes tube: The developed plate revealed the bones of the hand. In 1896, Henri Becquerel discovered the existence of natural radioactivity, which he demonstrated by exposing a photographic plate wrapped in black paper by laying crystals of a uranium compound on top of the paper. The exposed plate displayed emanations from the uranium that were similar to the X rays discovered by Roentgen.

Many uses were found for both natural and artificial radiation, but unfortunately, the consequences of human exposure to radiation were not immediately understood. One of the worst examples of occupational radiation poisoning involved young women who painted dials on watch faces using radioactive paint. The first dial painter to die of radium poisoning was a young woman who had been working at U.S. Radium in New Jersey for only 3 years; her death in 1922 was followed by that of a number of her coworkers. All the early deaths involved necrosis of the jawbone (the painters used their lips to maintain a fine point on the brush) and rampant infections; others died of anemia, bone cancer, or multiple myelomas. Working with artificial radiation also proved dangerous: for instance, Clarence Dally, chief assistant to Thomas Edison, repeatedly exposed his hands to X rays in the course of his experimental work. After a few years, Dally began to suffer burns and hair loss, followed by ulcers and cancerous sores, and ultimately had both arms amputated. Radiologists, who in the early years of their profession were exposed to high levels of radiation on a daily basis, suffered higher rates of cancer, infertility, and birth defects than the general public, and hand amputations were common among that occupational group.

Health Effects

The health effects of radiation are generally related to the type and amount of exposure. There are two broad categories of health effects: stochastic and nonstochastic. Stochastic health effects are associated with long-term, low-level exposure to radiation; increased exposure increases the probability of these effects, but does not influence their type or severity. Cancer is an example of a stochastic health effect: Ionizing radiation may break chemical bonds in atoms and molecules in the body and thus disrupt the control processes that regulate cell growth. Ionizing radiation can also cause changes in the DNA that may lead to genetic and teratogenic mutations.

Nonstochastic effects are caused by exposure to high levels of radiation and are more severe if the exposure is greater. The term *acute* is often used to characterize this type of exposure and the subsequent health effects. Nonstochastic effects include burns and radiation sickness; symptoms of the latter include nausea, weakness, hair loss, and diminished organ function. Cancer patients being treated with radiation typically receive high doses for a short period of time and often experience acute radiation effects.

Regulation

Most regulations regarding permissible exposure are based on the "linear no-threshold theory" that states that there is no totally safe amount of radiation exposure and that the danger increases directly with the dosage. This theory has been challenged, in particular by some scientists who believe that low doses of radiation may be beneficial, but is still reflected in, for instance, standards set by the U.S. Federal Government. The term *radiation dose* refers to the amount of radiation absorbed in the body and is measured in a unit called the *rem* (roentgen equivalent man).

In the United States, radiation safety policies are set by the Environmental Protection Agency (EPA), while execution of these policies are assigned to different agencies. For instance, the U.S. Nuclear Regulatory Commission (USNRC) regulates nuclear power plants and the disposal of radioactive waste, the Mine Safety and Health Administration regulates the exposure of miners to radon and gamma rays, and the Food and Drug Administration develops standards for radioactive material concentrations in food, devices that emit ionizing radiation, and medical devices used in radiation therapy. The 1999 USNRC regulations set dose limits at 0.1 rem/year for the general public, 5.0 rem/year for persons with occupational exposure, and 0.5 rem/year for pregnant women.

Chernobyl

In 1986, explosions within a reactor at the nuclear power plant in Chernobyl, Ukraine, led to large releases of radioactive materials into the atmosphere. These materials were deposited all over Europe, particularly in Belarus, Ukraine, and the Russian Federation. This accident provided a unique natural experiment in the effects of radiation exposure on human health. The WHO conducted a series of meetings in the years 2003 to 2005 to review scientific evidence on health effects of the Chernobyl accident and compare it with results from studies of other situations involving high radiation exposure, such as survivors of the atomic bombs dropped on Japan during World War II.

The WHO concluded that the only type of cancer that clearly increased after the Chernobyl accident and that could be directly attributed to radiation exposure from that accident was thyroid cancer. A large increase in thyroid cancer was found among people who lived in the most contaminated areas who were children or adolescents at the time of the accident. This was due to the radioactive iodine released from the reactor, which was deposited in pastures where the cows grazed. Children who consumed the milk produced by theses cows would get affected. A general iodine deficiency in the local diet exacerbated this problem. An increase in leukemia was found among the Chernobyl liquidators (people involved in containing and cleaning up the radioactive debris, many of whom received acute doses of radiation) but not among residents of the contaminated areas.

Increased mortality is expected over the lifetime of people exposed to radiation from the Chernobyl accident, but it is too early to test those predictions against actual mortality rates among residents of the contaminated areas. Among liquidators, 134 were diagnosed with acute radiation sickness (ARS) and 28 died due to ARS in 1986. No effects on fertility or adverse pregnancy outcomes were found that could be attributed to the Chernobyl accident.

—*Sarah Boslaugh*

See also Birth Defects; Cancer; Environmental and Occupational Epidemiology; Natural Experiment

Further Readings

Agency for Toxic Substances and Disease Registry. (1999). *Toxicological profile for ionizing radiation*. Atlanta, GA: Author. Retrieved December 13, 2006, from http://www.atsdr.cdc.gov/toxprofiles/tp149.html.
Nadakavukaren, A. (2000). *Our global environment: A health perspective* (5th ed.). Prospect Heights, IL: Waveland Press.
World Health Organization. (2006). *Health effects of the Chernobyl accident: An overview* (Fact Sheet No. 303).

Geneva, Switzerland: Author. Retrieved December 13, 2006, from http://www.who.int/mediacentre/factsheets/fs303/en/index.html.

Random-Digit Dialing

Random-digit dialing (RDD) is a method used to select participants for telephone surveys and for related purposes such as selecting control group subjects in case-control studies. The basis of RDD is the random generation of telephone numbers that are used to contact potential survey respondents or study participants. Several major U.S. Federal Government public health surveillance projects use RDD, including the Behavioral Risk Factor Surveillance System (BRFSS) and the National Immunization Survey (NIS). RDD does not require the use of telephone directories and has the advantage of including as potential respondents households with unlisted numbers or who have recently moved or changed phone service; failure to include these types of households can seriously bias the sample. However, RDD has the disadvantage that many of the numbers generated may not be in use or may be nonresidential leading to wasted time and effort.

RDD can be a cost-effective method of selecting subjects in an area where telephone ownership is nearly universal. However, it shares with all telephone-based survey methods the disadvantage that households that do not have telephones generally differ systematically from those who do (e.g., in terms of income, education, and other measures of social capital) and these differences can introduce bias into a study. This can be a major concern in some geographical areas; for instance, in parts of the rural Southern United States, as many as 40% of renter households do not have a telephone. In addition, calculating response rates may be more difficult in RDD surveys than in surveys that used a published telephone directory as a sampling frame.

List-assisted RDD can increase the efficiency of the sampling process. The basis of list-assisted RDD is limiting the randomly generated numbers to groups of numbers, known as 100-blocks, which are known to be in use and contain a high proportion of residential numbers. Each telephone number in the United States is made up of 10 digits—the area code (first three digits), the prefix (the next three digits), and the suffix (the last four digits). The first eight digits are sometimes collectively called 100-blocks because they define sets of 100 telephone numbers with the same first eight digits. Lists of these 100-blocks for the geographical area to be sampled, as well as lists of working phone numbers, may be purchased by firms that specialize in providing this information. Comparing the randomly generated numbers to a list of known business numbers and eliminating those that do not also have a residential listing can further improve efficiency, as can use of a machine to detect the dial tone that precedes the "number not in service message" and eliminating these numbers from the sample.

The increasing popularity of cell phones, in particular the increase in households that do not also have a "land line" (traditional phone) has introduced several other issues. Because cell phone numbers have not traditionally been included in telephone surveys, households with only a cell phone (about 7% of U.S. households in 2005) are excluded from the possibility of participation. In addition, concerns such as safety (a person could answer his or her cell phone while driving, which could lead to an accident), cost to the respondent (because cell phones contacts often include a charge for receiving incoming calls), and low yield (because cell phones are disproportionately owned by children and adolescents) are issues that must be dealt with.

—*Sarah Boslaugh*

See also Bias; Health Disparities; Social Capital and Health; Study Design; Survey Research Methods

Further Readings

Glaser, S. L., & Stearns, C. B. (2002). Reliability of random digit dialing calls to enumerate an adult female population. *American Journal of Epidemiology, 155*(10), 972–975.

Link, M. W., Battaglia, M. P., Frankel, M. R., Osborn, L., & Mokdad, A. H. (2006). Addressed-based versus random-digit-dial surveys: Comparison of key health and risk indicators. *American Journal of Epidemiology, 164*(10), 10191025.

Voigt, L. F., Davis, S., & Heuser, L. (1992). Random digit dialing: The potential effect on sample characteristics of the conversion of nonresidential telephone numbers. *American Journal of Epidemiology, 136*(11), 1393–1399.

RANDOMIZATION

Randomization is a term used in clinical trials to denote a scheme for assigning study subjects to treatment groups using methods that are independent of the individual subjects' characteristics. Typically, when randomization is used, each participant has an equal chance of assignment to each study group or treatment group. Many characteristics of study subjects may affect the relationship of treatment and outcome; some of these are known to the researcher in advance, some are not known. By randomization we hope to sort people with these characteristics equally between the treatment groups. Randomization should also yield equal distributions of characteristics that affect the outcome in ways that the researcher did not anticipate.

The effectiveness of randomization is evaluated through comparing the resulting treatment groups on baseline characteristics and demographics. If a subject characteristic is found unequally distributed between treatment groups despite randomization, it should be treated as a potential confounder in the analysis.

The effectiveness of randomization is sensitive to the size of the study population. A large study population will increase the chances that randomization will be successful in yielding equivalent distributions of participant characteristics; a smaller population is more susceptible to unequal assignment to groups through chance.

The unit of randomization may be the individual study subjects, or it may be larger groups. The unit of randomization may be groups such as clinic, hospital, neighborhood, town, city, or other social groupings. In this case, the entire group would be randomly assigned to one treatment group. For example, in a trial of the effectiveness of smoking-cessation messages, entire communities may be randomly assigned to different types of smoking-cessation messages.

Methods for implementing randomization include using a random number generator to assign a number to each subject with a set method of allocating specific numbers to particular treatments. For example, a random number generator is used to assign the numbers 0.1, 0.3, 0.8, 0.4, 0.3 to the first five study subjects and by prior decision those with an odd number are assigned to the active treatment and those with an even number are assigned to the control treatment.

Study Subjects 1, 2, and 5 would be assigned to the active treatment, while Subjects 3 and 4 would be assigned to the control treatment.

Some methods used to assign subjects to groups are not as truly random and should be used with caution if at all. For example, if clinic is held 4 days a week, subjects who come in on Monday or Wednesday may be assigned to one treatment, while those who come in on Tuesday or Thursday are assigned to the other treatment. This method may create effective randomization if there is no relationship between the day of the week and other subject characteristics, but the burden of establishing this rests on the researcher.

Nonrandomized trials may have problems with selection bias if patients are assigned to the treatment group according to some characteristic. In an early trial of cardiac care units (CCUs), heart attack patients who were deemed at greater risk were preferentially sent to the CCU rather than the comparison, the standard treatment. In the analysis, the CCU was found to have higher mortality than the standard treatment, but the comparison was skewed by the more serious condition of the patients assigned to the CCU compared with those who received the standard treatment.

—*Sydney Pettygrove*

See also Bias; Clinical Trials; Confounding

Further Readings

Friedman, L., Furberg, C. D., & DeMets, D. L. (1999). *Fundamentals of clinical trials* (3rd ed.). New York: Springer.
Piantadosi, S. (2005). *Clinical trials: A methodologic perspective* (2nd ed.). New York: Wiley-Interscience.

RANDOM VARIABLE

A variable whose observed values may be considered as outcomes of a stochastic or random experiment is called a *random variable*. The values of such a variable in a particular sample cannot be anticipated with certainty before the sample is gathered. Random variables are commonly classified as qualitative or categorical, discrete, or continuous.

A random variable is defined as a qualitative or categorical variable if its set of possible values do not represent numerical information. For example, gender is a categorical variable. Suppose that among 100 patients, there are 65 females and 35 males, and let X be the sex of a randomly chosen patient among these 100 patients. Then X is a qualitative *random variable*, and the values of X are "Female" and "Male" with 65% and 35% chance to be chosen, respectively. Even if numeric values, such as 0 and 1, are used to code gender in a data set, it remains a categorical variable because the values represent membership in a category rather than a measured quantity.

A random variable is discrete if its set of possible values is countable. If only two values are possible, such as alive versus dead, it may also be called a binomial random variable. For example, a new technique, balloon angioplasty, is being widely used to open clogged heart valves and vessels. The balloon is inserted via a catheter and is inflated, opening the vessel; thus, no surgery is required. Suppose that among untreated people with heart-valve disease, about 50% die within 2 years, and experience with balloon angioplasty suggests that approximately 70% treated with this technique live for more than 2 years. We can define X as the number of patients who will live more than 2 years, among the next five patients treated with balloon angioplasty at a hospital. Then, X constitutes a *discrete random variable*, which can take on the values 0, 1, 2, 3, 4, or 5.

To make an inference about the population from our sample data, we need to know the probability associated with each value of the variable that is called its *probability distribution*. Probability calculations are relatively simple for discrete variables and are often displayed in tabular form, as presented below. The *probability distribution* for a *discrete random variable* X displays the probability $P(x)$ associated with each value of x. This display can be presented as a table, a graph, or a formula. To illustrate, consider the above example; all possible values of X are 0, 1, 2, 3, 4, and 5. The probability distribution is a binomial distribution with $n=5$ and $p=0.7$ that can be given by the formula:

$$P(X=k) = \frac{n!}{k!(n-k)!}(0.7)^k(0.3)^{n-k},$$

$$k = 0, 1, 2, \ldots, 5.$$

It may also be displayed as shown in Table 1.

Table 1	Probability Distribution for Discrete Random Variable X
X	$P(x)$
0	0.00243
1	0.02835
2	0.13230
3	0.30870
4	0.36015
5	0.16807

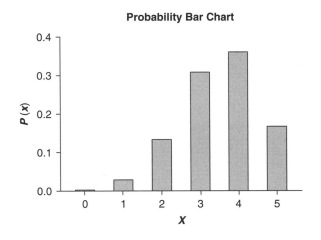

Figure 1 Bar Chart Displaying Probability Distribution for Discrete Random Variable X

Or, it may be presented graphically as a bar chart, as shown in Figure 1.

The properties of discrete random variables are as follows:

- The probability associated with every value of x lies between 0 and 1.
- The sum of the probabilities for all values of x is equal to 1.
- The probabilities are additive, that is, $P(X \geq 4)$ is the same $P(X=4) + P(X=5)$.

A random variable is defined as continuous if its set of possible values is an entire interval on the number line, that is, if it can take any value within a range rather than only a discrete set of values such as was specified in the previous example. Of course, any measuring device has a limited accuracy and therefore a continuous scale may in practice be something of an abstraction. Some examples of continuous random variables are the height of an adult male, the weight of a newborn baby, a patient's body temperature, and the survival time of a patient following a heart attack.

To describe the distribution of a continuous random variable, a probability density function $f(x)$ is used, which has three properties:

1. The total area under the probability density curve is 1.

2. $P\{a \leq X \leq b\} = $ Area under the probability density curve between a and b.

3. $f(x) \geq 0$ for all x.

Unlike the description of a discrete probability distribution, the probability density $f(x)$ does not represent the probability that the random variable will exactly equal the value x. Instead, a probability density function relates the probability of a value falling within the range between a and b, that is, the areas of the curve over that interval. The probability that $X = x$ for a continuous random variable is always equal to 0.

The last statement may need some clarification. In the birthweight example, $P\{X = 8.5\} = 0$ probably seems shocking. Does this mean that no child can have a birth weight of 8.5 lb? No. To understand it, we need to recognize that the accuracy of every measuring device is limited, so that here the number 8.5 is actually indistinguishable from all numbers in an interval surrounding it, say [8.495, 8.505], and the area under the curve between this interval is no longer 0.

There are many useful continuous random variables, each with a specific distribution or set of distributions described by mathematical functions that allow us to compute probabilities regarding specific values. The most famous of these distributions is the normal distribution, also called the bell curve, Z distribution or Gaussian distribution, which plays a special role in statistical theory (through the Central Limit Theorem) as well as in practice.

—*Renjin Tu*

See also Binomial Variable; Central Limit Theorem; Normal Distribution; Sampling Distribution; Z Score

Further Readings

Devore, J., & Peck, R. (2004). *Statistics: The exploration and analysis of data* (5th ed.). Belmont, CA: Duxbury Press.
Johnson, R. A., & Bhattacharyya, C. K. (2005). *Statistics principles and methods* (5th ed.). New York: Wiley.

RATE

A rate is a measure of change in one quantity with respect to change in another. As used in epidemiology, this typically refers to an incidence rate, where the numerator is the number of new events and the denominator is total person-time at risk. This is one of the key measures of occurrence of disease in populations and gives an estimate of how fast disease or death is happening in a given population.

An example calculation of an incidence rate can be done using data from Table 1. A total of three events occurred, and the total person-time at risk summed over all population members is $30 + 17 + 22 + 11 + 20 = 100$ person-years, giving a rate of 3/100 or 0.03 per year. In calculating a rate, events counted in the numerator should be those occurring among people contributing person-time to the denominator. Likewise, the denominator should include only person-time during which any events experienced by the subject would be counted in the numerator. Sometimes the denominator can be estimated as average population size times follow-up time for a relatively short period of time with stable population level. For example, this is often done for an annual mortality rate in a geographic area, such as a state.

Some properties of incidence rates include the following:

- They range from 0 to infinity.
- Units are (time) − 1, where any unit of time can be used.

Table 1   Data for Sample Calculation of Rate

Person ID#	Total Years of Follow-Up	Event
01	30	N
02	17	Y
03	22	Y
04	11	N
05	20	Y

- The actual measure depends on the unit of time used in the denominator.

For example, the following are equivalent:

$$1\frac{\text{Event}}{\text{Person} - \text{year}} = 0.083\frac{\text{Events}}{\text{Person} - \text{month}}$$
$$= 10\frac{\text{Events}}{\text{Person} - \text{decade}}.$$

The same rate may arise through alternate scenarios involving different lengths of follow-up time and population sizes. For example, following 100 people for an average of 1 year each and observing three events would give an incidence rate of 0.03 per year. The same rate of 0.03 per year would also be calculated if three events were observed among only five people followed for an average of 20 years, as shown in the example above.

Incidence rates are occasionally reported in terms of change in a unit other than person-time—for example, motorist fatality rates per person-mile or aviation events per pilot-flight hour. The rates given simply per unit time as opposed to per unit person-time may be referred to as absolute rates.

The term *rate* has sometimes been used in a more general sense to refer to proportions or ratios. The concept of rate as different from risk (a proportion) was elucidated in the 19th century by William Farr. Farr reported vital statistics for England and contrasted cholera with tuberculosis. The former had a higher *rate* of death among patients, because the disease could be quickly fatal; whereas the latter had a higher *risk* of death, since a greater percentage of those falling ill would eventually succumb to the disease. Even so, use of terminology such as *attack rate* and *prevalence rate* for measures that are technically proportions still persists.

Incidence rate is also known as incidence density, person-time rate, and force of morbidity or mortality.

—Keely Cheslack-Postava

See also Incidence; Mortality Rates; Person-Time Units; Proportion; Ratio

Further Readings

Elandt-Johnson, R. C. (1975). Definition of rates: Some remarks on their use and misuse. *American Journal of Epidemiology, 102*(4), 267–271.

Morabia, A. (2004). Epidemiology: An epistemological perspective. In A. Morabia (Ed.), *A history of epidemiologic methods and concepts* (pp. 3–125). Basel, Switzerland: Birkhauser Verlag.

Rothman, K. J., & Greenland, S. (1998). Measures of disease frequency. In K. J. Rothman & S. Greenland, *Modern epidemiology* (2nd ed., pp. 29–46). Philadelphia: Lippincott Williams & Wilkins.

RATIO

A ratio is an expression of the magnitude of one quantity in relation to another. Ratios are typically expressed by two numbers separated by a colon, for instance, 4:3, read as "four to three" and meaning that there are four units of the first items for every three units of the second item. Ratios do not require that the two numbers have common units and in fact are typically used to express the relationship between two quantities consisting of different units. For instance, the ratio of male to female patients in a hospital might be expressed as 2:1, meaning there were twice as many male patients as female patients or that there were two male patients for every one female patient.

The concept of ratio has to be clearly distinguished from the definitions of proportion and of rate. A ratio is a fraction in which the numerator is not necessarily a part of the denominator or, in other words, in a ratio the numerator is not necessarily included in the population defined by the denominator. In contrast, in a proportion the numerator by definition is included in the denominator. Taking the hospital example again, if the ratio of male to female patients is 2:1, in order to express this as a proportion we must introduce the unit of "patient" (as opposed to male patient and female patient) to be able to make the statement that proportion of male patients among all patients is 66.7% or two thirds; in this case of the proportion, male patients are included in both the numerator and denominator of the fraction. Ratios are distinguished from rates because ratios do not include a measure of time in the denominator.

The main properties of ratios are that they are greater than zero, they may or may not be greater than 100, and may or may not have units. Ratios may also be expressed as percentages. Ratios are commonly used in epidemiology and public health: For instance, the risk ratio, also known as relative risk, is used to express the risk of a person developing a condition given a particular exposure, relative to those lacking the exposure. Odds ratios similarly express the odds of developing a condition given an exposure, compared with those who do not have the exposure. Both the risk ratio and odds ratio are dimensionless.

Ratios are also used in epidemiology to express availability of services or cases of disease for a particular population. For instance, a commonly reported measure of health care availability is the number of hospitals or hospital beds per 10,000 people, which is calculated by dividing the number of hospitals or beds by the population size and multiplying by 10,000. Obviously, the numerator in these cases are hospitals or hospital beds, and the denominator in both cases are people, so they do not have a common unit. Similar examples include the per capita income: that is, the total income earned during a year by a group of people divided by the number of people (units = dollars per capita); and the mortality (or death) rate: that is, the number of deaths during a specified period divided by the number of persons at risk of dying during this period (units = deaths per 100 people; larger units such as per 10,000 people can be used for rare diseases or when mortality is rare). Note that the terms *ratio* and *rate* are sometimes used interchangeably, particularly when speaking of statistics such as the number of hospitals per 10,000 people. However, many epidemiologists prefer to reserve the term *rate* to refer to numbers expressed per unit time, such as infections per year.

—Carlos Campillo

See also Proportion; Rate

Further Readings

Armitage, P., & Berry, G. (1994). *Statistical methods in medical research.* London: Macmillan.
Daniel, W. W. (2004). *Biostatistics: A foundation for analysis in the health sciences.* New York: Wiley.

Receiver Operating Characteristic (ROC) Curve

The receiver operationg characteristic (ROC) curve is a two-dimensional measure of classification performance depicting the trade-off between sensitivity and specificity. It is used in the analysis of a diagnostic test or screening test that classifies experimental units into two categories such as diseased (D) or non-diseased ($\bar{D}$). Screening and laboratory test results are usually reported as a continuous variable. For example, the risk variable serum concentration of creatine phosphokinase for myocardial infarction (D) is approximately normally distributed varying from less than 100 units/ml to greater than 4,000 units/ml. The serum concentration of creatine phosphokinase for those without myocardial infarction ($\bar{D}$) also has an approximate normal distribution but has a different mean (see Figure 1). Suppose that we dichotomize the serum concentration by some cutpoint so that values above it represent positive ($+$) test results and values below it represent negative ($-$) test results. We may now define the following misclassification rates: *false-positive rate* $P(+|\bar{D})$ is the probability of classifying a noncase as positive, *true-positive rate (sensitivity)* $P(+|D)$ is the probability of classifying a case as positive, *false-negative rate* $P(-|D)$ is the probability of classifying a case as negative, and *true-negative rate (specificity)* $P(-|\bar{D})$ is the probability of classifying a noncase as negative. As shown in the table below, different cutpoints lead to tests with different levels of misclassification rates. For example, when the cutoff value of the serum concentration is chosen to be 5.4, calculation from the two normal distributions gives $P(+|D) = .725747$ (see the shaded area in Figure 1), $P(-|D) = .27425$, $P(-|\bar{D}) = 991802$, and $P(+|\bar{D}) = .008198$ (see the small double-shaded area in Figure 1). Note that if we lowered the cutoff value, we would decrease the false-negative rate, but we would also increase the false-positive rate. Similarly, if we raised the cutoff value, we would decrease the false-positive rate, but we would increase the false-negative rate (see Figure 1).

An ROC curve is obtained by plotting the false-positive rate ($1-$ specificity) against the true-positive rate (sensitivity) for a series of cutpoints defined by the test (see Figure 2). It shows the trade-off between the true-positive rate and the false-positive rate of a test (any increase in sensitivity will be accompanied by a decrease in specificity and conversely). In statistical terminology, it is the plot of Type I error against the power. This ROC plot is representative of those plotting one conditional distribution function against another found to be useful in epidemiology and other health sciences, which includes plotting the posttest

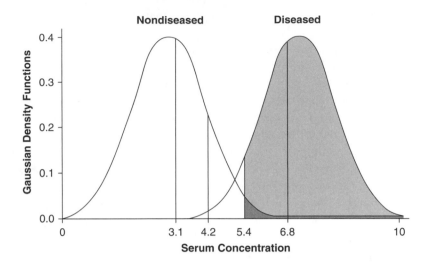

Figure 1   Distribution of Serum Concentration: Diseased Versus Nondiseased

probability of disease given the test is positive against the pretest probability of disease, plotting the positive predictive value against the point prevalence rate, and plotting the total time on test against the distribution function of the duration time. The closer the curve follows the left-hand border and then the top border of the ROC space, the more accurate the test. The closer the curve comes to the 45° diagonal of the ROC space, the less accurate the test. The slope of the tangent line at any point on the ROC curve may be accurately estimated by spline interpolation and differentiation. The slope of the tangent line at a cutpoint gives the likelihood ratio (LR) for that value of the test. So, by choosing the slope of the tangent to the ROC curve to equal the LR that will minimize the total cost of making false-positive and false-negative errors, one can identify the optimal cutoff values. Such LR turns out to be the ratio of the product of the net cost of treating nondiseased patients and the pretest probability of no disease to the product of the net benefit of treating diseased patients and the pretest probability of disease.

The area under the curve (AUC) is a measure of test accuracy, namely, a measure of how well the risk variable discriminates a disease state. If you take a random person from the nondiseased population and obtain a value X for the serum concentration and a random person from the diseased population and get a score of Y, then the area under the ROC curve represents $P\{Y > X\}$. This implies that the more apart the distribution for the diseased is from the distribution for the nondiseased, the more accurate is the

test. In other words, the accuracy of the test depends on how well the test separates the group being tested into those with and without the disease in question. AUC = 1, which corresponds to the left and top border of the ROC space, represents a perfect test, AUC = .5, which corresponds to the 45° diagonal of the ROC space, represents a random (hence useless) test, namely that the risk variable is completely independent of disease so that the probability of detecting disease will be the same for those with and without disease (the two distributions—one for the diseased and the other for the nondiseased—of the risk variable completely overlap). Here is a rough guide for classifying the accuracy of a diagnostic test using AUC:

96% to 100% = excellent

90% to 96% = very good

80% to 90% = good

70% to 80% = fair

60% to 70% = poor

50% to 60% = useless

Construction of ROC Curve

Suppose the serum concentrations for both diseased and nondiseased populations are normally distributed with the same variance but different means. They are transformed into $N(3,1)$ and $N(7,1)$ distributions in Figure 1. We first choose a series of cutpoints on the

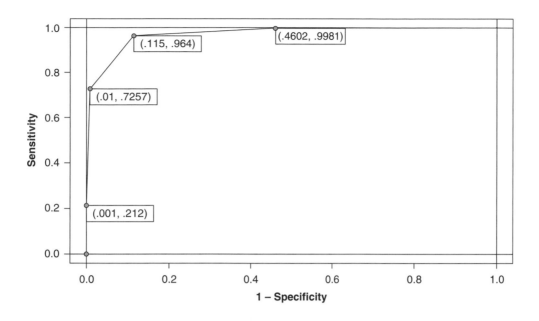

Figure 2   ROC Curve for Serum Creatine Phosphokinase

serum concentration 3.1, 4.2, 5.4, and 6.8 and erect vertical lines at these cutpoints in Figure 1. We then compute the corresponding sensitivity and false-positive rate (1 − specificity) for each cutpoint from the two normal distributions. These are the areas from each vertical cutpoint line to the right tails of the two respective normal curves. The two shaded areas in Figure 1 correspond to the sensitivity = 0.725747 and 1 − specificity = 0.008198 when cutoff value is chosen to be 5.4. The results for the four chosen cutoff values are as shown below:

Serum Concentration	Sensitivity	1 − Specificity
3.1	0.998134	0.460172
4.2	0.964070	0.115070
5.4	0.725747	0.008198
6.8	0.211855	0.000072

The data given in the last two columns (1 − specificity, sensitivity) are then graphed to obtain the ROC curve with 1 − specificity on the horizontal axis and sensitivity on the vertical axis as shown in Figure 2. These data are also used to compute the area under the ROC curve, where Area = (1 + .998134) × (1 − .460172)/2 + (.96407 + .725747) × (.11507 − .008198)/2 + (.725747 + .211855) × (.008198 − .000072)/2 + (.211855 × .000072)/2 = .972, by the trapezoidal rule, which, according to the criteria stated above, is considered to be excellent. This means that the relative ordering of the serum concentration of creatine phosphokinase has a 97.2% probability of correctly distinguishing a person with myocardial infarction from a normal person. A more accurate estimate of the area may be obtained by cubic spline interpolation and integration. When data on frequencies of various categories of the risk variable defined by the cutpoints for both the diseased and the nondiseased samples are available, sensitivity $P(+|D)$ and specificity $|P(-|\bar{D})$ can be estimated directly from these data as, $\#(+, D)/\#(D)$ and $\#(-, \bar{D})/\#(\bar{D})$, respectively, where $\#(x)$ stands for the number of x. These estimates can then be used to construct the empirical ROC curve by plotting the estimates of 1 − specificity versus the estimates of sensitivity. The resulting empirical curve may then be smoothed by smoothing splines.

Finally, the construction of two-dimensional ROC curve described above can also be generalized to construct the three-dimensional ROC surface just as plane geometry has been generalized to solid geometry.

—*John J. Hsieh*

See also Life Tables; Likelihood Ratio; Normal Distribution; Screening; Sensitivity and Specificity; Type I and Type II Errors; Z Score

Further Readings

Biggerstaff, B. J. (2000). Comparing diagnostic tests: A simple graphic using likelihood ratios. *Statistics in Medicine, 19*(5), 649–663.

Egan, J. P. (1975). *Signal detection theory and ROC analysis.* New York: Academic Press.

Hanley, J. A., & McNeil, B. J. (1982). The meaning and use of the area under a receiver operating characteristic (ROC) curve. *Radiology, 143*, 29–36.

Zweig, M. H., & Campbell G. (1993). Receiver-operating characteristic (ROC) plots: A fundamental evaluation tool in clinical medicine. *Clinical Chemistry, 39*(4), 561–577.

REED, WALTER

(1851–1902)

Walter Reed was a surgeon in the U.S. Army who significantly contributed to knowledge of the etiology and epidemiology of yellow fever. Reed's work is significant in that he focused on the means of disease transmission rather than a specific disease agent and, in doing so, greatly reduced infection rates. His yellow fever experiments also established the important role of the "healthy volunteer" in epidemiologic research and contributed greatly to the formalization and documentation of informed consent. Reed was born in Belroi, Virginia, and became a medical officer in the U.S. Army after graduating from the University of Virginia medical school. He remained in the military for the remainder of his life.

During the Spanish-American War, yellow fever killed thousands of soldiers in Cuba—more than died in battle—and continued to threaten troops occupying the island as well as individuals throughout North and South America. For several decades, scientists and local physicians had proposed that yellow fever was mosquito borne, but the insect's exact role was unclear. In 1900, Surgeon General George Sternberg established the Yellow Fever Commission under Reed's direction, and Reed went to Cuba.

Because there was no animal model in which to study yellow fever, identifying the exact mode and source of transmission required humans. Reed and his colleagues designed an experiment in which common house mosquitoes (now known as *Aedes aegypti*) that had fed on yellow fever patients were allowed to bite noninfected individuals. Reed's colleague suggested that the research team serve as the first group of subjects; after two physicians became ill (and one eventually died), Reed decided to forego self-experimentation. Instead, healthy volunteers (primarily soldiers and native Cubans) were recruited and separated into two groups—those who would be bitten and those who would be exposed to soiled bedding from patients (another potential suspect). The theory that yellow fever is transmitted by mosquitoes and not direct contact with an infected individual was confirmed.

Reed's research was recognized by Congress, and his reputation as a heroic researcher and the bravery of his colleagues were celebrated for decades. After conducting malaria research in Cuba, he returned to Washington, D.C., to teach pathology and bacteriology at the Army Medical School and the George Washington University Medical School. Reed's health began to decline following an appendectomy; in 1902, he died of peritonitis and was buried in Arlington National Cemetery. Named in his honor, Walter Reed General Hospital in Washington, D.C., opened on May 1, 1909. In 1951, the hospital was renamed the Walter Reed Army Medical Center, now the premier military medical facility in the eastern United States.

—Emily E. Anderson

See also Ethics in Human Subjects Research; Informed Consent; Insect-Borne Disease; Yellow Fever

Further Readings

Bean, W. B. (1982). *Walter Reed: A biography.* Charlottesville, VA: University of Virginia Press.

Pierce, J. R., & Writer, J. (2005). *Yellow Jack: How yellow fever ravaged America and Walter Reed discovered its deadly secrets.* Hoboken, NJ: Wiley.

Reed, W., & Agramonte, A. (1983). Landmark article. February 16, 1901: The etiology of yellow fever. An additional note. *Journal of the American Medical Association, 250*(5), 649–658.

Web Sites

Walter Reed Army Medical Center. http://www.wramc.amedd.army.mil.

REGRESSION

Many analyses of epidemiologic data are conducted using statistical methods common to other research fields, including the social and biologic sciences. In epidemiologic studies, however, the focus of the research question, and thus the methods used to study this question, tend to differ. The combination of human, social, environmental, and biological factors that may be present in epidemiologic studies can lead to a complexity not seen in large randomized trials or when the environment can be controlled. This entry discusses regression methods used in epidemiology and the conceptual framework that underlies these methods.

Predictive Analysis Versus Associative Analysis

Epidemiologic research questions tend to fall into two general categories: (1) What factors best explain or predict the occurrence of another factor (or outcome)? (2) What is the association between exposure(s) and outcome(s)? The analytic methods used for these research questions are known as predictive or associative, respectively.

Regression analysis is used for both analysis of prediction and association. However, the selection of factors included in the model differs based on the type of analysis performed. While most statistics books focus on measures of prediction, epidemiologic studies are primarily concerned with questions of association. Because measuring associations is the most common use of regression analysis in epidemiology, this methodology is the focus of this entry. Analysis for questions of prediction will primarily be discussed to provide a contrast on how analysis differs from that for estimating measures of association.

Prediction

Research questions focused on prediction take two main forms. They may seek to identify any factors that may influence the detection of a health outcome, or they may seek to identify which of the factors are most predictive of development of the health outcome in affected individuals.

An example of the first use of predictive analysis is the identification of victims of intimate partner violence. A study may be done to identify indicators of partner violence victimization for women seen in a primary care setting. In such a study, a group of factors is found to identify victims. These include injuries, multiple nonspecific physical symptoms (e.g., pain, fatigue, headaches, diarrhea), and psychiatric diseases (e.g., depression, anxiety, post-traumatic stress disorder) as well as characteristics of the victim (e.g., young), perpetrator (e.g., young, excessive alcohol use), and relationship (e.g., wife makes more money than husband). Many of these factors are common among women seen in primary care (e.g., young age, depression). The more characteristics a woman has that were identified as predictive in regression, the more likely that she is a victim of partner violence. This analysis had no interest in identifying the "best" predictor, but in understanding what factors, alone or in combination, predict partner violence so that these factors can be communicated to both physicians and patients. Some of the factors so identified may be outcomes rather than causes of partner violence, but this is not a concern when the purpose of the study is to identify potential victims of partner violence rather than make causal statements about it.

The goal of the second type of predictive model is to identify the most important factors that predict the outcome. For example, it is known that infection with Hepatitis C virus is a risk factor for development of liver cancer. However, not all individuals who are infected with Hepatitis C virus develop this cancer. Now that we can test for Hepatitis C, it may help understand what factors best predict liver cancer among those infected. It is then necessary to examine these other factors, which may include coinfection with Hepatitis B virus, gender, viral genotype, liver enzyme level, use of alcohol or tobacco, and environmental and occupational exposures. Using predictive modeling, we can identify which factors best predict development of liver cancer and then monitor the group with these characteristics more carefully to identify early disease and focus care to more aggressively reduce risk of liver cancer. Here, we are interested in identifying factors that are predictive of liver cancer, not how the factors are associated with or cause cancer.

Measures of Association

Questions of association focus on the estimation of the strength of association between an exposure, or exposures, and an outcome. Studying associations in this way helps inform us about the causes of disease, hospitalization, death, and other health-related outcomes. While a strong association does not mean that the exposure caused the outcome, establishing that an association exists is a critical piece of information to assess potential causality. Examples of studies that focus on association include measurement of the association between location of work within a chemical plant and the risk of developing cancer, between infection with a particular microorganism and development of a clinical disease, and between exposure to airborne dust and development of asthma.

In epidemiology, we are most often focused on identifying causal relationships, that is, determining the association between potential exposures (i.e., risk factors) and an outcome(s). Because other factors can complicate this association, particularly confounders and effect modifiers, regression analysis is a valuable tool to estimate the association when the relationship is complex; that is, confounders or effect modifiers exist.

Regression Analysis to Estimate Measures of Association

Although stratified analysis may be used to examine confounders, this approach quickly becomes problematic when many confounders exist. Many 2×2 tables need to be generated and analyzed, and as the number of tables grows, so does the potential for zero values in the table cells, which can lead to a poor estimate of association strength. Multivariate regression methods may be used to study these associations while taking into account all the potential confounders. Logistic, log-binomial, Poisson, and linear regression are discussed here to provide insight into these methods.

Regression Model Format

Most regression equations model the relationship between an outcome measure and a function (e.g., logit, log) of a linear combination of the independent factors and regression parameters. In studies designed to estimate the measure of association, the independent variables are made up of the exposure(s), potential confounders, and interaction terms for potential effect modifiers. The key difference in analysis between studies of prediction and studies of association is variable selection. For studies measuring associations, classic stepwise regression techniques are not appropriate; rather, variables need to be assessed with regard to their role as potential effect modifiers and confounders.

In a regression analysis, all information about association between exposure and outcome is stored in the slopes (β) of factors that contain the exposure term. Consider the following general combination of independent factors for a study:

1. $\beta_0 + \beta_1 \times E$

2. $\beta_0 + \beta_1 \times E + \beta_2 \times C_1 + \beta_3 \times C_2 + \beta_4 \times C_3$

3. $\beta_0 + \beta_1 \times E + \beta_2 \times C + \beta_3 \times M + \beta_4 \times E \times M$

4. $\beta_0 + \beta_1 \times E + \beta_2 \times C_1 + \beta_3 \times C_2 + \beta_4 \times C_3 + \beta_5 \times M_1 + \beta_6 \times M_2 + \beta_7 \times E \times M_1 + \beta_8 \times E \times M_2$

where

β (beta) is the regression coefficient

E is a dichotomous exposure ($1 =$ exposed, $0 =$ not exposed)

Cs are potential confounders: C_1 is dichotomous ($1 =$ present, $0 =$ absent), C_2 is dichotomous ($1 =$ present, $0 =$ absent), C_3 is continuous

Ms are potential effect modifiers: M_1 is dichotomous ($1 =$ present, $0 =$ absent), M_2 is continuous

Typically, a model including all factors of interest is created and fit to the data. The exception to this approach is when there is substantial collinearity; that is, the factors overlap a great deal causing mathematical problems in estimating βs.

For a model with a dichotomous exposure factor as the sole independent variable (Model 1), the measure of association between the exposure and outcome is simply the $\exp(\beta_1)$, that is, the odds ratio (in a logistic regression model), relative risk (in a log-binomial model), or rate ratio (in Poisson regression).

For studies where the measure of association may be confounded but no effect modification exists (Model 2), the measure of association is also estimated simply by $\exp(\beta_1)$; however, this estimate is different from the estimate from Model 1, as it is adjusted by the potential confounders during the iterative process used to estimate βs. To determine if the potential confounders are, in fact, confounders in the study, each one is removed, the model is rerun without that factor, and $\exp(\beta_1)$ (i.e., the odds ratio for the exposure) is examined to determine if it has changed compared with its value when the potential confounder was in the model. If $\exp(\beta_1)$ for the exposure is about the same whether the potential confounder is included in the model or not, then it is not a confounder in this study. If $\exp(\beta_1)$ for the exposure does change between the two models, then the potential confounder is a confounder in this study, and it must remain in the model to remove the effects of confounding associated with it. How much does $\exp(\beta_1)$ need to change to provide evidence of confounding? The answer is "it depends." Some epidemiologists use a 10% rule; that is, if the $\exp(\beta_1)$ changes by 10% or more between the two models, then the factor removed is a confounder. Others use a more subjective rule based on the study measures; that is, determine if the change is meaningful in the interpretation of the association between exposure and outcome. Still others do not believe it is appropriate to remove any potential confounder that was considered based on the literature, even if it is not a confounder for the study.

Usually, if potential effect modifiers exist, they are assessed first. Assessing effect modification is done by evaluating βs for the interaction terms. Epidemiologists focus on βs and not the p values for decision making, because the p value is affected by factors besides strength of association, such as sample size. As is discussed below, effect modification exists if there is a different association identified between exposure and outcome based on a third factor—for example, when the association between gender and risk of asthma onset is modified by age. For measures of association between an exposure (dichotomous) and outcome, the odds ratio (logistic regression), relative risk (log-binomial), and rate ratio (Poisson regression) is different for young children than for adolescents. In Model 3, with one dichotomous exposure and one dichotomous potential effect modifier, the odds ratio, relative risk, and rate ratios are estimated by

Modifier $= 0$ Measure of association $= \exp(\beta_1)$.

Modifier $= 1$ Measure of association $= \exp(\beta_1 + \beta_4)$.

It should be noted that βs are adjusted for the other factors in the model (i.e., the confounder and main effect of the modifier). These adjustments are done during the iterative process that is used to estimate βs.

To determine if M is actually an effect modifier, we assess if $\beta_4 = 0$. If β_4 is about equal to zero, then there is no effect modification, and the estimated association is about $\exp(\beta_1)$ for each level of M. A large p value (i.e., one that is not statistically significant) could occur for two reasons: (1) $\beta_4 \sim 0$, that is, no

effect modification is evident or (2) there are not sufficient data to assess effect modification (β_4 appears different than 0, but there is a relatively small sample size in some of the modifier levels, so the estimate β_4 lacks precision). Thus, p values need to be considered in conjunction with the actual βs to understand if no effect modification exists or if insufficient data are available to adequately assess effect modification.

Logistic Regression

Logistic regression is the most popular regression analysis method used in epidemiology today. Computer programs for widespread use were developed in the 1970s to respond to the data analysis needs of the Framingham Study. Now, user-friendly statistical software for logistic regression is widely available for researchers.

Models and Formulae

At the heart of logistic regression is the odds ratio, which is exactly what the name implies: a ratio of two odds. In fact, logistic regression provides a direct method to compute adjusted odds ratios, adjusting for confounders. In a case-control study, the exposure odds are calculated; that is, the odds of cases being exposed versus the odds of controls being exposed. In a cohort study or randomized trial, the incidence odds are computed; that is, the odds of the outcome among the exposed and the odds of the outcome among the not exposed. Fortunately, the model looks the same and the odds ratios are calculated similarly regardless of the study design. In logistic regression, the probability of a specific outcome, $P(Y = 1)$, is modeled as a function of the factors of interest (i.e., exposure(s), confounder(s), and effect modifier(s)) and regression parameters. In its simplest form, with only one dichotomous exposure factor (E, with $1 =$ exposure and $0 =$ no exposure), the model is as follows:

$$P(Y = 1 | E = 1) = \frac{\exp(\beta_0 + \beta_1)}{1 + \exp(\beta_0 + \beta_1)}.$$

The odds ratio is then

$$OR = e^{\beta_1}.$$

Regression analysis is typically not conducted with just a dichotomous exposure and outcome, because this can be done more simply using a 2×2 table, but is useful when a model includes multiple confounders. For instance, a model might include E as the exposure of interest (1 = exposed and 0 = not exposed) and C_1 and C_2 as potential confounders. Thus,

$$P(Y=1) = \frac{\exp(\beta_0 + \beta_1 E + \beta_2 C_1 + \beta_3 C_2)}{1 + \exp(\beta_0 + \beta_1 E + \beta_2 C_1 + \beta_3 C_2)}.$$

The adjusted odds ratio between exposure and outcome is

$$aOR = e^{\beta_1}.$$

The simplicity of this formula is due to the fact that the adjustment of β, and thus the odds ratio, is done during the iterative process used to estimate βs. Thus, β is adjusted for all the other factors that are included in the model.

Logistic Regression Model Assumptions

The following are the assumptions made with this model:

- The outcome variable is binomial.
- All observations must be independent and identically distributed, or the dependence between observations must be taken into account in the analysis (for instance, by using generalized estimating equations).
- The sample size is large (or an exact program is used, such as LogXact). The suggested guidelines for adequate sample size typically range from 10 to 15 cases per independent variable.
- The factors are linear in the logit scale.
- The model fits the data.

Advantages and Disadvantages

The main advantages of logistic regression are its natural fit to study data from public health and medical research and ease of use due to widely available software. Compared with other types of modeling with categorical outcomes, logistic regression is not prone to issues with the outcome data such as the problem of overdispersion, sometimes seen with Poisson regression, and the problem of estimates existing outside the appropriate boundary parameter, as can happen with log-binomial regression.

However, because the output of logistic regression is the odds ratio, the standard warnings governing the use of this measure apply, most notably the overestimation of the relative risk when the outcome is common, usually defined as greater than 10% for each set of characteristics (i.e., each covariate pattern). When the outcome is mathematically rare, the odds ratio is a good estimate of the relative risk.

Poisson Regression

Poisson regression is most commonly used when data exist as counts of events per a unit of measure (e.g., time, area). Cohort studies and randomized trials that estimate rates because of different follow-up times for participants will typically use Poisson regression to estimate adjusted rate ratios. Also, while data can exist as rates (e.g., number of deaths per month), the use of rates is not required for Poisson regression. Nonrate measures of risk (e.g., number of nurses colonized with methicillin-resistant *Staphylococcus aureus* in hospital wards) also often follow a Poisson distribution and can be modeled using this technique.

Poisson regression can also be used to estimate adjusted relative risks of studies of common outcomes (i.e., when more than 10% of the participants develop the outcome). In this case, all participants must be followed for the same length of time, a requirement for the direct estimation of relative risk. However, in this case a robust approach is needed to compute confidence intervals. This is the approach suggested by Spiegelman and Hertzmark (2005).

Models and Formulae

Poisson regression models the natural logarithm of the expected value of the outcome, $\mu = E(Y)$, as a linear combination of regression parameters and independent factors. For example, a single dichotomous exposure, E, with two confounders, C_1 and C_2, can be expressed as

$$\log(\mu) = \beta_0 + \beta_1 E + \beta_2 C_1 + \beta_3 C_2.$$

The adjusted rate ratio between exposure and outcome is

$$aRR = e^{\beta_1}.$$

Given a Poisson model, the probability of the dependent variable being equal to a given value (k) can be calculated as

$$P(Y=k) = [(e^{-\mu}) \times \mu^k]/k!$$

Model Assumptions

The following are the assumptions made with this model:

- The outcome variable is distributed Poisson.
- All observations must be independent and identically distributed, or the dependence between observations must be taken into account in the analysis (such as using generalized estimating equations).
- The expected value of the dependent variable $E(Y)$ is equal to the variance of the dependent variable $\text{Var}(Y)$.
- The model fits the data.

Checking Model Assumptions

Independence of observations can be maintained through the use of appropriate study design and data collection, ensuring that observations collected are independent. The fit of the regression model is evaluated through analysis of residuals. Overdispersion can be evaluated by checking the ratios of the goodness-of-fit statistics (deviance and Pearson χ^2) to the degrees of freedom for the analysis. Values much greater than 1 may be indicative of overdispersion.

Advantages and Disadvantages

Poisson regression is most commonly used when the data under study exist as individual counts, such as the number of cases of illness in different communities. Poisson regression, with robust estimation for confidence intervals, is also useful to estimate relative risk directly when the outcome is common.

The defining characteristics of the Poisson distribution can lead to an estimation problem. Poisson distributions by definition have their variance equal to their mean. However, a real data set may have variance in the observed data that is greater than the theoretical variance calculated in the regression model, a condition known as overdispersion, which is indicative of inadequate model fit and may indicate the need to use other modeling techniques, such as log-binomial. Using standard Poisson regression with overdispersed data may result in confidence intervals that are too wide. In this case, it is possible to modify the regression model to incorporate robust error variances into the Poisson regression.

Log-Binomial Regression

Log-binomial regression, similar to logistic regression, models a binomial outcome. However, in log-binomial regression the log of the proportion of interest is modeled, as opposed to the log odds or logit. Since the proportion is directly modeled, the final result from log-binomial regression is a direct measure of the relative risk. Log-binomial regression is, therefore, particularly useful for estimating relative risk when the need to control for multiple confounders exists.

Models and Formulae

Log-binomial regression models the log of the outcome under study as a linear combination of regression parameters and independent factors. For example, a single dichotomous exposure, E, with two confounders, C_1 and C_2, can be expressed as

$$\log(Y) = \beta_0 + \beta_1 E + \beta_2 C_1 + \beta_3 C_2.$$

The adjusted relative risk between exposure and outcome is

$$aRR = e^{\beta_1}.$$

Using the above equation as an example, the probability of a positive outcome ($Y = 1$) can be calculated as

$$P(Y = 1 | X - x_i) = \left[e^{(\beta_0 + \beta_1 E + \beta_2 C_1 + \beta_3 C_2)} \right].$$

Model Assumptions

The following are the assumptions made with this model:

- The outcome variable is binomial.
- All observations must be independent and identically distributed, or the dependence between observations must be taken into account in the analysis (such as using generalized estimating equations).
- The sample size is large or exact methods are used.
- The data fit the model.
- The estimates are within the boundaries of the parameter space.

Advantages and Disadvantages

Because the log proportion is used, as opposed to the logit in logistic regression, direct measurements of risk proportions and relative risk can be made using log-binomial regression.

While odds can range between 0 and ∞, proportions can only range between 0 and 1. When parameter estimates are at or near the boundary of the parameter space, there is a possibility of the estimates exceeding the limits of a proportion with log-binomial modeling. This indicates a failure of the model to fit the data properly within the bounds of log-binomial regression, possibly requiring modeling with a different technique.

Linear Regression

Linear regression differs from the previously described regression modeling techniques in that it is used to model outcomes that are continuous, as opposed to categorical. The measure of association calculated from linear regression is also different, yielding the correlation coefficient as opposed to the relative risk, rate ratio, or odds ratio. The expected value of Y can be directly determined through the straightforward model.

Models and Formulae

Linear regression directly models the expected value of the dependent variable as a linear combination of regression parameters and independent factors. For example, a single exposure, E, with two confounders, C_1 and C_2, can be expressed as

$$E(Y) = \beta_0 = \beta_1 E + \beta_2 C_1 + \beta_3 C_2.$$

Based on least squares analysis, the correlation between independent and dependent variables can be calculated using Pearson's correlation coefficient and R^2. The measure R^2 provides an estimate of the amount of variation in the data that is explained through the regression line and ranges from 0 (none of the variation is explained by the regression line) to 1 (all data points lie exactly on the regression line).

Model Assumptions

The following are the assumptions made with this model:

- The outcome variable is continuous.
- A predicted value of Y can be calculated for each set of x_is based on the regression line, and each of these predicted values of Y has a defined mean and variance.
- All observations must be independent and identically distributed or the dependence between observations must be taken into account in the analysis (such as using generalized estimating equations).
- The relationship between $E(Y|x_i)$ for all x_i is a straight line function.
- The predicted value of Y calculated for any x_i is normally distributed.
- The variance of the predicted value of Y calculated for any x_i is homoscedastic, meaning that the variance of Y for each x_i is the same.

Checking Model Assumptions

Independence of observations can be maintained through the use of appropriate study design and data collection, ensuring that observations collected are independent. Homoscedasticity can be evaluated by plotting the residuals as a function of the independent variable(s) and observing if the spread of the data points does not widen as the independent variables' values increase. The fit of the regression model, including evaluations of normality, is evaluated through analysis of residuals.

Advantages and Disadvantages

Linear regression is a straightforward technique to perform and to interpret. It is very robust in its ability to handle continuous outcome measures as long a there is one mode that does not fall on an extreme of the parameter space. Given a set of regression coefficients, for any combination of x_i, the expected value of Y can be directly calculated. Also, the level of correlation between dependent and independent variables can be directly determined.

The main disadvantage of linear regression is its inability to study categorical outcomes. As many epidemiologic data are in this form (e.g., persons have the outcome of interest or they do not), the application of linear regression is limited. However, for studies with continuous measures as an outcome (e.g., blood pressure), linear regression is an extremely useful technique.

Model Fit: Influence and Outliers

It is always important to understand the fit of the model to the data. Several questions are posed to determine if the model is a "good" one. Does the model fit the data overall? Does the overall fit change significantly when factors are added or dropped? Are there cases in the study that exert an undue influence on the final model, and thus the final estimate(s) of the measure of association between exposure(s) and outcome? If so, which are they? What is the association without these influential cases? Are there subgroups of cases that the model does not describe well, and if so, which cases?

Assessing the model fit usually has three components: (1) overall fit, (2) influential cases, and (3) outliers. Most researchers spend substantial time selecting terms for a model before assessing the fit of the model to the data. This is a problematic approach because if the first version of the model does not fit the data, decisions based on this model are flawed. Thus, it is important to determine if the first model reasonably fits the data before making decisions on effect modification and confounding and subsequently estimating the measure of association of interest. Overall fit of the model is typically assessed with some form of a chi-square test comparing the observed data and the expected values based on model estimates. If these are similar, then the model is deemed to fit reasonably well. If not, then the model is not a good fit overall and finding a model that does fit the data is the first order of business.

Assessment of the influence of individual cases on the overall outcome in linear regression is performed by dropping one individual case at a time and refitting the model. Cases that produce the largest difference in the parameters of interest (i.e., those relating to the exposure factors) when dropped are identified as the most important influential effects, which require further investigation. The measure of association is also assessed with these individuals included in the analysis and excluded to examine their influence.

In an analysis modeling categorical outcomes with categorical independent factors, it is possible that many individuals have exactly the same values on exposure, confounders, and modifiers. Thus, when assessing influence instead of dropping individuals one at a time, all individuals with the same characteristics are removed and the model refit with the remaining participants. Again, the difference in estimates with and without the group being evaluated is compared and their influence is estimated by the difference in the parameter estimates of interest between the two models. When there are many individuals with the same characteristics, then the group may be

influential simply due to its size. This is not a matter of concern. Only when a small group (e.g., 1, 2, or 3 individuals) exerts strong influence on the model is influence considered a problem.

Outliers are individuals that are not well described by the model. That is, the reported measures of association between exposure and outcome are not typical for the outliers. Outliers often provide interesting information about the association and how it varies. For example, it is possible that effect modification by ethnicity exists but that the sample size in a minority group is not sufficient to estimate it with any precision. When fitting a model to the entire population, members of a minority in the study may thus be identified as outliers. Noting for whom the model does not fit is important for the overall interpretation of the study results. Additionally, outliers may provide information that can lead to further study to understand a more complex relationship between exposures and outcomes.

Data Analysis Example

To illustrate the points made above, an example of quantitative data analysis is presented here. Briefly, it is an examination of the number of cesarean sections occurring in two regions of a state to determine the reason for the higher level of births by cesarean section in one region versus the other.

For reference, Table 1 displays the results of the crude exposure-outcome analysis along analyses stratified on three available covariates—number of comorbidities experienced (categorized as 0 to 1 or 2 or more), whether Medicaid benefits were used (yes or no), and age (16 to 17 years, 18 to 34 years, and 35 to 49 years).

Trying to determine associations across many different stratified analyses can be difficult. According to the stratified analysis discussed above, number of comorbidities and use of Medicaid benefits appear to be effect modifiers, but the level of confounding seen by age is not as clear. To further examine the influence of age, Medicaid use, and number of comorbidities, the data were analyzed using multivariate regression modeling. For purposes of illustration, models were generated using logistic regression, log-binomial regression, Poisson regression, and Poisson regression with a robust error variance to account for overdispersion. Table 2 displays the results of modeling with interaction terms included to account for effect modification by number of comorbidities and use of Medicaid benefits, as well

Table 1   Crude and Stratified Tabular Results for Analysis of Association Between Hospital Location in Two Regions of a State and Deliveries by Cesarean Section

| | Region A | | | | Region B | | | | | |
| | Cesarean | | Vaginal | | Cesarean | | Vaginal | | | |
Delivery Type	N	%	N	%	N	%	N	%	OR (95% CI)	RR (95% CI)
Crude	6,918	28.1	17,740	71.9	2,717	17.1	13,147	82.9	1.89 (1.80, 1.98)	1.64 (1.57, 1.70)
Age										
16–17	64	15.5	349	84.5	32	7	424	93	2.43 (1.55, 3.80)	2.21 (1.48, 3.30)
18–34	4,856	26.3	13,631	73.7	2,037	16.1	10,598	83.9	1.85 (1.75, 1.96)	1.63 (1.56, 1.71)
35–49	1,998	34.7	3,760	65.3	648	23.4	2,125	76.6	1.74 (1.57, 1.93)	1.48 (1.38, 1.60)
Medicaid Benefits										
No	1,058	20.5	4,104	79.5	1,836	15.9	9,703	84.1	1.36 (1.25, 1.48)	1.29 (1.20, 1.38)
Yes	5,860	30	13,636	70	881	20.4	3,444	79.6	1.68 (1.55, 1.82)	1.48 (1.39, 1.57)
Comorbidities										
2 or more	1,976	27.5	5,222	72.6	1,005	19.5	414	80.5	1.56 (1.43, 1.70)	1.41 (1.31, 1.50)
0 or 1	4,942	28.3	12,518	71.7	1,712	16	9,007	84	2.08 (1.95, 2.21)	1.77 (1.69, 1.86)

Table 2   Comparative Results of Regression Modeling Examining the Association Between Hospital Location in Two Regions of a State and Deliveries by Cesarean Section

| | | Regression Type | | | |
| | | Logistic | Log-Binomial | Poisson | Poisson* |
Medicaid Benefits	Comorbidities	OR (95% CI)	RR (95% CI)	RR (95% CI)	RR (95% CI)
No	0 or 1	1.83 (1.68, 2.00)	1.58 (1.48, 1.69)	1.58 (1.47, 1.71)	1.58 (1.48, 1.69)
No	2 or more	1.40 (1.25, 1.56)	1.27 (1.16, 1.38)	1.27 (1.15, 1.40)	1.27 (1.17, 1.38)
Yes	0 or 1	1.53 (1.40, 1.68)	1.41 (1.31, 1.53)	1.42 (1.30, 1.54)	1.42 (1.31, 1.53)
Yes	2 or more	1.17 (1.05, 1.30)	1.13 (1.04, 1.23)	1.14 (1.03, 1.25)	1.14 (1.04, 1.24)

Notes: Analyses include controlling for confounding by age. Asterisk (*) indicates Poisson regression with robust error variance.

as controlling for confounding by age. Table 3 displays the results of modeling with interaction terms included to account for effect modification by number of comorbidities and use of Medicaid benefits, with no other covariates controlled for.

Results for log-binomial regression, Poisson regression, and Poisson regression with robust error variance (Poisson* in the table) are very similar to

each other. Overestimates of variance seen in Poisson regression are not large, but are accounted for when Poisson regression with robust error variance is used.

The odds ratio values obtained from logistic regression modeling are similar to odds ratios generated from multiple stratified tabular analysis, just as the relative risk values obtained from log-binomial, Poisson, and Poisson with robust error variance

Table 3 Comparative Results of Regression Modeling Examining the Association Between Hospital Location in Two Regions of a State and Deliveries by Cesarean Section

Medicaid Benefits	Comorbidities	Regression Type			
		Logistic	*Log-Binomial*	*Poisson*	*Poisson* *
		OR (95% CI)	*RR (95% CI)*	*RR (95% CI)*	*RR (95% CI)*
No	0 or 1	1.82 (1.67, 1.98)	1.58 (1.47, 1.69)	1.58 (1.46, 1.70)	1.58 (1.47, 1.69)
No	2 or more	1.40 (1.25, 1.56)	1.27 (1.17, 1.38)	1.27 (1.15, 1.40)	1.27 (1.17, 1.38)
Yes	0 or 1	1.50 (1.37, 1.65)	1.39 (1.29, 1.50)	1.39 (1.28, 1.52)	1.39 (1.29, 1.50)
Yes	2 or more	1.15 (1.03, 1.28)	1.12 (1.03, 1.22)	1.12 (1.02, 1.23)	1.12 (1.03, 1.22)

Notes: Analyses do not include controlling for confounding by age. Asterisk (*) indicates Poisson regression with robust error variance.

regression modeling are similar to relative risks generated from multiple stratified tabular analysis. The results suggest that age does not need to be adjusted for in the analysis as the results are similar with and without adjusting for age. It should also be noted that logistic regression provides odds ratio estimates that overestimate relative risks (or prevalence ratios in this case). Thus, logistic regression should not be used for this analysis as the outcome (cesarean section) occurs too frequently for the odds ratio to be a reasonable estimate of the prevalence ratio.

—*Robert Bednarczyk and Louise-Anne McNutt*

See also Causation and Causal Inference; Effect Modification and Interaction; Logistic Regression; Study Design

Further Readings

Agresti, A. (2002). *Categorical data analysis* (2nd ed.). Hoboken, NJ: Wiley-Interscience.

Barros, A. J. D., & Hirakata, V. N. (2003). Alternatives for logistic regression in cross-sectional studies: An empirical comparison of models that directly estimate the prevalence ratio [Electronic version]. *BMC Medical Research Methodology*, 3(21). Retrieved August 8, 2007, from http://www.biomedcentral.com/content/pdf/1471-2288-3-21.pdf.

Hardin, J. W., & Hilbe, J. M. (2002). *Generalized estimating equations*. Boca Raton, FL: Chapman & Hall.

Hosmer, D. W., & Lemeshow, S. (2000). *Applied logistic regression* (2nd ed.). Hoboken, NJ: Wiley-Interscience.

Kleinbaum, D. G., & Klein, M. (2002). *Logistic regression: A self-learning text* (2nd ed.). New York: Springer.

Kleinbaum, D. G., Kupper, L. L., Muller, K. E., & Nizam, A. (1998). *Applied regression analysis and other multivariable methods* (3rd ed.). Pacific Grove, CA: Duxbury Press.

McNamee, R. (2005). Regression modeling and other methods to control confounding. *Journal of Occupational and Environmental Medicine*, 62, 500–506.

McNutt, L. A., Wu, C., Xue, X., & Hafner, J. P. (2003). Estimating the relative risk in cohort studies and clinical trials of common outcomes. *American Journal of Epidemiology*, 157, 940–943.

Rothman, K. J., & Greenland. S. (1998). *Modern epidemiology* (2nd ed.). Philadelphia: Lippincott Williams & Wilkins.

SAS FAQ. (n.d.). *How to estimate relative risk in SAS using Proc Genmod for common outcomes in cohort studies?* Retrieved March 8, 2007, from http://www.ats.ucla.edu/STAT/SAS/faq/relative_risk.htm.

Spiegelman, D., & Hertzmark, E. (2005). Easy SAS calculations for risk of prevalence ratios and differences. *American Journal of Epidemiology*, 162(3), 199–200.

Stokes, M. E., Davis, C. S., & Koch, G. G. (2000). *Categorical data analysis using the SAS system* (2nd ed.). Cary, NC: SAS Institute.

Wacholder, S. (1986). Binomial regression in GLIM: Estimating risk ratios and risk differences. *American Journal of Epidemiology*, 123(1), 174184.

Web Sites

LogXact Overview: http://www.cytel.com/Products/LogXact.

RELATIONAL DATABASE

By far the most common use for computers during most of their existence has been to create and store databases. From large databases that manage a bank's account information to the common e-mail program, databases are the engines behind most of the software in use today. In simple terms, a database is computer software that contains organized data. The data are structured to allow a user to search for specific data, reorder the data, and create reports containing specified parts of the data. For the epidemiologist, a relational database can provide a tool to manage and maintain large data sets, create reports, and prepare basic statistical analyses.

In the earliest mainframe computers, databases were complex to create and maintain and remained the province of trained professionals. When the desktop or personal computer appeared in the 1980s, database software was introduced that allowed individuals without a background in computer science to create and use databases. Ashton Tate's dBASE was the first major commercial database software to be widely used on those early desktop computers. With the evolution of the graphic interface within Microsoft's Windows operating system and Apple's Macintosh computer, it became even simpler for noncomputer professionals to create their own database systems. Currently, the two dominant database systems on desktop computers are Microsoft Access and Filemaker Pro. These two programs offer both the database software and integrated tools to create data displays and reports and allow users to write basic computer programs necessary for data management, even for users with little or no experience in database design.

A structure of a database is referred to as a "schema." The basic structure is made up of *records*, each of which contains *fields*. To use the analogy of a patient's medical form, each form containing information about an individual patient is a record. The data on the form are contained within different fields, such as name, address, age, and gender. The database itself is comparable with a file cabinet that contains all the patient records. In this type of database, referred to as a "flat file," all the data are self-contained and could just as well be maintained on a spreadsheet as on a relational database.

The limitation of the flat file is that it may be inconvenient to have all the information about a given patient in a single flat file. For instance, you may want to keep a record of each of a patient's visits, to record specific information about that visit (such as blood pressure, temperature, height, and weight), to add a new field to a single flat file for each of these

	A	B	C	D	E
1	Dr. Lionel Schmerz				
2					
3	Patient Records				
4					
5	Patient _ID	DOB	Gender	1st Visit	
6	1	04-May-56	F	01-Aug-05	
7	2	15-Mar-53	M	03-Sep-05	
8	3	27-Mar-53	M	10-Oct-04	
9	4	17-Jun-90	F	08-May-05	
10	5	20-Dec-63	F	08-Jan-05	
11	6	09-Jun-42	M	09-Jul-04	
12	7	08-Apr-62	F	07-Sep-05	
13	8	17-Mar-59	M	28-Jan-05	
14	9	08-May-62	F	19-Aug-05	
15	10	05-Nov-68	F	08-Dec-05	

Figure 1   Spreadsheet With Patient Records

Note: In this spreadsheet, each row contains data for a specific patient, and each column contains data of a specific type.

variables on each visit would be awkward. Neither do you want to reenter basic information about patients, such as their age and insurance company, each time they have an office visit. Another reason to not store all information in a single flat file is that certain information needs to be kept confidential. For instance, you would not want information about a patient's HIV status to be accessible to a staff member who needs to use the patient file only to perform billing operations. By using a *relational* database model, multiple databases, also referred to as "tables," can be linked so that different types of information can be entered into different tables, yet all the information about a single record, for instance, a particular patient, is linked and can be combined to create different reports. For instance, you might have one table that records basic demographic and contact information for each patient (age, home address, etc.) and a second table that records information about individual patient visits. Both would be linked by an identification number unique to a particular patient. This is referred to as a "one-to-many" relationship, because one patient record may be linked to multiple visit records. The visits database can display the patient information from the patient file, and because this information is linked rather than reentered, the likelihood of error is reduced. By extension, other tables can be created containing data about drugs prescribed, treatments administered, insurance payments, and so on. These tables can all be linked to and can use data from the original patient information table.

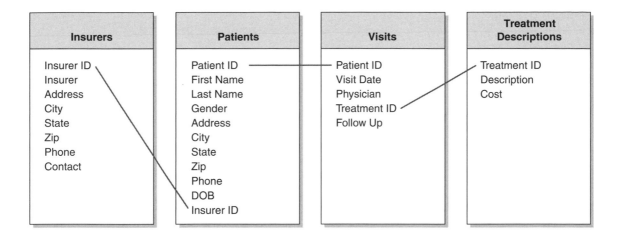

Figure 2   Database Structure

Related tables are linked through the use of a *key field*. The key field contains data unique to an individual record, a patient ID number, for example. When a new record is created in a related table, the key field data are entered in that record and provide the link back to the appropriate record in the first table.

When designing a database, particular attention must be paid to creating a proper structure from the outset. For example, names should always be separated (parsed) and entered in two fields (for first name and last name) rather than as a single name field. With a single name field, it would be impossible to sort (reorder) the data by last name, a serious limitation. Since it is difficult to restructure data after it has been entered, it is important that the structure be correct from the start.

Relational database software has many capabilities beyond just storing and displaying information. For instance, queries may be performed that allow the user to create customized reports, and built-in functions allow the computation of many basic statistics. Charts and form letters can also be produced directly from information stored in the database Access and Filemaker Pro that have features that allow a user to create data displays that incorporate both data and graphics elements. Data entry forms can be created with elements such as drop-down lists or check boxes in a particular field to speed up data entry and minimize entry errors. Relational database software also includes data-processing functions similar to that available in spreadsheets that can calculate and display arithmetic and statistical results.

Database software can import data from a wide variety of sources, so data can be added easily to an existing system. The data can then be searched, reordered (sorted), and extracted for use in other programs. For example, it would be simple to search a database of patient records to identify all those pertaining to women above 50 years of age, and then export those records (with data from multiple tables) for analysis in a dedicated statistics package such as SAS.

Multiuser databases allow multiple users to use the databases simultaneously, so that one user can enter new records while another searches the data and creates reports, all working simultaneously on the same set of tables. Multiuser capabilities can be limited to just the internal network of an office or extended to the entire world via the Internet, greatly facilitating multisite research projects.

Multiuser databases must be configured with certain security issues in mind, especially when they contain confidential information such as patient records or Social Security numbers. Through the use of account names and passwords, each user can be allotted specific privileges so that one user may only view data but not change it, while another can only enter new data but not change existing entries. Security settings can also prevent a specific user from viewing data in certain fields while allowing them to work on others.

—Daniel Peck

See also Data Management; Spreadsheet

Further Readings

Chase, K. (2005). *Access 2003 for starters: The missing manual*. Sebastopol, CA: O'Reilly Media.

Hernandez., M. J. (2003). *Database design for mere mortals: A hands-on guide to relational database design*. Upper Saddle River, NJ: Addison-Wesley.

Hester, N. (2006). *Filemaker Pro 8: Visual QuickStart guide*. Berkeley, CA: Peachpit Press.

RELIABILITY

The issue of reliability (i.e., repeatability or reproducibility) is crucial in selecting and developing the most appropriate item, scale, or instrument. Reliability refers to the extent to which an instrument or the measurements of a test will consistently produce the same result, measure, or score if applied two or more times under identical conditions. A technique is reliable, or has achieved a high level of agreement, if it yields consistent results on repetition. If repeated measurements produce different results, and the entity being measured is assumed to not have changed, the instrument would be considered unreliable.

Methods of Assessing or Estimating Reliability

There are a variety of methods for estimating instrument reliability. DeVellis classifies these methods into two categories: (1) the type of instrument (observer or external source vs. self-report) and (2) time instrument applied or method (single administration or multiple administration). Reliability is estimated in one of four ways:

1. *Internal Consistency.* This estimation is based on the correlation among the variables comprising the set or the homogeneity of the items comprising a scale (usually estimated with Cronbach's alpha).

2. *Split-Half Reliability.* This estimation is based on the correlation of two equivalent forms of the scale (usually estimated with the Spearman-Brown coefficient).

3. *Test-Retest Reliability.* This estimation is based on the correlation between scores from two (or more) administrations of the same item, scale, or instrument for different times, locations, or populations, when the two administrations do not differ in other

relevant variables (usually estimated with the Spearman-Brown coefficient).

4. *Interrater Reliability.* This estimation is based on the correlation of scores between/among two or more raters who rate the same item, scale, or instrument (usually estimated with intraclass correlation, of which there are six types discussed below).

These four reliability estimation methods are sensitive to different sources of error and are not necessarily mutually exclusive. Therefore, the reliability scores measured using these methods should not be expected to be equal nor need they lead to the same results. All reliability coefficients are forms of correlation coefficients and are thus sample dependent. In other words, another sample may well result in a different estimate.

Internal Consistency Reliability

Cronbach's coefficient alpha is the classic form of internal consistency reliability and is widely used as a measure of reliability. Cronbach's alpha can be interpreted as a measure of mean intercorrelation among item responses obtained at the same time. Cronbach's alpha is influenced by the number of items in a scale, so alpha will increase as the number of items in the scale increases, if new items have the same average intercorrelation of items. There are no absolute standards for knowing when reliability is adequate, but an often-used rule of thumb is that alpha should be at least .70 for a scale to be considered adequate, and many researchers require a cutoff of .80 for a "good scale."

Cronbach's α is defined as

$$\frac{N}{N-1}\left(\frac{\sigma_X^2 - \sum_{i=1}^{N} \sigma_{Y_i}^2}{\sigma_X^2}\right),$$

where N is the number of items, σ_X^2 is the variance of the observed measure, and $\sigma_{Y_i}^2$ is the variance of sum of the items.

Cronbach's α is closely related to the correlation among items, and when evaluating whether an individual item should be retained in a scale, it is good to look at the squared multiple correlation, R^2 for an item when it is predicted from all other items in the scale. The larger this R^2, the more the item is contributing to internal consistency. The lower the R^2, the more the researcher should consider dropping it. Note that a scale with an acceptable overall Cronbach's α may have some items with a low R^2. *The Kuder-Richardson (KR20) coefficient* is a special version of Cronbach's α for items that are dichotomous.

Split-Half Reliability

Split-half reliability measures equivalence among two measurement instruments or between two halves of the same instrument. It is related to the concept of parallel-forms reliability, in which two different measurement instruments, which are assumed to be equivalent, are administered twice to the same people. Spearman-Brown split-half reliability coefficient, also called the *Spearman-Brown prophecy coefficient*, is used to estimate full test reliability based on split-half reliability measures. The Spearman-Brown "prophecy formula" predicts what the full-test reliability would be, based on half-test correlations. This coefficient will be higher than the half-test reliability coefficient. This coefficient is usually equal to and easily calculated by hand as twice the half-test correlation divided by the quantity 1 plus the half-test reliability.

$$r_{SB1} = (k \times r_{ij})/[1 + (k-1) \times r_{ij}],$$

where

$r_{SB1} =$ the Spearman-Brown split-half reliability,

$r_{ij} =$ the Pearson correlation between forms i and j, and

$k =$ total sample size divided by sample size per form (k is usually 2).

As with other split-halves measures, the Spearman-Brown reliability coefficient is highly influenced by alternative methods of sorting items into the two forms, which is preferably done randomly. Random assignment of items to the two forms should ensure equality of variances between the forms, but this is not guaranteed and should be checked by the researcher.

Test-Retest Reliability

Test-retest reliability, which measures the temporal stability or stability over time, is administering the same test to the same subjects at two points in time. In other words, test-retest reliability is replicating the measurement and computing the correlation coefficient to see how constant the scores remain from one occasion to another. Statistically, test-retest reliability is treated as a variant of split-half reliability and also uses the Spearman-Brown coefficient.

Test-retest methods, as an appropriate way of gauging reliability, are subject to several restrictions. Among these restrictions are the following: (1) it must be assumed that the underlying phenomenon or the true score has not changed; (2) if the scale itself is unreliable for a single administration, test-retest reliability cannot be evaluated; and (3) there are no carry-over effects, that is, the scores from the second episode of testing are not influenced by the subject's memory (or physical traces, such as drugs remaining in the bloodstream) from the first episode. Researchers using test-retest reliability must weigh and understand the special validity concerns to make informed judgments when designing a measurement or evaluative study.

Interrater Reliability

Interrater reliability is a method of determining how well raters agree in their judgment of some event; it is often reviewed to evaluate agreement among several individuals assigned to review medical charts, for instance. Interrater reliability is evaluated by having two or more raters or interviewers administer the same form to the same people or evaluate the same objects (such as medical charts) to establish the extent of consensus on use of the instrument by those who administer it. Raters should be as blind as possible to expected outcomes of the study and should be randomly assigned. There are different ways to calculate interrater agreement; for dichotomous items, the most common choices are simple percent agreement and kappa, which is percent agreement corrected for the amount of agreement expected by chance alone. For continuous data, consensus is measured by *intraclass correlation* (ICC); note that the term *ICC* is sometimes applied to percent agreement and kappa also.

The guidelines for choosing the appropriate form of the ICC varies depending on whether a one-way or two-way analysis of variance (ANOVA) is suitable, whether the differences between the judges' mean ratings are relevant, and whether reliability is to be measured based on an individual rating or the mean of several ratings. ICC may be conceptualized as the ratio of between-groups variance to total variance and is interpreted similarly to Kappa. Shrout and Fleiss (1979) have defined six kinds of ICC:

1. *ICC(1,1)*. Used when each subject is rated by multiple raters, raters assumed to be randomly assigned to subjects, all subjects have the same number of raters; one-way (random targets are the grouping variable) single measure reliability.

2. *ICC(2,1)*. Used when all subjects are rated by the same raters, who are assumed to be a random subset of all possible raters; a two-way random effects model single measure reliability.

3. *ICC(3,1)*. Used when all subjects are rated by the same raters, who are assumed to be the entire population of raters; two-way mixed effects model single measure reliability.

4. *ICC(1,k)*. Same assumptions as for ICC(1,1) but reliability is for the mean of *k* ratings; one-way model single and average measure reliability.

5. *ICC(2,k)*. Same assumptions as for ICC(2,1) but reliability is for the mean of *k* ratings; a two-way random effects model average measure reliability.

6. *ICC(3,k)*. Same assumptions as for ICC(3,1) but reliability is for the mean of *k* ratings. This additionally assumes no subject by judges interaction; the two-way mixed effects model average measure reliability.

—*Kevin Robinson*

See also Bias; Item Response Theory; Kappa; Response Rate; Validity

Further Readings

Carmines, E. G., & Zeller, R. A. (1979). *Reliability and validity assessment.* London: Sage.

Cronbach, L. J. (1951). Coefficient alpha and the internal structure of tests. *Psychometrika, 16,* 297–334.

DeVellis, R. F. (2003). *Scale development: Theory and applications* (2nd ed.). Thousand Oaks, CA: Sage.

Nunnaly, J. (1978). *Psychometric theory.* New York: McGraw-Hill.

Shrout, P. E., & Fleiss, J. L. (1979). Intraclass correlations: Uses in assessing rater reliability. *Psychological Bulletin, 2,* 420–428.

REPRODUCTIVE EPIDEMIOLOGY

Reproductive epidemiology is the study of reproduction-related morbidity, mortality, and other health issues in males and females. The topics covered in reproductive epidemiology include development and physiology of reproductive systems and functions, conception, pregnancy, birth outcomes, and maternal morbidity and mortality.

Measures of Reproductive Health

The number of measures of reproductive health is substantial. Several select indicators commonly used in reproductive epidemiologic studies are described below.

Maternal Mortality

Maternal mortality is defined by the World Health Organization (WHO) as the death of a woman during pregnancy or within 6 weeks of termination of pregnancy from any cause related to or aggravated by the pregnancy or its management. The causes of the death can be categorized into direct and indirect obstetric deaths. Direct obstetric death is caused by complications of pregnancy, delivery, or the puerperium (the period immediately after childbirth and lasting about 6 weeks, during which the mother's body returns to its prepregnant condition). The five major causes of direct obstetric deaths worldwide are hemorrhage, complications of unsafe abortion, eclampsia, infection, and obstructed labor. Indirect obstetric death results from previously existing conditions or conditions physiologically aggravated by the pregnancy. Common examples of such conditions are malaria, anemia, HIV/AIDS, and cardiovascular disease. Non-obstetric deaths include other deaths during but not caused by the pregnancy, such as those caused by accidents or by intentional acts not caused directly by the pregnancy (e.g., murder). According to a report jointly prepared by the WHO, UNICEF (United Nations Children's Fund), and UNFPA (United Nations Population Fund), there were 529,000 maternal deaths in 2000, of which more than 99.5% occurred in developing regions. Three commonly used measures related to maternal mortality are the maternal mortality rate, maternal mortality ratio, and lifetime risk of maternal death.

Maternal Mortality Rate

The maternal mortality rate is calculated as the number of maternal deaths in a given period per 1,000 women of reproductive age (usually 15–49 years of age) during the same time period and reflects the frequency with which women are exposed to mortality risk through fertility.

Maternal Mortality Ratio

This is a measure of the risk of death associated with pregnancy. It is calculated as the number of maternal deaths during a given time period per 100,000 live births during the same time period. In other words, the numerator is the number of maternal deaths multiplied by 100,000, and the denominator is the number of live births. This measure is often referred to as a rate, although it is really a ratio.

Lifetime Risk of Maternal Death

The lifetime risk of maternal death is the probability that a woman will die from complications of pregnancy or childbirth at some point during her reproductive years. It is a cumulative risk across a woman's reproductive years and is often used as an index of risk faced by women in developed and developing countries.

Infant Mortality

The infant mortality rate (IMR) is defined as the rate per 1,000 live births at which babies less than 1 year of age die. It is calculated by dividing the number of infant deaths in a given year by the number of live births in the same given year. The IMR is often used to compare the general health and well-being of populations within and between countries and is sometimes considered a proxy or indicator of the quality of health care available to the relevant population. Comparing different countries' IMRs can sometimes be difficult when different definitions of "live birth" are employed. For example, the WHO defines a live birth as any born human being who demonstrates independent signs of life, including breathing, voluntary muscle movement, or heartbeat. Some European states and Japan, however, only count as live births those in which an infant breathes at birth, thereby causing their IMRs to be somewhat lower and their perinatal mortality rates to be somewhat higher than in settings using other definitions. Excluding high-risk infants from the denominator or numerator in reported IMRs also makes comparing rates problematic.

The IMR has declined steadily over the past several decades in the United States, from a national average of 26.0 per 1,000 live births in 1960 to 6.9 per 1,000 live births in 2000, but large racial and ethnic disparities persist. In 2000, the IMR among whites in the United States was 5.7 per 1,000 live births, compared with 14.1 per 1,000 live births for African Americans. Reducing the IMR overall and closing gaps between white and minority IMRs are national objectives put forth in *Healthy People 2010*. In the United States and other western nations, common causes of infant death include congenital malformations, preterm birth and low birthweight, sudden infant death syndrome, problems related to pregnancy complications, and respiratory distress syndrome.

Differences in IMRs are also evident among developed versus developing countries. The United Nations estimated the 2000 IMR among developed countries to be 8 per 1,000 live births, compared with 62 per 1,000 live births for less developed countries. The causes of IMR in developing countries tend to be different as well and include infectious disease, communicable disease, and dehydration.

Pregnancy Outcomes

Low Birthweight

Low birthweight is typically divided into three categories: low birthweight, very low birthweight, and extremely low birthweight. Low birthweight is defined as weight at birth of $\leq 2{,}500$ g (5.5 lb), very low birthweight refers to babies born weighing $\leq 1{,}500$ g, and extremely low birthweight is defined as weight at birth of $\leq 1{,}000$ g. It is estimated that in 2000, more than 20 million infants (approximately, 15.5% of all live births worldwide) were low birthweight. Prevalence of low birthweight varies substantially by countries' development status. The prevalence of low birthweight is approximately 7.0% in developed countries, 16.5% in developing countries, and 18.6% in the least developed countries. Low birthweight is associated with child physical growth and psychosocial development and with chronic medical conditions later in life. Measurement error is not a major concern for birthweight in developed countries because birthweight can be measured accurately; however, it can be of substantial concern in developing countries since most babies are not born in a medical setting and therefore not often weighed at birth.

Pregnancy Loss

Pregnancy loss refers to the loss of a pregnancy before birth and may occur through miscarriage (sometimes referred to as "spontaneous abortion"), termination, or stillbirth. Early pregnancy loss occurs prior to 20 weeks of completed gestation, before a fetus can survive outside the womb. Miscarriage occurs in approximately 15% to 20% of all pregnancies, most commonly within the first 13 weeks of pregnancy. Some miscarriages occur before a woman even realizes she is pregnant, even before missing a menstrual period, so the true number of miscarriages is probably significantly underestimated. The cause of miscarriage is frequently unknown, but chromosomal abnormalities in the fetus, maternal health problems such as infections (e.g., bacterial vaginosis) or chronic disease (e.g., diabetes or lupus), maternal lifestyle behaviors (e.g., smoking, substance use), or uterine impairments can be contributing factors. Chromosomal abnormalities are more common among women above 35 years of age, which places these women at higher risk of miscarriage compared with younger women.

Infertility

Infertility refers to the phenomenon of couples who try to conceive but fail to have a pregnancy for more than a year. Rather than the number of live births, infertility denotes reproductive capacity. Studies of infertility need to be cautious of case ascertainment as infertility diagnosis is prone to selection bias. For instance, women or couples who seek infertility care may differ from those who choose not to try to conceive (and may not ever realize they are infertile) or who cannot afford to obtain infertility diagnosis or treatment. Couples with infertility problems may have no apparent clinical symptoms and may appear to be healthy otherwise. Psychosocial factors and personal choices also can be significant influences and should be considered when measuring infertility.

Offspring Morbidity

The survival rate of newborns, including infants with low birthweight and those born as a result of assisted reproductive technology, has increased dramatically over the past two decades. This is particularly true in developed countries. The increased survival of newborns with some medical conditions (e.g., birth defects, extremely low birthweight) may lead to a higher prevalence of infant morbidity because those infants are at high risk for morbidity and mortality, and previously they would not have survived the birth process.

Some researchers have studied whether later health outcomes are influenced in utero. David Barker was one of the first to propose these notions in what is known as "Barker theory" or the "fetal origins hypothesis." Barker hypothesized that biophysiologic programming occurs at certain critical periods of fetal development, thereby strongly influencing health in later life. Since then, many studies have tested the programming hypothesis, exploring causal relationships between fetal and childhood exposures and adult chronic disease. Barker's hypothesis could help explain some of the socioeconomic and racial disparities in chronic illnesses such as cardiovascular disease and hypertension, although lifestyle and other environmental influences may also play a role.

Some researchers have critiqued studies based on fetal programming theory, citing methodological concerns such as selection bias, failure to assess and control for potential confounding, ecologic fallacy, and so on. Recent studies, however, have continued to find evidence supportive of the association between exposures and experiences in utero with adult blood pressure and certain cause-specific mortalities. Research based on fetal programming theory can be difficult to conduct due to challenges such as recall bias related to exposure, gene and environment interaction, expense of long-term follow-up, loss to follow-up, and determination of causality.

Health Disparities

Although some of the disparities in reproductive health are related to biological differences between populations, many are due to inequality in health care availability, social and cultural issues, and differences in lifestyle. The following are some of the areas in which health disparities are often addressed through reproductive epidemiologic studies.

Preventive Care

Preventive services in reproductive health include education, screening, treatment for sexually transmitted diseases (STDs) and sexually transmitted infections (STIs), preconceptional and prenatal care, and counseling concerning lifestyle factors such as smoking and drinking alcohol. Preconceptional and early comprehensive prenatal care can reduce the risk of pregnancy- and birth-related complications. Contraceptive practice can lengthen intervals between pregnancies to protect the health of the mother and her children. Despite its importance, the relation between the number of prenatal care visits and pregnancy outcomes is not linear. Research evidence suggests that receiving less (or no) and more than the recommended number of prenatal care visits all are associated with poor pregnancy outcomes. Receiving more than the recommended amount of prenatal care could reflect a problematic pregnancy, whereas receiving less or no prenatal care is likely due to barriers or lack of knowledge of its importance. Some common barriers a woman and her family (especially her partner) face in obtaining appropriate preventive care services include health care unavailability, lack of health insurance and underinsurance, lack of transportation, and lengthy waiting time for care. As with many other chronic conditions, unhealthy lifestyle (e.g., substance abuse, obesity) is associated with many adverse reproductive health outcomes in women and men. Education and policy can play important roles in promoting healthy behaviors, which in turn improves reproductive health.

Infectious Diseases

STIs or STDs are those that are typically transmitted between people by sexual contact, such as vaginal or anal intercourse, or oral sex. Other possible routes of transmission include birth, breastfeeding, blood transfusions, or sharing intravenous needles. Many people with STIs, especially women, are asymptomatic and unaware of their condition but are still able to spread infection. For women, regular Papanicolaou (Pap) screening can help identify asymptomatic and symptomatic STIs, allowing treatment that could help prevent serious complications, such as pelvic inflammatory disease and infertility.

The incidence of STIs is high in most of the world, despite the existence of effective protection (e.g., condoms), diagnosis, and treatment. In the United States, more than 2.8 million new cases of chlamydia were diagnosed in 2005, the rate of gonorrhea was 115.6 per 100,000, and the syphilis rate increased 11.1% between 2004 and 2005. As is the case with many reproductive health issues, socioeconomic and racial/ethnic disparities are evident in STI infection rates. For various reasons, funding for STI prevention and treatment is insufficient, and in many parts of the world, frank discussion of issues related to sexual behavior is not common.

Some STIs, such as chlamydia and gonorrhea, are easily treated with antibiotics, while others, such as herpes and HIV/AIDS, either cannot be cured currently or are difficult to treat. Recently, advances have been made in developing a prophylactic vaccine for females and males to protect against human papillomavirus, the virus that is responsible for the majority of cervical cancer cases.

Sociocultural Factors

Although women and men have the right to determine the course of their reproductive lives, numerous sociocultural factors may prevent them from being able to do so. These factors vary across different countries or regions and may differ within the same country. Politics and religion may influence how an individual experiences or manages his or her reproductive health. Other factors, such as insurance coverage for access to birth control and emergency contraception, pregnancy termination or abortion, and general reproductive health care, also play influential roles.

Nutrition

Evidence indicates that maternal excess body mass and body fat are associated with menstrual disorders, infertility, pregnancy complications, and pregnancy outcomes. Currently, more than 60% of U.S. women of childbearing age are either obese or overweight. In 2003, there were about 4 million live births in the United States. This suggests that more than 2 million children were born to mothers who were obese or overweight in the United States in 2003 alone. Researchers have begun to investigate pregnancy as a catalyst for maternal obesity after childbirth; however, the findings are inconclusive. Given the current obesity epidemic observed in developed countries, further investigation of obesity-related reproductive health problems is greatly needed. Findings from this research will inform the public and health providers and guide the development of intervention strategies and effective prevention programs. In contrast, many poor maternal health conditions and adverse birth outcomes in developing countries are more frequently due to poor or undernutrition. Examples of these health conditions and birth outcomes include hypertensive disorders, anemia and infection during pregnancy, low birthweight, maternal depletion, and neural tube defects. When body mass index (BMI: weight in kilograms divided by height in meters squared) is used as an indicator or proxy of nutrition, both underweight (< 18.5 BMI) and obese (≥ 30 BMI) status are risk factors for poor maternal health conditions and birth outcomes. A great disparity exists between the health and nutritional status of populations living in the developing and developed world. For example, low BMI (< 18.5), a known predictor of poor pregnancy outcome, is prevalent in 34% of women of childbearing age in south Asia and in 18% of women of childbearing age in sub-Saharan Africa in contrast to a prevalence of 4% in women of childbearing age from the developed world.

Large disparities in many reproductive health outcomes continue to exist between disadvantaged and higher socioeconomic groups within the same country, between different racial and ethnic populations, and between lower- and higher-resource countries. Most of the disparities can be attributed to poverty, lack of education, and ineffective or nonexistent policies. To eliminate the inequities, collaborative efforts from communities, governmental agencies, and the global society are needed.

Key Study Design and Measurement Issues

As with research on most rare diseases, researchers exploring uncommon reproductive conditions may consider adopting a case-control study design to obtain a satisfactory sample size that would permit detection of an effect in a more efficient way with given resources and time. However, information bias (e.g., recall bias) and measurement errors can be a concern. Case-case study design can be carried out in the situation in which data were collected for cases only. For example, the Autism Genetic Resource Exchange is a large collaborative gene bank for which biosamples are collected only from families of children with autism. One can analyze the data by comparing cases with and without a perinatal exposure of interest and their autism subtype diagnosis or genetic traits. The prospective

cohort study design is ideal for studying the effect of an early exposure that does not manifest until later in life. This approach, however, can be very costly and impractical. One way to handle the problems of prospective cohort studies, such as long follow-up time and low occurrence of cases or events, is to select a cohort that is at high risk of disease. For example, autism is one of the most heritable neuropsychiatric disorders. To investigate whether perinatal suboptimality is related to autism, one can recruit a cohort that consists of mothers who have a child with autism and are planning or intending to have another pregnancy in the near future.

Some methodologic considerations that occur more often in reproductive epidemiologic research than in chronic or infectious disease research are worthy of mention. First, some reproductive health studies may need to consider the couple as a unit rather than as two individuals. For example, the decision to conceive, ideally, involves decisions made by both partners. Second, the heterogeneity in risk of the individuals comprising the couple needs to be considered; focus should not be given only to the female, for instance. Third, researchers must remember that pregnancy outcomes can be competing. For example, a research interest is to investigate a specific exposure and infant mortality. Epidemiologists need to recognize that pregnancy outcomes, such as early pregnancy loss, spontaneous abortion, miscarriage, stillbirth, neonatal, postneonatal, and infant mortality compete with one another, and to bear in mind that a harmful exposure artificially observed as "protective" for infant mortality is not addressed if early pregnancy loss or spontaneous abortion occurred beforehand.

Public Health Implications

Reproductive epidemiologic research has made great contributions in terms of informing treatment approaches and policy making aimed at improving human reproductive health. A noteworthy example is periconceptional folic acid supplementation to prevent neural tube defects. While progress has been made in many areas, including advances in tools for measuring environmental toxicants and genotyping in reproductive health research, disparity issues remain and must be addressed. Some of the reproductive health disparities that persist are those between men and women, between populations in developing versus developed countries, between wealthy and impoverished persons, and across racial and ethnic groups.

The breadth of reproductive epidemiologic research needs to expand to understand etiologic risks more fully. Instead of solely measuring perinatal factors and immediate birth outcomes, the expansion should address the time prior to the periconception period and assess long-term maternal and child health impacts that occur later in life. Because reproduction involves both males and females, both male and female reproductive function warrants continuous investigation.

Some reproductive health issues are influenced heavily by politics (e.g., contraception and abortion), some are more influenced by familial and cultural factors (e.g., intimate partner violence), while others depend on the individual's financial status, access to health care, and reproductive history (e.g., assisted reproductive technology). As a consequence, the social and biologic context of reproduction will sustain its epidemiologic study.

—*Li-Ching Lee, Deborah L. Dee, and Amy Tsui*

See also Birth Defects; Fertility, Measures of; Fetal Death, Measures of; Gestational Age; Maternal and Child Health Epidemiology; Newborn screening programs; Oral Contraceptives; Preterm Birth; Sexually Transmitted Diseases

Further Readings

Centers for Disease Control and Prevention. (2007). *Trends in reportable sexually transmitted diseases in the United States, 2005: National surveillance data for chlamydia, gonorrhea, and syphilis.* Retrieved February 12, 2007, from http://www.cdc.gov/std/stats/trends2005.htm.

Maternal Mortality in 2000: Estimates developed by WHO, UNICEF and UNFPA. (2004). *Department of reproductive health and research World Health Organization.* Geneva, Switzerland: WHO.

National Center for Health Statistics. (2002). Infant, neonatal, and post neonatal mortality rates by race and sex: United States, 1940, 1950, 1960; 1970, and 1975-2000 (Table 34). *National Vital Statistics Report, 50*(15), 100–101. Retrieved February 12, 2007, from http://www.cdc.gov/nchs/fastats/pdf/nvsr50_15tb34.pdf.

Walboomers, J. M., Jacobs, M. V., Manos, M. M., Bosch, F. X., Kummer, J. A., Shah, K. V. et al. (1999). Papillomavirus is a necessary cause of invasive cervical cancer worldwide. *Journal of Pathology, 189*, 12–19.

Weinberg, C. R., & Wilcox, A. J. (1998). Reproductive epidemiology. In J. R. Rothman & S. Greenland (Eds.), *Modern epidemiology* (2nd ed., pp. 585–608). Philadelphia: Lippincott-Raven.

Winer, R. L., Hughes, J. P., Feng, Q., O'Reilly, S., Kiviat, N. B., Holmes, K. K., et al. (2006). Condom use and the risk of genital human papillomavirus infection in young women. *New England Journal of Medicine, 354*, 2645–2654.

Web Sites

World Health Organization, Sexual and Reproductive Health: http://www.who.int/reproductive-health/index.htm.

RESPONSE RATE

A study's response rate is an important gauge for the quality of data collection. The response rate, in its most basic form, refers to the proportion of people eligible for a study who actually enroll and participate. In fact, despite the name, the response rate is a proportion rather than a rate.

Although the concept is simple, the computation of response rates can be complex, and the use of multiple formulas diminishes the ability to compare studies by degree of nonresponse. Any comparison of response rates between studies requires knowledge of the study designs, sampling frames, modes of study recruitment, and formulas for computing response rates.

The American Association for Public Opinion Research (AAPOR) has attempted to standardize response rates for surveys conducted by mail or random-digit dialing by offering guidance on different computation methods. For example, calculating response rates for cases in a case-control study are reasonably straightforward because a list of cases is likely available (e.g., incident cases of a specific cancer received by a cancer registry). Thus, a simple proportion of the individuals with incident disease who agree to participate in the study can be computed. For controls selected from the general population, response rates need to combine information about who could be contacted, and among who could be contacted, who agrees to participate. The response rate for controls can be computed using one of the AAPOR standard formulas. Cohort studies and randomized trials tend to sample from defined subpopulations with a complete list of eligible participants or clinical settings with methods that allow for straightforward response rate computation.

It is widely recognized that response rates for all study types have decreased. This decrease may correlate with the increase in (and dislike of) telemarketing, overscheduled lifestyles, and lack of trust in government, academia, and medicine to use time efficiently and effectively. The Behavioral Risk Factor Surveillance System is a national random-digit-dial (RDD) telephone survey that collects information about health behaviors and health care access and is administered by the Centers for Disease Control and Prevention in conjunction with the states. This survey provides an example of the decrease in response rates over the past two decades. The BRFSS response rate declined from 71% in 1993 to 51% in 2005.

Response Rates for Telephone Surveys With Random Samples

Telephone surveys have their own set of issues regarding response rates. Not all telephone numbers belong to households; some belong to businesses. Because many people use technology to screen phone calls, it may not be possible to separate those who refuse to participate from those who are simply unavailable (for instance, not at home). Those who answer may not provide information to determine if an eligible person for the study resides at home, and some eligible people refuse to participate. The computation of a response rate for RDD telephone surveys requires multiple levels of information. The RDD response rate typically comprises two elements: the contact rate and the cooperation rate, both of which are really proportions (not rates). The *contact rate* is the proportion of nonbusiness numbers dialed resulting in households reached. The *cooperation rate* (sometimes called the *participation rate*) is the proportion of contacted eligible units resulting in completed interviews. While it may seem simple to construct numerators and denominators for these proportions, the myriad formulas take into account the almost 20 ways a phone call may or may not result in an eligible household or person being contacted. When comparing response rates in an assessment of data collection quality, it is clearly important to take into account the formulas used.

Response Rates in Clinical Settings

Studies conducted in clinical settings have the major advantage of having convenient sampling options. Consecutive sampling, for example, considers every patient to be eligible from the beginning of the study period until the end if they meet specific criteria (e.g., age, diagnosis). Thus, a list of all patients in the order of their appointments would constitute the sampling frame. The response rate is simply the proportion of eligible patients who agreed to participate in the study. This type of simple computation is possible for all studies where a list of eligible individuals can be developed, either before the study starts or throughout the study (e.g., a daily list of patients who have medical appointments).

The Target Response Rate

What response rate would convey good coverage of the target population? The answer is "it depends." The higher the response rate, the better it is. Historically, a response rate of 80% or more was required to establish scientific validity. However, the decline in response rates over the past two decades has eroded this standard. Some researchers have resorted to the inherently flawed "same as other studies" standard as justification for their response rates.

Because response rates are declining for both telephone and mailed surveys, researchers are studying the implications of low response rates. This research is in its infancy and, not surprisingly, has generated mixed results. Studies that compared low-response telephone surveys with higher-response interview surveys found similar response patterns for the major components, such as health behaviors and access to health care. Such a comparison conducted for the BRFSS found that it provided very similar estimates as the National Health Interview Survey, which has a response rate of about 90%. Other studies identified the potential for bias due to nonresponse. For example, in a study of response to telephone surveys on domestic violence, individuals who had experienced domestic violence were more likely to participate than those who had no such experience. In general, individuals who have a particular interest in the study topic are more likely to participate than others. The implication is that disease or events may be overestimated by studies with a particular focus; such a possibility must be carefully considered when evaluating the findings.

Reasons for Nonresponse

Many reasons for nonresponse exist, only some of which can be controlled by the researcher. Today's lifestyle is busier than ever, and people are more careful in assessing survey requests, selecting only those with the highest value for themselves, their families, and the community. Trust is an issue, especially for telephone surveys; potential respondents may evaluate whether they believe the request comes from a scientific study or a telemarketer, for instance. Another issue is conflict between a common RDD protocol that prohibits leaving a message on an answering machine, and the custom of some families to not answer the phone unless they know who is calling.

Once contact is made with an eligible individual, several factors can affect willingness to participate. Longer surveys will garner fewer participants than those projected to take little time (e.g., 5 min or less). Interviewers themselves have a good deal of impact on response, as rapport is or is not established within seconds. Thus, untrained interviewers or those with an unfamiliar accent may be less likely to elicit cooperation. For mailed surveys, visual appeal and ease of completion are important factors in determining likelihood of response.

Methods to Improve Response Rates

Several methods are known to improve response rates. In-person recruitment and interviews tend to be more successful than telephone recruitment, which tends to be more effective than mail surveys. It is not yet clear where Web-based recruitment and survey may fall in terms of response. Recent information suggests that response rates may be reasonably high for some Web-based surveys, but if surveys flood the Web, response rates are likely to drop just as they did with RDD and mailed surveys.

Because in-person recruitment and interview tends to be expensive and logistically difficult, it is important to maximize the quality of alternative methods. Several relatively simple and cost-effective methods can improve response rates:

- First, establish credibility. Clarifying the purpose of the research and the organization conducting the research can greatly encourage participation.
- Send a postcard, letter, or e-mail to inform individuals of the upcoming study and evoke their interest before surprising them with a telephone call or mailed survey. Provide a phone number as part of the information to allow potential participants to ask questions in advance.
- Use reminder messages to encourage participation and improve response.
- The use of incentives is now normative. Incentives range from trinkets to cash. The amount needs to be carefully weighed for usefulness and the risk of coercion.
- Keep the survey simple and pleasant.

Sampling in special populations (e.g., medical clinics) requires constant attention to improve and maintain high response rates while protecting privacy. It is critical that good surveys and sampling plans be designed to maximize response rates. Studying a sample of nonrespondents compared with participants will help interpret the results of studies and inform the reader about the data quality.

—*Shazia Hussain and Louise-Anne McNutt*

See also Bias; Interview Techniques; Questionnaire Design; Random-Digit Dialing; Sampling Techniques

Further Readings

Langer, G. (2003). About response rates: Some unresolved questions. *Public Perspective*, pp. 16–18. Retrieved August 8, 2007, from http://www.ropercenter.uconn.edu/pubper/pdf/pp14_3c.pdf.

Nelson, D. E, Powell-Griner, E., Town, M., & Kovar, M, G. (2003). A comparison of national estimates from the National Health Interview Survey and the Behavioral Risk Factor Surveillance System. *American Journal of Public Health, 93*(8), 1335–1341.

Schmidt, L., Morton, S. C., Damberg, C., & McGlynn, E. A. (1998). An overview of methods for conducting surveys. In E. A. McGlynn, C. Damberg, E. A. Kerr, & R. H. Brook (Eds.), *Health information systems: Design issues and analytic applications* (pp. 189–212). Santa Monica, CA: RAND. Retrieved August 8, 2007, from http://www.rand.org/pubs/monograph_reports/MR967/mr967.chap8.pdf.

Smeeth, L., & Fletcher, A. E. (2002). Improving the response rates to questionnaires. *British Medical Journal, 324,* 1168–1169.

RICKETTS, HOWARD
(1871–1910)

Howard Taylor Ricketts was an American pathologist and an ambitious pioneer of infectious disease who became renowned as the first to establish the identity of the infectious organism that causes Rocky Mountain spotted fever. The groundbreaking efforts of Ricketts and his research team was one of the earliest collaborations between physicians and entomologists, and the results have had an enormous impact on the often interdisciplinary field of epidemiology. His findings opened new pathways of knowledge in understanding the etiology of diseases.

Ricketts was born in Findley, Ohio. He completed his undergraduate degree in zoology at the University of Nebraska and went on to Northwestern University where he attained his medical degree. While working as a professor of pathology at the University of Chicago, he became interested in the mysterious and widely feared disease that was causing a very high fever and spots on the skin and was killing people who were spending a great deal of time outdoors. In 1906, Dr. Ricketts devoted his research on the discovery of the etiology of Rocky Mountain spotted fever. He characterized the basic epidemiologic features of the disease, including the role of tick vectors.

His definitive studies in the endemic area of Montana's Bitterroot Valley (where the disease was especially virulent) found that Rocky Mountain spotted fever was caused by a microorganism now called *Rickettsia rickettsii*. These unique microorganisms have both bacterial and viral characteristics and are pathogenic in humans. Ricketts demonstrated that Rocky Mountain spotted fever is not only transmitted by wood ticks but also caused by a bloodborne bipolar bacillus. Although he observed a small bacillus, Rickets was unable to culture a causal agent. His work suggested that bacterial diseases could be biologically passed from pests to people in his published findings in 1909, "A Micro-Organism Which Apparently Has a Specific Relationship to Rocky Mountain Spotted Fever: A Preliminary Report."

Through a series of groundbreaking investigations, now considered landmark epidemiological achievements, Ricketts used noninfected guinea pigs as hosts for ticks carrying the disease, and afterward the guinea pigs developed the infection. He proved that a nonfilterable virus, not protozoa, was the etiologic agent for Rocky Mountain spotted fever. Ricketts was quite devoted to his research and was known to inject himself with pathogens on several occasions to measure their effect.

Four years later, he showed that typhus is caused by a similar organism carried by lice. Tragically, Dr. Ricketts died of typhus (another rickettsial disease) in Mexico in 1910 at the age of 39, shortly after completing his remarkable studies on Rocky Mountain spotted fever. His death came only a few days after he isolated the organisms he believed caused typhus. The two organisms Ricketts discovered were the first of what were later shown to be an unusual genus of virus-like bacteria—the *Rickettsiae*. He is now remembered as one of the great martyrs of epidemiologic research.

—Sean Nagle

See also Etiology of Disease; Insect-Borne Disease; Parasitic Diseases

Further Readings

Heyneman, D. (2001). The blight of the Bitterroot, the Mysterious Rocky Mountain Spotted Fever, and the significant role of Wilson and Chowning: A commentary. *Wilderness and Environmental Medicine*, *12*(2), 118–120. Retrieved August 8, 2007, from http://www.wemjournal.org/pdfserv/ i1080-6032-012-02-0118.pdf.

Ricketts, H. T. (1909). A microorganism which apparently has a specific relationship to Rocky Mountain spotted fever. *Journal of the American Medical Association*, *52*, 379–380.

ROBUST STATISTICS

Maximum likelihood (ML) is the most widely used approach for statistical inference. Although it has the advantage of employing straightforward calculations, the ML approach lacks robustness, giving rise to spurious results and misleading conclusions. Researchers in epidemiology and a variety of other experimental and health sciences are becoming increasingly aware of this issue and are informed about the available alternatives for more reliable inference.

Concept of Robustness

What is robustness? Although it is intuitively clear what robustness should be, there is no unique statistical definition, in part because of the diverse aspects of robustness. The generally accepted notion is that a robust statistical procedure should be insensitive to changes not involving the parameters, but sensitive to changes in model parameters. For example, the ML approach is the most powerful for detecting changes in the parameters under the model. However, it is generally sensitive to model assumptions, yielding biased estimates and incorrect inference when the study data depart from the model. A robust procedure aims to provide good power under the model, while still yielding reliable estimates when data drift away from the model.

To elucidate the basic idea, consider a relatively simple problem of comparing two independent groups. The most common procedure is the *t* test developed based on ML under normal distribution assumption. This procedure compares the two sample means for evidence of group differences. If the data are normally distributed for both groups, the difference statistic between the two group means has a *t* distribution, providing the basis for inference (i.e., *p* values and confidence intervals). In many applications, however, data often deviate from the normal model. Such departures from normality can affect both the estimate and inference. For example, the difference statistic may severely over- or underestimate the true group difference in the presence of outliers, giving rise to biased estimates. In many applications, the difference statistic may be unbiased, but the skewness and sparseness in the data distribution may seriously affect the sampling distribution of the statistic, making inference based on the *t* distribution incorrect. Thus, a robust procedure must address either one or both issues.

Robustness Approaches

A common cause of bias in the estimate is outliers (observations that are exceptionally large or small). Although the sample mean is easy to interpret and work with, it is sensitive to such outlying observations. The common approach to address the effect of outlier is the use of order statistics. By ordering the observations from the smallest to the largest, we can define estimates that are not influenced, or are less influenced, by outliers. For example, the trimmed

mean is the sample mean calculated based on the data after removing a certain percentage of observations in the smallest and largest range of the order statistic. Alternatively, one may downweight such outliers to lessen their effect. For example, the winsorized mean is the sample mean after replacing a fraction of the lowest and highest values by the next values counting inward from the extremes, respectively. The sample median is yet another common robust estimate based on the order statistic. Thus, for comparing two groups, we can also form a difference statistic by using any of these robust estimates.

Although these order statistic-based estimates are all more robust than the sample mean, they are not widely used in real study applications. First, these estimates contain a subjective element regarding what constitute outliers and how they are treated. For example, the trimmed and winsorized means involve subjective decisions for trimming and downweighting observations. Second, order statistic-based estimates often give rise to very complex sampling distributions even for univariate outcomes. As a result, existing methods do not apply to cohort and longitudinal studies, which are becoming increasingly popular in epidemiologic and other health-related research. Thus, for most real study applications containing outliers, two sets of analyses are usually performed to examine their effect; one that includes all data and the other that leaves out the outliers. In cases where the outliers have substantial effect on inference, investigation is conducted to determine the nature of their occurrence and whether they should be included in the analysis. Such sensitivity analysis is easy to perform and bypasses the technical difficulties for inference using the order statistic-based estimates.

Even in the absence of outliers, inference based on ML may still be wrong if the distribution assumptions are violated. For example, in the two-group comparison case, if the data from one or both groups are skewed or heavily tailed, the difference statistic generally does not follow the *t* distribution. Thus, although the statistic may be unbiased, the *t* distribution is no longer appropriate for inference. The two most popular alternatives are the asymptotic theory-based large sample and permutation-based exact inference. While large sample procedures require large sample size for valid inference, exact methods apply without this restriction.

The estimating equations (EE) approach is the most widely used large sample procedure. Rather than relying on the likelihood for inference as with the ML approach, the EE constructs estimates and sampling distributions based on a set of estimating equations. Since the equations can be set up without any distribution assumption, this approach provides valid inference regardless of the data distribution. The EE approach applies to many commonly used models such as multiple regression, logistic, and log-linear models. Its extension to longitudinal (or panel) data and other types of clustered data, known as the generalized estimating equations (GEE), has been widely used in biomedical, epidemiologic, behavioral, and social science research.

For data with relatively small sample sizes, large sample procedures may not be applicable; in such cases, exact methods provide an alternative for inference. Exact methods are developed based on the permutation distribution of a test statistic under the null hypothesis. Fisher's exact test for analysis of a 2×2 contingency table is the most familiar example of this approach for discrete outcomes. We can also readily apply such methods to the two-group comparison problem in our example. Under the null hypothesis of no between-group difference, the two groups have the same distribution. Thus, group membership does not matter and can be arbitrarily mixed or permuted between the two groups. By calculating the difference statistic for all possible permutations, we obtain the permutation distribution of the statistic under the null hypothesis and use it like a sampling distribution for inference. Even for small sample size and a simple problem such as two-group comparison, it is difficult to find the exact permutation distribution because of the astronomically large number of permutations and formidable computing problems. In practice, we often approximate the permutation distribution by considering 1,000 to 5,000 different permutations. Such a Monte Carlo implementation generally provides reasonably good results.

Discussion

Robust estimate and robust inference are related, but differ in both concept and application. Estimate robustness is concerned with locally contaminated data such as outliers, while inference robustness addresses global distribution assumptions such as normality. For example, when comparing two groups using the median or trimmed mean, we may still assume normality, in which case inference may still be wrong if the normal model is violated. On the other hand, although inference based on EE is robust against violations of distribution assumptions, it can still be wrong if EE-based estimates are seriously biased, as in the presence of outliers.

We may also apply robust inference to robust estimates. For example, instead of large sample inference, we can compare two-group medians using exact inference. This combination of robust estimate and inference is robust against not only outliers, but data distributions as well.

Rank statistics offer another approach to address robustness. However, as rankings of observations have no direct relationship with the scale of the data, such methods are generally used to provide inference rather than modeling data as the EE and GEE procedures do. For example, the Mann-Whitney-Wilcoxon rank sum test is only used to compare whether there is a shift in location between two otherwise identical distributions. It does not provide any information regarding the distributions or features of the distributions such as mean, median, and standard deviation.

Although EE and GEE are widely used for robust inference for cross-sectional and longitudinal (or panel) data, applications of robust estimates are largely limited to relatively simple, cross-sectional data analyses. In addition, specialized software such as StatXact by Cytel Inc. are often required, as most major statistical packages, including SAS, Splus, SPSS, and STATA, do not provide support for inference based on robust estimates. Alternatively, user-written and supported functions may also be used and are often available free of charge. For example, a set of Splus programs for performing robust analyses, including the median, trimmed, and winsorized mean, can be downloaded from www.apnet.com/updates/ireht.htm.

—Wan Tang, Qin Yu, and Xin Tu

See also Fisher's Exact Test; Nonparametric Statistics; Panel Data

Further Readings

Diggle, P. J., Heagerty, P. J., Liang, K. Y., & Zeger, S. L. (2002). *Analysis of longitudinal data.* New York: Oxford University Press.

Efron, B., & Tihshirani, R. J. (1998). *An introduction to the Bootstrap.* Boca Raton, FL: Chapman & Hall.

Wilcox, R. R. (1977). *Introduction to robust estimation and hypothesis testing.* San Diego, CA: Academic Press.

ROCHESTER EPIDEMIOLOGY PROJECT

The Rochester Epidemiology Project (REP) is a population-based medical records linkage system that was established by Leonard T. Kurland in 1966. It exploits the geographic isolation of Olmsted County in southeastern Minnesota from other urban centers so that almost all medical care for residents of the county (or the central city of Rochester) is delivered within the community. Care is mainly provided by Mayo Clinic and Olmsted Medical Center. Mayo Clinic is a major referral center but has always provided primary, secondary, as well as tertiary care to local residents. It employs a dossier (or unit) medical record for each individual containing the details of every admission to its two affiliated hospitals (St. Marys and Rochester Methodist), every outpatient office or clinic visit, all emergency room and nursing home care, all laboratory results, all pathology reports including autopsies, and all correspondence concerning each patient.

Mayo Clinic now holds medical histories on more than 6.3 million unique individuals (including referral patients); less than a 1,000 of these dossiers have been lost over the past century. The records of the other providers have also been maintained and are available for use in approved research studies. These original and complete (inpatient and outpatient) records that span each person's entire period of residency in the community are easily retrievable for study because Mayo has maintained, since 1910, extensive indices based on clinical and histologic diagnoses and surgical procedures. With continuous support from the NIH for the past 40 years, the REP created similar indices for the records of the other providers of medical care to county residents, most notably Olmsted Medical Center with its affiliated Olmsted Community Hospital.

The result is a unique medical record system capable of addressing research questions in a community population with more than 5.2 million person-years of experience from 1950 through 2005. These detailed data, accumulated over a long period of time, have provided the basis for almost 1,700 studies by investigators inside and outside Mayo. Most of these studies could not have been carried out as efficiently anywhere else. Complete ascertainment of diagnosed cases supports descriptive studies of the incidence and outcomes of diverse diseases and diagnostic/therapeutic procedures. Inception cohorts with verified exposures can be identified for long-term retrospective (historical) cohort studies, and the local community can be enumerated and sampled for population-based cross-sectional and case-control studies. Due to the nature of the database, the main focus has been on clinical risk factors and clinical outcomes; because of the contemporary documentation available, these are much more accurately ascertained compared with self-report. The population of Olmsted County was 124,000 in 2000 and is largely white (99% in 1950, 90% in 2000). Except for a higher proportion of the working population in the health care industry, its population resembles U.S. whites generally. Judged by previous studies of a variety of chronic diseases, results can probably be extrapolated to that population.

—*Lee Joseph Melton III*

See also Administrative Data; Biomedical Informatics; Clinical Epidemiology

Further Readings

Melton, L. J., III. (1996). History of the Rochester Epidemiology Project. *Mayo Clinic Proceedings, 71,* 266–274.

RURAL HEALTH ISSUES

The definition of a rural area is complex. According to the U.S. Census Bureau, rural areas are all territories, populations, and housing units not classified as urban. An urban area is defined as one with a total population of at least 2,500 for urban clusters or at least 50,000 for urbanized areas. Rural areas can be located in both metropolitan and nonmetropolitan areas. According to the 2000 census, 21% of the U.S. population (60 million people) live in rural areas.

Many of the health challenges faced by rural America, including chronic illnesses such as hypertension and diabetes, are similar to those faced by all Americans; however, populations in rural areas also have unique health concerns. This entry discusses some of these concerns, including occupational health, environmental health, and access to health care and also addresses the health of minority groups and migrant workers in rural areas.

Occupational Hazards

Agriculture, fisheries, logging, mining, hunting, and trapping are among the common industries found in rural areas. These industries include the most hazardous occupations for occupational morbidity and mortality. All the above industries require heavy physical labor under demanding weather and environmental conditions. The National Institute of Occupational Safety and Health estimates that 4.5 million people work in agriculture, of whom 23% are minorities. Although agricultural workers make up less than 3% of the U.S. total labor force, they suffer 12% of fatal workplace injuries. In addition to the higher mortality, about 500 agricultural workers experience disabling injuries daily, and 5% of these injuries result in permanent impairment.

The types of occupational hazards that result in increased morbidity and mortality include machinery-related deaths and injuries, noise exposure leading to hearing loss, vibratory exposure leading to neurovascular degeneration of the hands, and the risk of blindness from flying objects. Respiratory irritants can result in asthma, farmer's lung, silo-filler's disease, black lung disease, asbestosis, and asphyxiation. Working with animals can result in zoonotic diseases. In the fisheries industry, there is the risk of drowning or capsizing vessels; in the mining industry, there is the risk of mine collapse. In all these industries, there is physical isolation that results in increased stress and depression.

Environmental Hazards

In addition to the above occupational exposures, there are environmental hazards as well. Rural populations face exposure to chemicals and pesticides, lack of clean drinking water, lack of hand-washing facilities and toilets, temperature extremes, and exposure to zoonotic (animal) diseases. Outside labor with more exposure to sunlight increases the risk of skin cancers.

Pesticides are known to cause a multitude of acute and chronic problems. The EPA estimates that 1.2 billion pounds of pesticides are used annually in the United States, 76% in agriculture. If pesticides seeped into groundwater, they could easily contaminate 90%

of rural America's supply of drinking water. Some minor effects of pesticides include eye and nose irritation, fatigue, nausea, and diarrhea. Pesticides can cause human reproductive and developmental toxicity, infertility, neural tube defects, and limb reduction defects. They have also linked pesticides to neurobehavioral problems, Parkinson's disease, depression, and many types of skin problems. Chemical and pesticide exposure can increase risks of non-Hodgkins lymphoma, leukemia, prostate, and stomach and brain cancers.

Health-Related Behaviors

Lifestyle choices such as alcohol and tobacco use are seen in higher proportions in rural areas. In both rural adults and youth, alcohol abuse, alcohol dependence, tobacco use, and illegal drug use are more common than in their urban counterparts. Forty percent of rural 12th graders reported using alcohol while driving compared with 25% in urban areas.

In rural areas, there is an increased use of smokeless tobacco and smoking of homemade or unfiltered cigarettes. Approximately, 28% of rural high school students state that they regularly smoke some type of tobacco. Eleven percent of urban teens report daily tobacco use. Rural 8th graders are twice as likely to smoke cigarettes than their urban counterparts.

Although illegal drug use is common in rural areas, production of amphetamine has increased in isolated rural areas where it is more likely to go unnoticed. In 1999, there were 300 times more seizures of methamphetamine labs in Iowa than in New York and New Jersey combined.

Access to Health Care

Providing health care in rural areas of the United States poses different challenges than in urban areas, because rural populations tend to be poorer, are more likely to travel greater distances to obtain health care, and are less likely to have health insurance. Other issues relating to health care access include inflexible work schedules, loss of pay, language and cultural barriers, poverty, and lack of both public and private transportation.

Access to health care and funding for health care in rural areas are major concerns. Although certain groups of populations have insurance coverage, many do not. The government provides Medicare for the elderly, Medicaid for those in extreme poverty, and government-sponsored children's health insurance plans for some children. However, during any given year, approximately 15% to 20% of the rural population below age 64 is without health insurance. If you live in a rural area, odds are 80% higher that you will be uninsured.

For those patients seeking health care (with or without insurance), physicians are still difficult to access. Approximately, 75% of all rural counties are considered health care professional shortage areas. There are limited numbers of physicians and specialists per capita. Only about 10% of all physicians practice in rural areas, despite the fact that nearly 25% of the population lives in rural areas. Medicare payments to rural hospitals and physicians are dramatically less than those to their urban counterparts for equivalent services. This correlates closely with the fact that more than 470 rural hospitals have closed in the past 25 years. Since rural hospitals rely on government funding, budget cuts in Medicaid and Medicare make it difficult for many hospitals to continue operations.

Individuals below the age of 64 who work typically do not qualify for government health insurance. Many of the employment opportunities in rural areas are either self-employed or blue-collar jobs, neither of which provides health insurance. These populations are responsible for purchasing private health insurance that can dramatically decrease their monthly income. Instead, many chose to forego health insurance and hope that they will never need to use medical facilities. Many patients without health insurance do not seek regular preventive medical care and only seek care in emergency situations. This lack of preventive care hinders their overall health and quality of care, as well as raising final costs to both the patient and to society. The Institute of Medicine estimates that the United States loses $65 to $130 billion annually because of poorer health and earlier death of those that lack health insurance.

Migrant Farmworkers

The definition of a migrant farmworker is someone who changes residences during the year to accommodate crop harvests. Although the total number of migrant farmworkers is unknown, it is estimated that there are between 2.5 million and 4 million working in the United States. An increasing number of these farmworkers are born outside the United States. In 1998, 89% of migrant farmworkers were Hispanic and 50% admitted that they lacked legal documentation. The health of migrant farmworkers is an important issue in rural health. Not only do these workers harvest and package fresh produce for the United States but their health affects their families, their local communities, and the population at large.

Migrant workers are also exposed to a variety of environmental and occupational hazards, including exposure to extreme temperatures and pesticides. Some of the health issues that affect this population include living in remote isolated areas that do not have health care facilities, increased distance from health care providers, limited choices of providers, poverty, transportation difficulties, inflexible work schedules, discrimination, and language and cultural barriers. They are often housed in crowded living conditions that allow the spread of infectious disease, particularly in populations that have inadequate immunization. Rubella, varicella, and tuberculosis are easily spread in these conditions. Intestinal parasites are common among agricultural workers and may be either imported from their country of origin or may be secondary to polluted water sources within the United States. Their work is often physically demanding and repetitive, and they often suffer from sleep deprivation and separation from family, which may lead to alcohol and drug abuse, violence, and boredom. Prostitution, an additional source of income for some, increases the spread of disease. Lack of experience with machinery and tools can increase injuries. The management of chronic conditions such as hypertension or diabetes is especially challenging in a mobile population, and migrant farmworkers may also be unavailable to obtain the results of preventive screening tests such as pap smears or mammograms. Needs-based programs such as Medicaid, WIC (Women, Infants, Children), and food stamps are rarely used by migrant farmworkers. Approximately 50% of this population has never visited a dentist.

Minority Groups

American Indians and Alaska Natives (AI/AN)

There are approximately 3.3 million AI/AN in the United States, and a higher percentage live in rural areas (including reservations) as compared with the general population. This population has a higher rate of chronic disease than the average population. Cardiovascular disease, hypertension, and diabetes mellitus are leading causes of morbidity and mortality in this population. Cancer is also higher in this population, with the top cancers including lung, breast, prostate, and colon cancer with lower overall cancer survival rates. AI/AN are three times more likely to die from diabetes as compared with all U.S. races.

The great epidemic among this population is injuries, both intentional and unintentional. Unintentional injuries are the leading cause of death for AI/AN up to 45 years of age. Motor vehicle accidents make up half of all unintentional injuries. The associated factors are alcohol abuse, speeding, and substandard road conditions. There is also a twofold increase in other unintentional injuries such as drowning, falls, poisoning, and burns as compared with the normal population. There are high risks of suicide believed to be associated with loss of traditional culture and exposure to the Western culture. Only 50% of males will reach their 45th birthday.

With improvements in both health care and access to health care, life expectancy has improved dramatically but still lags behind that of the general population. This improvement was primarily seen through sharp reductions in infant mortality. The Indian Health Service (IHS) provides a nationally integrated system of lifetime health care for this population. In addition to providing health care to approximately 1.8 million AI/AN, the IHS provides education, outreach activities and opportunity for tribal involvement in developing and managing programs to meet their health needs.

African Americans

Nearly, 90% of rural African Americans live in the southeastern United States. This population faces higher rates of chronic illness and injury-related mortality and has lower levels of participation in health-promoting behaviors than their urban counterparts. Recent studies have shown that those living in the southeast suffer from higher rates of diabetes, stroke, and obesity. African American populations in rural areas also experience high rates of teenage pregnancy, alcoholism, and uncontrolled blood pressure. Many of these health problems are attributed to lower socioeconomic status, poorer diets, greater risk of occupational injury, higher levels of stress, and less access to health care. Many African Americans also face limited opportunity for quality education and employment.

The Road to Improvement

There are multiple areas for improvement in the health of rural populations. Main areas include increasing safety in the workplace, improving standards regarding environmental exposure, increasing access to health care, and increasing education on the prevention of disease.

Programs such as those of the U.S. Department of Labor's Mine Safety and Health Administration (MSHA) have decreased injuries in the workplace for miners through stricter guidelines and workplace standards. This agency enforces compliance with mandatory safety and health programs required by the 1977 Mine Safety and Health Act. MSHA also aims to prevent or decrease illness and injury on the job through training programs for workers and mine inspectors, technical assistance to miners and mine operators, and efforts to encourage employers to provide safer equipment and more education for the mining community.

Community health programs must stress preventive measures, such as screening and monitoring for chronic illness (especially hypertension and diabetes) and providing public health education and information on issues such as prenatal care, symptom management for chronic illness, diet, exercise, and tobacco use. An often-undervalued resource for youth in rural communities is the cooperative extension service. This service provides education aimed toward pregnant teens and youth development and discusses a multitude of topics, including sex education, ATOD (alcohol, tobacco, other drugs) use, smoking prevention, and nutrition. The 4-H program encourages citizenship, leadership, and teaches life skills to teenagers in rural areas.

Access to health care and increasing the number of insured patients needs to be at the top of the list to improve rural health. Improved health status among rural Americans would reduce health care expenditures, and it would improve the quality of life and productivity of the population. Although the Health Service Corp and the IHS have increased the number of physicians in rural areas, more needs to be done to recruit and retain physicians in these areas to provide needed medical assistance.

—Amanda Bush Flynn

See also African American Health Issues; Environmental and Occupational Epidemiology; Geographical and Social Influences on Health; Health Disparities; Immigrant and Refugee Health Issues; Native American Health Issues; U.S. Public Health Services

Further Readings

Coward, R., Davis, L., Gold, C., Smiciklas-Wright, H., Thorndyke, L., & Vondracek, F. (2006). *Rural women's health: Mental, behavioral, and physical issues.* New York: Springer.
Glasgow, N., Morton, L., & Johnson, N. (Eds). (2004). *Critical issues in rural health.* Ames, IA: Blackwell.
Loue, S., & Quill, B. (Eds). (2001). *Handbook of rural health.* New York: Kluwer Academic.
Straub, L., & Walzer, N. (Eds.). (1992). *Rural health care: Innovation in a changing environment.* Westport, CT: Praeger.

Web Sites

Indian Health Service, U.S. Dept of Health and Human Services: http://www.ihs.gov.
Mine Safety and Health Administration, U.S. Department of Labor: http://www.msha.gov.
National Health Service Corps, U.S. Dept of Health and Human Services, Health Resources and Services Administration: http://nhsc.bhpr.hrsa.gov.
National Industry for Occupational Safety and Health: http://www.cdc.gov/niosh/homepage.html.
National Rural Health Association: http://www.nrharural.org.

RUSH, BENJAMIN
(1745–1813)

Acknowledged as a father of modern psychiatry as well a signatory of the Declaration of Independence, Benjamin Rush modeled a social activist's tireless approach to public health issues in early American society, while becoming the most famous physician and medical educator of his generation. As a boy in Byberry Township outside Philadelphia, Rush was a student at West Nottingham Academy (now the oldest boarding school in the country) under Reverend Samuel Finley, who subsequently became the president of the College of New Jersey (now Princeton University). Although initially intent on becoming a lawyer, Rush switched to medicine. He attended medical school in England, graduating from the medical department of the University of Edinburgh in 1768. During his time abroad, Rush attended medical lectures in Paris, where he befriended Benjamin Franklin, who became a benefactor. Later, he also developed close relationships with John Adams and Thomas Jefferson.

Medicine and Politics

On his return to the United States, Rush was appointed Professor of Chemistry at the College of Philadelphia and launched a public career as a political activist and advocate of colonial rights. As a physician, he practiced extensively among the poor. In 1771, Rush published essays on slavery, temperance, and health. In 1774, he delivered the annual guest lecture at the Philosophical Society, titled "Natural History of Medicine Among the Indians of North America." Two years later, after the adoption of the Declaration of Independence, he was elected to Congress. The same year, he married Julia Stockton, daughter of another signatory of the Declaration, and together they had 13 children. Indiscreet criticism of George Washington, however, somewhat sullied his reputation and led him to resign a medical post in the Continental Army. Nonetheless, he attended the wounded at various Revolutionary War battles while retaining his medical posts in Philadelphia.

In 1793, Rush was credited with overcoming the yellow fever epidemic in his home city, during which he treated over a 100 patients a day. A founder of Dickinson College, Rush was also a strong advocate of public education, including education of women. Rush served as Professor of Medical Theory and Clinical Practice at the University of Pennsylvania for 22 years, and from 1799 until his death, he was also Treasurer of the U.S. Mint. In 1803, Rush succeeded Benjamin Franklin as President of Pennsylvania Society for the Abolition of Slavery.

Health Beliefs and Publications

Rush's most important publications include *An Inquiry Into the Effects of Ardent Spirits on the Human Mind and Body* (1784), *Medical Inquiries and Observations* (a five-volume set, last published in 1806), *Essays, Literary, Moral, and Philosophica* (1798), *Sixteen Introductory Lectures* (1811), and *Diseases of the Mind* (1812, 5th ed., 1835). He also edited several other medical books. Some of Rush's medical ideas, such as his beliefs about the value of bloodletting and purging, have proved to be ill founded. On the other hand, he sensed the dangers of tobacco use and is recognized as the first physician to define alcohol dependence, or what he termed *inebriety*, as a disease.

—Merrill Singer

See also Alcohol Use; Tobacco; Yellow Fever

Further Readings

D'Elia, D. (1966). Dr. Benjamin Rush and the American medical revolution. *Proceedings of the American Philosophical Society, 110*(4), 227–234.

Powell, J. (1965). *Bring out your dead: The great plague of yellow fever in Philadelphia in 1793.* New York: Time.

Shryock, R. (1972). *Medicine and society in America: 1660–1860.* Ithaca, NY: Cornell University Press.

S

SAMPLE SIZE CALCULATIONS AND STATISTICAL POWER

Sample size determination and prospective power analysis are important factors in planning a statistical study, because a study executed with an inappropriate sample size may result in wasted resources. If the sample is too small, the inference goal may not be achieved and true effects may not be detected, and if it is too large, money and resources have been unnecessarily expended, and subjects may have been exposed unnecessarily to a drug or the treatment. Conversely, with an optimal sample, the investigator has increased chances of detecting true effects without wasting resources or exposing subjects to unnecessary risk. For this reason, many funding agencies required sample size determinations to be supported by statistical power analysis. To illustrate, the National Institutes of Health (NIH) Policy Manual (NIH, 1988) states that requests for approval from the Office of Management and Budget to conduct epidemiological studies should include a discussion of sample size and statistical power analysis, among other things. In general, a power of at least 80% is considered satisfactory.

The process of determining the optimum sample size that will give adequate power to detect effects is a task that involves the entire research team. Several factors influence the statistical power of the study and consequently the required sample size. The factors include the hypothesis to be tested, the probability model to test the hypothesis, the significance level α, and a guess on the variance and effect size; that is, in the simplest terms, the expected difference between groups based on scientific considerations. Because some of the factors that influence the statistical power of the study have to be guessed, the statistical power should be tested under different scenarios of sample size, assumptions, and study conditions. For example, if it is important to detect a relative risk of 3, then power analysis should also include a range of neighboring values such as 2 and 4.

There are many formulas available for sample size calculations, although some of the commonly used formulas are based on approximations that assume that large sample sizes will be used in the study. In 1989, in an article titled "How Appropriate Are Popular Sample Size Formulas?," Kupper and Hafner (1989) discuss the use of some of the formulas that have large-sample approximation and recommend the use of formulas that consider statistical power. In epidemiological studies that plan to test hypotheses, it is very important to select a formula that will consider power. Note that not all the formulas consider power estimates. Generally speaking, power analysis is important in obtaining a balance between Type I and Type II errors.

Statistical Power

The concept of power is analogous to the concept of error type. The significance level α is the probability of Type I error—that is, the probability of finding a statistically significant difference by chance—when it does not truly exist. The power is $1 - \beta$, where β is the probability of Type II error. Recall that the Type II error is the probability of not finding a statistically significant difference when it exists. Therefore, the power is the probability that the null hypothesis will be rejected given that the alternative hypothesis is true. This means that a study with low power will not be able to detect significant effects. Thus, power analysis has the objective of balancing Type I and Type II errors.

The statistical power will depend on the level at which the significance was fixed. For example, imagine that the significance level is fixed at 0.01 instead of 0.05. That will require a larger confidence level $(1 - \alpha)$ of 99% instead of 95%. It will be harder to find significance with 99% than it would be with 95%, and therefore, the statistical power of the study will be lower.

The approach taken in a power analysis to define the optimum sample size depends on the nature of the data (e.g., Are the variables continuous, binary, or ordinal?) and the statistical test or model that will be used. For example, for comparisons of means with t tests and analysis of variance (ANOVA), power can be approximated using the noncentral t distribution or noncentral F distribution. With categorical data, for comparisons of proportions in contingency tables with Pearson chi-square tests, power can be approximated using the noncentral chi-square distribution. Agresti (2002) and O'Brien and Muller (1993) discuss methods of statistical power analysis for many other tests such as the t test of correlated means, generalized linear models, and logistic regression. Statistical power analysis is an active area of statistical research and better approaches to power calculations are being developed, in particular for more complex models such as specific mixed models. Another approach to power calculation are methods based on simulation: This approach is a particularly effective tool for verifying if the approximations chosen are reasonable and for performing calculations in cases where good approximations are not yet available.

Examples of Calculations

Two-Sample t Test

Suppose that one plans to test the difference between the means of two groups, $\mu_1 - \mu_2$. For example, the null hypothesis can be that there is no difference between the means, $\mu_1 - \mu_2 = 0$, and that it can be assumed that the parameters μ_1 and μ_2 have a common standard deviation, σ. In this case, the power calculation will involve the noncentral t distribution, where the power will be the probability

$$1 - p(z \le t(df) * - \delta),$$

where z is the standard normal random variable, $t *$ is the t distribution critical value, at the selected significance level α, with degrees of freedom df (which is equal to the total sample $- 2$), and the noncentrality parameter δ defined as

$$\delta = \frac{|\mu_1 - \mu_2|}{\sigma} \left(\frac{1}{n_1} + \frac{1}{n_2} \right)^{-1/2}.$$

Note that if $\mu_1 = \mu_2$, then the noncentrality parameter δ will be 0. This is equivalent to the null hypothesis. The larger the noncentrality parameter δ is, the higher the departure from the null hypothesis and the power.

Imagine the following numerical example. An investigator is planning a study with two groups consisting of 45 subjects in each group. He or she wants to be able to detect a difference of at least 9 points $(\mu_1 - \mu_2 = 9)$ in the group means, at 5% confidence level. He or she has a guess that the standard deviation will be equal to 15. From a table, he or she obtains the value of $t *$ (upper tail probability $= \alpha = 0.05$ and $df = 45 + 45 - 2 = 88$) of 1.99. The statistical power of the study will be

$$1 - p(z \le t * - \delta)$$

$$= 1 - p\left(z \le 1.99 - \frac{9}{15} \left(\frac{1}{45} + \frac{1}{45} \right)^{-1/2} \right) \approx 0.8.$$

The study has a statistical power of 80%. Therefore, if all the assumptions hold, the study will correctly reject the null hypothesis at 5% significance level in 80% of all possible samples.

Analysis of Variance

The power test for the one-way ANOVA is fairly similar to the power test for the two-sample t test, except that instead of the noncentral t distribution, the noncentral F distribution will be used. Consider that one plans to test the null hypothesis that the mean of I groups is the same, $\mu_1 = \mu_2 = \cdots = \mu_i$, and that we can assume a common standard deviation σ. Let I be the total number of groups, N be the total sample size, and n_i and μ_i be the sample size and the mean of each group, respectively. In this case, the power will be probability

$$p(F(df_{\text{hypothesis}}, df_{\text{error}}, \lambda) \ge F(df_{\text{hypothesis}}, df_{\text{error}}) *),$$

where $F(df_{hypothesis}, df_{error})*$ is the F distribution critical value at the selected significance level α and $F(df_{hypothesis}, df_{error}, \lambda)$ is the noncentral F distribution value with degrees of freedom $df_{hypothesis}(= I - 1)$ and $df_{error}(= N - 1)$, and the noncentrality parameter λ defined as

$$\lambda = \frac{\sum n_i(\mu_i - (N^{-1} \sum n_i\mu_i))^2}{\sigma^2}.$$

Similar to δ, if all the means are equal, then the noncentrality parameter λ will be zero; and the larger the noncentrality parameter λ is, the higher the departure from the null hypothesis and the power.

To illustrate, imagine that the investigator is now planning a study with three groups consisting of 30 subjects in each group. His or her null hypothesis is that there is no difference in the group means (H_0: $\mu_1 = \mu_2 = \mu_3$), at a 5% significance level. Based on his or her experience, he or she guesses that the means are $\mu_1 = 55$, $\mu_2 = 60$, and $\mu_3 = 65$, with a standard deviation of 15.

From a table, he or she obtains the value of $F*$ (upper tail probability $= \alpha = 0.05$, $df_{hypothesis} = 3 - 1 = 2$ and $df_{error} = 120 - 1 = 119$) of 3.07, $\lambda = 6.67$, and the power of the study will be

$$p(F(2, 119, 6.67) \geq 3.07) \approx 0.62.$$

The study's statistical power of 62% would probably be considered low, and the investigator may opt to increase the sample size.

Pearson Chi-Square Tests of Independence

Imagine that one plans to have a contingency table with two levels of exposure versus levels of severity of a certain disease. One plans to test the null hypothesis (H_0) that there is independence between levels of exposure to a virus and levels of disease severity. Let π represent the true proportion in each of the cells in the contingency table, and let $\pi(H_0)$ represent the proportions under the null hypothesis. If the sample is large, the power calculation can use the noncentral chi-square distribution as discussed by Alan Agresti, where the power will be the probability

$$p(\chi^2(df, \lambda) > \chi^2(df)*),$$

where $\chi^2(df)*$ is the chi-square distribution critical value at the selected significance level α, $\chi^2(df, \lambda)$ is

the noncentral chi-square distribution, and the noncentrality parameter λ is defined as

$$\lambda = \frac{\sum n_i[\pi_i - \pi_i(H_0)]^2}{\pi_i(H_0)}.$$

To illustrate, imagine that the investigator is now planning a study with four groups consisting of 50 subjects in each group. The proportion of subjects with disease is expected to be 0.05, 0.12, 0.14, and 0.20 in each of the groups. For each group, the proportion of subjects without disease will be $1 -$ the proportion of subjects with disease, 0.95, 0.88, 0.86, and 0.8, respectively. Because the sample size is equal for all the four groups, the expected proportion can be calculated by summing the proportions of subjects with disease and dividing by 4. In this case, $\pi(H_0)$ for subjects with disease is equal to 0.1275, and $\pi(H_0)$ for subjects without disease is equal to 0.8725. Using the formula, he or she estimates λ to be approximately 5.158. From the table, he or she obtains the value of $\chi^2(df)*$ (upper tail probability $= \alpha = 0.05$, $df = 4 - 1 = 3$) of 7.81, and the power of the study will be

$$p(\chi^2(3, 5.158) > 7.81) \approx 0.45.$$

The study's statistical power of 45% would probably be considered low, and the investigator may opt to increase the sample size.

Packages and Programs

It is often more convenient to use commercial software packages designed for power calculations and sample size determination than to write customized code in statistical packages such as SAS or R to do the calculations. There are many packages available that perform sample size analyses. Some packages are specific for power analysis and sample sizes calculation, such as PASS®, nQuery Advisor®, and SamplePower from SPSS. SAS includes two procedures (POWER and GLMPOWER) that estimate power for many different statistical tests. Additionally, UnifyPow is a freeware SAS module/macro (written by Ralph O'Brien) that performs power analysis (but requires that SAS be available on the user's computer), and it is available at www.bio.ri.ccf.org/UnifyPow.

—*Ana W. Capuano*

See also Hypothesis Testing; Sampling Techniques; Study Design; Type I and Type II Errors

Further Readings

Agresti, A. (1990). *Categorical data analysis.* New York: Wiley.

Castelloe, J. (2000). *Sample size computations and power analysis with the SAS system.* Paper presented at the proceedings of the 25th annual SAS User's Group International Conference [Paper 265-25], Cary, NC: SAS Institute.

Kupper, L. L., & Hafner, K. B. (1989). How appropriate are popular sample size formulas? *American Statistician, 43*(2), 101–105.

National Institutes of Health. (1988, December). *NIH policy manual. Chapter 1825: Information collection from the public.* Retrieved April 16, 2007, from http://www1.od.nih.gov/oma/manualchapters/management/1825.

O'Brien, R. G. (1998). *A tour of UnifyPow: A SAS module/macro for sample-size analysis.* Paper presented at the proceedings of the 23rd annual SAS Users Group International Conference (pp. 1346–1355). Cary, NC: SAS Institute.

O'Brien, R. G., & Muller, K. E. (1993), Unified power analysis for *t*-tests through multivariate hypotheses. In L. K. Edwards (Ed.), *Applied analysis of variance in behavioral science* (chap. 8, pp. 297–344). New York: Marcel Dekker.

Whitehead, J. (1993). Sample size calculations for ordered categorical data. *Statistics in Medicine, 12*, 2257–2271.

SAMPLING DISTRIBUTION

The sampling distribution of a statistic, S, gives the values of S and how often those values occur. The sampling distribution is a theoretical device that is the basis of statistical inference. One use is to determine if an observed S is rare or common.

Creating a Sampling Distribution

Recall that a statistic describes the sample and a parameter describes the population. First, one has the population. Then, one takes a random sample of size n from the population and finds the value of S. This value is the first value of the sampling distribution of the statistic. Take another random sample of size n from the population; find the value of S. This value is the second value of the sampling distribution. This is repeated. The resulting collection of Ss is the sampling distribution of S. Figure 1 gives a visual representation of the process of creating a sampling distribution. The S value varies from sample to sample.

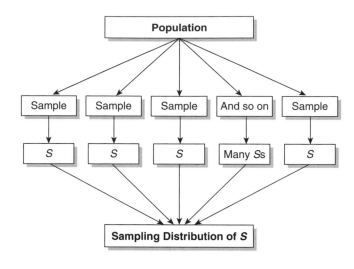

Figure 1   Model of Creating a Sampling Distribution

The sampling distribution of S enables one to see that variability.

The population size is either finite or infinite or large enough to be considered "infinite." When the population size is finite, that is, small, then a proper random sample would be taken from the population *without replacement.* So the number of possible random samples from the population of size N is

$$\binom{N}{n} = \frac{N!}{n!(N-n)!}.$$

Example 1: Finite Population

Example 1 (created by author for this article) contains $N = 6$ items (presented in Table 1), and suppose we are interested in a sample size of 3, $n = 3$, so there are

$$\binom{6}{3} = \frac{6!}{3!(6-3)!} = 20$$

unique random samples from the data set. The population median is 6, the population mean is 5.8, and the population standard deviation is 2.4.

Table 2 contains the 20 unique samples as well as the values for the following statistics: sample mean, sample median, and sample standard deviation. Figure 2 shows

Table 1   Example 1: Finite Population

2	4	5	7	8	9

Table 2   The 20 Possible Random Samples of Size 3 and the Values of Three Statistics

Sample	Median	Mean	St. Dev.	Sample	Median	Mean	St. Dev.
2 4 5	4	3.7	1.5	4 5 7	5	5.3	1.5
2 4 7	4	4.3	2.5	4 5 8	5	5.7	2.1
2 4 8	4	4.7	3.1	4 5 9	5	6.0	2.6
2 4 9	4	5.0	3.6	4 7 8	7	6.3	2.1
2 5 7	5	4.7	2.5	4 7 9	7	6.7	2.5
2 5 8	5	5.0	3.0	4 8 9	8	7.0	2.6
2 5 9	5	5.3	3.5	5 7 8	7	6.7	1.5
2 7 8	7	5.7	3.2	5 7 9	7	7.0	2.0
2 7 9	7	6.0	3.6	5 8 9	8	7.3	2.1
2 8 9	8	6.3	3.8	7 8 9	8	8.0	1.0

the sampling distributions of the sample mean, sample median, and sample standard deviation. Notice that the sample distributions are centered on the associated parameter; that is, the sampling distribution of the median is centered on 6, and the same is true for the mean (centered at 5.8) and standard deviation (centered at 2.4). Also, notice that there is variability in the sampling distributions. This variability is known as *sampling variability*—the variability that is induced by the act of taking a random sample. The value of a statistic does not equal the value of the parameter (typically) but varies around the parameter.

By looking at the sampling distribution, one can determine if an observed statistic is rare or common. For example, suppose one takes a random sample of three items and finds that the sample mean is 4 or

below. If the random sample is from the original population, then the chance of observing an $\bar{x}$ equal to 4 or less is $1/20 = 0.05$. So there is only a 5% chance that the random sample is from the original population.

Example 2: Infinite Population, Quantitative Values

In most situations, the size of the population is infinite or large enough; therefore, when one takes random samples from the population, one can take the sample with replacement and then take a large number of samples.

In Example 2, the population has an exponential distribution with mean and standard deviation equal to 3, and the median is $2.0794 = -3 \ln(0.5)$. Figure 3 gives

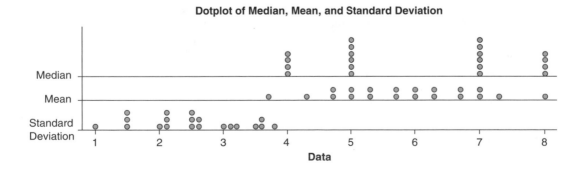

Figure 2   Sampling Distributions for the Median, Mean, and Standard Deviation, Finite Population

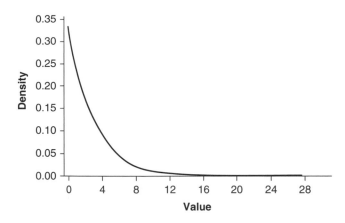

Figure 3 Exponential Population With Mean = 3

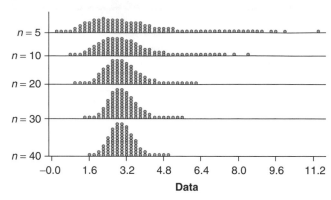

Figure 4 Sampling Distribution of the Mean

Note: Each symbol represents up to 136 observations.

the density function of the population. The sampling distributions given in Figures 4, 5, and 6 were created by taking 10,000 samples of size *n*. The associated statistics were found, and then those statistics were used in the sampling distribution. This process is repeated for five different sample sizes, 5, 10, 20, 30, and 40.

For all three statistics, one observes that the variability of the distributions decreases as the sample size increases. Intuitively, this makes sense because as one has more items in a sample one would expect that the statistic should vary less, that is, the statistic becomes more consistent.

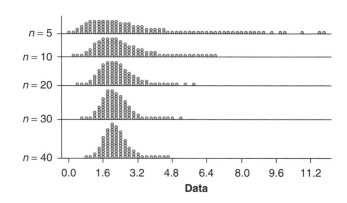

Figure 5 Sampling Distribution of the Median

Note: Each symbol represents up to 141 observations.

Sampling Distribution of Common Statistics

Sampling Distribution of the Sample Mean

The *central limit theorem* explains that if the population has a finite population mean, μ, and a finite population standard deviation, σ, then

- The population mean of the sampling distribution of the sample mean is μ.
- The population standard deviation of the sampling distribution of the sample mean is $\sigma/\sqrt{n}$.
- The sampling distribution of the sample mean converges to a normal distribution as *n* is increased.

Sampling Distribution of the Sample Proportion

The sample proportion is the main statistic of interest with categorical data. The population has a population

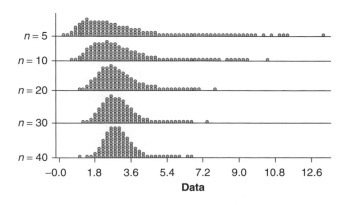

Figure 6 Sampling Distribution of the Standard Deviation

Note: Each symbol represents up to 111 observations.

proportion, p, which measures the proportion or probability of a "success." The sampling distribution of the sample proportion has the following properties:

- The population mean of the sampling distribution is p.
- The population standard deviation of the sampling distribution is $\sqrt{p(1-p)/n}$.
- As the sample size increases, the sampling distribution converges to a normal distribution.

Although one has seen visually the creation of sampling distribution in this entry, statisticians do not solely rely on visual images. The proofs of the sampling distribution of the sample mean and sample proportion are not based on graphs but are based on statistical theory. Statisticians use a variety of tools, such as the moment generating function or characteristic functions and expected values, to determine the distribution of the statistic. However, the key to understanding sampling distributions is not in the statistical theory. The key is understanding that the sampling distribution of S gives the possible values of S and how often S takes those values. In the real world, one does not have multiple samples from a population. Instead, one has a single sample and a single statistic. But by making assumptions about the population, one is able to test those assumptions based on the single sample:

- If the population assumption is true, then one can determine the sampling distribution of S.
- Using this sampling distribution, one determines whether the observed S from the random sample is common or rare.
- If S is rare, then one's assumptions about the population may not be true.
- If S is common, then one does not have sufficient evidence against the assumptions.

—*Marjorie E. Bond*

Author's Note: All data for this article were created by the author for this entry or simulated using Minitab.

See also Central Limit Theorem; Confidence Interval; Hypothesis Testing

Further Readings

Agresti, A., & Franklin, C. (2007). *Statistics: The art and science of learning from data.* Upper Saddle River, NJ: Pearson Prentice Hall.

Moore, D. S. (2007). *The basic practice of statistics* (4th ed.). New York: W. H. Freeman.

SAMPLING TECHNIQUES

Proper scientific sampling is an important element in the study of populations. The population of interest may be a general population, such as all people in the United States 18 years of age or older, or a targeted subpopulation, such as people in the United States 18 years of age or older living in poverty or living in urban areas. Many epidemiologic studies involve gathering information from such populations. The population of interest in such studies may be specific—such as physicians, people in homeless shelters, people with a specific chronic disease—or may involve any population that can be accurately defined. Drawing an appropriate sample of the target population is the foundation on which such studies must be built. An improper sample can negate everything that the study wishes to discover. This entry describes different techniques that can be used for drawing a proper sample and when they are most appropriate. The Further Readings section provides a more in-depth look at the specific statistical properties of various sampling techniques, such as variance estimation and the approximation of required sample sizes.

Simple Random Samples

Any discussion of sampling techniques must begin with the concept of a simple random sample. Virtually all statistics texts define a simple random sample as a way of picking a sample of size n from a population of size N in a manner that guarantees that all possible samples of size n have an equal probability of being selected. From an operational standpoint, consider a list of N population members. If one used a random number generator to assign a random number to each of the N population members on the list and then selected the n smallest numbers to make up one's sample of size n, this would constitute a valid simple random sample. If one replicated this process an infinite number of times, each possible sample of size n would be expected to be selected an equal number of times. This then meets the definition of a true simple random sample. Many statistical software packages contain a sampling module that usually applies this type of simple random sampling.

It is important to point out that virtually all statistical procedures described in textbooks or produced as output of statistical software programs assume simple random sampling was performed. This includes the estimation of means, variances, standard errors, and confidence intervals. It is also assumed in the estimation of standard errors around regression coefficients, correlation coefficients, odds ratios, and other statistical measures. In other words, the development of statistical estimation is built around the concept of simple random sampling. This does not imply that proper statistical estimates cannot be derived if simple random sampling was not performed, but that estimates derived by assuming simple random sampling may be incorrect if the sampling technique was something different.

In practice, it is usually the case that simple random sampling will lead to the best statistical properties. It usually will be found to produce the smallest variance estimates and smallest confidence intervals around estimates of interest. It also leads to the least analytic complexity as again all statistical software programs can handle simple random sampling without any problem. It must be noted that a simple random sample will not always produce the best statistical properties for estimation, but that in practice this usually will be the case.

The question then arises as to why other sampling techniques are ever used. The answer is that while simple random sampling may be shown to generally have the best statistical properties, it also frequently may be the most expensive to conduct, may at times be impossible to do, and frequently will not address all the goals of a particular study. In these instances, more complex sampling techniques must be investigated.

Systematic Samples

A systematic sample is the sampling technique that is closest to simple random sampling in nature. A systematic sample is generally defined as an interval sampling approach. From a list or other device that defines a target population, first select a random number between 1 and m. Then starting with this random number, take every mth element into the sample. As an example, one may want to draw a systematic sample of 100 elements from a target population of 1,000 elements. In this case, m could be set to 10. Drawing a random number between 1 and 10 might lead to the

number 7. The resulting systematic sample would then be the elements from the original list that were numbered 7, 17, 27, 37, . . . , 997. There are many instances in practice that could be seen as practical applications of such an interval sampling technique. Examples are drawing a sample of files from file cabinets, telephone numbers from the page of a telephone book, housing units on a specific city block, or every mth patient who visits a clinic on a specific day. In practice, it may be more practical to implement a systematic sampling procedure than to draw a simple random sample in these types of instances.

In general, systematic samples usually can be assumed to behave similarly to simple random samples for estimation purposes. Still, great care must be taken to make sure a systematic bias does not result. As an example, consider a proposed study of people in homeless shelters. On a given night, it is decided to take a systematic sample of every third bed in every shelter in a city. From the people placed into these beds, assessments would be made concerning the medical condition and needs of these people. Suppose it was discovered that in numerous shelters beds are arranged as triple-decked bunk beds. Furthermore, the practice in these shelters is to place the most physically impaired people in the bottom bunks, the less impaired in the middle bunks, and the healthiest in the top bunks. In this instance, taking every third bed would result in a completely biased sample. If systematic samples are to be used, it is critical to examine such potentially unforeseen biases that may result from the interval selection.

Complex Random Samples

The term *complex sample* is generally used to mean any sampling technique that adds a dimension of complexity beyond simple random sampling. Three of the most common forms of complex samples will be discussed. They are stratified samples, cluster samples, and samples selected with probability proportionate to size.

Stratified Samples

Suppose the population of interest can be divided into nonoverlapping groups. Examples of such a situation are states into counties, physicians into primary specialties, hospitals into size (measured by number of beds), or patients into primary clinical diagnosis. The groups in these instances are referred to as strata. The identifying characteristic is that every member of the target population is found in one and only one of the strata. If one is not only interested in studying the whole population but also interested in comparing strata, then stratified sampling is the best sampling technique. For example, suppose one wants to study physicians and make estimates about the characteristics of how they spend their time and the degree of difficulty of their practices. One might also want to be able to compare physicians across specialties. If one were to draw a simple random sample of physicians from some list (such as AMA membership), one would find that there are many more internists than cardiologists, as one example. The resulting simple random sample would either not contain enough cardiologists to be able to accurately compare them to internists or the size of the original simple random sample would have to be so large to ensure that there are enough cardiologists that the study is not feasible. In instances such as these, stratified sampling is the better approach. The original population can be broken into strata by primary specialty. Within each stratum, a simple random sample of physicians can be drawn. The size of the samples within each stratum can be controlled to guarantee that comparisons across strata can be accurately performed. This type of approach can be used in many similar settings. In theory, the resulting stratified sample may even have better sample characteristics, such as smaller variance estimates. In practice, it should be expected that this is not the case.

Cluster Samples

At times, the population of interest can be more easily located by knowing that they reside in naturally nonoverlapping groups. The groups are of no particular interest to the study, but they serve as a mechanism to more easily identify or find the population members that are desired. In these instances, the groups are known as clusters. Many examples exist in practice. If a study wants to sample households within a city to investigate the possible presence of environmental risk factors that can adversely affect the health of household residents, one possibility is to get a list (if it exists) of all households in the city and then to draw a simple random sample of households. If this is done, the cost of sending interviewers across all parts of the city, usually to examine a single house here and another there, can be very expensive. If it is

recognized that household residents are in one and only one city block, then the city can be initially divided into nonoverlapping city blocks. A simple random sample of city blocks can be drawn and then a simple random sample of households within each selected block. This makes it far more efficient and less expensive to examine the sample households as they are in groups or clusters of close proximity. These blocks (or clusters) have no intrinsic interest to the study but simply serve as a mechanism for more efficiently getting to the households of interest.

This type of sampling technique is called cluster sampling. It is frequently used in practice as it usually reduces costs. Sampling college students within colleges, residents or interns within hospitals, and patients within physician practices are just a few examples. Although this sampling may be necessary, it frequently increases estimated sample variances and standard errors because variables that are to be measured can be correlated within the clusters. The higher the amount of correlation, the larger the increase in estimated standard errors. This must be factored in and compared with the estimated cost savings to determine if cluster sampling is advisable.

Probability Proportionate to Size Samples

Sampling done proportionate to some measure of size may sometimes be preferable to simple random sampling where each element of a population has an equal probability of being selected into the sample. An example can serve best. Suppose a sample of college students is the goal. Since there is no list that contains all college students in the country, it is necessary to sample college students by initially sampling colleges. Each college does have a list of its own students. Drawing a simple random sample of colleges can be done using a list of all accredited colleges. However, because a random sample of students is the ultimate goal and colleges can have radically different sizes in terms of number of students, a random sample of these colleges would not yield the desired result. In fact, a closer look shows that approximately 50% of the college students in the country can be found in approximately 15% of the colleges. There are a great many small colleges, and it takes many of them to equal the student body of a large state university. In this instance, drawing a simple random sample of colleges would lead to a disproportionately large sample of students from small colleges. This is not reflective of how students are distributed. A better sampling technique in such instances is sampling proportionate to size. In this instance, the number of students at a college can serve as a measure of size, and colleges are selected using this measure. As a result, the larger the college, the higher the probability its students will be selected. This more closely resembles the actual distribution of students across colleges. If simple random samples of students of equal size are then selected from within each selected college, it can be shown that each student in the original population had an equal probability of being included in the sample. Again, many examples exist, including sampling hospitals using number of beds or surgical procedures as a measure of size, sampling patients in a hospital by length of stay, and sampling census blocks within a city using the estimated number of people with a specified characteristic (e.g., above 65 years of age) as a measure of size. Care must be taken with this approach as measures of size that are in error can lead to biases in the sample.

Summary

The complex sampling techniques just specified can be used alone or in conjunction. For example, the country can be divided into strata by using states; then, within each state, a sample of clusters (e.g., colleges or hospitals) can be drawn using probability proportionate to size sampling and then simple random sampling can be used within each cluster. Whenever complex sampling techniques are used, they *must* be reflected in the resulting statistical analysis. Failure to do so undermines the validity of any stated statistical result. Fortunately, many statistical software programs have modules for handling complex sample designs. The design must be entered correctly into such software programs to get the appropriate results. In practically all cases, failure to do so will result in estimated variances and standard errors that are too small. This in turn leads to potentially stating that results are statistically significant when they are not.

The techniques specified are all probability sampling techniques. Nonprobability samples, such as volunteer samples and convenience samples, cannot be used to make population estimates as they lack the statistical foundation. For clinical trials, volunteers can be randomly assigned to treatment and control groups. Comparing these groups can then result in a valid analysis of the treatment but only in the context of the initial volunteer sample. How volunteers differ from the population in general will be a potential unknown. The techniques mentioned here do not handle all sampling situations but are the most common that are used. In any truly complicated study, the advice of a sampling statistician should always be sought.

—*Anthony Roman*

See also Questionnaire Design; Randomization; Study Design; Target Population

Further Readings

Cochran, W. G. (1977). *Sampling techniques*. New York: Wiley.

Groves, R. M., Fowler, F. J., Jr., Couper, M. P., Lepkowski, J. M., Singer, E., & Tourangeau, R. (2004). *Survey methodology*. New York: Wiley.

Kish, L. (1995). *Survey sampling*. New York: Wiley.

SCATTERPLOT

The scatterplot is a graphical technique that is often used to explore data to get an initial impression of the relationship between two variables. It is an important component of descriptive epidemiology and can be helpful in providing clues as to where further exploration of the data may be valuable. It gives a sense of the variability in the data and points to unusual observations. The scatterplot is most frequently used when both the variables of interest are continuous.

To create a scatterplot, the value of the y variable, the dependent variable, is plotted on the y axis against the corresponding value of the x variable, the independent variable, which is plotted on the x axis. This is done for each data point. The resulting plot is a graphical description of the relationship between the two variables. In other words, it is a visual description of how y varies with x. See Figure 1 for an illustration of a scatterplot. The circled diamond corresponds to a data point with a value of 53 in. for height and 80 lb for weight.

Besides being an important technique that allows epidemiologists to get a visual description of the data, aiding in the detection of trends that may exist between two variables, the scatterplot is a useful tool as an initial step in the determination of the type of

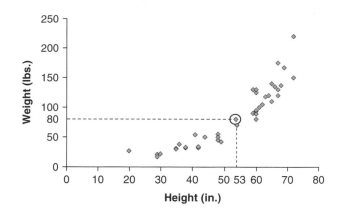

Figure 1   Weight and Height in U.S. Children Aged
0 to 17 Years

Source: Data from random selection of 43 points from Centers for Disease Control and Prevention, National Center for Health Statistics, State and Local Area Integrated Telephone Survey, National Survey of Children's Health (2003).

model that would best explain the data. For example, if the relationship appears linear, linear regression may be appropriate. If, however, the relationship does not appear linear, a different type of regression or the inclusion of a term such as the quadratic term or a spline term may be more appropriate.

Another use of the scatterplot is to explore the relationship between two predictor, or independent, variables. If two predictor variables appear to be highly correlated, this may be an indication that they are collinear. In other words, they may be providing the same information to the model. Adding both variables to the model, therefore, is giving redundant information and may result in inflated standard errors, reducing the precision of the model. For this reason, it is of value to understand how predictor variables are related. The scatterplot is one way to begin to explore this.

The scatterplot can be used when both the variables of interest are not continuous; however, there are other types of graphs that may be preferable and give a better depiction of the data. Box-and-whisker plots are of value when comparing binary or categorical data. Bar charts are useful not only for ordinal data but also for categorical data.

In short, the scatterplot is an important tool to use, especially in the beginning stages of data exploration, to describe the data. It provides insight into how variables are related to each other, what steps should be taken next in the data analysis process, and

allows for checks as to whether or not model assumptions are met.

—Rebecca Harrington

See also Bar Chart; Box-and-Whisker Plot; Collinearity; Dependent and Independent Variables; Inferential and Descriptive Statistics

Further Readings

Tukey, J. (1977). *Exploratory data analysis.* Reading, MA: Addison-Wesley.

SCHIZOPHRENIA

Schizophrenia is a disorder of psychotic intensity characterized by profound disruption of cognition and emotion, including hallucinations, delusions, disorganized speech or behavior, and/or negative symptoms. This entry reviews the epidemiology of schizophrenia, along with its natural history and risk factors. It focuses on the period since the review by Yolles and Kramer in 1969, concentrating on results that are most credible methodologically and consistent across studies, and on the most recent developments.

Descriptive Epidemiology

The most credible data on the epidemiology of schizophrenia come from registers, including inpatient and outpatient facilities for an entire nation, in which the diagnosis is typically made carefully according to the standards of the World Health Organization's *International Classification of Diseases* and in which treatment for schizophrenia in particular and health conditions in general is free (e.g., Denmark). The global point prevalence of schizophrenia is about 5 per 1,000 population. Prevalence ranges from 2.7 per 1,000 to 8.3 per 1,000 in various countries. The incidence of schizophrenia is about 0.2 per 1,000 per year and ranges from 0.11 to 0.70 per 1,000 per year. The incidence of schizophrenia peaks in young adulthood (15 to 24 years, with females having a second peak at 55 to 64 years). Males have about 30% to 40% higher lifetime risk of developing schizophrenia than females.

Natural History

The onset of schizophrenia is varied. In 1980, Ciompi found that about 50% of cases had an acute onset and about 50% had a long prodrome. About half of the individuals had an undulating course, with partial or full remissions followed by recurrences, in an unpredictable pattern. About one third had a relatively unremitting course with poor outcome; and a small minority had a steady pattern of recovery with good outcome. Several studies have shown that negative symptoms and gradual onset predict poor outcome. There is variation in the course of schizophrenia around the world, with better prognosis in the so-called developing countries. Although there is a long literature on the relation of low socioeconomic position to risk for schizophrenia, it seems likely that the association is a result of its effects on the ability of the individual to compete in the job market. Recent studies suggest that the parents of schizophrenic patients are likely to come from a higher, not lower, social position.

Some individuals with schizophrenia differ from their peers even in early childhood in a variety of developmental markers, such as the age of attaining developmental milestones, levels of cognitive functioning, neurological and motor development, and psychological disturbances, but no common causal paths appear to link these markers to schizophrenia. Minor physical anomalies, defined by small structural deviations observed in various parts of the body (e.g., hands, eyes, and ears), are more prevalent in individuals with schizophrenia and their siblings as compared with the rest of the population. This evidence on developmental abnormalities is consistent with the hypothesis that schizophrenia is a neurodevelopmental disorder, with causes that may be traced to early brain development.

Risk Factors

A family history of schizophrenia is the strongest known risk factor, with first-degree relatives having about 5- to 10-fold relative risk and monozygotic twins having about 40- to 50-fold relative risk. In addition to family history, there are several risk factors that have been identified in the past 50 years, including complications of pregnancy and birth, parental age, infections and disturbances of the immune system, and urban residence.

It has been long known that individuals with schizophrenia are more likely to be born in the winter. This risk factor is interesting in part because it is indisputably not genetic in origin. The relative risk is approximately a 10% increase for those born in the winter compared with those born in the summer. The effect exists in both hemispheres, with more births during the winter in the Southern Hemisphere, which does not coincide with the beginning of the calendar year. One possible explanation is that winter months coincide with seasonal peaks in infectious agents (e.g., influenza) that may affect prenatal development. Many studies have reported a doubling of odds for developing schizophrenia among those with a birth complication (e.g., preeclampsia). Recently, several population-based studies have provided strong evidence about the role of paternal age, rather than maternal age, in schizophrenia.

A series of ecological studies suggested that persons whose mothers were in their second trimester of pregnancy during a flu epidemic had a higher risk for schizophrenia. Prenatal infection as a risk factor is consistent with the neurodevelopmental theory of schizophrenia. Consistent evidence shows that individuals with antibodies to *Toxoplasma gondii* (the parasite that causes toxoplasmosis) have higher prevalence of schizophrenia. A relatively small but consistent literature indicates that persons with schizophrenia have unusual resistance (e.g., rheumatoid arthritis) or susceptibility (e.g., celiac disease) to autoimmune diseases. A single weakness in the immune system in schizophrenic patients may explain both the data on infections and the results on autoimmune disorders, with ongoing studies examining this hypothesis.

In the 1930s, Faris and Dunham showed that admissions for schizophrenia in and near Chicago, Illinois, tended to come from the city center, with decreasing rates among individuals living in zones of transition (the less central part of the city; zones of transition are characterized by mixed-use [commercial and housing] and is a transition to the primarily residential areas that would be even further removed from the city center), a pattern not seen in manic depression. The relative risk of schizophrenia is about two to four times higher for those born in urban areas. Additionally, evidence suggests that schizophrenia is a disease of relatively recent origin. While identifiable descriptions of manic depression have been found during the time of Galenic medicine in the 2nd century AD, descriptions of schizophrenia are vague and rare. There appears to be an upward trend in schizophrenia over four centuries, with a doubling or quadrupling of the prevalence. Many of the possible explanations for the rise in prevalence of schizophrenia with modernization parallel the explanations for the higher risk in urban areas—animals in the household, crowding in cities, and difficulty formulating a life plan when the future is uncertain.

As late as a quarter century ago, the epidemiology of schizophrenia was nearly a blank page. The only risk factors that seemed strong and consistent were the conditions of lower social class in life and the family history of schizophrenia. Since that time, there has been considerable progress delineating a more or less consistent picture of the descriptive epidemiology and the natural history of schizophrenia. In the future, concerted efforts will be made to study risk factors in combination. Such efforts will make the prospects for prevention more targeted and effective.

—*Briana Mezuk and William W. Eaton*

See also Child and Adolescent Health; Neuroepidemiology; Psychiatric Epidemiology

Further Readings

Brown, A., & Susser, E. (2002). In utero infection and adult schizophrenia. *Mental Retardation and Developmental Disabilities Research Reviews, 8,* 51–57.

Cannon, M., Jones, P., & Murray, R. (2002). Obstetric complications and schizophrenia: Historical and meta-analytic review. *American Journal of Psychiatry, 159,* 1080–1092.

Ciompi, L. (1980). The natural history of schizophrenia in the long term. *British Journal of Psychiatry, 136,* 413–420.

Eaton, W. W., & Chen, C.-Y. (2006). Epidemiology. In J. A. Lieberman, T. Scott Stroup, & D. O. Perkins (Eds.), *The American Psychiatric Publishing textbook of schizophrenia* (pp. 17–37). Washington, DC: American Psychiatric Publishing.

Faris, R., & Dunham, W. (1939). *Mental disorders in urban areas.* Chicago: University of Chicago Press.

Murray, R. W., & Lewis, S. W. (1987). Is schizophrenia a neurodevelopmental disorder? *British Medical Journal (Clinical Research Edition), 295,* 681–682.

Torrey, E. F., Miller, J., Rawlings, R., & Yolken, R. H. (1997). Seasonality of births in schizophrenia and bipolar disorder: A review of the literature. *Schizophrenia Research, 7,* 1–38.

Yolles, S., & Kramer, M. (1969). Vital statistics. In L. Bellak (Ed.), *The schizophrenic syndrome* (pp. 66–113). New York: Grune & Stratton.

SCREENING

Screening is the process of systematically searching for preclinical disease and classifying people as likely or unlikely to have the disease. It involves using a reasonably rapid test procedure, with more definitive testing still required to make a diagnosis. The goal of screening is to reduce eventual morbidity or mortality by facilitating early treatment. Mass or population screening targets a whole population or population group. Clinical use of screening tests for diseases unrelated to patient symptoms is referred to as opportunistic screening. This entry discusses the general principles related to mass screening and study designs for the evaluation of screening programs.

Screening is primarily a phenomenon of the 20th century (and beyond). Early screening tended to deal with communicable diseases, such as tuberculosis and syphilis, and had as a goal reducing transmission as much as treatment for the individual's sake. As the public health burden associated with these diseases was reduced in developed countries, the practice of screening evolved to focus on chronic diseases, such as cancer and diabetes, and risk factors for coronary heart disease. Screening programs related to infant and child development, such as newborn screening for genetic and metabolic disorders or vision and lead screening in children, have also become a routine part of public health practice. Newer or emerging concepts include prenatal screening and testing for genetic susceptibility to diseases such as cancer.

Criteria for Screening

The criteria for an ethical and effective screening program were first outlined by Wilson and Jungner in 1968. Their list has been reiterated and expanded over the years and remains pertinent even today. Meeting a list of criteria does not guarantee the success of a screening program, and on the other hand, there may be utility in programs that do not meet every guideline. However, the following are important considerations.

Disease

The disease should represent a significant public health problem because of its consequences, numbers affected, or both. Additionally, the natural history of the disease must include a *preclinical detectable period*. This is a period of time when it is feasible to identify early disease using some existing test, but before the onset of symptoms that would otherwise lead to diagnosis. This preclinical detectable period should be of long enough duration to be picked up by tests at reasonably spaced time intervals. This is why screening is generally applied for chronic conditions that develop slowly. In an acute disease with rapid onset, even if a short preclinical detectable period exists, testing would need to be extremely frequent to pick it up before symptomatic disease developed. Finally, there should be a treatment for the disease available that improves outcome and is more effective when given earlier.

Screening Test

Practically, the screening test should be relatively simple and quick to carry out, acceptable to the population receiving it, and not prohibitively expensive. It should also be sensitive, specific, and reliable. Having high sensitivity means that there will be few cases of the disease that get "missed"—and miss the opportunity for early treatment. High specificity means that there are few false positives—that is, people without the disease who may undergo further testing and worry needlessly. Although both are ideally high, a trade-off between sensitivity and specificity may occur, especially for tests, such as a blood glucose test for diabetes, where a positive or negative result is determined by dichotomizing a continuous measure. The sensitivity and specificity can only be determined if there is an accepted "gold standard" diagnostic test to define true disease status. Although considered properties of the test, sensitivity and specificity can differ according to population characteristics such as age.

Population

When a population subgroup is targeted for screening, it should be one where the disease is of relatively high prevalence. Higher prevalence of disease results in a higher positive predictive value, which means that there will be fewer false positives. Also, the number of screening tests administered per case identified is lower, improving cost and resource efficiency. For example, the U.S. Preventive Services Task Force recommends screening for syphilis in high-risk groups, such as those engaging in risky sexual behavior or incarcerated populations, but recommends against routinely screening those who are not at increased risk. Screening in a high-risk population is sometimes referred to as *selective screening*.

System

Screening should occur within a system where follow-up testing to confirm disease presence is available for all persons who test positive, and treatment is available to those in whom disease is confirmed. Screening persons who will not have access to these services may not be acceptable ethically, as they will be subjected to the psychological consequences of a positive result without the presumed benefit of early treatment. As a corollary, the screening program should be economically feasible as a part of total health care expenditures within the system. Finally, screening for many disorders should be a continuing process with tests repeated at regular intervals.

Evaluation of Screening Programs

Despite the intuitive appeal of finding and treating disease early, screening programs cannot simply be assumed effective. Because a positive screening result may produce worry for the individual or family, a risk of side effects from diagnostic testing and treatment, and the expenses involved, screening may not be warranted if it does not result in decreased morbidity or mortality. Data may not exist prior to the inception of a screening program to fully evaluate all criteria, and the effectiveness of a program may vary over time or across populations. Therefore, evaluating programs or methods is an important function of epidemiology related to screening. Several different types of study design may be used.

Ecologic studies compare disease-specific mortality rates or indicators of morbidity between screened and unscreened populations, defined, for example, by geographic area or time period before versus after the screening program began. Outcomes between areas with different per capita screening frequencies could also be compared. Such studies may be relatively simple to conduct, especially if outcome data have already been systematically collected (i.e., vital statistics). However, because individual-level data are not collected, it is not shown whether those with better disease outcomes are actually the ones who participated in screening.

Case-control studies can be used to compare cases dying from the disease or having an otherwise "poor" outcome (e.g., cancer that has metastasized) with controls drawn from all members of the source population without the outcome (death or advanced disease). This control group can include persons with the disease who have not developed the outcome. Exposure status is then defined by screening history. Another strategy for study design is to classify newly diagnosed cases as exposed or not according to screening history and then followed up to death or other defined outcome.

Several types of bias may arise in observational studies of screening. Selection bias may occur because those who choose to participate in screening are different from those who refuse and may tend to have other behaviors in common that affect disease risk. *Lead time bias* happens when a survival time advantage appearing in screen-detected cases is actually because they have by definition been diagnosed earlier in the course of illness than the cases detected due to symptomatic disease. *Length bias* can occur if cases with a long preclinical detectable period tend to have a slower-progressing or less fatal disease variant. Since these cases are also more likely to be detected through screening, the screen-detected group of cases may have better outcomes even if treatment has no effect. *Overdiagnosis* involves disease diagnosis, in the screening group only, of persons truly without disease or with disease that would never become symptomatic within the natural lifespan. This has been advanced as an explanation for cancer screening trials that have found more disease in screened groups but then failed to find any difference in mortality.

Due to the biases inherent in observational studies, randomized trials, where subjects are randomly assigned to be screened (or not), are typically considered the optimal study design. However, a large sample size and long follow-up period may be required to observe a sufficient number of events. Additionally, feasibility is limited to situations where participants and their physicians are willing to go along with randomization. This may not be the case if a test has become generally accepted, even if its effectiveness is not proven.

—*Keely Cheslack-Postava*

See also Negative Predictive Value; Newborn Screening Programs; Positive Predictive Value; Preclinical Phase of Disease; Prevention: Primary, Secondary, and Tertiary; Sensitivity and Specificity

Further Readings

Gordis, L. (2004). The epidemiologic approach to the evaluation of screening programs. In *Epidemiology* (3rd ed., pp. 281–300). Philadelphia: Elsevier Saunders.

Morabia, A., & Zhang, F. F. (2004). History of medical screening: From concepts to action. *Postgraduate Medical Journal*, 80, 463–469.

Morrison, A. S. (1998). Screening. In K. J. Rothman & S. Greenland (Eds.), *Modern epidemiology* (2nd ed., pp. 499–518). Philadelphia: Lippincott Williams & Wilkins.

Parkin, D. M., & Moss, S. M. (2000). Lung cancer screening. Improved survival but no reduction in deaths: The role of "overdiagnosis." *Cancer*, 89, 2369–2376.

U.S. Preventive Services Task Force. (2004, July). *Screening for syphilis infection: Recommendation statement.* Rockville, MD: Agency for Healthcare Research and Quality. Retrieved December 8, 2006, from http://www.ahrq.gov/clinic/3rduspstf/syphilis/syphilrs.htm.

Wilson, J. M. G., & Jungner, G. (1968). *Principles and practice of screening for disease.* Geneva, Switzerland: World Health Organization.

SECONDARY DATA

Researchers in epidemiology and public health commonly make a distinction between *primary data*, data collected by the researcher for the specific analysis in question, and *secondary data*, data collected by someone else for some other purpose. Of course, many cases fall between these two examples, but it may be useful to conceptualize primary and secondary data by considering two extreme cases. In the first case, which is an example of *primary data*, a research team collects new data and performs its own analyses of the data so that the people involved in analyzing the data have some involvement in, or at least familiarity with, the research design and data collection process. In the second case, which is an example of *secondary data*, a researcher obtains and analyzes data from the Behavioral Risk Factor Surveillance System (BRFSS), a large, publicly available data set collected annually in the United States. In the second case, the analyst did not participate in either the research design or the data collection process, and his or her knowledge of those processes come only from the information available on the BRFSS Web site and from queries to BRFSS staff.

Secondary data are used frequently in epidemiology and public health, because those fields focus on monitoring health at the level of the community or nation rather than at the level of the individual as is typical in medical research. In many cases, using secondary data is the only practical way to address a question. For instance, few if any individual researchers have the means to collect the data on the scale required to estimate the prevalence of multiple health risks in each of the 50 states of the United States. However, data addressing those questions have been collected annually since the 1980s by the Centers for Disease Control, in conjunction with state health departments, and it is available for download from the Internet. Federal and state agencies commonly use secondary data to evaluate public health needs and plan campaigns and interventions, and it is also widely used in classroom instruction and scholarly research.

There are both advantages and disadvantages to using secondary data. The advantages relate primarily to the fact that an individual analyst does not have to collect the data himself or herself and can obtain access through a secondary data set information much more wide-ranging than he or she could collect alone. Specific advantages of using secondary data include the following:

- *Economy*, because the analyst does not have to pay the cost of data collection
- *Speed and convenience*, because the data are already available before the analyst begins to work
- *Availability of data from large geographic regions*, for instance, data collected on the national or international level
- *Availability of historical data and comparable data collected over multiple years*, for instance, the BRFSS data are available dating back to the 1980s, and certain topics have been included every year
- *Potentially higher quality of data*, for instance, the large surveys conducted by federal agencies such as the Centers for Disease Control commonly use standardized sampling procedures and professional interviewers in contrast to many locally collected data sets that represent a convenience sample collected by research assistants.

The disadvantages of using secondary data relate primarily to the potential disconnect between the analyst's interests and the purposes for which the data were originally collected and the analyst's lack of familiarity with the original research design and data collection and cleaning processes. These disadvantages include the following:

- *Specific research questions may be impossible to address through a secondary data set*, either because the relevant data were not collected (because it was not germane to the original research project) or because it was suppressed due to confidentiality concerns (e.g., home addresses of respondents).
- *Data may not be available for the desired geographic area or time period.* This is of particular concern to researchers studying a small geographic area, such as a neighborhood within a city, or to those who are interested in specific time periods, such as immediately before and after a particular historic event.
- *Different definitions or categories* than what the analyst desires may have been used for common constructs such as race and ethnicity, and certain constructs may not have been recognized at the time of the survey—for instance, same-sex marriage.
- *Potential lack of information about the data collection and cleaning process* may leave the analyst uninformed about basic concerns such as the response rate or the quality of the interview staff. In some cases, some of this information is available, in others it is not, but in any case every research project has its idiosyncrasies and irregularities that affect data quality and the lack of information about these details may lead the analyst to reach inappropriate conclusions using the data.

Primary and secondary data analyses are not in competition with each other. Each has its place within the fields of epidemiology and public health, and the most useful approach is to choose the data to be analyzed for a particular project based on what is most appropriate for the primary research questions and based on the resources available.

There are many sources of secondary data in epidemiology and public health that are easily accessible. The best-known sources are the data from large-scale governmental-sponsored surveys, such as the BRFSS, which are available on the Internet and may be accessed through the CDC Wonder Web site or through the Web site of the relevant agency. Claims records and other data relating to the Medicare and Medicaid systems are also available, with certain restrictions. Secondary data may also be accessed through clearinghouses that collect data from other sources, including private researchers, and make it available for use, such as that of the Interuniversity Consortium for Social and Political Research located at the University of Michigan. Vital statistics data (records of births, deaths, marriages, divorces, and fetal deaths) are often available at the local or state level, and some of this information is available at the national level as well. Access to private administrative data, for instance, claims records of insurance companies, must be negotiated with the company in question.

—*Sarah Boslaugh*

See also Centers for Disease Control and Prevention; National Center for Health Statistics

Articles on individual secondary data sets and sources of data can be located through the Reader's Guide.

Further Readings

Boslaugh, S. (2007). *Secondary data sources for public health: A practical guide*. New York: Cambridge University Press.

Web Sites

Centers for Disease Control Wonder: http://wonder.cdc.gov.
Interuniversity Consortium for Social and Political Research: http://www.icpsr.umich.edu.

SELF-EFFICACY

In 1977, Albert Bandura introduced the concept of self-efficacy, which is defined as the conviction that one can successfully execute the behavior required to produce a specific outcome. Unlike efficacy, which is the power to produce an effect (i.e., competence), self-efficacy is the belief that one has the power to produce that effect. Self-efficacy plays a central role in the cognitive regulation of motivation, because people regulate the level and the distribution of effort they will expend in accordance with the effects they are expecting from their actions. Self-efficacy is the focal point of Bandura's social-cognitive theory as well as an important component of the health belief model.

Theories and models of human behavior change are used to guide health promotion and disease prevention efforts. Self-efficacy is an important psychosocial concept for epidemiologists to understand because it influences study participants' behavior, intervention uptake, and potential for long-term

program maintenance. Ignoring the role that psychosocial concepts, such as self-efficacy, play in intervention efforts may cause study effects to be misinterpreted and project results to be misattributed. For instance, individuals participating in a smoking cessation program may be given solid smoking cessation strategies, social support, and alternative stress reduction activities, but if they do not believe that they can stop smoking—that is, if they lack self-efficacy—the program will be less successful. On the other hand, if a smoking cessation expert recognizes that overcoming an individual's lack of self-efficacy to stop smoking is critical to his or her quitting, the program could readily be designed with this factor in mind, and the program evaluation could determine the success of raising self-efficacy. Understanding self-efficacy can shed light on the determinants of health and disease distributions.

Factors Influencing Self-Efficacy

Bandura points to four sources affecting self-efficacy—experience, modeling, social persuasions, and physiological factors. Experiencing mastery is the most important factor for deciding a person's self-efficacy; success raises self-efficacy, failure lowers it. During modeling, an individual observes another engage in a behavior; when the other succeeds at the behavior, the observing individual's self-efficacy will increase—particularly if the observed person is similar in meaningful ways to the person doing the observation. In situations where others are observed failing, the observer's self-efficacy to accomplish a similar task will decrease. Social persuasions relate to encouragement and discouragement. These can be influential—most people remember times where something said to them severely altered their confidence. Positive persuasions generally increase self-efficacy, and negative persuasions decrease it. Unfortunately, it is usually easier to decrease someone's self-efficacy than it is to increase it. Physiologic factors play an important role in self-efficacy as well. Often, during stressful situations, people may exhibit physical signs of discomfort, such as shaking, upset stomach, or sweating. A person's perceptions of these responses can markedly alter his or her self-efficacy. If a person gets "butterflies in the stomach" before public speaking, a person with low self-efficacy may take this as a sign of his or her inability, thus decreasing efficacy further. Thus, it is how the person interprets the physiologic response that affects self-efficacy rather than the physiologic response per se.

Self-Efficacy: Influences on Beliefs and Behavior

Self-efficacy can enhance human accomplishment and well-being in numerous ways. It may influence the *choices* people make because individuals tend to select tasks in which they feel competent and avoid those in which they are not. Self-efficacy may also determine how much effort to expend, how long to persevere, and how resilient to be when faced with adverse situations. The higher the sense of efficacy, the greater the effort, persistence, and resilience a person will generally demonstrate. Self-efficacy can also influence an individual's thought patterns and emotional reactions. High self-efficacy helps create feelings of calm or competence in approaching difficult tasks and activities. Conversely, people with low self-efficacy may believe that things are tougher than they really are, a belief that fosters anxiety and stress and may serve to narrow problem-solving capacity. Self-efficacy can also create a type of self-fulfilling prophecy in which one accomplishes only what one believes one can accomplish. It is not unusual for individuals to overestimate or underestimate their abilities; the consequences of misjudgment play a part in the continual process of efficacy self-appraisals. When consequences are slight, individuals may not need to reappraise their abilities and may continue to engage in tasks beyond their competence. Bandura argued that strong self-efficacy beliefs are the product of time and multiple experiences; therefore, they are highly resistant and predictable. Weak self-efficacy beliefs, however, require constant reappraisal. Both, of course, are susceptible to a powerful experience or consequence.

—*Lynne C. Messer*

See also Health Behavior; Health Belief Model; Intervention Studies

Further Readings

Glanz, K., Lewis, F. M., & Rimer, B. K. (Eds.). (1997). *Health behavior and health education.* San Francisco: Jossey-Bass.

SENSITIVITY AND SPECIFICITY

In medicine, diagnostic tests are administered to patients to detect diseases so that appropriate treatments can be provided. A test can be relatively simple, such as a bacterial culture for infection, or a radiographic image to detect the presence of a tumor. Alternatively, tests can be quite complex, such as using mass spectrometry to quantify many different protein levels in serum and using this "protein profile" to detect disease. Screening tests are special cases of diagnostic tests, where apparently healthy individuals are tested with the goal of diagnosing certain conditions early, when they can be treated most effectively and with higher success. For example, in the United States, annual screening mammograms are recommended for healthy women aged 40 years and older to facilitate early detection of breast cancer.

Whether for diagnosis or screening, the objective is to use some kind of a test to correctly classify individuals according to their true disease state. Sensitivity and specificity are two related measures used to quantify the performance of a screening or diagnostic test compared with the true condition or disease state. The test yields a binary result for each individual, positive for the presence of a condition or negative for its absence, which is compared with the true disease state for the same individuals. In practice, since the true disease state cannot always be identified with absolute certainty, a gold standard test that also yields a binary result (presence or absence of a condition) is considered the true status for an individual. For example, screening tests conducted among pregnant women to measure the chance of a child having birth defects usually take results from an amniocentesis as the gold standard, since the true status of the infant may not be determined until birth. In most cases, the amniocentesis results reflect the truth with extremely high probability.

A comparison of diagnostic or screening test results with the true disease state (or gold standard test results) can be displayed in a 2×2 table, as in Table 1.

Sensitivity, calculated as $a/(a + c)$, gives the proportion of individuals who truly have the disease for whom the test gives a positive result. Sensitivity is also sometimes referred to as the "true positive fraction" or "true positive rate." That is, among those individuals in whom the condition is truly present, sensitivity reflects how often the test detects it.

Table 1 True Disease State and Screening Test Result

Screening Test Result	True Disease State or Gold Standard Result		Total
	Positive (D+)	Negative (D–)	
Positive (T+)	a	b	a + b
Negative (T–)	c	d	c + d
Total	a + c	b + d	a + b + c + d

Notes: Cell a = number of true positives; Cell b = number of false positives; Cell c = number of false negatives; Cell d = number of true negatives.

Specificity, calculated as $d/(b+d)$, gives the proportion of those individuals who truly do not have the disease for whom the test gives a negative result—the true negatives. That is, for those individuals in whom the disease or condition is truly absent, specificity reflects how often the test gives a negative result. Closely related to specificity is the proportion of false-positive test results, which is calculated as $b/(b+d)$ or $1 -$ specificity. In the health sciences literature, sensitivity, specificity, and false-positive rate are usually reported as a percentage rather than as proportions (i.e., they are multiplied by 100).

Sensitivity and specificity are also interpretable as conditional probabilities. Sensitivity is the probability of a case having a positive test given that the case truly has the disease. Sensitivity is the probability of a case having a negative test given that the disease is truly absent. Both can be represented mathematically as

$$\text{Sensitivity} = \Pr(T + |D+),$$
$$\text{Specificity} = \Pr(T - |D-),$$

where T represents the test result (either positive or negative) and D represents the true disease state (either with or without disease). Because these are each probabilities for a given disease state, they are not dependent on the prevalence (probability) of the disease in a population. In the context of the cells displayed in Table 1, this means that sensitivity and specificity do not require that $(a+c)/(a+b+c+d)$ and $(b+d)/(a+b+c+d)$ represent the proportions of those with and without disease in the population of interest. For example, one could still estimate sensitivity and specificity for a test that detects a rare condition even if equal numbers of individuals with and without the condition were assessed. In fact, the strategy of enrolling equal numbers of $D+$ and $D-$ individuals is quite common in some of the early stages of diagnostic test development.

Ideally, a screening or diagnostic test would maximize both sensitivity and specificity. However, there is usually a trade-off between the two measures for any given test. For many tests, the result is a numeric value rather than simply positive or negative for a disease. A culture may provide bacterial counts or a laboratory assay may provide serum protein concentration levels, for example. Still other tests may be reported as ordinal categories, such as breast cancer tumors, which are classified as Stage 0, 1, 2, 3, or 4 based on their size, cell types, and lymph node involvement. These continuous or ordinal results may be translated to a binary classification of "positive" or "negative" for a disease by establishing a cutpoint such that values on one side of the cutpoint (usually higher) are interpreted as positive and values on the other side (usually lower) are interpreted as negative. In the case of tumor staging, a binary classification may be used to designate "severe" versus "less severe" forms of cancer. Body mass index (BMI), which is computed by dividing an individual's weight (in kg) by the individual's height (in m) squared, is a widely used method to diagnose whether a person is overweight or obese. Typically, individuals with BMI values between 25 and 29.9 are considered overweight, while those with BMI values of 30 or greater are considered obese. It is important to note that BMI is an indirect measure of true body composition—a complex relationship between lean mass (i.e., muscle) and fat mass. However, lean and fat mass measures are difficult to obtain compared with weight and height. Therefore, BMI, when used in the context of overweight and obesity, is used as an easily obtainable measure of body fat, as is frequently used to diagnose overweight and obesity.

Altering a cutpoint that designates a positive versus a negative result on a diagnostic test will alter the sensitivity and specificity of that test. If a cutpoint is lowered for a test in which a score over the cutpoint is interpreted as having the disease, the test may identify more people with the disease with a positive test (increased sensitivity), but included in those positive tests will be a greater number of people without the disease (higher proportion of false positives, which implies decreased specificity). It is estimated that approximately 65% of people in the United States are overweight or obese when the BMI > 25 definition is used. If we lower the cutpoint from 25 to, say, 24, we would classify more individuals as overweight. Using this classification, we may correctly classify some individuals as overweight and who were missed using the standard classification, increasing the specificity. However, we may also increase the number of false positives; that is, we may mistakenly classify some individuals who have high lean mass, rather than fat mass, relative to their height as overweight. On the other hand, if we increased the cutpoint to diagnose overweight to 27 or 28, we would classify fewer people as overweight and have fewer false-positive results. However, we would potentially miss diagnosing some overweight individuals who could benefit from treatments or lifestyle changes that may help lower body fat and reduce risk for future medical conditions related to overweight and/or obesity.

When considering what the ideal sensitivity and specificity of a particular diagnostic or screening test should be, one must consider the "costs" (not necessarily strictly monetary) of failing to identify someone who truly has the disease compared with the "cost" of falsely identifying a healthy person as having the disease. When the consequence of missing a person with the disease is high, as is the case with rapidly fatal or extremely debilitating conditions, then sensitivity should be maximized, even at the risk of decreasing specificity. Falsely identifying someone as diseased in this instance has less dire consequences than failing to identify a diseased person. However, when the consequence of wrongly classifying someone as diseased is greater than the risk of failing to identify a diseased person, as in the case of a slowly progressing but highly stigmatizing condition, then one would prefer to maximize specificity even in the face of decreasing sensitivity.

Predicted Values

Once test results are known, a patient or medical professional may wish to know the probability that the person truly has the condition if the test is positive or is disease free if the test is negative. These concepts are called positive and negative predicted values of a test and can be expressed probabilistically as $\Pr(D+|T+)$ and $\Pr(D-|T-)$. Unlike sensitivity and specificity, positive and negative predicted values cannot always be computed from a fourfold table such as Table 1, as they are dependent on the prevalence of disease in the population of interest. Only if $(a+c)/(a+b+c+d)$ and $(b+d)/(a+b+c+d)$ accurately reflect the proportions of those with and without disease in the population can the fourfold table can be used to estimate the predicted values. In such cases where this holds true, the positive predicted value (PPV) can be computed as $a/(a+b)$, and the negative predicted value (NPV) can be computed as $c/(c+d)$. However, the PPV and the NPV can always be obtained by using Bayes's theorem. If one can obtain estimates of sensitivity and specificity for a particular test, and, from another source, estimate the prevalence of disease in a population of interest, Bayes's theorem yields the following:

$$PPV = \frac{\text{Sensitivity} \times \text{Prevalence}}{(\text{Sensitivity} \times \text{Prevalence}) + (1 - \text{Sensitivity}) \times (1 - \text{Prevalence})}$$

and

$$NPV = \frac{\text{Sensitivity} \times (1 - \text{Prevalence})}{\text{Sensitivity} \times (1 - \text{Prevalence}) + (1 - \text{Sensitivity}) \times (1 - \text{Prevalence})}.$$

All else being equal, the lower the prevalence of disease (i.e., rare conditions), the lower the proportion of true positives among those who test positive; that is, the PPV will be lower if a condition is rare than if it is common, even if the test characteristics, sensitivity and specificity, are high. Screening pregnant women for a rare condition such as Down syndrome (trisomy 21), whose prevalence in the United States is approximately 9.2 per 10,000 live births (0.0092), results in more false positive than true positive tests despite the fact that the screening tests have adequate sensitivity (75% or higher) and excellent specificity (95% or higher).

Receiver Operating Characteristic Curves

As previously noted, binary classifications are frequently derived from numerical or ordinal test results via a cutoff value. When this is the case, the performance of different cutoff values can be assessed using a receiver operating characteristic (ROC) curve. ROC curves are plots of the true-positive fraction of a test (sensitivity) versus the false-positive fraction (1 − specificity) across the entire spectrum of observed test results. An example of an ROC curve for a simulated diagnostic test that is measured on a continuum is presented in Figure 1. Test 1 (bold line in Figure 1) has higher sensitivity for certain false-positive fractions than Test 2 (dotted line). However, both tests have low, but comparable, sensitivity when false-positive fractions are 0.10 and lower.

The area under the ROC curve can range from 0.5, which represents results from an uninformative test, whose results are the same as flipping a coin to make a diagnosis, to 1.0, which represents a perfectly discriminative test with 100% sensitivity and 100% specificity. The area under the ROC curve for BMI as a test for obesity (obtained via direct measures of body fat) is in the range of 0.8 for adult men and above 0.9 for adult women.

The areas under ROC curves are an appropriate summary index to compare performance of the multiple diagnostic tests for the same condition. The area under the ROC for Test 1 in Figure 1 is 0.81, but only 0.74 for Test 2, leading us to prefer Test 1 over Test 2. Like sensitivity, specificity, and predicted values, the area under the ROC curve also has a probabilistic interpretation—the probability that a randomly selected pair of individuals with and without disease or condition is correctly classified. Thus, ROC curves, which are simply graphical representations of sensitivity and specificity, are extremely helpful in illustrating the trade-off between increasing sensitivity and increasing the proportion of false positives (or decreasing specificity).

—*Jodi Lapidus*

See also Bayes's Theorem; Clinical Epidemiology; Evidence-Based Medicine; Receiver Operating Characteristic (ROC) Curve

Further Readings

Loong, T. W. (2003). Understanding sensitivity and specificity with the right side of the brain. *British Medical Journal, 327,* 716–719.
Rosner, B. (1999). *Fundamentals of biostatistics* (5th ed., chap. 3). Pacific Groove, CA: Duxbury Press.

Sentinel Health Event

A sentinel health event is the occurrence of a specific health condition, or the occurrence of an adverse outcome to a medical intervention, which signals that (a) the incidence of a condition or disease has exceeded the threshold of expected cases, (b) changes are occurring in the health levels of a population, or (c) the quality of medical care may need to be improved. Each of these circumstances may indicate the presence of a broader public health problem, and each requires epidemiologic investigation and intervention.

For example, the occurrence of a single case of smallpox anywhere in the world would signal the recurrence of a disease that has been eradicated in the wild, indicating that a highly unusual and unexpected event has occurred that requires immediate

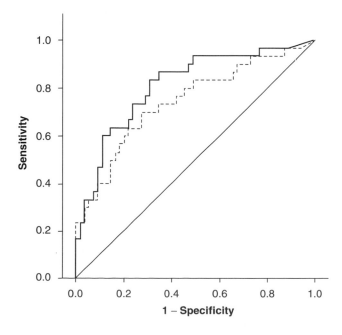

Figure 1   Receiver Operating Characteristic Curve for Simulated Diagnostic Tests That Are Reported as a Numerical Value

Note: Diagonal reference line represents an uninformative test.

investigation. Likewise, an increase in the incidence of birth defects in a community that has had a stable incidence over time also indicates that the health level of that population has changed, possibly due to a change in the environment or due to a common exposure, which also warrants investigation. And when physicians began seeing cases of Kaposi's sarcoma, a very rare cancer seen almost exclusively in older men of Mediterranean or eastern European extraction, occurring in young American men, this was the harbinger of the presence of an entirely new condition, human immunodeficiency virus infection.

Sentinel health events have also been defined for use in monitoring health care settings for potential problems in health care quality. In this setting, the sentinel health event is an illness, disability, or death that was otherwise preventable or avoidable, except for a problem in health care delivery or quality. An increase in postoperative infections in a particular hospital or specific ward may indicate a problem involving individual operating room staff, ventilation systems, sterilization equipment, or other systems involved in the treatment and care of surgical patients.

To be able to identify when conditions or occurrences are unusual, good baseline information is required. Public health surveillance systems are used to gather such baseline data for a given population and facilitate the monitoring of sentinel health events.

—*Annette L. Adams*

See also Applied Epidemiology; Bioterrorism; Epidemic; Field Epidemiology; Notifiable Disease; Outbreak Investigation; Public Health Surveillance

Further Readings

Gregg, M. B. (Ed). (2002). *Field epidemiology* (2nd ed.). New York: Oxford University Press.

Teutsch, S. M., & Churchill, R. E. (2000). *Principles and practice of public health surveillance* (2nd ed.). New York: Oxford University Press.

SEQUENTIAL ANALYSIS

Sequential analysis refers to a statistical method in which data are evaluated as they are collected, and further sampling is stopped in accordance with a predefined stopping rule as soon as significant results are observed. This contrasts to classical hypothesis testing where the sample size is fixed in advance. On average, sequential analysis will lead to a smaller average sample size compared with an equivalently powered study with a fixed sample size design and, consequently, lower financial and/or human cost.

Sequential analysis methods were first used in the context of industrial quality control in the late 1920s. The intensive development and application of sequential methods in statistics was due to the work of Abraham Wald around 1945. Essentially, the same approach was independently developed by George Alfred Barnard around the same time.

Interestingly, sequential analysis has not been frequently used in epidemiology despite the attractive feature of allowing the researcher to obtain equal statistical power at a lower cost. In 1962, Lila Elveback predicted a great increase in the application of sequential methods to problems in epidemiology in the coming few years; however, the prediction has not come true. The reluctance to apply sequential methods might be attributed to the fact that making a decision following every observation is complicated. Furthermore, in epidemiological studies, complex associations among outcome variable and predictor variables (rather than simply the primary outcome) are often a major interest and need to be determined in a relatively flexible multivariable modeling framework in light of all available data, while sequential analysis usually requires a well-defined and strictly executed design. Nevertheless, sequential analysis could be appropriately applied to some of the epidemiology research problems where the data are monitored continuously, such as in the delivery of social and health services and disease surveillance.

Wald's Sequential Probability Ratio Test

Sequential analysis is a general method of statistical inference. Wald's sequential probability ratio test (SPRT) is one of the most important procedures for hypothesis testing in sequential analysis. Its application is suitable for continuous, categorical, or time-to-event data, and the test includes sequential t tests, F tests, or χ^2 tests, among others. Generally, the test is performed each time a new observation is taken. At each step, the null hypothesis is either rejected or accepted, or based on predefined criteria, the study continues by taking one more observation without drawing any conclusions. In practice, Wald's SPRT need not be started with the first observation, but after a certain number of observations have been taken, since small sample size often does not provide enough evidence to reject or accept the null hypothesis. Sequential estimation procedures have also been developed to allow the estimation of confidence intervals in sequential sampling. Since binomial data are frequently encountered in public health and epidemiology applications, Wald's SPRT for binomial proportions is shown here.

Suppose that null hypothesis $H_0: p = p_0$ versus alternative hypothesis $H_1: p = p_1 \, (> p_0)$ is tested here. The criterion for accepting or rejecting the null hypothesis is given by two parallel straight lines. The lines are functions of p_0, p_1, Type I error (α), Type II error (β), and the number of total observations to date:

$$d_l = \beta_{01} + \beta_1 N \text{ (lower line)},$$

$$d_u = \beta_{02} + \beta_1 N \text{ (upper line)},$$

where N is the number of total observations, and

$$\beta_1 = \frac{\log\left(\frac{1-p_0}{1-p_1}\right)}{\log\left[\left(\frac{p_1}{p_0}\right)\left(\frac{1-p_0}{1-p_1}\right)\right]},$$

$$\beta_{01} = -\frac{\log\left(\frac{1-\alpha}{\beta}\right)}{\log\left[\left(\frac{p_1}{p_0}\right)\left(\frac{1-p_0}{1-p_1}\right)\right]},$$

and

$$\beta_{02} = \frac{\log\left(\frac{1-\beta}{\alpha}\right)}{\log\left[\left(\frac{p_1}{p_0}\right)\left(\frac{1-p_0}{1-p_1}\right)\right]}.$$

The power of a test is defined as $1 - \beta$. The repeated testing of hypothesis was incorporated in the construction of Wald's SPRT so the Type I error is preserved at the level of α. The commonly accepted value for α is 0.05; for β, 0.10 or 0.20 is typically used, which translates to 90% or 80% power. At each new observation, d_l and d_u are calculated based on prespecified values of p_0, p_1, α, and β. Denote the number of cases as d, then if $d \leq d_l$, the null hypothesis is accepted; if $d \geq d_u$, the null hypothesis is rejected; otherwise, sampling is continued, until the null hypothesis is rejected or accepted. The regions are illustrated in Figure 1. The smaller the

difference between p_0 and p_1, the greater the number of observations needed.

One example of using Wald's SPRT is monitoring of a breast screening program for minority women to determine whether the program was reaching its target population. The information was to be collected over time, and it was the researcher's goal to have 95% of the screened women to be African American since 95% of the target area residents were African American. If not and if at least 90% of the screened women were African American, it would indicate that the women in the target population were not being adequately reached. For this problem, the hypotheses could be set up as follows:

H_0: the program adequately reached its target population ($p_0 = 5\%$, proportion of non–African American women screened).

H_1: the program did not adequately reach its target population ($p_1 = 10\%$).

Note that $p_1 > p_0$. Given $\alpha = 0.05$ and $\beta = 0.10$, Wald's SPRT could be performed based on the methods described above, and the study continued until enough women were observed to draw a conclusion.

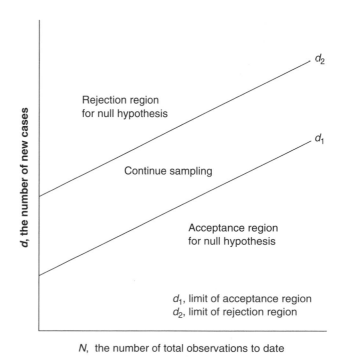

Figure 1 Graphical Illustration of Wald's Sequential Probability Ratio Test

Group Sequential Design

Sequential methods seemed initially to be an attractive solution to achieve the scientific and ethical requirements of clinical trials. However, sequential analysis was designed to perform a hypothesis testing after data on each new case were collected, which do not work well for clinical trials. A modified sequential method, called *group sequential design*, was developed for clinical trials, in which the accruing efficacy data are monitored at administratively convenient intervals and treatments are compared in a series of interim analyses. Important decisions concerning the future course of the study are made along the way, such as early stopping for futility or benefit, sample size readjustment, or dropping ineffective arms in multiarm dose-finding studies. Investigators may also stop a study that no longer has much chance of demonstrating a treatment difference. This method has now been routinely used in clinical trials. A well-known example is the hormone therapy trials of Women's Health Initiatives, where two treatment arms were stopped earlier because it was decided that the risks exceeded the benefits.

—Rongwei (Rochelle) Fu

See also Clinical Trials; Hypothesis Testing; Type I and Type II Errors

Further Readings

Bakeman, R., & Gottman, J. M. (1997). *Observing interaction: An introduction to sequential analysis.* New York: Cambridge University Press.

Howe, H. L. (1982). Increasing efficiency in evaluation research: The use of sequential analysis. *American Journal of Public Health, 72,* 690–697.

Wald, A. (1946). Sequential tests of statistical hypotheses. *Annals of Mathematical Statistics, 16,* 117–186.

Whitehead, J. (1997). *The design and analysis of sequential clinical trials* (2nd Rev. ed.). Chichester, UK: Wiley.

SEVERE ACUTE RESPIRATORY SYNDROME (SARS)

Severe acute respiratory syndrome (SARS) is a severe atypical pneumonia resulting from infection with a novel coronavirus, the SARS coronavirus (SARS-CoV). SARS is thought to have first occurred in humans in Guangdong province, China, in November 2002. International recognition of SARS occurred in March 2003 after many persons infected at a Hong Kong hotel seeded outbreaks of SARS in several countries and areas within days of each other. On March 12, 2003, the World Health Organization (WHO) issued a global alert regarding an acute respiratory syndrome of unknown aetiology and 3 days later issued an emergency travel advisory. By July 2003, cases of SARS had been identified in 29 countries and areas on most continents resulting in at least 774 deaths and 8,096 probable cases of SARS reported to the WHO. Global collaboration, coordinated by the WHO, was vital for the rapid identification of the causative agent, and prompt detection and isolation of cases, strict adherence to infection control procedures, vigorous contact tracing, and implementation of quarantine measures proved effective in containing the global outbreak.

The emergence of SARS provided a major scientific and public health challenge and resulted in rapid scientific achievements, a speedy epidemiological response, and international collaboration. Although SARS appears to be contained, the threat of another global outbreak remains as SARS may reemerge from unidentified animal reservoirs, laboratories that store the virus, or via undetected transmission within the human population. The epidemiology of SARS serves as a reminder of the global nature of infectious diseases and their continuing threat. The lessons learned provide a useful template for future international public health preparedness and response strategies.

Global Spread

The rapid global spread of SARS from the southern Chinese province of Guangdong was amplified by international air travel and "superspreading" events. A superspreading event may be defined as a transmission event whereby one individual with SARS infects a large number of persons. In February 2003, an infected physician from Guangdong who had treated SARS patients flew to Hong Kong and stayed in the Metropole Hotel, where he infected at least 14 hotel guests and visitors. Several of these infected individuals subsequently seeded outbreaks in Hanoi, Hong Kong, Singapore, Toronto, and elsewhere. Such superspreading events were reported from all sites with sustained local transmission before the implementation of strict hospital infection control measures. Although several theories have been proposed to explain why superspreading events occurred, such as patient immune status, underlying disease, higher level of viral shedding at the peak of infection or other environmental factors, a definitive reason has not been identified, and further research is required to explain this phenomenon.

On July 5, 2003, the WHO declared that the last known chain of human-to-human transmission had been broken and that the global SARS outbreak was contained. By this time, the global cumulative total of probable cases was 8,096, with 774 deaths. Mainland China, Hong Kong, and Taiwan accounted for 92% of all cases and 89% of all deaths. Globally, most cases (21%) occurred in health care workers and their close contacts; however, secondary community transmission did occur in particular—the Amoy Gardens outbreak in Hong Kong in March 2003 where more than 300 residents were infected.

In the current postoutbreak period, 17 SARS cases have been reported. Six cases of laboratory-acquired infection have been reported from China, Singapore, and Taiwan. One of the laboratory-acquired cases in China resulted in seven additional cases. In addition to the laboratory-acquired cases, a further four community-acquired cases were reported from Guangdong province, China.

Origin of SARS

The actual reservoir of SARS-CoV in nature is unknown; however, it is suggested that SARS-CoV originated from a wild animal reservoir in mainland China, supported by a number of factors. Masked palm civets and raccoon dogs in animal markets in China had a SARS-CoV almost identical to that seen in SARS patients. Additionally, more than one third of the early SARS patients in Guangdong were involved in either the trade or preparation of food from wild animals in markets. Furthermore, there was a much higher seroprevalence of SARS-CoV among wild animal handlers than among controls in Guangdong. Further surveillance on animals is needed to help understand the reservoir in nature that led to the SARS outbreak.

Transmission of SARS

The incubation period for SARS is between 3 and 10 days, with a median of 4 to 5 days. However, it may be as long as 14 days. The SARS-CoV is transmitted predominately through droplets from the respiratory tract of the infected person, particularly when coughing, sneezing, and even speaking. The risk of transmission is highest when there is close face-to-face contact. SARS-CoV transmission is believed to be amplified by aerosol-generating procedures such as intubation or the use of nebulizers. The detection of SARS-CoV in fecal as well as respiratory specimens indicates that the virus may be spread by both fecal contamination and via respiratory droplets. SARS-CoV also has the ability to survive on contaminated objects in the environment for up to several days and therefore transmission may occur via fomites. Although SARS spreads rapidly around the world as a result of international travel, relatively few cases were acquired by this route.

Efficient environments for transmission of the SARS-CoV were health care facilities and households, leading to a preponderance of SARS cases who were either health care workers or household contacts of cases. Several risk factors may account for this. In the health care setting, close contact is required to care for severely ill patients. Additionally, efficiency of transmission appears to be directly related to the severity of the illness, and those more severely ill are more likely to be hospitalized. Furthermore, patients with SARS-CoV appear to be most infectious during the second week of their illness, and although transmission can also occur during the first week, they are more likely to present to hospital as their clinical condition worsens, usually during the second week. In Singapore, the secondary attack rate among household members of SARS cases was approximately 6%. The risk factors associated with household transmission included older age of the index case and non–health care occupation of the index case. Interestingly, there were no reports of transmission from infected children to other children or to adults.

Diagnostic Criteria and Treatment

The WHO issued updated case definitions for SARS during the outbreak using a combination of clinical signs and symptoms together with epidemiologic factors to assist in the identification of hospital cases. These have been revised in the postoutbreak period and include radiographic and laboratory findings. To date no consistently reliable rapid test is available for SARS-CoV.

Sudden onset of fever is the most common initial symptom of SARS and may also be associated with headache, myalgia, malaise, chills, rigor, and gastrointestinal symptoms. However, documented fever did not occur in some cases, particularly the elderly.

Although a variety of treatment protocols have been tested, at present sufficient evidence is not available to recommend any specific therapy for the treatment of SARS.

Prognostic Factors

Factors associated with a poor prognosis or outcome (i.e., admission to an intensive care unit or death) included advanced age, coexisting illness such as diabetes or heart disease, and the presence of elevated levels of lactate dehydrogenase or a high neutrophil count on admission. Clinically, compared with adults and teenagers, SARS-CoV infection was less severe in children (< 12 years) and had a more favorable outcome. Additionally, preterm and term infants born to women infected with SARS-CoV were not found to be clinically affected or shedding the virus after birth.

Prevention and Control

In the absence of a vaccine, the most effective way to control a viral disease is to break the chain of human-to-human transmission. This was achieved for SARS using the traditional public health methods of early case detection and isolation, strict infection control measures, contact tracing, and quarantine measures. The SARS outbreak also clearly demonstrated the effectiveness of international collaboration.

Early identification of SARS cases is crucial in making it possible to initiate appropriate precautions, and studies of transmission show this to be a critical component in controlling any future outbreaks of SARS. However, clinical symptoms alone are not enough to diagnose SARS, especially as these are nonspecific in the early stages and cases may present during seasonal outbreaks of other respiratory illnesses. Furthermore, SARS-CoV laboratory tests have limited sensitivity when used in the early stages of illness. However, most SARS cases could be linked to contact with SARS patients or a place where SARS transmission was known or suspected. Transmission was also interrupted by the use of stringently applied infection control precautions, including the appropriate use of personal protective equipment. The relatively long incubation period of SARS facilitated contact tracing, the implementation of quarantine measures, and the institution of control measures for contacts who developed illness. Other measures were also instituted, including closing hospitals and schools, wearing masks in public, banning public gatherings, screening inbound and outbound international travelers, and issuing travel advisories. There is a need to fully evaluate the effectiveness of these measures.

—Karen Shaw and Babatunde Olowokure

See also Epidemic; Outbreak Investigation; Zoonotic Disease

Further Readings

Chowell, G., Fenimore, P. W., Castillo-Garsow, M. A., & Castillo-Chavez, C. (2003). SARS outbreaks in Ontario, Hong Kong and Singapore: The role of diagnosis and isolation as a control mechanism. *Journal of Theoretical Biology, 224*, 1–8.

Goh, D. L.-M., Lee, B. W., Chia, K. S., Heng, B. H., Chen, M., Ma, S., et al. (2004). Secondary household transmission of SARS, Singapore [Electronic version]. *Emerging Infectious Diseases.* Retrieved March 7, 2006, from http://www.cdc.gov/ncidod/EID/vol10no2/03-0676.htm.

Hui, D. S. C., Chan, M. C. H., Wu, A. K., & Ng, P. C. (2004). Severe acute respiratory syndrome (SARS): Epidemiology and clinical features. *Postgraduate Medical Journal, 80*, 373–381.

Mackenzie, J., & Olowokure, B. (2006). Biocontainment and biosafety issues. In *SARS: How a global epidemic was stopped* (pp. 234–240). Manila, Philippines: World Health Organization, Western Pacific Region.

Olowokure, B., Merianos, A., Leitmeyer, K., & Mackenzie, J. (2004). SARS. *Nature Reviews. Microbiology, 2*, 92–93.

Riley, S., Fraser, C., Donnelly, C. A., Ghani, A. C., Abu-Raddad, L. J., Hedley, A. J., et al. (2003). Transmission dynamics of the etiological agent of SARS in Hong Kong: Impact of public health interventions. *Science, 300*, 1961–1966.

Shaw, K. (2006). The 2003 SARS outbreak and its impact on infection control practice. *Public Health, 120*, 8–14.

World Health Organization. (2003). *SARS breaking the chains of transmission, 2003.* Retrieved March 7, 2006, from http://www.who.int/features/2003/07/en.

World Health Organization. (2003). *WHO consensus on the epidemiology of SARS.* Retrieved March 7, 2006, from http://www.who.int/csr/sars/archive/epiconsensus/en.

World Health Organization. (2003). *World Health Report. Chapter 5: SARS: Lessons from a new disease.* Retrieved March 7, 2006, from http://www.who.int/whr/2003/chapter5/en/print.html.

SEXUALLY TRANSMITTED DISEASES

Sexually transmitted diseases (STDs), also commonly referred to as sexually transmitted infections (STIs), are primarily spread through the exchange of bodily fluids during sexual contact. STDs may also be transmitted through blood-to-blood contact and from a woman to her baby during pregnancy or delivery (congenital transmission). Exposure to STDs can occur through any close exposure to the genitals, rectum, or mouth. Unprotected sexual contact increases the likelihood of contracting an STD. Abstaining from sexual contact can prevent STDs, and correct and consistent use of latex condoms reduces the risk of transmission. STDs include gonorrhea, chlamydia, genital herpes, syphilis, human papillomavirus or genital warts, lymphogranuloma venereum, trichomoniasis, bacterial vaginosis, human immunodeficiency virus (HIV), which causes AIDS, and hepatitis B. Other infections that may be sexually transmitted include hepatitis C, cytomegalovirus, scabies, and pubic lice. Having an STD increases the risk of becoming infected with HIV if one is exposed to HIV. Most STDs can be treated and cured, though important exceptions include HIV and genital herpes. Successful treatment of an STD cures the infection, resolves the clinical symptoms, and prevents transmission to others. HIV is not currently curable and can cause death. Genital herpes symptoms may be managed, but genital herpes is a recurrent, lifelong infection.

STDs remain a major public health concern due to their physical and psychological effects, as well as their economic toll. The Centers for Disease Control and Prevention (CDC) estimates that 19 million new infections occur each year, almost half of them among young people aged 15 to 24 years. Women, especially young women, ethnic minorities, and men who have sex with men (MSM) are often most affected by STDs (except chlamydia). The following are descriptions of key features associated with STDs.

Gonorrhea

Gonorrhea is caused by the bacterium *Neissera gonorrheae* and can be spread during vaginal, anal, or oral sex, as well as from a woman to her newborn during delivery regardless of whether the mother is symptomatic at the time. Gonorrhea can affect the urethra, rectum, throat, pelvic organs, and, in rare cases, conjunctiva, as well as the cervix in women. Colloquially referred to as the "clap" or the "drip," the incubation period is usually 2 to 5 days but may take up to 30 days to become visible. Gonorrhea is symptomatic in approximately 50% of infected individuals and possible symptoms include painful urination, abnormal discharge from the penis or vagina, genital itching or bleeding, and, in rare cases, sore throat or conjunctivitis. In women, symptoms may also include lower abdominal pain, fever, general tiredness, swollen and painful Bartholin glands (opening of the vaginal area), and painful sexual intercourse. In men, symptoms can include discharge from the penis that is at first clear or milky and then yellow, creamy, excessive, and sometimes blood tinged. If the infection disseminates to sites other than the genitals, possible symptoms include joint pain, arthritis, and inflamed tendons.

Left untreated, gonorrhea may cause complications to the female reproductive system, including pelvic inflammatory disease (PID), which can result in an increased risk of infertility (a danger that increases with subsequent episodes), tubo-ovarian abscess, inflammation of the Bartholin glands, ectopic (tubal) pregnancy, chronic pelvic pain, and, in rare occurrences, Fitz-Hugh-Curtis syndrome (inflammation of the liver). Left untreated in men, complications can include urethritis (infection of the urethra), epididymitis (inflammation and infection of epididymis), prostatitis, and infertility. If gonorrhea is not treated, complications may arise from disseminated gonococcal infection and include fever, cellulites, sepsis, arthritis, endocarditis (inflammation of the heart valves and the chambers of the heart), and meningitis.

Diagnosis of gonorrhea involves a medical history; physical exam, including a pelvic or genital exam; and collection of a sample of body fluid or urine. Discovered early and treated before complications arise, gonorrhea causes no long-term problems. Antibiotic treatment is recommended for individuals who have a positive gonorrhea test or who have had sex partners within the past 60 days who tested positive.

Chlamydia

Chlamydia is caused by the bacterium *Chlamydia trachomatis* and is the most common STD/STI in the United States. Chlamydia infects the urethra of men and the urethra, cervix, and upper reproductive organs of women. It may also infect the rectum, throat, pelvic organs, and conjunctiva. Chlamydia can be passed from mother to newborn during vaginal delivery and, in rare instances, during Caesarean delivery. Symptoms develop in only about 10% of those with chlamydia. In women, symptoms include painful urination, cloudy urine, abnormal vaginal discharge, abnormal vaginal bleeding during intercourse or between periods, irregular menstrual bleeding, genital itching, lower abdominal pain, fever and general tiredness, swollen and painful Bartholin glands, and conjunctivitis. In men, symptoms include painful urination or itching during urination, cloudy urine, watery or slimy discharge from the penis, crusting on the tip of the penis, a tender anus or scrotum, and conjunctivitis. Complications in women include cervicitis (inflammation of the cervix), urethritis, endometritis, inflammation of the Bartholin glands, PID, pelvic abscess, infertility, and Fitz-Hugh-Curtis syndrome. Complications in men include urethritis, epididymitis, prostatitis, and infertility. Complications in both sexes include conjunctivitis, inflammation of the mucous membrane of the rectum (proctitis), and Reiter's syndrome, which is caused by a bacterial infection and results in varied symptoms, including joint and eye inflammation.

Chlamydia is diagnosed with a medical history; physical exam, including a pelvic or genital exam; and collection of body fluid or urine. Discovered early and treated before complications arise, chlamydia causes no long-term problems. Antibiotic treatment is recommended for individuals who have a positive chlamydia test or who have had sex partners within the past 60 days who tested positive. Because of the high incidence of chlamydia in the United States, the CDC recommends annual screening for sexually active women up to the age of 25 years and for women above the age of 25 years who engage in high-risk sexual behaviors. Health professionals are obligated to report a positive diagnosis to the State Health Department for the purposes of notification of sexual partner(s).

Genital Herpes

Genital herpes is a lifelong, recurrent viral infection caused by herpes simplex virus type 2 (HSV-2) and less frequently by herpes simplex virus type 1 (HSV-1). At least 50 million persons in the United States have genital HSV infection, and most exhibit minimal or no symptoms. HSV-1, which more commonly causes infections of the mouth and lips ("fever blisters"), can also be transmitted to the genitals through oral-genital (during oral outbreaks) or genital-genital contact. The painful multiple ulcerative lesions that typically characterize those infected with genital herpes are often absent. Most persons with genital herpes have mild or unrecognized infections. Although they are not aware of their condition, those with undiagnosed HSV are still contagious, as the virus periodically "sheds" in the genital tract. The majority of genital herpes infections are transmitted by persons who are unaware of infection or who are aware but asymptomatic when transmission occurs. Visible symptoms usually occur within 2 weeks of transmission and include blisters or ulcers on or around the penis, vagina, and anus. Outbreaks of genital ulcers typically last 2 to 4 weeks during the first clinical episode and several weeks to months during subsequent episodes, which are often less severe. Although the infection remains in the body indefinitely, outbreaks tend to decrease over a period of years.

Clinical diagnosis of genital herpes is insensitive and nonspecific and thus should be confirmed through laboratory testing. Isolation of the HSV in a cell culture is the preferred virologic test in patients who present with genital ulcers or other lesions. Because false-negative HSV cultures are common, especially in patients with recurrent infection or with healing lesions, type-specific serologic tests are useful in confirming a clinical diagnosis of genital herpes. Laboratory testing can be used to diagnose persons with unrecognized infection, which in turns allows for the treatment of sex partners. Distinguishing between HSV serotypes is important and influences prognosis and treatment since HSV-1 (which is responsible for about 30% of first-episode outbreaks) causes less frequent recurrences.

There is no cure for genital herpes, and the virus may be transmitted during asymptomatic periods. The burden caused by the lack of a cure, recurrence of outbreaks, and the possibility of transmission to sexual partners causes some people with genital herpes to experience recurrent psychological distress. Antiviral chemotherapy is the mainstay of management and offers clinical benefits to most symptomatic patients. Systematic antiviral drugs partially control the symptoms and signs of herpes episodes when used to treat both first clinical and recurrent episodes, or when used as daily suppressive therapy. However, these drugs neither eradicate the latent virus nor affect the risk, frequency, or severity of recurrences after the drug is discontinued. Consequently, counseling regarding the natural history of genital herpes, sexual and perinatal transmission, and methods of reducing transmission is integral to clinical management. Persons with genital herpes should be informed that sexual transmission of HSV could occur during asymptomatic periods and that it is important to abstain from sexual activity when lesions or prodromal symptoms are present. The risk for neonatal HSV infection should be explained to both men and women.

Syphilis

Syphilis is caused by the bacterium *Treponema pallidum*, which is transmitted by vaginal, anal, or oral contact with the infected individual's open ulcers during the primary stage and mucus membrane or other sores during the secondary and latent stages. Syphilis may also be passed from mother to baby during pregnancy or labor and delivery. The CDC and the U.S. Prevention Services Task Force strongly recommend that all pregnant women be screened for syphilis because of the severe health consequences of congenital syphilis. The development of syphilis occurs in four stages—primary, secondary, latent, and tertiary stages. During the *primary stage*, the individual develops an often painless ulcer at the transmission site within 10 to 90 days after exposure. Ulcers mainly occur on the external genitals (men), inner or outer part of the vagina (women), or rectum. Ulcers usually last from 28 to 48 days and heal without treatment, leaving a thin scar. The *secondary stage* may begin before ulcers occurring in the primary stage have healed and is characterized by a rash that appears between 4 and 10 weeks after the development of the ulcer and consists of reddish brown, small, solid, flat, or raised skin sores that may mirror common skin problems. Small, open sores that may contain pus or moist sores that look like warts may develop on the mucous membranes. The skin rash usually heals without scaring in 2 to 12 weeks. Symptoms occurring during this stage include fever, sore throat, physical weakness or discomfort, weight loss, patchy hair loss, swelling of the lymph nodes, and nervous system symptoms such as headaches, irritability, paralysis, unequal reflexes, and irregular pupils. During the primary and secondary stages, the person is highly contagious. After secondary-stage symptoms subside, the person enters the *latent stage* and has no symptoms for a period of time ranging from 1 year to 20 years, although about

20% to 30% of individuals have a relapse during this period. If the syphilis infection is left untreated, the latent stage is followed by the *tertiary stage*, during which serious blood vessel and heart problems, mental disorders, gummata (large sores inside the body or on the skin), blindness, nerve system problems, and death may occur. Complications during this stage also include cardiovascular syphilis, which affects the heart and blood vessels, and neurosyphilis, which affects the brain or the brain lining.

The two definitive methods for diagnosing early syphilis are dark-field examinations and direct fluorescent antibody tests of lesion exudiate or tissue in the adjacent area. A presumptive diagnosis is possible with the use of two types of serologic tests: nontreponemal tests (e.g., Venereal Disease Research Laboratory test and rapid plasma reagin test) and treponemal tests (e.g., fluorescent treponemal antibody absorbed test and *T. pallidum* particle agglutination test). The use of only one type of serologic test is insufficient for diagnosis, because false-positive nontreponemal test results may occur due to various medical conditions. Penicillin G, administered parenterally, is the preferred drug treatment of all stages of syphilis, though dosage and length of treatment depend on the stage and clinical manifestations of the disease. The efficacy of penicillin for the treatment of syphilis is well established, and almost all treatments have been supported by case series, clinical trials, and 50 years of clinical experience.

Human Papillomavirus

Human papillomavirus (HPV) is the name of a group of approximately 100 related strains of a virus, more than 30 of which are sexually transmitted. HPV can affect the vulva, lining of the vagina, and the cervix of women; the genital area—including the skin of the penis—of men; and the anus or rectum of both men and women, which in turn may result in anal warts (it is not necessary to have had anal sexual contact to contract anal warts). HPV affects approximately 20 million people in the United States, and at least 50% of sexually active men and women will acquire genital HPV at some point in their lives. By the age of 50 years, at least 80% of women will have acquired genital HPV infection. The virus itself lives in the skin or mucous membranes, and most infected people are asymptomatic and unaware of the infection. Some people develop visible genital warts or have precancerous changes in the cervix, vulva, anus, or penis. Genital warts may appear around the anus, penis, scrotum, groin, or thighs of men and on the vulva, in or around the vagina, and on the cervix of women. Most infections clear up without medical intervention. Although no HPV test is currently available for men, there exists a test to detect HPV DNA in women. A Pap test is the primary cancer-screening tool for cervical cancer or precancerous changes in the cervix, many of which are related to HPV. All types of HPV can cause mild Pap test abnormalities, and approximately 10 to 30 identified HPV types can lead, in rare cases, to cervical cancer. Pap tests used in U.S. cervical cancer-screening programs are responsible for greatly reducing deaths from cervical cancer. For 2004, the American Cancer Society (ACS) estimated that about 10,520 women will develop invasive cervical cancer and about 3,900 women will die from the disease. Certain types of HPV have also been linked to cancer of the anus and penis in men. The ACS estimates that about 1,530 men will be diagnosed with penile cancer in the United States in 2006. This accounts for approximately 0.2% of all cancers in men. The ACS estimates that about 1,910 men will be diagnosed with anal cancer in 2006, and the risk for anal cancer is higher among gay and bisexual men and men with compromised immune systems, including those with HIV.

There is currently no cure for HPV. The recently developed HPV vaccine has been shown to be effective in protecting against four strains of HPV. The HPV vaccine is targeted toward preventing cervical cancer and has been approved for women aged 9 to 26 years. The vaccine is nearly 100% effective in preventing precancerous cervical changes caused by two strains of HPV. These two strains cause 70% of all cervical cancers and most vaginal and vulvar cancers. It is also somewhat effective in protecting against two other HPV strains that are responsible for 90% of all cases of genital warts. The vaccine is not effective in women who are already infected with HPV and is most effective if given before women become sexually active.

Lymphogranuloma Venereum

Lymphogranuloma venereum (LGV) is caused by a type of *Chlamydia trachomatis* and is transmitted by genital or oral contact with infected fluid. The *first stage* of the disease occurs 3 days to 3 weeks after infection, during which a small, painless vesicle

appears on the genitalia, anus, or mouth. This vesicle soon develops into an ulcer and goes away in a few days without treatment. Some men develop a node or bubonulus ("bubos") at the base of the penis, which may rupture or form draining sinuses or fistulas. The next stage, which occurs 7 to 30 days after the primary lesion resolves, is called regional lymphangitis. The lymph nodes that drain the area of original infection become swollen, tender, and painful. With mouth or throat infections, LGV can produce bubos under the chin, in the neck, or in the clavicular region. The bubos transform from hard and firm to softer masses, accompanied by reddened skin, which will sometimes rupture or form draining sinuses or fistulas. The patient may also suffer from fever, chills, headache, stiff neck, loss of appetite, nausea, vomiting, muscle and joint pains, or skin rashes. Women may suffer from lower abdominal or back pain. Those with rectal infections may have mucoid discharge from the anus. Late complications of LGV include elephantiasis (grotesque swelling due to lymphatic blockages) of the genitals, other genital deformities, ulcerative lesions (especially of the vulva), perianal abscesses, rectal strictures, fistulas, and large perianal swellings known as lymphrrhoids. LGV causes ulcers, which can increase the risk of contracting HIV infection.

LGV rarely occurs in the United States and other industrialized countries. However, recent outbreaks of LGV proctitis in MSM in the Netherlands and other European countries in 2003, and a handful of cases in New York City, have raised concerns in the United States. White, HIV-infected MSM constitute the majority of patients diagnosed with LGV proctitis, and preliminary findings suggest that the main mode of transmission was unprotected anal intercourse. Men and women may be asymptomatic and unknowingly transmit LGV. Men can spread infection while only rarely suffering long-term health problems. Women are at high risk of severe complications of infection, including acute salpingitis and PID, which can lead to chronic pain, ectopic pregnancy, and infertility. LGV is sensitive to a number of antibiotics, including erythromycin, tetracyclins, doxycyclin, and sulfadiazine. Infected lymph nodes must often be drained through aspiration, and fistulas or other structural problems may require surgery. Technology for LGV testing is not currently commercially available. In U.S. states that lack laboratory capacity to perform LGV diagnostic testing, specimens may be submitted to the CDC.

Bacterial Vaginosis

Bacterial vaginosis (BV) is a condition where the normal balance of bacteria in the vagina is disrupted and there is an overgrowth of harmful bacteria. It is estimated that approximately 16% of pregnant women have BV, and it is the most common vaginal infection in women of childbearing age. Little is known about what causes BV or how it is transmitted. It is believed that some behaviors such as having a new sex partner, having multiple sex partners, douching, and using an intrauterine device for contraception can upset the normal balance of bacteria in the vagina and put women at increased risk. BV may spread between two female partners.

Symptoms of BV include a vaginal discharge—which is white-gray, thin, with an unpleasant odor—burning during urination, and itching around the outside of the vagina. Some women with BV report no signs or symptoms, and in most cases, BV causes no complications. Serious risks do exist, however, and include increased susceptibility to HIV infection if exposed to the HIV virus, increased chance of passing HIV to a sex partner if infected with the HIV virus, increased development of PID following surgical procedures such as a hysterectomy or an abortion, increased risk of complications during pregnancy, and increased susceptibility to other STDs. Although BV will sometimes clear up without treatment, all women with symptoms of BV should be treated to avoid complications such as PID. Treatment is especially important for pregnant women.

Trichomoniasis

Trichomoniasis is caused by the single-celled parasite *Trichomonas vaginalis* and affects the vagina in women and the urethra in men. Trichomoniasis is sexually transmitted through penis-to-vagina intercourse or vulva-to-vulva contact. Women can acquire the disease from infected men or women, while men usually contract it only from infected women. Most men with trichomoniasis are asymptomatic, although some may experience temporary irritation inside the penis, mild discharge, or slight burning after urination or ejaculation. Some women have symptoms, including vaginal discharge that is frothy, yellow-green, and has a strong odor; discomfort during intercourse and urination; irritation and itching of the genital area; and, in rare cases, lower abdominal pain. Symptoms usually appear in women within 5 to 28 days of exposure.

For both sexes, trichomoniasis is diagnosed by physical examination and laboratory test, although the parasite is harder to detect in men. Trichomoniasis can usually be cured with a single dose of an orally administered antibiotic. Although the symptoms of trichomoniasis in men may disappear within a few weeks without treatment, an asymptomatic man can continue to infect or reinfect a female partner until he has been treated. Therefore, both partners should be treated concurrently to eliminate the parasite.

—Roy Jerome

See also HIV/AIDS; Hepatitis; Partner Notification; Sexual Risk Behavior

Further Readings

American Cancer Society. (2006, June 8). *HPV vaccine approved: Prevents cervical cancer*. American Cancer Society News Center. Retrieved June 19, 2006, from http://www.cancer.org/docroot/NWS/content/NWS_1_1x_HPV_Vaccine_Approved_Prevents_Cervical_Cancer.asp.

Centers for Disease Control and Prevention. (2002, May 10). Sexually transmitted disease treatment guidelines, 2002 [Electronic version]. *Morbidity and Mortality Weekly Report*, *51*(RR-6), 13–36, 44–47. Retrieved June 19, 2006, from http://www.cdc.gov/std/treatment/default-2002.htm.

Centers for Disease Control and Prevention. (2004). *Bacterial vaginosis: Fact sheet*. Retrieved May 15, 2006, from http://www.cdc.gov/std/bv/STDFact-Bacterial-Vaginosis.htm.

Centers for Disease Control and Prevention. (2004). *Genital herpes: Fact sheet*. Retrieved May 15, 2006, from http://www.cdc.gov/std/Herpes/STDFact-Herpes.htm.

Centers for Disease Control and Prevention. (2004). *Genital HPV infection: Fact sheet*. Retrieved May 15, 2006, from http://www.cdc.gov/std/HPV/STDFact-HPV.htm.

Centers for Disease Control and Prevention. (2004). *Trichomonas infection: Fact sheet*. Retrieved May 15, 2006, from http://www.cdc.gov/ncidod/dpd/parasites/trichomonas/factsht_trichomonas.htm.

Centers for Disease Control and Prevention. (2005, November). *Trends in reportable sexually transmitted diseases in the United States, 2004*. Retrieved May 15, 2006, from http://www.cdc.gov/std/stats04/trends2004.htm.

Centers for Disease Control and Prevention. (2006). *Lymphogranuloma Venereum (LGV) Project: Information sheet*. Retrieved June 19, 2006, from http://www.cdc.gov/std/lgv/LGVinf05–22–2006.pdf.

Centers for Disease Control and Prevention. (2006). *Viral hepatitis B: Fact sheet*. Retrieved May 15, 2006, from http://www.cdc.gov/ncidod/diseases/hepatitis/b/fact.htm.

Hook, E. W. (2004). Syphilis. In L. Golman, & D. Ausiello (Eds.), *Cecil textbook of medicine* (22nd ed., Vol. 2, pp. 1923–1932). Philadelphia: Saunders.

Low, N. (2004). Chlamydia (uncomplicated, genital). *Clinical Evidence, 11,* 2064–2072.

Peipert, J. F. (2003). Genital chlamydial infections. *New England Journal of Medicine, 349,* 2424–2430.

Quest Diagnostics. (2005). *Chlamydia.* Retrieved May 15, 2006, from http://www.questdiagnostics.com/kbase/topic/ major/hw146904/descrip.htm.

Quest Diagnostics. (2005). *Gonorrhea.* Retrieved May 15, 2006, from http://www.questdiagnostics.com/kbase/topic/ major/hw188975/descrip.htm.

Quest Diagnostics. (2005). *Syphilis.* Retrieved May 15, 2005, from http://www.questdiagnostics.com/kbase/topic/major/ hw195071/descrip.htm.

van de Laar, M. J., Gotz, H. M., de Zwart, O., van der Meijden, W. I., Ossewaarde, J. M., Thio, H. B., et al. (2004). Lymphogranuloma venereum among men who have sex with men: Netherlands, 2003–2004 [Electronic version]. *Morbidity and Mortality Weekly Report, 53,* 985–988.]

Weinstock, H., Berman, S., & Cates, W. (2004). Sexually transmitted diseases among American youth: Incidence and prevalence estimates, 2000. *Perspectives on Sexual and Reproductive Health, 36,* 6–10.

World Health Organization. (1995). Sexually transmitted diseases. In *Teaching modules for continuing education in human sexuality: Vol. 8.* (pp. 5–40). Manila, Philippines: Author.

World Health Organization. (2000). *Guidelines for surveillance of sexually transmitted diseases.* New Delhi: Author.

Sexual Minorities, Health Issues of

The health of sexual minorities represents a broad and rapidly expanding area of public health research and concern. Encompassing people who are lesbian, gay, bisexual, and transgender (LGBT), sexual minorities are diverse populations who have struggled with issues of sexuality, identity, and gender amidst historic and continuing stigma, fear, and discrimination. Consequently, while possessing the same basic health needs as the general population, LGBT people face additional health issues related to social discrimination, behavioral risk factors, and unique medical conditions. The diversity of these populations spans race, ethnicity, age, education, socioeconomic position, geography, political affiliation, and the degree to which individuals identify and interact with other LGBT people. From all indications, sexual minorities exist wherever there are human societies. This entry examines health outcomes among LGBT people, including the impact of disparities in their access to health care. It also discusses methodological issues related to research on these populations.

Over the past 25 years, since the birth of the modern gay rights movement following the "Stonewall Riots" in New York City in 1969, LGBT people have experienced growing acknowledgment of their basic human rights throughout the world. Facilitated in large measure by the activism of LGBT people themselves, this has led to increased awareness of persistent health disparities among and between these populations, including rates of HIV/AIDS among gay and bisexual men and certain types of cancers among lesbians. However, conducting epidemiological research on LGBT people is complicated by several issues, including varying definitions of the most basic terms (such as *homosexual*), reluctance of LGBT people to identify themselves as such or participate in research due to stigma, and a history of differing priorities and conflicts between LGBT people and the medical and social science communities.

Definitions of Terms and Conceptual Issues

To consider the health issues of sexual minorities first requires a clarification of terms and an appreciation for the subject's conceptual complexity. While there is no complete agreement over language, broadly speaking, *sexual orientation* refers to a person's sexual and romantic attraction to other people. This term is increasingly favored over *sexual preference*, which implies that attraction is merely a choice and not an inherent personal characteristic. Individuals whose sexual orientation is to people of the opposite sex are *heterosexual* and those whose orientation is to people of the same sex are *homosexual*, with women who are primarily attracted to other women referred to as *lesbians* and men who are primarily attracted to other men referred to as *gay*. Individuals who are attracted to both men and women are *bisexual*, and depending on the person, this attraction may be felt equally toward both sexes or it may be stronger or different toward one or the other. It is important to note that sexual orientation is not the same as sexual identity or behavior, and one does not necessarily imply the other.

Transgender is an umbrella term referring to people who do not fit to traditional or customary notions of *gender*—the sociocultural norms and beliefs that define what it means to be a man or a woman. In general, society assigns an individual's gender role at birth based on one's genitals, but some people identify more strongly with the opposite gender (e.g., natal females who identify as men, natal men who identify as women) or with a variance that falls outside dichotomous gender constructions (e.g., individuals who feel they possess both or neither genders, including those with ambiguous sex characteristics). Some transgender people are *transvestites* or cross-dressers, primarily men who dress in women's clothing for erotic or other personal interests; others may "do drag" for fun, entertainment, or personal expression. Many of these people are comfortable with their natal gender. Other transgender people may be *transsexuals*, people who pursue medical interventions such as the use of hormones of the opposite sex and/or surgeries to align their bodies more closely with their interior sense of self. Still others reject any categorization of their gender or sexuality. Transgender people may identify as male or female independent of their anatomy or physiology and may be heterosexual, homosexual, bisexual, or nonsexual.

At the individual level, sexuality and gender reflect attractions, behaviors, and identities that develop throughout the life course, influenced by both biological and psychosocial factors such as family and culture. For example, a man may engage repeatedly in sexual activities with other men but neither acknowledge participation in homosexual behavior nor identify as gay. A woman may enter into an emotionally fulfilling intimate relationship with another woman that involves temporary identification as a lesbian but at a future time enter into exclusive long-term relationships with men, at no time seeing herself as bisexual. Another individual may present as anatomically female but personally identify as a transgender gay man. These examples illustrate the need for health professionals to approach the subjects of gender and sexuality with few assumptions and perspectives open to the needs of the clients within their cultural contexts.

The health of LGBT people may be affected by social conditions characterized by stigma, fear, rejection, prejudice, discrimination, and violence. *Heterosexism* is unconscious or deliberate discrimination that favors heterosexuality, such as the assumption that everyone is heterosexual or the extension of social privileges or an elevated social status based on heterosexual identity, behaviors, or perceived heterosexual

orientation. *Homophobia*, *biphobia*, and *transphobia* describe the respective hatred and fear of homosexuals, bisexuals, and transgender people. These fears and prejudices operate at all levels of society to varying degrees and at various times, interacting with and exacerbating the effects of racism, sexism, and class-based discrimination. These biases may account for a large degree of the disparity in health outcomes observed among LGBT populations, although research is currently insufficient to determine this conclusively.

Consequently, whether working with individuals or populations, many health professionals find it useful to apply an ecological framework to better comprehend LGBT health issues, taking time to identify, articulate, and address both needs and assets among interpersonal, community, and societal factors. For example, LGBT stigma and discrimination can influence the determination and funding of research priorities, the design and implementation of prevention and intervention programs, the development of standards of care, and the use of culturally appropriate services. This discrimination can be expressed directly through exposures to violence, humiliation, or suboptimal care and indirectly through invisibilization and marginalization of LGBT health concerns and treatment. However, taking an assets-based approach, these inequities can be mitigated by inclusive and supportive policies, education, research, and training; community empowerment; and by drawing on the resources, resilience, and participation of LGBT people themselves.

Outcomes

Prevalence estimates of same-sex attractions, identities, and behaviors range between approximately 1% and 13% of the general population. In a 1994 national study of U.S. adults, Laumann, Gagnon, Michael, and Michaels found 8% of respondents reported same-sex attractions; 2% identified as gay, lesbian, or bisexual; and 7% reported having engaged in same-sex behaviors. These data appeared congruent with data from national population-based samples of France and the United Kingdom the following year. Prevalence estimates of transgender individuals are much less certain; there are no reliable data for the U.S. population. Outside the United States, transgender estimates range from 0.002% to 0.005%, with some transgender activists estimating prevalence of "strong transgender feelings" (without sexual reassignment) at 0.5%, or 1 of every 200 persons. LGBT estimates, where they exist, vary across studies due to a variety of factors, including definitions and use of terms, sampling methodologies, data analyses, age (youth vs. adults), location (rural vs. urban), and cultural contexts. These gaps and inconsistencies in knowledge suggest the need for more routine, rigorous, and inclusive population-based sampling, as done during censuses, risk-behavior surveys, and disease surveillance and reporting.

It may be useful to categorize LGBT health outcomes among three areas of concern. First, sexual minorities may experience risks or exposures unique to the population of interest, such as hormone use among transsexuals or anal sex among men who have sex with men. Second, the risk or exposure may not be unique to the population but exists at a prevalence higher than that found in the general population, such as substance abuse or depression. Third, the risk or exposure may neither be unique nor exist in greater proportion, but the issue warrants an approach that is particularly attentive or culturally sensitive, such as screening of sexually transmitted diseases (STDs) among bisexuals, reproductive services among lesbians, or routine medical examinations among transsexuals.

Stigmatizing social conditions, particularly among youth, racial/ethnic minorities, and transgender individuals, contribute to a number of health disparities shared to varying degrees among LGBT populations. These include access and use of programs and services, mental health issues, and exposures to violence. For example, the Women's Health Initiative, a U.S. sample of 96,000 older women, found that lesbians and bisexual women were significantly more likely to be uninsured compared with heterosexual women (10%, 12%, and 7%, respectively). Uninsured levels appear highest among transgender people, disproportionately so among people of color (21% to 52% among studies), and most health care related to transgender issues is not covered by insurance, making transgender health care personally very expensive. Adolescents are the most uninsured and underinsured among all age groups, and LGBT youths perhaps face the greatest barriers to appropriate, sensitive care.

Social stigma is a stressor with profound mental health consequences, producing inwardly directed feelings of shame and self-hatred that give rise to low self-esteem, suicidality, depression, anxiety, substance abuse, and feelings of powerlessness and despair that limit health-seeking behaviors. According to findings documented in the report, Healthy People 2010

Companion Document for LGBT Health, homosexually active men report higher rates of major depression and panic attack compared with men who report no homosexual behavior, and homosexually active women report higher rates of alcohol and drug dependence compared with women who report no homosexual behavior. In New Zealand, LGBT youths were found to be at higher risk for major depression, generalized anxiety disorder, and conduct disorders than were non-LGBT youths. Among 515 transsexuals sampled in San Francisco in 2001, Clements-Nolle and colleagues reported depression among 62% of the transgender women and 55% of the transgender men; 32% of the sample had attempted suicide. While the earliest studies of alcohol and other substance use among lesbians and gay men suggested alarmingly high rates, subsequent studies describe elevated rates among LGBT populations as a function of socially determined factors, including age, race/ethnicity, socioeconomic position, and prior exposures to trauma and violence.

These more recent studies demonstrate the focus and refinement that is now taking place in the field of LGBT public health research, providing unprecedented opportunities to comprehend health issues within specific populations. For example, studies suggest that lesbians and bisexual women are at higher risk for breast cancer compared with heterosexual women due to higher rates of risk factors, including obesity, alcohol consumption, having never given birth, and lower rates of breast cancer screenings. Similarly, lesbians and bisexual women may also be at higher risk for gynecologic cancers because they receive less frequent gynecologic care. Among men who have sex with men, in addition to higher rates of HIV/AIDS—particularly among racial/ethnic minorities—gay and bisexual men are at increased risks for other STDs, including syphilis, gonorrhea, chlamydia, human papillomavirus, and hepatitis A, B, and C. Cross-sex hormone use among transsexuals, including long-term use of estrogen and testosterone, presents potential health risks that are poorly documented at this time, including possible cancers of the breast and ovaries. Because of transphobia, transgender people may be reluctant to provide a full health history to their medical providers or they may be flagrantly denied care. These experiences contribute to absence of treatment or delayed treatments, such as cancer screenings, or to informal and medically unsupervised procedures, such as unregulated hormone therapy or the cosmetic use of injectable silicone.

Access

Access refers to the ways that LGBT health concerns are or are not addressed at various levels of society, from government and institutional policies and resources to the individual practices of health professionals. For example, following the removal of homosexuality from the American Psychiatric Association's *Diagnostic and Statistical Manual of Mental Disorders* in 1974, the mental health profession reversed its long-held position that regarded homosexuality as a psychopathology and emerged as one of the most important advocates for the normalization and acceptance of same-sex attraction. By the beginning of the 21st century, the American Public Health Association had acknowledged the special health concerns of LGBT populations with a policy statement on the need for research on gender identity and sexual orientation and a subsequent journal issue wholly dedicated to the topic in 2001. The U.S. government signaled similar support with publication of an Institute of Medicine report on lesbian health in 1999 and the inclusion of gays and lesbians in *Healthy People 2010*, the 10-year blueprint for public health produced by the U.S. Department of Health and Human Services. In turn, these policies potentially influence research, funding, and programs that directly affect the lives and well-being of LGBT people and their families.

However, to be effective, resources and a proactive political agenda must be mobilized to enact findings and recommendations. A provider motivated to do more for LGBT health can do little with insufficient funding or a hostile or indifferent environment. A client can't seek health services that don't exist, or he or she is less willing to do so if he or she has either experienced stigma or anticipates a stigmatizing environment. For these reasons, advocates have advanced guidelines and standards of care for LGBT people, including provider guidelines from the U.S. Gay and Lesbian Medical Association and the seminal transgender standards of care from the World Professional Association for Transgender Health (formerly the Harry Benjamin International Gender Dysphoria Association). At their most basic, these guidelines encourage providers to promote open, honest, and trusting relationships with LGBT individuals that facilitate optimal delivery of care and services. Recommendations include (1) *the creation of a welcoming environment*, including provider participation in LGBT referral programs and displays of media, brochures, and a nondiscrimination policy inclusive of sexual orientation and gender identity/expression in a multicultural context; (2) *use of inclusive forms, languages, and discussions* that does not assume the individual's identity, orientation, behavior, and relationship status; (3) *development of a written confidentiality policy* that outlines the types of information collected and how that information is protected and shared; and (4) *training and evaluation of staff* to maintain standards of respect, sensitivity, and confidentiality toward LGBT patients, clients, and personnel. Given the ubiquitous and diverse nature of LGBT populations and their varied health concerns, it is incumbent on the ethical health professional to anticipate and prepare for the presence of sexual minorities, remaining especially sensitive to the ways LGBT people may have experienced prior discrimination and trauma from the health care system.

Methodologies

Until very recently, little research specifically detailing LGBT health issues existed, as social stigma discouraged scientific careers dedicated to LGBT health, the allocation of resources, and the publication of findings in reputable sources. This maintained a cycle of silence: Without valid information, it was difficult to demonstrate need; with no demonstrated need, it was difficult to justify LGBT research.

Beginning in the early 1980s, with the advent of HIV/AIDS primarily among white, middle-class, gay-identified men in the United States and western Europe, LGBT individuals began to organize themselves into groups, such as the AIDS Coalition to Unleash Power, to protest seeming government indifference to this emerging epidemic. These actions spurred revolutionary changes in institutional research protocols, including improved access to clinical trials and faster approval of new treatments. As research agendas began to focus on HIV risks among men who have sex with men and other sexual minorities (albeit more slowly and to a lesser degree), government and academia established collaborative partnerships with community-based LGBT organizations, such as Gay Men's Health Crisis in New York City and the Howard Brown Health Center in Chicago. Over the succeeding 25 years, this catalyzed the development of a research infrastructure more amenable to address LGBT health issues than at any other time in history.

While HIV/AIDS remains one of the most widely studied health concerns among these populations, the field of research in LGBT health has expanded in breadth and depth to encompass the social, behavioral, biomedical, and policy dimensions across a wide range of issues. This diversity presents numerous ethical and methodological challenges that, in turn, provide rich opportunities for innovation, discussion, and refinement. Alluding to the complexities described previously, it is essential that researchers clarify terms during the collection, analysis, and reporting of data regarding sexual and gender orientations, identities, and behaviors. For example, behavioral risk surveys that ask "Are you a lesbian?" potentially miss same-sex behavior unless the question "Do you have sex with men, women, or both?" is specifically asked, and this same survey may miss past experience unless a time frame is specifically assigned. A form that provides only for "male" or "female" gender identities, or allows descriptions of relationship status based on heterosexual concepts of marriage, fails to capture potentially relevant data and tacitly devalues the contributions of LGBT participants.

Social stigma and the relatively small numbers of LGBT people create difficulties when data are collected using traditional probability sampling methods such as random household- or telephone-based surveys. Individuals may be reluctant disclosing such personal information when other household members may be present or they may not trust the researchers, potentially providing biased, unreliable responses. Additionally, securing a representative, statistically significant sample size may prove expensive. Consequently, LGBT research has historically relied on samples of convenience, using targeted, venue-based, or snowball sampling methods that are nonrandom and therefore difficult to generalize to the larger populations of interest. These limitations have led to the development of time-space (or time-location) sampling and respondent-driven sampling, two probability sampling methods specifically designed to reach hidden or rare populations.

Many advocates recommend a participatory research model (also known as participatory action research) that involves LGBT community members themselves in the development, implementation, and analysis of research conducted on these populations. The traditional researcher enters into a partnership with diverse representatives of the populations of interest, who work together to identify the research question, develop and implement the research plan, collect and analyze data, and disseminate results, including among the populations under investigation. In turn, the research partnership serves to educate and empower participating communities, as the experience builds capacity among community members and findings help guide policies, programs, and further research. As outlined in the 2007 groundbreaking text, *The Health of Sexual Minorities*, one such model is Fenway Community Health, a comprehensive, community-based health center that integrates care, education, and research for lesbian, gay, bisexual, and transgender populations throughout the greater Boston area.

—*Carey V. Johnson and*
Matthew J. Mimiaga

See also Community-Based Participatory Research; Ethics in Health Care; Ethics in Public Health; Health Disparities; HIV/AIDS

Further Readings

Conway, L. (2002, December). *How frequently does transsexualism occur?* Retrieved February 11, 2007, from http://www.lynnconway.com.

Dean, L., Meyer, I. H., Robinson, K., Sell, R. L., Sember, R., Silenzio, V. M. B., et al. (2000). Lesbian, gay, bisexual, and transgender health: Findings and concerns. *Journal of the Gay and Lesbian Medical Association, 4,* 102–151.

Dunn, P., Scout, W. J., & Taylor, J. S. (Eds.). (2005). *Guidelines for care of lesbian, gay, bisexual and transgender patients.* San Francisco: Gay and Lesbian Medical Association.

Gay and Lesbian Medical Association and LGBT Health Experts. (2001). *Healthy People 2010 companion document for lesbian, gay, bisexual and transgender (LGBT) health.* Retrieved January 24, 2007, from http://www.glma.org/_data/n_0001/resources/live/HealthyCompanionDoc3.pdf.

Gross, M. (Ed.). (2003). Special issue devoted to lesbian, gay, bisexual and transgender public health. *American Journal of Public Health, 93,* 857–1012.

Harry Benjamin International Gender Dysphoria Association. (2001). *The standards of care for gender identity disorders* (6th version). Düsseldorf, Germany: Symposium Publishing.

Laumann, E. O., Gagnon, J., Michael, R. T., & Michaels, S. (1994). *The social organization of sexuality: Sexual practices in the United States.* Chicago: University of Chicago Press.

Meyer, I. H. (Ed.). (2001). Special issue devoted to lesbian, gay, bisexual, and transgender public health. *American Journal of Public Health, 91,* 856–991.

Meyer, I. H., & Northridge, M. E. (Eds.). (2007). *The health of sexual minorities.* New York: Springer.

Solarz, A. (Ed.). (1999). *Lesbian health: Current assessment and directions for the future.* Washington, DC: National Academy Press.

U.S. Department of Health and Human Services. (2000). *Healthy People 2010: Understanding and improving health* (2nd ed.). Washington, DC: Government Printing Office.

Weitze, C., & Osburg, S. (1996). Transsexualism in Germany: Empirical data on epidemiology and application of the German Transsexuals' Act during its first ten years. *Archives of Sexual Behavior, 25,* 409–425.

SEXUAL RISK BEHAVIOR

Sexual risk behaviors constitute a range of sexual actions that increase individuals' risk for bacterial and viral sexually transmitted infections (STIs), including the human immunodeficiency virus (HIV), and for unintended pregnancy. Increased sexual risk results from a combination of the specific sexual behavior and the level of protective action used. Contextual factors, such as drug and alcohol use, can also influence the level of risk involved. While abstinence and autoeroticism are the only truly effective methods of preventing unintended pregnancy and STIs, various risk-reduction strategies exist. Ultimately, sexual behaviors fall on a risk continuum, which depends on the sexual behavior and the protective action employed.

Sexual Behaviors and Associated Risk

Sexual behaviors comprise a wide array of acts ranging from minimal contact to penetration. Abstinence from vaginal intercourse is the only completely effective method for preventing unintended pregnancy. Abstinence from oral, vaginal, and anal intercourse, as well as autoeroticism (otherwise known as masturbation)—fulfilling individual sexual needs without a partner—is the only truly effective means for preventing STIs. When more than one individual is involved in a sexual act, sexual behaviors fall along a continuum of risk. At the low end of the risk continuum are behaviors that consist of minimal physical contact, including kissing, frottage (rubbing against the body of another individual), and fondling.

Oral sex, the act of orally stimulating the penis, vagina, or the anus (termed anilingus or rimming), is toward the middle of the risk continuum when no barrier method is used. While the risk for STI transmission during oral sex is lower than the risk associated with vaginal or anal sex, the risk is still present. The theoretical risk of STI transmission from *oral-penile* contact is present due to infected preejaculate or semen, penile fissures, open sores on the penis, bleeding gums, or open sores in the mouth. The theoretical risk from *oral-vaginal* contact is present due to infected vaginal fluid or blood from menstruation, open sores in the vulva or vagina, or bleeding gums or open sores in the mouth. The theoretical risk from *oral-anal* contact is present due to infected blood in fecal matter, anal fissures, open sores in the anal area, or if infected blood from the mouth enters the rectal lining.

Vaginal-penile intercourse is at the high end of the risk continuum when no barrier method is used. The consequences of unprotected vaginal intercourse include STIs, including HIV, and unintended pregnancy. The risk of HIV transmission from unprotected vaginal intercourse is present for either partner due to infected semen, infected vaginal fluid or menstrual blood, or open sores in the vulva or vagina. STI transmission also occurs through these pathways; however, certain STIs can be transmitted solely through contact with mucosal surfaces or infected skin.

While unprotected insertive anal intercourse is at the high end of the risk continuum, the riskiest sexual behavior is unprotected receptive anal intercourse. The risk consequences of unprotected anal intercourse are HIV and other STIs. The risk of infection is present in methods used without a barrier due to infected semen (including preejaculate), open sores in the anus, or tears in the lining of the anus.

Factors That Increase Sexual Risk

Several factors can place individuals at increased risk for the consequences of sexual behaviors, including substance use and sex with multiple or anonymous partners.

Individuals who use substances (including drugs and/or alcohol) prior to and/or during sexual activity place themselves at higher risk for engaging in sexual behaviors that may expose them to HIV and other STIs, including abandoning barrier methods. Furthermore, individuals addicted to mood-altering substances may trade sexual acts for money or drugs, increasing the associated risks.

Having multiple sexual partners also increases the risk for consequences associated with sexual behaviors because it increases the likelihood of having a sexual encounter with an infected partner. This is also the case for individuals having sexual relations with anonymous partners or partners with unknown STI status without protection.

Prevalence of Sexual Risk Behaviors

Although various studies have examined sexual risk behaviors, the definitions and questions used to measure these behaviors have been inconsistent. Furthermore, nationally representative studies are dated. These issues make it difficult to assess prevalence on a national level and to ascertain how pervasive the problem currently is. The lack of such data may be partly attributable to the difficulty in defining and measuring these behaviors due to the sensitive nature of the topic.

Prevalence data on sexual risk behaviors have focused less on the general adult population and more so on specific populations, including men who have sex with men (MSM) and adolescents. National-level data from the United States have estimated the prevalence of alcohol and/or drug use directly prior to sexual encounters at, on average, between 52% and 85% among MSM and between 20% and 31% among high school students. Additionally, having multiple sexual partners (operationalized differently in different studies) has been estimated at 11% for the general population of adults, between 26% and 50% for MSM, and 14% for high school students. Finally, the estimated prevalence of condom use at last sexual intercourse has been estimated to be between 19% and 62% in the general adult population (dependent on level of commitment with the sexual partner), 55% to 77% of MSM living in urban areas, and 51% to 65% of sexually active high school students. It is important to note that these assessments include individuals involved in mutually exclusive relationships.

Physical Consequences of Sexual Risk Behavior

The physical consequences of unprotected vaginal intercourse are unintended pregnancy and the transmission of STIs. The consequences of unprotected oral and anal intercourse are STIs, which can be either bacterial or viral. Bacterial STIs can be both treated and cured. The most common bacterial STIs in the United States include bacterial vaginosis, chlamydia, gonorrhea, pelvic inflammatory disease, syphilis, and trichomoniasis.

Viral STIs can be treated but are incurable. Once infected with a viral STI, an individual will always be infected, and although they are not always symptomatic, they always remain at risk for infecting others. The most common viral STIs in the United States include HIV; herpes simplex viruses type 1 and type 2; hepatitis A, B, and C; and human papillomavirus (also known as genital warts).

Risk Reduction

For sexually active individuals, various methods exist to reduce risk associated with sexual behavior, including physical barrier methods, chemical methods, and monogamy. Physical barrier methods to prevent pregnancy and STIs include male condoms and female condoms. When used correctly (i.e., using a new condom for each sexual encounter) and consistently, male latex condoms have been demonstrated to be a highly effective form of protection against unintended pregnancy and HIV. Condoms have also been shown to provide high levels of protection against some STIs, including gonorrhea, chlamydia, and trichomoniasis. Condoms afford less protection against genital ulcer STIs, including herpes, chancroid, and syphilis, because they may be transmitted via contact with mucosal surfaces or infected skin not covered by a condom.

For individuals with allergies to latex, male condoms are also manufactured in polyurethane. These condoms have also been shown to be highly effective in preventing unintended pregnancy, HIV, and other STIs. However, the breakage and slippage rate among polyurethane male condoms has been shown to be significantly higher, making them a slightly inferior physical barrier method.

Natural skin condoms, which are made out of animal tissue, have been shown to be effective in preventing unintended pregnancy but not in preventing HIV or other STIs. Because these condoms are made of animal membrane, they may be porous, potentially allowing viruses to pass through.

The female condom is another form of physical barrier method that is manufactured out of polyurethane. These condoms line the vagina to form a protective barrier to prevent STI acquisition and unintended pregnancy. The female condom may also be placed on the penis for use as a barrier method during vaginal or anal sex. The female condom has been shown to be as effective as male condoms in preventing unintended pregnancy and the transmission of HIV and other STIs.

For additional protection, condoms may be used with chemical barriers such as spermicide, a chemical agent that immobilizes sperm to prevent pregnancy, and/or microbicide, a chemical agent that prevents the transmission of HIV and other STIs. Nonoxynol-9, a spermicide that has in vitro activity against some STIs, is the active ingredient in the majority of over-the-counter contraceptive products. Research has demonstrated that Nonoxynol-9 is not effective alone as a preventive method for STIs. Furthermore, some evidence has shown that repeated use can create genital or anal lesions, thereby increasing the risk of STI acquisition.

A third method for risk reduction is mutual monogamy, when sexual partners only have sexual relations with one another. Because having sexual encounters with multiple partners dramatically increases the risk for STI transmission, mutual monogamy can eliminate the risk, if both partners are uninfected.

—Margie Skeer and Matthew J. Mimiaga

See also HIV/AIDS; Partner Notification; Sexually Transmitted Diseases

Further Readings

Centers for Disease Control and Prevention. (2000). *HIV/ AIDS update: Preventing the sexual transmission of HIV, the virus that causes AIDS: What you should know about oral sex.* Retrieved June 20, 2006, from http:// www.cdcnpin.org/Updates/oralsex.pdf.

Centers for Disease Control and Prevention. (2001). Prevalence of risk behaviors for HIV infection among adults: United States, 1997. *Morbidity and Mortality Weekly Report, 50,* 262–265.

Centers for Disease Control and Prevention. (2002). Trends in sexual risk behaviors among high school students: United States, 1991–2001. *Morbidity and Mortality Weekly Report, 51,* 856–859.

Holmes, K. K., Levine, R., & Weaver, M. (2004). Effectiveness of condoms in preventing sexually transmitted infections. *Bulletin of the World Health Organization, 82,* 454–461.

Minnis, A. M., & Padian, N. S. (2005). Effectiveness of female controlled barrier methods in preventing sexually transmitted infections and HIV: Current evidence and

future research directions. *Sexually Transmitted Infections, 81,* 193–200.

Van Damme, L. (2004). Clinical microbicide research: An overview. *Tropical Medicine and International Health, 9,* 1290–1296.

SF-36® HEALTH SURVEY

The SF-36® Health Survey is a 36-item questionnaire used to assess patient-reported health-related quality-of-life outcomes. The SF-36® Health Survey measures eight domains of health:

1. Physical functioning
2. Role-Physical
3. Bodily pain
4. General health
5. Vitality
6. Social functioning
7. Role-Emotional
8. Mental health

It yields an eight-scale profile of norm-based scores (one for each of the eight domains of health) as well as physical and mental health component summary scores, a self-reported health transition rating, a response consistency index (RCI), and a preference-based health utility index (SF-6D).

The SF-36® Health Survey is a generic measure proven to be useful for comparing general and specific populations, comparing the relative burden of diseases, differentiating the health benefits produced by a wide range of different treatments, screening individual patients, and predicting health care costs, mortality, and other important outcomes. Adapted for use in more than 90 country/language versions, it is available in standard (4-week recall) or acute (1-week recall) forms. It has been successfully administered to persons 14 years and older using self-administration by paper and pencil, Internet, telephone, interactive voice response, and personal digital assistant, as well as interviewer-administered forms. Cited in more than 7,500 publications, including approximately 1,000 published randomized clinical trials, the SF-36® Health Survey is part of the "SF (or short-form) family" of instruments representing an international benchmark for health outcomes measurement generally accepted by the Food and Drug Administration as valid measures of health outcomes that can be used in clinical studies.

Background

With roots in the landmark Health Insurance Experiment (HIE) and Medical Outcomes Study (MOS), the SF-36® Health Survey was constructed to be a comprehensive yet practical measure that achieves reductions in response burden without sacrificing psychometric standards of reliability, validity, and measurement precision.

The HIE's main goal was to construct the best possible scales for measuring a broad array of functional status and well-being concepts for group-level longitudinal analyses of data from children and adults. Results from data collected between 1974 and 1981 clearly demonstrated the potential of scales constructed from self-administered surveys to be reliable and valid tools yielding high-quality data for assessing changes in health status in the general population.

The MOS was a 4-year longitudinal observational study from 1986 through 1990 of the variations in practice styles and of health outcomes for more than 23,000 chronically ill patients. It provided a large-scale test of the feasibility of self-administered patient questionnaires and generic health scales among adults with chronic conditions, including the elderly, and attempted to answer two questions resulting from the HIE: (1) Could methods of data collection and scale construction such as those used in the HIE work in sicker and older populations? (2) Can more efficient scales be constructed?

The eight health domains represented in the SF profile were selected from 40 domains that were included in the MOS. The health domains chosen represented those most frequently measured in widely used health surveys and believed to be most affected by disease and health conditions. The SF-36® Health Survey was first made available in "developmental" form in 1988 and released in final original form in 1990 by its principal developer, John E. Ware Jr., Ph.D.

In 1991, the SF-36® Health Survey was selected for the International Quality of Life Assessment (IQOLA) Project, an organized effort to expand the use of health status instruments worldwide. The goal was to develop validated translations of a single health status questionnaire that could be used in multinational clinical studies and other international studies of health. By 1993, 14 countries were represented in the IQOLA Project. Interest in developing translations of the tool continued such that it had been translated for use in more than 90 country/language versions by 2006.

SF-36® Health Survey (Version 2)

Although the original SF-36® Health Survey form proved to be useful for many purposes, 10 years of experience revealed the potential for improvements. A need to improve item wording and response choices identified through the IQOLA Project, as well as a need to update normative data, led to development of the SF-36® Health Survey (Version 2).

In 1998, the SF-36® Health Survey (Version 2) was made available with the following improvements: (1) improved instructions and item wording; (2) improved layout of questions and answers; (3) increased comparability in relation to translations and cultural adaptations, and minimized ambiguity and bias in wording; (4) five-level response options in place of dichotomous choices for seven items in the Role-Physical and Role-Emotional scales; and (5) simplified response options for the Mental Health and Vitality scales. Without increasing the number of questions, improvements make the survey easier to understand and complete and substantially increase the reliability and validity of scores over a wider range, thereby reducing the extent of floor and ceiling effects in the role performance scales.

The SF-36® Health Survey (Version 2) is part of the "SF family" of patient-reported outcomes measures for adults—including the SF-8™ Health Survey, SF-12® Health Survey, SF-12® Health Survey (Version 2), SF-36® Health Survey, and DYNHA® Generic Health Assessment (a dynamic or "computerized adaptive" instrument)—which are all cross-calibrated and scored on the same norm-based metric to maximize their comparability.

Scales and Component Summaries

Physical Functioning (PF)

The content of the 10-item PF scale reflects the importance of distinct aspects of physical functioning and the necessity of sampling a range of severe and minor physical limitations. Items represent levels and kinds of limitations between the extremes of physical activities, including lifting and carrying groceries; climbing stairs; bending, kneeling, or stooping; and walking moderate distances. One self-care item is included. The PF items capture both the presence and extent of physical limitations using a three-level response continuum.

Role-Physical (RP)

The four-item RP scale covers an array of physical-health-related role limitations in the kind and amount of time spent on work, difficulties performing work, and level of accomplishment associated with work or other usual activities.

Bodily Pain (BP)

The BP scale is composed of two items: one pertaining to the intensity of bodily pain and one measuring the extent of interference with normal work activities due to pain.

General Health (GH)

The GH scale consists of five items, including a general rating of health ("excellent" to "poor") and four items addressing the respondent's views and expectations of his or her health.

Vitality (VT)

This four-item measure of vitality was developed to capture ratings of energy level and fatigue.

Social Functioning (SF)

This two-item scale measures the effects of health on quantity and quality of social activities and, specifically, the impact of either physical or emotional problems on social activities.

Role-Emotional (RE)

The three-item RE scale covers mental-health-related role limitations assessing time spent on, level of accomplishment associated with, and level of care in performing work or other usual activities.

Mental Health (MH)

The five-item scale includes one or more items from each of four major mental health dimensions (anxiety,

depression, loss of behavioral/emotional control, and psychological well-being).

Reported Health Transition (HT)

The survey includes a general health item that requires respondents to rate the amount of change they experienced in their health in general over a 1-year period. This item is not used to score any of the eight multi-item scales or component summary measures but provides information about perceived changes in health status that occurred during the year prior to the survey administration.

Physical and Mental Component Summary (PCS and MCS)

The aggregate of the scales is referred to as "component" summaries because the scales were derived and scored using principal components analysis. Although they reflect two broad components or aspects of health—physical and mental—*all* the eight scales are used to score *both* component summary measures.

All items, scales, and summary measures are scored so that a higher score indicates a better health state.

Norm-Based Scoring

The SF-36® Health Survey originally produced eight scales with scores ranging from 0 to 100 and norm-based PCS and MCS scores. The improved SF-36® Health Survey (Version 2) produces norm-based scores for all eight scales and the two component summaries, easing interpretation and score comparability.

Norm-based scoring linearly transforms the scales and summary measures to have a mean of 50 and a standard deviation of 10 in the 1998 U.S. general population. Thus, scores above and below 50 are above and below the average, respectively, in the 1998 U.S. general population. Also, because the standard deviation is 10, each one-point difference or change in scores has a direct interpretation; that is, it is one tenth of a standard deviation or an effect size of 0.10.

Scoring Software

Scoring instructions for the eight scales, the PCS and MCS measures, the reported HT item, and the optional RCI are published in the *User's Manual for the SF-36® Health Survey (Version 2)*, Second

Edition. QualityMetric offers scoring services for Version 2 and the other SF instruments through the QualityMetric Health Outcomes™ scoring software. Among the features of the software is its ability to remove bias in estimates of scores for those having one or more missing responses and to enable score estimation for virtually all respondents regardless of the amount of missing data. In addition, the scoring software conducts data quality evaluations (i.e., data completeness, responses outside range, response consistency index, percentage of estimable scale scores, item internal consistency, item discriminant validity, scale reliability) and allows users of the SF-36® Health Survey (Versions 1 and 2) to make direct comparisons of scores across data sets that use different versions of the SF surveys and to published norms obtained on either form.

Reliability and Validity

Years of empirical research have demonstrated the reliability and validity of the SF-36® Health Survey, which is summarized in several user's manuals and thousands of articles. For the SF-36® Health Survey (Version 2), this tradition was continued by retaining item content from the original survey, making past empirical work on the reliability and validity of the tool generalizable to the SF-36® Health Survey (Version 2).

Evidence of the survey's internal, alternative forms and test-retest (Version 1) reliability has been documented in peer-reviewed articles and the *User's Manual for the SF-36® Health Survey (Version 2)*, Second Edition. To summarize, internal consistency (Cronbach's alpha) estimates using data from the 1998 U.S. general population ranged from .83 to .95 across the eight scales and summary component measures (internal consistency reliability estimates for the summary components take into account the reliability of and covariances among the scales), all exceeding the recommended minimum standard (.70) for group-level comparison of scores. Overall, reliability estimates for general population subgroups are also favorable and higher for component summary estimates than the eight scales. Studies of the reliability of alternative forms indicate that the SF-36® Health Survey (Version 2) is a comparable yet improved version of the original. Correlations (ranging from .76 to .93) between scales and related DYNHA domain item banks corrected for item overlap provide further evidence of alternative forms' reliability. Formal studies

of the test-retest reliability of the SF-36® Health Survey (Version 2) have not yet been conducted, but studies of the original tool's scales indicate reliability that exceeds the recommended standard for measures used in group comparisons. Because four of the scales were improved and the other four scales remained unchanged during the development of the SF-36® Health Survey (Version 2), reliability estimates reported in the original tool's studies may be interpreted as representing the lower limits of scale reliabilities for the SF-36® Health Survey (Version 2).

Evidence of the tool's *construct validity* has been documented in studies involving factor analysis, item-scale correlations, interscale correlations, correlations of the scales with the component summary measures and the SF-6D, and known-groups comparisons. *Criterion validity* has been demonstrated through the correlations of each scale with the theta score for its associated DYNHA® item bank. Data on the likelihood of future events (e.g., job loss, psychiatric treatment) based on scale score ranges also provide evidence of criterion validity. *Content validity* has been shown through a comparison of the SF-36® Health Survey's (Version 2) coverage of health domains to the health domain coverage of other general health surveys. The validity of the tool is fully documented in the *User's Manual for the SF-36® Health Survey (Version 2)*, Second Edition, and further documented in peer-reviewed articles by the developer and in numerous studies from the research literature (Versions 1 and 2).

Interpretation

Generally, interpretation of the SF-36® Health Survey's profile begins by determining if the norm-based scores for the PCS and MCS measures deviate from what is considered the "average" range for the general U.S. population. This is followed by an examination of the scale scores to make a similar determination. Each of these decisions is based on separate, empirically based individual patient- and group-level guidelines. Unlike previous presentations of the SF profile, the current profile now begins with a presentation of the results of the PCS and MCS measures, emphasizing the importance of first considering findings from these more general measures of health status (see Figure 1). It also facilitates interpretation by immediately establishing what the general burden of illness or effects of treatment are (i.e., physical or mental) before examining the more specific scales. As

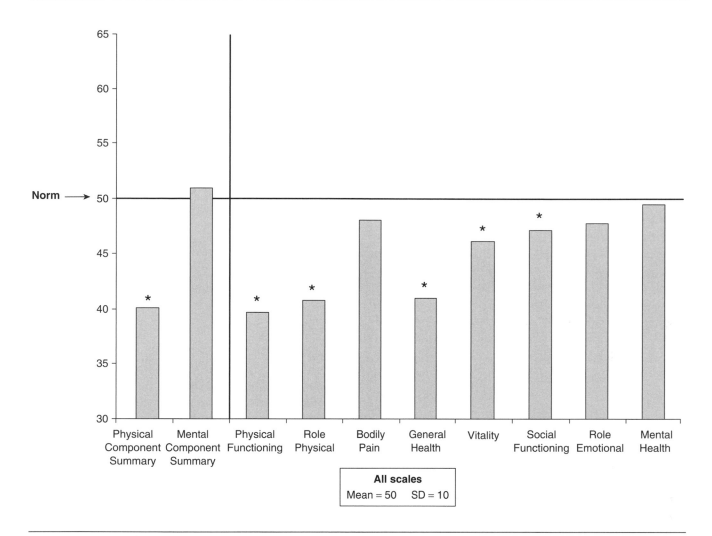

Figure 1   SF-36® Health Survey Profile of Norm-Based Scores (Adult Asthma Sample)

Source: Adapted from Okamoto, Noonan, DeBoisblanc, and Kellerman (1996).

Note: Norm significantly higher.

their labels suggest, the PCS and MCS scores provide a summary of the respondent's health status from both a broad physical health perspective and a broad mental health perspective, respectively.

In addition, the application of measure- or scale-specific standard errors of measurement allows one to determine, within specific levels of confidence, intervals in which the respondent's true score on every measure and scale falls. Guidelines for interpreting high and low scores on the PCS and MCS measures and on each scale, guidelines for determining the minimally important difference, score cutoffs for determining the likelihood of the presence of a physical or mental disorder, and U.S. general population norms

for age, gender, age-by-gender, and combined groups for both the standard and acute forms are provided in the *User's Manual for the SF-36® Health Survey (Version 2)*, Second Edition.

Applications

Applications of the SF-36® Health Survey (Versions 1 and 2) include the following:

- Clinic-based evaluation and monitoring of individual patients
- Population monitoring

- Estimating the burden of disease (by standardizing questions, answers, and scoring, reliable and valid comparisons can be made to determine the relative burden of different conditions in several domains of health)
- Evaluating treatment effects in clinical trials
- Disease management and risk prediction (i.e., the ability to predict health outcomes, hospitalization, future medical expenditures, resource use, job loss and work productivity, future health, risk of depression, use of mental health care, future health, and mortality)
- Cost effectiveness
- Enhancing patient-provider relations
- Providing direct-to-consumer information (i.e., educating the public about medical conditions, their symptoms and effects, and potential treatment options; prompting recognition or detection of personal health problems that may benefit from clinical consultation, thereby encouraging more appropriate care seeking, case finding, and physician-patient dialogue; and promoting self-care and compliance with treatment regimens)

—Diane M. Turner-Bowker,
Michael A. DeRosa, and John E. Ware Jr.

Note: Joint copyright for the SF-36® Health Survey, SF-36® Health Survey (Version 2), SF-12® Health Survey, SF-12® Health Survey (Version 2), and SF-8® Health Survey is held by QualityMetric Incorporated (QM), Medical Outcomes Trust, and Health Assessment Lab. Licensing information for SF-tools is available from www.qualitymetric.com/products/license. Those conducting unfunded academic research or grant-funded projects may qualify for a discounted license agreement through QM's academic research program, the Office of Grants and Scholarly Research.

SF-36® and SF-12® are registered trademarks of Medical Outcomes Trust. DYNHA® is a registered trademark, and SF-8® and QualityMetric Health Outcomes® are trademarks of QualityMetric Incorporated.

See also Functional Status; Global Burden of Disease Project; Measurement; Missing Data Methods; Quality of Life, Quantification of

Further Readings

Gandek, B., & Ware, J. E., Jr. (Eds.). (1998). Translating functional health and well-being: International quality of life assessment (IQOLA) project studies of the SF-36 Health Survey [Special issue]. *Journal of Clinical Epidemiology, 51*(11).

Okamoto, L. J., Noonan, M., DeBoisblanc, B. P., & Kellerman, D. J. (1996). Fluticasonepropionate improves quality of life in patients with asthma requiring oral corticosteroids. *Annals of Allergy, Asthma and Immunology, 76,* 455–461.

Ware, J. E., Jr. (2000). SF-36 Health Survey update. *Spine, 25,* 3130–3139.

Ware, J. E., Jr., & Kosinski, M. (2001). *SF-36 Physical & Mental Health Summary Scales: A manual for users of version 1* (2nd ed.). Lincoln, RI: QualityMetric.

Ware, J. E., Jr., Kosinski, M., Bjorner, J. B., Turner-Bowker, D. M., & Maruish, M. E. (2006). *User's manual for the SF-36® Health Survey (Version 2)* (2nd ed.). Lincoln, RI: QualityMetric.

Ware, J. E., Jr., & Sherbourne, C. D. (1992). The MOS 36-Item Short-Form Health Survey (SF-36). I. Conceptual framework and item selection. *Medical Care, 30,* 473–483.

Ware, J. E., Jr., Snow, K. K., Kosinski, M., & Gandek, B. (1993). *SF-36® Health Survey: Manual and interpretation guide.* Boston: Health Institute.

Web Sites

Further information about tools from the SF family of instruments is available from http:// www.qualitymetric.com or http://www.sf36.org.

The sf36.org Web site is a community forum for users of the SF tools and offers news, events, online discussion, and a searchable database of SF publications.

SICK BUILDING SYNDROME

Sick building syndrome (SBS) is a term applied to a situation in which some or all the people occupying a building (usually working or living in it) experience unpleasant health and comfort effects such as headache; dizziness; nausea; irritated eyes, nose, or throat; dry cough; or skin irritation. The term is sometimes applied to the symptoms themselves also. These effects may be localized to a part of the building or be present throughout. The definition of SBS requires that the symptoms disappear soon after leaving the building and that they cannot be ascribed to a specific cause or illness. SBS is differentiated from building-related illness, which describes diagnosable illness whose cause can be attributed to airborne contaminants within a building. SBS is usually assumed to be caused by poor indoor air quality (IAQ). It was first identified in the 1970s, and a 1984 report by the World Health Organization suggested that up to 30% of new and remodeled buildings may have problems with IAQ sufficient to cause health symptoms. Inadequate building ventilation is the most common cause; the appearance of SBS in the mid-1970s has often been attributed to decreased ventilation standards for commercial buildings to increase energy efficiency during the oil embargo of 1973. Chemical contaminants are also potential contributors to SBS; these include volatile organic compounds emitted by carpeting, upholstery, cleaning agents, and other sources and combustion products including particulate matter and carbon monoxide produced from heating devices such as fireplaces and stoves. Biological contaminants such as molds, pollen, viruses, bacteria, and animal or bird droppings can also contribute to SBS.

Investigation of SBS requires first ascertaining whether the complaints are actually due to IAQ; if so, the investigation will gather information about the building's ventilation, heating and air conditioning system, possible sources of internal contaminants, and possible pathways for exterior pollutants to enter the building. Air sampling alone rarely provides sufficient information to solve the problem, because in SBS buildings contaminant concentration levels rarely exceed existing standards. The most common solutions to SBS include removing a known source of pollution, increasing ventilation rates and air distribution, and adding air cleaning devices.

SBS is a difficult condition to study because its symptoms are commonplace and could have many causes, such as allergies or stress, and may be influenced by psychological factors, such as dislike of a job or workplace. In addition, because many different aspects of the indoor environment can contribute to SBS, it is often difficult to identify the cause or causes for a particular case, and extensive renovations may fail to solve the problem. There is also a natural opposition between the interests of building owners and occupants in a case of suspected SBS. The occupants may believe SBS is causing their health symptoms and demand building inspections and modifications, while the owner may not believe that the building is the cause of their symptoms and may therefore be reluctant to pay for any inspections or alterations. Because of the aforementioned difficulties in verifying SBS and identifying its cause, the "truth of the matter" may never be unequivocally determined. In addition, some clinicians believe that SBS is not a meaningful term and should be abandoned, while others have argued that investigations into SBS should include evaluation of psychological and social as well as physical, environmental, and biomedical factors.

—*Sarah Boslaugh*

See also Environmental and Occupational Epidemiology; Pollution

Further Readings

Stenberg, B., & Wall, S. (1995). Why do women report "sick building symptoms" more often than men? *Social Science and Medicine, 40*, 491–502.

Thorn, A. (1998). The sick building syndrome: A diagnostic dilemma. *Social Science and Medicine, 47*, 1307–1312.

U.S. Environmental Protection Agency. (n.d.). *Indoor air facts no. 4 (revised): Sick building syndrome (SBS)*. Retrieved August 9, 2007, from http://www.epa.gov/iaq/pubs/sbs.html.

SIGNIFICANCE TESTING

See HYPOTHESIS TESTING

SIMPSON'S PARADOX

Simpson's paradox is an extreme form of confounding, where the association between two variables in a full group is in the opposite direction of the association found within every subcategory of a third variable. This paradox was first described by G. U. Yule in 1903 and later developed and popularized by E. H. Simpson in 1951.

By way of example, consider a new drug treatment that initially appears to be effective, with 54% of treated patients recovering, as compared with 46% of patients receiving a placebo. However, when the sample is divided by gender, it is found that 20% of treated males recover compared with 25% of placebo males, and 75% of treated females recover as compared with 80% of placebo females. So the apparent paradox is that the drug is found to be more effective than the placebo in the full group but less effective than the placebo in each of the two gender-specific subgroups that fully comprise the combined group.

The key to unraveling this puzzle involves the gender confound—differing numbers of patients of each gender receiving the treatment versus placebo, combined with differing overall recovery rates for males versus females. Table 1 shows that in this example males are 1.6 times more likely to receive the placebo than the treatment, whereas females are 1.6 times

Table 1 Recovery Rates

	Treatment	Placebo
Male	10/50 (20%)	20/80 (25%)
Female	60/80 (75%)	40/50 (80%)
All patients	70/130 (54%)	60/130 (46%)

more likely to receive the treatment than the placebo. At the same time, females are more than three times as likely to recover as males within both the treatment group and the placebo group. In other words, females are relatively easy to cure. So the fact that the placebo is more effective than the treatment in both groups is obscured when the groups are combined, due to the disproportionate number of easy-to-cure females in the treatment group.

In this particular example, it would be commonly agreed that the correct conclusion involves the subgroup-specific results—the drug is not effective—and that the apparent effectiveness found in the combined group is merely a statistical artifact of the study design due to the gender confound.

Simpson's paradox can be problematic when not recognized, leading to naive and misleading conclusions regarding effectiveness or other relations studied. Perhaps more ominously, knowledge of Simpson's paradox can be intentionally used to present or emphasize results that support a desired conclusion, when that conclusion is not valid. More generally, Simpson's paradox has been shown to have implications for the philosophical study of causation and causal inference. In practical terms, it is prudent for both researchers and research consumers to be on guard for this potentially perilous paradox.

—*Norman A. Constantine*

See also Confounding; Ecological Fallacy

Further Readings

Malinas, G., & Bigelow, J. (2004, Spring). Simpson's paradox. In E. N. Zalta (Ed.), *The Stanford encyclopedia of philosophy*. Retrieved August 30, 2006, from http://plato.stanford.edu/archives/spr2004/entries/paradox-simpson.

Reintjes, R., de Boer, A., van Pelt, W., & Mintjes-de Groot, J. (2000). Simpson's paradox: An example from hospital epidemiology. *Epidemiology, 11*, 81–83.

Simpson, E. H. (1951). The interpretation of interaction in contingency tables. *Journal of the Royal Statistical Association, 13*, 238–241.

Wainer, H., & Brown, L. M. (2004). Two statistical paradoxes in the interpretation of group differences: Illustrated with medical school admission and licensing data. *American Statistician, 58*, 117–123.

SKEWNESS

If a person says that there is a car parked "askew" in a lined parking space, then we know the car is not parked straight and is closer to one side than the other. This common usage of the idea of skewness carries over into the statistical definition. If a statistical distribution is skewed, then more of the values appear in one end of the distribution than the other. Skewness, then, is a measure of the degree and direction of asymmetry in a distribution. Skewness is also called the third moment about the mean and is one of the two most common statistics used to describe the shape of a distribution (the other is kurtosis). Skewed distributions have values bunched at one end and values trailing off in the other direction. The most commonly used measure of skewness is the Pearson coefficient of skewness.

There are three types of skewness: right, left, or none. Often, these are referred to as positive, negative, or neutral skewness, respectively. Often, people are confused about what to call the skewness. The name of the type of skewness identifies the direction of the longer tail of a distribution, not the location of the

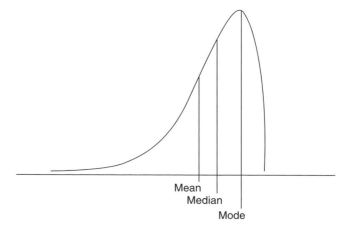

Figure 1 Negatively Skewed Distribution

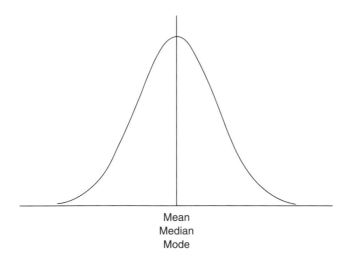

Figure 2   Neutrally Skewed Distribution

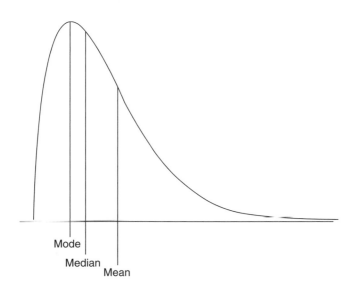

Figure 3   Positively Skewed Distribution

larger group of values. If a distribution is negatively or left skewed, then there are values bunched at the positive or right end of the distribution, and the values at the negative or left end of the distribution have a longer tail. If a distribution is positively or right skewed, then there are values bunched at the negative or left end of the distribution, and the values at the positive or right end have a longer tail.

The most commonly known distributions and their type of skewness are given in Table 1.

Often, skewness is used to help assess whether a distribution being studied meets the normality

Table 1   Common Distributions With Type of Skewness

Distribution	Type of Skewness
Normal	Neutral
Student's t	Neutral
Uniform	Neutral
Exponential	Positive
Laplace	Neutral
Weibull	Depends on the parameter values; may be negative, neutral, or positive

assumptions of most common parametric statistical tests. While the normal distribution has a skewness of 0, it is important to realize that, in practice, the skewness statistic for a sample from the population will not be exactly equal to 0. How far off can the statistic be from 0 and not violate the normality assumption? Provided the statistic is not grossly different from 0, then that decision is up to the researcher and his or her opinion of an acceptable difference. For most typically sized samples, values of the Pearson coefficient of skewness between -3 and $+3$ are considered reasonably close to 0. To accurately measure the skewness of a distribution, sample sizes of several hundred may be needed.

If a researcher determines that the distribution is skewed, then reporting the median rather than or along with the mean provides more information about the central tendency of the data. The mean is sensitive to extreme values (those skewed), while the median is robust (not as sensitive).

—*Stacie Ezelle Taylor*

See also Inferential and Descriptive Statistics; Kurtosis; Measures of Central Tendency; Normal Distribution

Further Readings

Joanes, D. N., & Gill, C. A. (1998). Comparing measures of sample skewness & kurtosis. *Journal of the Royal Statistical Society: Series D (The Statistician), 47,* 183–189.

Keller, D. K. (2006). *The Tao of statistics: A path to understanding (with no math).* Thousand Oaks, CA: Sage.

Sleep Disorders

An estimated 70 million people in the United States suffer from sleep problems, and more than half of those with sleep problems have a sleep disorder that is chronic. The four most prevalent sleep disorders are insomnia, obstructive sleep apnea, narcolepsy, and periodic limb movements in sleep, with sleep apnea accounting for nearly 80% of all sleep diagnoses in sleep centers in the United States. About 30 million American adults have frequent or chronic insomnia. Approximately 18 million have obstructive sleep apnea, but only 10% to 20% have been diagnosed. An estimated 250,000 people have narcolepsy, and more than 5% of adults are affected by periodic limb movements in sleep syndrome. Sleep disorders have major societal impacts. Each year, sleep disorders, sleep deprivation, and excessive daytime sleepiness (EDS) add approximately $16 billion annually to the cost of health care in the United States and result in $50 to $100 billion annually in lost productivity (in 1995 dollars). According to the National Highway Traffic and Safety Administration, 100,000 accidents and 1,500 traffic fatalities per year are related to drowsy driving. Nearly two thirds of older Americans have sleep difficulties, and the prevalence of sleep problems will increase as the older adult population increases. The 1990s has seen a significant increase in our awareness of the importance of diagnosing and treating sleep disorders. The prevalence rates, risk factors, and treatment options will be reviewed for each of the four major sleep disorders.

Insomnia

Insomnia is the most commonly reported sleep complaint across all stages of adulthood. An estimated 30 million American adults suffer from chronic insomnia, and up to 57% of noninstitutionalized elderly experience chronic insomnia. In the United States, total direct costs attributable to insomnia are estimated at $12 billion for health care services and $2 billion for medications. Emerging evidence suggests that being female and old age are two of the more common risk factors for the development of insomnia; other predisposing factors include excess worry about an existing health condition, lower educational level, unemployment, and separation or divorce. Insomnia is comorbid with anxiety and depressive disorders and may lead to the development of psychiatric disorders. Insomnia is correlated with high levels of medical use and increased drug use, as well as increased psychosocial disruption including poor work performance and poor memory.

Insomnia Treatments

Traditional management of insomnia includes both pharmacologic and nonpharmacologic treatments. Current guidelines suggest that chronic insomnia be treated with a combination of nonpharmacologic interventions, such as sleep hygiene training, relaxation training, stimulus control training, cognitive-behavioral therapy, or sleep restriction/sleep consolidation therapy, and pharmacologic interventions. Medications prescribed for insomnia range from newer agents such as zolpidem, zaleplon, and eszoplicone to older agents such as antidepressants (e.g., amitriptyline or trazodone) and benzodiazepines (e.g., clonazepam, lorazepam). Medications are not typically indicated for long-term treatment of insomnia, except for a medication recently approved by the Food and Drug Administration, eszoplicone.

Obstructive Sleep Apnea

Obstructive sleep apnea (OSA) is a medical condition characterized by repeated complete (apnea) or partial (hypopnea) obstructions of the upper airway during sleep. It is prevalent in 2% to 4% of working, middle-aged adults, and an increased prevalence is seen in the elderly ($\sim 24\%$), veterans ($\sim 16\%$), and African Americans. Being an obese male is the number one major risk factor for OSA. The risk of OSA increases significantly with increased weight, and more than 75% of OSA patients are reported to be more than 120% of ideal body weight. Other risk factors that can contribute to OSA include anatomical abnormalities of the upper airway (e.g., large uvula, enlarged tonsils, large neck circumference). Estimates of health care costs for OSA patients are approximately twice that of matched, healthy controls. This cost difference is evident several years prior to the diagnosis. OSA is associated with a higher mortality rate.

Consequences of OSA

OSA is associated with several cardiovascular diseases, most notably hypertension, ischemic heart disease, heart failure, stroke, cardiac arrhythmias, and pulmonary hypertension. Compared with the general population, OSA patients have twice the risk for hypertension, three times the risk for ischemic heart disease, and four times the risk for cerebrovascular disease. The evidence supporting the link between OSA and hypertension is compelling, with OSA now officially recognized as an identifiable cause of hypertension. Alterations in sleep architecture cause sleep to be nonrestorative, resulting in mild to severe EDS. EDS and/or hypoxia due to OSA are associated with a number of neurocognitive, mood, and behavioral consequences, including lowered health-related quality of life, impaired cognitive performance, impaired driving ability (two to seven times increased risk of a motor vehicle accident), dysphoric mood, psychosocial disruption (e.g., more intensely impaired work performance and higher divorce rates), and disrupted sleep and impaired quality of life of spouses of OSA patients.

OSA Treatments

The goals of any OSA treatment are the elimination of breathing events and snoring, maintaining high blood oxygen levels, and improving symptoms. Categories of OSA treatments include medical devices (continuous positive airway pressure therapy and oral appliances), behavioral recommendations (weight loss, positional therapy), and surgical procedures. Nasal continuous positive airway pressure (CPAP) is the treatment of choice for this condition, with meta-analytic reports of numerous randomized controlled trials showing that CPAP improves both objectively and subjectively measured daytime sleepiness as well as health-related quality of life. CPAP has been shown to normalize sleep architecture and reduce blood pressure. Oral appliances (OAs) alter the oral cavity to increase airway size and improve patency. OAs reduce the number of apneas and hypopneas and reduce sleepiness levels. Weight loss helps reduce the number of apneas and hypopneas in obese OSA patients, reduces oxygen desaturations, and improves sleep architecture. Positional therapies, primarily indicated for mild sleep apnea, are based on the observation that most disordered breathing occurs in the supine (i.e., lying on the back) position, so the therapy encourages sleep in the prone (i.e., lying face downward) or side positions. There are a wide variety of surgical treatments that are now considered secondary treatments if other treatments do not work well or are not well tolerated.

Narcolepsy

Narcolepsy is a chronic neurological disorder caused by the brain's inability to regulate sleep-wake cycles normally. It is estimated that approximately 250,000 adult Americans are affected by narcolepsy. Narcolepsy is the most common neurological cause of EDS. Direct medical costs for narcolepsy can cost the patient more than $15,000 per year. The impact of narcolepsy is often more severe than that of other chronic diseases, such as epilepsy. Genetics may play a large role, with first-degree relatives having a 40-fold increased risk for narcolepsy. Men and women appear to be at equal risk.

The two most common symptoms of narcolepsy are EDS and cataplexy. Cataplexy is a sudden loss of muscle tone and strength, usually caused by an extreme emotional stimulus.

Narcoleptic patients also can experience sleep paralysis, falling asleep at inappropriate times (conversations, dinner), psychosocial problems, and EDS. EDS comprises both a strong background feeling of sleepiness and sometimes an irresistible urge to sleep suddenly. These sudden naps associated with narcolepsy can last minutes to an hour and occur a few times each day. Furthermore, as a consequence of EDS, patients with narcolepsy often report problems with inattention, blurred vision, cataplexy, poor memory, and driving without awareness (automatic behaviors).

Narcolepsy Treatments

Because narcolepsy is a chronic condition, treatment focuses on long-term symptom management through medications and behavioral treatments. Medications for treatment of narcolepsy are aimed at managing the daytime symptoms of the disorder. EDS can be reduced by a newer, nonamphetamine "wake promoting agent" named modafinil and by amphetamine derivatives (dexamphetamine, methylphenidate). Side effects from the amphetamine-type drugs are common and include tolerance, irritability, and insomnia. Drugs suppressing rapid eye movement sleep can help in reducing cataplexy; the newest one is xyrem (gamma-hydroxybutyrate). The goals of behavioral therapies are to promote behaviors that can alleviate daytime symptoms. The primary therapy is planned research showing that scheduled daytime naps are effective in helping reduce daytime sleepiness.

Periodic Limb Movements in Sleep

Periodic limb movements in sleep (PLMS) is a sleep phenomenon characterized by periodic episodes of repetitive and highly stereotyped limb movements. Periodic limb movements are defined by their occurrence in a series (four or more) of similar movements with a wide range of periods and duration between 0.5 and 5.0 s. It has been estimated that 5% of those below the age of 50 years will have PLMS, while more than 30% of individuals aged above 65 years may have a significant number of PLMS. PLMS may begin at any age although prevalence increases markedly in elderly healthy people. In patients with periodic limb movement disorder, insomnia and EDS are common complaints. There is significant overlap between PLMS and restless legs syndrome (RLS), with more than 80% of RLS patients having PLMS as well.

PLMS Treatments

Treatment of PLMS consists primarily of pharmacological and secondarily of nonpharmacological interventions. Pharmacological agents recommended for use include dopaminergic agents, anticonvulsants, opioids, and sedatives/hypnotics. Nonpharmacological treatment of PLMS primarily consists of advising the patient of good sleep hygiene.

—*Carl Stepnowsky and Joe Palau*

See also Aging, Epidemiology of; Hypertension; Obesity; Vehicle-Related Injuries

Further Readings

Buscemi, N., Vandermeer, B., Friesen, C., Bialy, L., Tubman, M, Ospina, M., et al. (2005, June). *Manifestations and management of chronic insomnia in adults.* Evidence Report/Technology Assessment No. 125. AHRQ Publication No. 05-E021-2. Rockville, MD: Agency for Healthcare Research and Quality. Retrieved August 9, 2007, from http://www.ahrq.gov/clinic/epcsums/insomnsum.pdf.

Chesson, A. L., Jr., Wise, M., Davila, D., Johnson, S., Littner, M., Anderson, W. M., et al. (1999). Practice parameters for the treatment of restless legs syndrome and periodic limb movement disorder. An American Academy of Sleep Medicine Report. Standards of Practice Committee of the American Academy of Sleep Medicine. *Sleep, 22,* 961–968.

Kushida, C. A., Littner, M. R., Hirshkowitz, M., Morgenthaler, T. I., Alessi, C. A., Bailey, D., et al. (2006). Practice parameters for the use of continuous and bilevel positive airway pressure devices to treat adult patients with sleep-related breathing disorders. *Sleep, 29,* 375–380.

National Center for Sleep Disorders Research and National Highway and Traffic Safety Expert Panel on Driver Fatigue and Sleepiness. (1998). *Drowsy driving and automobile crashes: Report and recommendations.* Washington, DC: Author.

Thorpy, M. (2001). Current concepts in the etiology, diagnosis and treatment of narcolepsy. *Sleep Medicine, 2,* 5–17.

SMALLPOX

Smallpox, a contagious disease produced by the variola virus (genus *Orthopoxvirus*), was eradicated in 1977. The word *smallpox* is believed to come from the Latin word *pocca* meaning "pouch," and *variola* from *varius* or *varus* meaning "spotted pimple." There were three subspecies of variola: variola major, intermedius, and minor. The milder form of the disease, variola minor, had a case-fatality rate of less than 1%, whereas the rate for variola major was 25% to 50%. Ten percent of the smallpox cases involved hemorrhagic smallpox that was quickly fatal.

Smallpox was found only in humans and was usually transmitted through droplet nuclei, dust, and fomites (inanimate objects such as blankets that can transmit germs). The incubation period was between 12 and 14 days, with the respiratory tract as the main site of infection. The prodrome, or early symptom of the development of smallpox, was a distinct febrile illness that occurred 2 to 4 days before eruptive smallpox. Rashes usually developed 2 to 4 days after being infected. The smallpox rash was centrifugal, found more on the head, arms, and legs than on the trunk area of the body. Smallpox was very disfiguring because crusts on the skin would form from the fluid and pus-filled spots on the body. Many who survived smallpox had bad scars on their face or were blinded. Because of the rash that formed in the majority of smallpox cases, surveillance of the disease was less problematic.

Common symptoms of smallpox were fever, headache, backache, malaise, and abdominal pain. The very young and very old were at higher risk of dying of smallpox. Exposure to smallpox usually occurred in either the family or hospital setting. Compared with chickenpox and measles, smallpox was not as infectious. Persons with smallpox were infectious from the time fever arose until the last scab separated; they were not infectious during the incubation period. A patient who survived smallpox was resistant to the infection.

The origin of the smallpox virus is thought to have been 3,000 years ago in India or Egypt. For a very long time, smallpox epidemics were quite common, annihilating populations. Smallpox wreaked havoc on the royal houses of Europe between 1694 and 1774, with Queen Mary II of England, Emperor Joseph I of Austria, King Luis I of Spain, Tsar Peter II of Russia, Queen Ulrike Elenora of Sweden, and King Louis XV of France all dying of the disease. In the 18th century, 1 out of every 10 children born in Sweden and France died from smallpox. Many Native American tribes were annihilated by the smallpox epidemic that occurred around 1837. The Native American tribes were introduced to smallpox through European settlement.

There were a number of ancient practices that were introduced to prevent smallpox. Worshippers could pray to a deity such as the Indian goddess of smallpox, Shitala Mata, or to the Chinese goddess of smallpox, T'ou-Shen Niang-Niang. Roman Catholic Europeans could pray to St. Nicaise, the patron saint of smallpox. There was also a widespread notion that red-colored objects could combat smallpox. The Red Treatment, as it was called, used red objects such as a red cloth hung in a room of smallpox victims in an attempt to prevent smallpox. Another method tried was inoculation of infectious matter from smallpox victims implanted into patients. It was not until 1796 that an English physician by the name of Edward Jenner (1749–1823) discovered a vaccination for smallpox.

Jenner discovered that immunity against smallpox was possible by injection of the cowpox virus into the system. He observed that a patient who had contracted coxpox by milking cows with cowpox lesions on their teats resisted variolation. Milkmaids had scars on their hands from previous cowpox infections, and Jenner noted that these women were immune from developing smallpox. He invented the vaccine and initiated a new field of medicine—preventative medicine. He successfully immunized an 8-year-old boy with a substance that was taken from a cowpox sore on the hand of a milkmaid, Sarah Nelmes. Jenner published his work *An Inquiry into the Causes and Effects of the Variolae Vaccinae, a Disease Known by the Name of Cox Pox* in 1798.

In 1966, the World Health Organization (WHO) led the Smallpox Eradication Program, an intensive effort to eradicate smallpox throughout the world. When the campaign started, smallpox was still found in 41 countries in the world. The eradication program focused on using a standardized vaccine and extensive public education. Furthermore, eradication was facilitated through active surveillance of cases that identified the location of the disease and through attempts to vaccinate all those who were in areas with widespread infection. Advances in technology helped the eradication efforts by making it possible to freeze-dry vaccines so that they did not need to be refrigerated. Other technological advances that aided in the eradication program included adaptation of the jet injector, which allowed for smallpox vaccine to be given intradermally starting in the early 1960s, and the development of the bifurcated needle in 1968.

In 1949, the last case of smallpox occurred in the United States. The last case of naturally occurring smallpox in the world was found in October 1977 in Somalia. Two cases associated with a virologic laboratory were reported in England in 1978. Since then, smallpox has no longer appeared in the world. In May 1980, at the 33rd World Health Assembly, the WHO declared victory in its fight for global eradication of smallpox. Smallpox was the first disease ever to be eradicated by humans.

There is growing concern that smallpox may be used by terrorists as a biologic weapon in warfare. Because of the threat, active duty service members continue to be vaccinated against smallpox. There are two remaining stocks of the smallpox virus: at the Centers for Disease Control and Prevention in Atlanta, Georgia, and at the Institute for Viral Preparations in Moscow, Russia. There is only a limited supply in the world of the smallpox vaccine, which protects against the smallpox virus for 10 years. Given that many of the historical cases of smallpox occurred at a time with significant population immunity from vaccination or having had the virus, the world population today is more susceptible to smallpox. Many countries are considering increasing their supply due to the threat of a biological terrorist attack using smallpox, for which there is no effective treatment.

—Britta Neugaard

See also Bioterrorism; Jenner, Edward; World Health Organization

Further Readings

Bazin, H. (2000). *The eradication of smallpox: Edward Jenner and the first and only eradication of a human infectious disease*. London: Academic Press.

Behbehani, A. M. (1988). *The smallpox story in words and pictures*. Kansas City: University of Kansas Medical Center.

Gorbach, S. L., Bartlett, J. G., & Blacklow, N. R. (Eds.). (2004). *Infectious diseases* (3rd ed.). Philadelphia: Lippincott Williams & Wilkins.

Hoeprich, P. D., Jordan, M. C., & Ronald, A. R. (Eds.). (1994). *Infectious diseases: A treatise of infectious processes* (5th ed.). Philadelphia: Lippincott.

Hopkins, D. R. (1988). Smallpox: Ten years gone. *American Journal of Public Health, 78*, 1589–1595.

SNOW, JOHN
(1813–1858)

John Snow has an unusual place in medical history because he is a seminal figure in two medical disciplines—anesthesiology and epidemiology. His contribution to the first field was to establish the chemical and biological principles underlying the administration of consistent dosages of anesthetic gases effectively and with minimal toxicity. In the latter field, he discovered how cholera—and, by extension, every form of intestinal infection—was transmitted. The process by which he discovered the fecal-oral and waterborne routes of disease communication was the first true model of epidemiologic investigation.

Snow's twin accomplishments were not unrelated. As the world's first practicing anesthesiologist, he was intimately familiar with the effects of gases on human physiology. This understanding made him skeptical of the then-reigning dogma that miasmas—hypothesized gaseous emanations from rotting material that were inhaled—could cause disease at a distance. As so often in science, the first step in developing a new hypothesis was recognition of the limitations of the old.

Snow had cared for cholera patients as a teenage apprentice in 1832. When cholera made its second appearance in Europe in 1848, he published a small pamphlet and a two-page paper on cholera transmission. He argued that cholera was fundamentally a disease of the intestinal system and that its major symptoms were the result of fluid loss. This led him to conclude that the "agent" of cholera was ingested.

He further reasoned, from much circumstantial evidence, that the "agent" was transmitted by accidental soiling of the hands by the colorless evacuations of cholera and that this transmission could be greatly multiplied if the evacuations found their way into water supplies.

The work that most epidemiologists recognize as Snow's signature achievement was undertaken during the third European epidemic, from 1854 to 1855. Snow examined mortality from cholera in two regions of London with overlapping water supplies. One water company (Lambeth) used the rural Thames above London as its source, while the other (Southwark and Vauxhall) took its water from the Thames downstream of the city's sewage effluent. Snow visited hundreds of houses in the region to determine their water supplies, enlisting the help of medical colleagues, including the public health official William Farr, and linking the source of water in each house to the number of deaths from cholera among its residents. He found that in the first weeks of the epidemic, death rates were 14 times higher in houses with water from Southwark and Vauxhall than in houses supplied by Lambeth. He also showed that in a major local outbreak in Soho, the source was almost certainly a shallow well supplying a widely used public pump on Broad Street. He persuaded local officials to remove the pump handle, but by then the outbreak was almost over. The well was later shown to have been fecal contamination from a leak from a nearby cesspool. Decades before the work of Pasteur and Koch, Snow speculated that the cholera "agent" could reproduce, that the duration of reproduction accounted for the incubation period, and that the agent probably had a structure like a cell.

Although to modern readers Snow seems eminently persuasive, his views on cholera were not widely accepted in his day. Cholera investigations later in the century, however, convinced many British and American physicians that water supplies were a central feature of cholera transmission.

—Nigel Paneth

See also Waterborne Diseases

Further Readings

Snow, J. (1848). *On the mode of communication of cholera*. London: Churchill.

Snow, J. (1848). On the pathology and mode of communication of cholera. *London Medical Journal*, 44, 745–752, 923–929.

Snow, J. (1855). *On the mode of communication of cholera* (2nd ed.). London: Churchill.

SOCIAL CAPITAL AND HEALTH

As a possible determinant of population health, social capital has emerged as a topic of growing interest in the epidemiologic literature. Epidemiologic studies have explored the potential protective effects of social capital on a variety of health outcomes. This entry highlights the conceptualization of social capital, hypothesized mechanisms for its health effects, and features of the empirical evidence on the relations between social capital and health to date, including the measurement of social capital.

Conceptualization

Unlike financial capital, which resides in people's banks and in property, and human capital, which is embedded in people's education and job skills, social capital has been conceptualized to exist in people's relations to one another—that is, within social networks.

Conceptualizations of social capital have ranged from definitions focusing on the resources within social networks that can be mobilized for purposeful actions to definitions that encompass both social structures and associated cognitive resources such as trust and reciprocity. In addition to being categorized according to structural and resource characteristics, social capital has been dichotomized into many forms, including formal versus informal social capital (e.g., participation in labor unions vs. family dinners), inward-looking versus outward-looking social capital (e.g., chambers of commerce vs. the Red Cross), and bonding versus bridging social capital.

The distinction between bonding social capital and bridging social capital has probably gained the most prominence in the social capital and health literature. Bonding social capital refers to social capital within relationships between individuals with shared identities such as race/ethnicity and gender, whereas bridging social capital corresponds to social capital in relationships between individuals who are dissimilar.

There is ongoing debate among social capital scholars as to the extent to which social capital is primarily an individual-level social network asset (i.e., dwelling within individuals' family and friend relationships), a collective or public good, or both. Furthermore, not all social capital can be considered an unqualified benefit for all. The sociologist Alejandro Portes recognized the potential for "negative externalities" of social capital that could harm individuals outside of a group, yet produce benefits, or "positive internalities," for group members. For example, among residents in a predominantly African American, racially segregated neighborhood, individuals may experience positive effects from their relationships with one another but suffer negative consequences from discriminatory practices by outside individuals of other races/ethnicities.

Hypothesized Mechanisms

Several mechanisms by which social capital may affect health have been proposed. These include the diffusion of knowledge about health promotion, influences on health-related behaviors through informal social control, the promotion of access to local services and amenities, and psychosocial processes that provide support and mutual respect. Each of these mechanisms is plausible based on separate theories and pathways. First, through the theory of diffusion of innovations, it has been suggested that innovative behaviors diffuse much faster in communities that are cohesive and high in trust. Informal social control may also exert influence over such health behaviors. In social-cognitive theory, one's belief in collective agency is tied to the efficacy of a group in meeting its needs. For example, a neighborhood high in social capital and trust would be expected to effectively lobby together for local services, such as adequate transportation and green spaces. Finally, psychosocial processes, including social support and trust, may buffer the harmful effects of stress or may have direct positive effects on health.

Empirical Evidence

With origins in political science and sociology, social capital was first introduced to the public health literature in the early 1990s. Interest on this topic subsequently expanded, and beginning in the late 1990s, there was a surge in the body of literature examining the associations between social capital and health outcomes.

This literature may be broadly classified according to the level at which the measure of social capital corresponds (i.e., the individual level, the collective level, or both), the domains captured in the measure, the health outcomes, and the study design applied (i.e., ecologic vs. multilevel).

To date, measures of social capital in epidemiologic studies have largely been based on individual-level indicators of interpersonal trust, norms of reciprocity, and associational memberships, as gathered through surveys administered to representative samples of individuals (primarily adults). To construct measures of social capital at the collective level, the level that has increasingly become the focus of much current research, researchers typically aggregate the individual-level measures by taking their mean value at the collective level of interest—that is, the neighborhood/community, metropolitan/municipal, state/provincial, or country level. Measures of collective social capital that are not derived from individual-level measures of social capital are more difficult to find and validate.

Early epidemiologic studies on social capital primarily focused on broad health outcomes, including life expectancy, all-cause mortality rates, and homicide rates. The more recent literature has explored associations with other outcomes, including general self-rated health and its components (e.g., physical and mental health), health behaviors such as physical activity and medication use, and specific diseases and conditions ranging from sexually transmitted diseases and obesity to behavioral problems in children and food security.

Many of the ecologic studies (i.e., studies in which only data at an area level and not individual level are compared) on social capital have determined significant and moderate associations between social capital and better population health outcomes, whereas "multilevel" analyses (incorporating both area- and individual-level characteristics) have generally found these associations to be more modest. A key disadvantage of ecological studies is the potential for ecological fallacy—that is, relationships between social capital and health at the collective level that may not necessarily translate to the individual level. *Multilevel analyses* can address this issue by modeling individual-level characteristics as well as area-level features simultaneously, and thus allowing for the distinction between population-level *contextual effects* of social capital from *compositional effects*

(i.e., health effects due to the sociodemographic and socioeconomic composition of areas), while further taking into account similarities between individuals within the same areas. Multilevel analyses have also revealed the presence of significant interactions between collective and individual levels of social capital and between collective social capital and individual-level characteristics such as race/ethnicity, gender, and income in their health effects. Importantly, these interactions support the notion that the benefits of collective social capital do not necessarily occur uniformly across subgroups of populations.

—Daniel Kim

See also Diffusion of Innovation; Health Disparities; Multilevel Modeling; Social Epidemiology

Further Readings

Kawachi, I., & Berkman, L. F. (2000). Social cohesion, social capital and health. In L. F. Berkman & I. Kawachi (Eds.), *Social epidemiology* (pp. 174–190). New York: Oxford University Press.

Kawachi, I., Kim, D., Coutts, A., & Subramanian, S. V. (2004). Commentary: Reconciling the three accounts of social capital. *International Journal of Epidemiology, 33*, 682–690.

Kim, D., Subramanian, S. V., & Kawachi, I. (2006). Bonding versus bridging social capital and their associations with self-rated health: A multilevel analysis of 40 US communities. *Journal of Epidemiology and Community Health, 60*, 116–122.

Lin, N. (2001). *Social capital: A theory of social structure and action.* New York: Cambridge University Press.

Portes, A. (1998). Social capital: Its origins and applications in modern sociology. *Annual Reviews of Sociology, 24*, 1–24.

Putnam, R. D. (2000). *Bowling alone.* New York: Simon & Schuster.

Putnam, R. D., & Goss, K. A. (2002). Introduction. In R. D. Putnam (Ed.), *Democracies in flux* (pp. 3–19). New York: Oxford University Press.

SOCIAL-COGNITIVE THEORY

Albert Bandura's social-cognitive theory (SCT) is the result of a revision and expansion of his social learning theory and advocates a model of triadic reciprocal determinism to explain a person's behavior in a particular context. That is, (1) external environment, (2) behavior, and (3) cognitive/biological/other personal factors all influence each other bidirectionally. Bandura notes that this is a change from previous models that advocate unidirectional causation of behavior being influenced by internal dispositions and/or environmental variables and that SCT does not dictate that the different sources of influence are of equal strength nor does all the influence necessarily take place simultaneously. In summary, (1) internal dispositions (biology, cognition, emotion, etc.) may influence behavior, and behavior may influence internal dispositions; (2) internal dispositions may influence environmental events/reactions, and environmental events may influence internal dispositions; and (3) behavior may influence environmental events, and environmental events may influence behavior. SCT has been applied to study a wide range of public health issues, including medication compliance, alcohol abuse, and immunization behavior, and many public health interventions are based on SCT or selected aspects of it.

SCT recognizes the importance of modeling as an influence on human behavior: It explains how individuals may acquire attitudes from people in the media, as well as from those in their social network. *Direct modeling* refers to observing and possibly imitating people in our networks engaged in certain favorable or unfavorable behaviors, such as watching a father fasten his seat belt as soon as he enters the car. *Symbolic modeling* refers to observing and possibly imitating such behaviors portrayed in the media, such as seeing one's favorite film star smoke cigarettes in movies and magazine photos. Symbolic modeling forms the basis for many public health campaigns in which a celebrity spokesperson endorses or is seen performing a health behavior (such as drinking milk) or condemns a behavior (such as smoking).

Whether modeling leads to changed behavior on the part of the observers depends on many other variables, including individuals' perceptions of the favorable or unfavorable consequences of the behavior, their *outcome expectancies* (i.e., what they think will happen if they perform the behavior), and individuals' perceived ability to carry out the behavior—that is, their *self-efficacy*.

Self-Efficacy in Social-Cognitive Theory

Perhaps the most studied construct in SCT is self-efficacy. A PsycInfo search with self-efficacy as a keyword resulted in 11,530 citations from 1967 to 2006. When "health" as a keyword is combined with the previous search, PsycInfo lists 2,422 citations from 1967 to 2006. Bandura (1986) defines self-efficacy as "people's judgments of their capabilities to organize and execute courses of action required to attain designated types of performances. It is concerned not with the skills one has but with the judgments of what one can do with whatever skills one possesses" (p. 391). In his 1997 book *Self-Efficacy: The Exercise of Control*, he makes it clear that the power to make things happen is very different from the mechanics of how things are made to happen. He emphasizes the importance of *personal agency* (acts done intentionally) and comments that the power to originate behaviors toward a particular goal is the key to personal agency. Beliefs in personal efficacy are what make up the human agency. If people think they have no power to produce certain results, then they will not even try. This concept has clear implications for health behaviors since it may help explain why many people may not even attempt the health promotion behaviors recommended by their health professionals, family members, the media, and so on, or if they do, they do not effectively set short-term subgoals to help them reach their long-term goals.

Interestingly, Bandura suggests that self-efficacy influences the development of competencies as well as the regulation of action. An example of self-efficacy's influence on development might be the neophyte jogger using perceived self-efficacy to dictate the type of situations chosen while learning and/or perfecting his or her skills (e.g., only jogging with others who are just starting or only jogging alone and not with others who may jog faster). Therefore, self-efficacy influences which activities we choose to engage in, our motivational level, and our aspirations.

Bandura differentiates self-efficacy from several other popular constructs in the health and behavioral sciences—*self-esteem*, *locus of control*, and *outcome expectations* (sometimes referred to as *response efficacy*). Perceived self-efficacy is concerned with judgments of personal capacity, whereas self-esteem is concerned with judgments of self-worth; locus of control is concerned with the perception of whether one's actions affect outcomes; and outcome expectations, as noted above, are concerned with the consequences of behaviors that are performed. While self-efficacy asks, "Can I do it?" (e.g., Can I get up early each morning and jog 3 miles?), outcome expectation or response efficacy asks, "If I do it, will it work?" (e.g., If I jog 3 miles each morning, will I lose weight?).

SCT, Self-Efficacy, and Health Behaviors

Salovey, Rothman, and Rodin (1998) remark that self-efficacy may change over time, and in fact, media campaigns, social support groups, and other entities often target our self-efficacy regarding health behaviors to convince us that we can eat more fruits and vegetables, increase our physical activity, lose weight, see our doctor for regular exams, and so on. They suggest that changes in our perceived self-efficacy may be more important than the original baseline levels in motivating and maintaining health behaviors. Salovey et al. further state that, as social scientists are finding with a variety of dispositional constructs, self-efficacy is domain specific rather than a generalized expectation. One may be high in perceived self-efficacy when it comes to adding more fruit to his or her diet but still low on perceived self-efficacy when it comes to increasing his or her physical activity. As has been found in the attitude-behavior consistency research, perceived self-efficacy best predicts behavior when it is measured in the same domain and at the same level of abstraction as the behavior of interest.

There is an impressive amount of research supporting the importance of perceived self-efficacy in predicting behavior in laboratory and field research and in experimental and correlational research. Salovey et al. note that social-cognitive theorists believe that the more skill that a health behavior requires the larger the role played by self-efficacy.

Effects of Perceived Self-Efficacy on Biological Reactions

Bandura notes that social-cognitive theorists view biological reactions to stress (increased blood pressure, etc.) as a result of a low sense of efficacy to exert control over aversive environmental demands. Therefore, if these individuals believe that they can effectively cope with stressors, they are not troubled by them; however, without such a belief system they experience increased distress and impaired performance. Several studies support this view, including research in which phobics' perceived coping efficacy was raised to different levels by modeling or mastery experiences. Those with higher levels of mastery showed less autonomic activation when exposed to the phobia stressor. He also reports on research

suggesting the importance of perceived self-efficacy in the management of pain and depression.

Self-Efficacy and Health Promotion

Bandura noted that research by DiClemente, Prochaska, Fairhurst, Velicer, Velasquez, and Rossi (1991) supported the reciprocal influence of behavior and cognition, as they found that perceived self-efficacy increases as people proceed from contemplation to initiation to maintenance of behavior change. He also emphasizes the importance of perceived self-efficacy in being resilient to the disheartening effects of relapses, a frequent problem with health enhancing and compromising behaviors (e.g., persons may start smoking again after abstaining for many weeks, or they may stop exercising after going to the gym on a regular basis for many weeks) and that these people may not even attempt preventive behaviors (e.g., breast self-exams to detect cancerous lumps early) or treatment (e.g., take their medication) since they do not believe they can be successful.

Bandura advocates incorporating self-efficacy-related arguments into health education/persuasive messages as preferable to trying to scare someone via the use of fear appeals into engaging in health-enhancing behavior or ceasing health-compromising behaviors. He observes that often public service campaigns address the efficacy of the method or treatment but ignore promoting personal efficacy. He advocates providing people with the knowledge about how to regulate their health behavior and helping them develop a strong belief in the personal efficacy to turn their concerns into preventive action. Both preexisting perceived self-efficacy as well as altered perceived self-efficacy predict health behavior. Again, part of this process is an emphasis on perseverance of effort and recovering from temporary relapses that often occur with entrenched health-compromising habitual behaviors such as smoking or overeating.

Self-Efficacy in Other Models of Health Behavior

Several issues are common to much research about self-efficacy and health behavior. Self-efficacy is similar to several constructs that have been used in other models of health behavior, including the construct of perceived behavioral control in Ajzen's theory of planned behavior and the protection motivation theory, which includes both self-efficacy and response efficacy. Unfortunately, these related constructs are often confused with self-efficacy when research is designed and measures developed. This problem is increased because many researchers develop their own measures of self-efficacy, which may actually tap one or more of these other related constructs as well. A meta-analysis by Holden found that more than 75% of the studies they reviewed used their own measures of self-efficacy that had not been validated independently, leaving the question open of what they were actually measuring. Therefore, many studies, whether or not they support the predictive ability of self-efficacy on some health behavior, may not be measuring self-efficacy in the way Bandura originally conceptualized the construct but may instead be assessing one or more of the related constructs.

—*Eddie M. Clark*

See also Health Behavior; Self-Efficacy

Further Readings

Bandura, A. (1977). Social efficacy: Toward a unifying theory of behavioral change. *Psychological Review, 84,* 191–215.

Bandura, A. (1986). *Social foundations of thought and action: A social cognitive theory.* Englewood Cliffs, NJ: Prentice Hall.

Bandura, A. (1992). Social cognitive theory. In R. Vasta (Ed.), *Six theories of child development: Revised formulations and current issues* (pp. 1–60). London: Jessica Kingsley.

Bandura, A. (1997). *Self-efficacy: The exercise of control.* New York: W. H. Freeman.

DiClemente, C. C., Prochaska, J. O., Fairhurst, S. K., Velicer, W. F., Velasquez, M. M., & Rossi, J. S. (1991). The process of smoking cessation: An analysis of precontemplation, contemplation, and preparation stages of change. *Journal of Consulting and Clinical Psychology, 59,* 295–304.

Holden, G. (1991). The relationship between self-efficacy appraisals in subsequent health related outcomes: A meta-analysis. *Social Work in Health Care, 16,* 53–93.

Rogers, R. W. (1975). A protection motivation theory of fear appeals and attitude change. *Journal of Psychology, 91,* 93–114.

Rogers, R. W. (1983). Cognitive and physiological processes in fear appeals and attitude change: A revised theory of protection motivation. In J. T. Cacioppo & R. E. Petty (Eds.), *Social psychophysiology* (pp. 153–156). New York: Guilford Press.

Salovey, P., Rothman, A. J., & Rodin, J. (1998). Health behaviors. In D. T. Gilbert, S. T. Fiske, & G. Lindzey (Eds.), *Handbook of social psychology* (4th ed., Vol. 2, pp. 633–683). Boston: McGraw-Hill.

Zanna, M. P., & Fazio, R. H. (1982). The attitude-behavior relation: Moving toward a third generation of research. In M. P. Zanna, E. T. Higgins, & C. P. Herman (Eds.), *Consistency in social behavior: The Ontario symposium* (pp. 283–301). Hillsdale, NJ: Erlbaum.

SOCIAL EPIDEMIOLOGY

Social epidemiology is a field that primarily focuses on the investigation of the social determinants of population distributions of health, disease, and well-being. In contrast to many other fields in epidemiology, social epidemiology places emphasis on the causes of incidence of disease (i.e., the "causes of causes"), which may be very different from the causes of individual cases of disease. This entry describes several fundamental concepts within the field of social epidemiology, including socioeconomic status, social networks, race/ethnicity, residential segregation, social capital, income inequality, and working conditions, and details how these factors have been conceptually and empirically related to health. The entry also briefly discusses some of the core statistical methods that have been applied.

Socioeconomic Status (SES)

Individual-Level SES

The concept of SES is commonly used in the social epidemiologic literature to refer to the material and social resources and prestige that characterize individuals and that can allow individuals to be grouped according to relative socioeconomic position (although it should be noted that the term *socioeconomic status* is a bit of a misnomer, as it appears to emphasize status over material resources). Individual-level SES is typically measured through querying one's income, education, and occupation in surveys. Significant gradients in all-cause and cause-specific mortality for a number of diseases, including coronary heart disease, according to individual SES were established in the classic Whitehall study of British civil servants more than two decades ago (with higher occupational grades being inversely associated with mortality). Similar relations between individual-level income and mortality have also been found among individuals in other countries, including the United States. Several possible mechanisms have been proposed for the presence of these gradients. These include material pathways (e.g., being able to afford more nutritious foods; having more knowledge about healthy behaviors through higher educational attainment; and having the ability to move into a richer neighborhood, which may provide a more conducive environment for healthy behaviors—as will be discussed further) and psychosocial pathways (e.g., fewer occupational demands relative to the degree of job control—as will also be later described).

Area-Level SES

There are conceptual reasons and empirical evidence to support the notion that the levels of socioeconomic resources and amenities across places in which people live affect the health of individuals, even after taking into account the SES of individuals. For instance, the availability of nutritious foods and green spaces plausibly vary across neighborhoods and, in turn, could influence individuals' diets and physical activity levels. Other characteristics of higher SES neighborhoods that might be relevant to health include the quality of housing and of health services; the presence or lack of "incivilities," such as graffiti and litter; and environmental hazards, such as air pollution and noise. Studies typically operationalize area-level SES by aggregating individual-level SES measures (e.g., by taking the median income of individual survey respondents within a neighborhood). A number of studies have found moderate yet statistically significant associations between neighborhood socioeconomic characteristics and one's risk of dying from cardiovascular disease and from any cause, with 1.1 to 1.8 times higher risks of these outcomes after controlling for one's SES. Other studies have reported significant inverse associations between neighborhood SES with chronic disease risk factors, including smoking, diet, physical activity, and hypertension, and with the incidence of coronary heart disease.

Social Networks

The importance of social networks (i.e., the web of social relationships surrounding an individual and the characteristics of individual ties) to health dates back to the late 19th century, when the sociologist Emile Durkheim showed that individual pathology was a consequence of social dynamics, by tying patterns of suicide to levels of social integration. During the 1950s, the anthropologists Elizabeth Bott and John Barnes developed the concept of "social networks" to understand social ties that extended beyond traditional categories such as kin groups, tribes, or villages. Later, in the mid-1970s, seminal work by the epidemiologists John Cassel and Sidney Cobb linked social resources and support to disease risk and was followed by a number of epidemiologic studies that consistently demonstrated that the lack of social ties predicted death from nearly every cause. These studies include the groundbreaking Alameda County Study in the late 1970s, which prospectively followed nearly 7,000 adults in Alameda County, California, over a 9-year period and found in both men and women a greater than two times greater risk of dying among those who lacked community and social ties, even after taking into account one's age, SES, and lifestyle risk factors such as smoking, physical activity, and obesity.

Psychosocial mechanisms by which social networks may produce its health effects include the provision of social support (e.g., emotional support or instrumental support such as money in times of need), social influence (i.e., interpersonal influence through the proximity of two individuals in a social network), social engagement (i.e., social participation that helps define and reinforce meaningful social roles), person-to-person contact (influencing exposure to infectious disease agents), and access to resources and material goods (e.g., job opportunities and access to health care and education). In turn, these psychosocial pathways have been hypothesized to affect health through health behavioral, psychological, and physiological pathways. For instance, individuals who are socially isolated may adopt unhealthy behaviors such as smoking, may develop negative emotional states such as poor self-esteem or depression, and may acquire prolonged stress responses such as an intermittently raised blood pressure, ultimately leading to hypertension.

Racial/Ethnic Disparities and Racial Residential Segregation

Race/ethnicity refers to the social categorization of individuals into groups, often according to shared ancestry and cultural characteristics, as well as arbitrary physical features such as skin color. Disparities in health along racial/ethnic lines are well established. For example, in the United States, African Americans have a substantially higher risk of dying from coronary heart disease, stroke, cancer, and diabetes compared with whites. Possible reasons for these disparities relate largely to racism (an ideology used to justify the unequal treatment of racial/ethnic groups considered as inferior by individuals and institutions) and to residential segregation along racial/ethnic lines. Racial discriminatory practices have been shown to affect access to and quality of health care received and educational and employment opportunities and through perceived racial discrimination may contribute to higher levels of stress and unhealthy behaviors.

Residential segregation by race/ethnicity refers to the segregation of racial/ethnic groups along subunits of a residential area. Because of the range of opportunities and resources that different neighborhood socioeconomic environments may provide, as discussed, this segregation into different neighborhood contexts can propagate the socioeconomic deprivation among particular racial/ethnic groups that have historically been disadvantaged (e.g., in the United States, African Americans and Native Americans compared with whites). During the first half of the 20th century, racial discriminatory practices through federal housing policies, bank lending practices, and the real estate industry worked to physically separate blacks from whites in residential areas. More recently, there has been evidence showing the "targeting" and saturation of low-income African American and other minority neighborhoods with fast food restaurants and, prior to tobacco legislation, the targeted advertising of cigarettes within minority neighborhoods. These patterns likely contributed to poorer eating habits and other unhealthy lifestyle behaviors. Several measures of residential segregation by race/ethnicity exist, such as the index of dissimilarity, which captures the percentage of a particular racial/ethnic group that would have to move to evenly distribute the racial/ethnic groups across a residential area.

Other Contextual Determinants of Health

Apart from area-level SES and residential segregation, both *social capital* and *income inequality* have gained

prominence in the social epidemiologic and public health literature as possible contextual determinants of population and individual health.

The application of *social capital* to the field of public health arose from prior theoretical and empirical work in the fields of sociology and political science. Definitions of the concept of social capital are varied, ranging from those focusing on the resources within social networks that can be mobilized for purposeful actions to definitions that include both social structures and associated cognitive resources (such as trust and reciprocity) to categorizations such as formal versus informal social capital (e.g., memberships in professional associations vs. outings with friends). A key distinction that cross-cuts these definitions is the level at which social capital exists—that is, the individual level (whereby social capital could take the form of individual-level networks and social support) versus the collective level (e.g., the neighborhood or state level). Several mechanisms by which collective social capital may affect health have been proposed. These include influencing the diffusion of knowledge about health promotion, affecting health-related behaviors through social norms, promoting access to local services and amenities, and psychosocial processes that provide support and mutual respect.

Over the last decade, the number of epidemiologic studies examining the associations between social capital and health outcomes has rapidly grown, primarily as a result of several ecologic studies (i.e., studies in which only data at an area level and not individual level are compared) that found significant inverse associations between social capital and broad health outcomes such as life expectancy, all-cause mortality rates, and homicide rates. More recently, the breadth of this literature has increased to explore associations with one's general self-rated health and its components (e.g., physical and mental health), health behaviors such as physical activity and medication use and specific diseases and conditions ranging from sexually transmitted diseases and obesity to behavioral problems in children and food security, in models additionally controlling for one's SES.

Like social capital, research interest and empirical work on *income inequality* has flourished over the past decade. Income inequality refers to inequality in the distribution of income within populations and has been postulated to have harmful effects on health. The original hypothesis arose from the inability of a country's gross domestic product to account for variations in average life expectancy among rich nations. Mechanisms have since been put forth, including negative health effects resulting from individuals' feelings of relative deprivation, the erosion of social capital, and underinvestments in public goods such as education and health care, as the interests of the rich diverge from those of the poor. Although a number of measures of income inequality have been constructed (such as the 90/10 ratio, which compares the household income at the 90th percentile with that at the 10th percentile), the most widely applied measure is the Gini coefficient. The Gini coefficient equals half the arithmetic mean of the absolute differences between all pairs of incomes in a population and ranges from 0 (perfect equality) to 1 (perfect inequality).

As with the social capital and health literature, initial studies on income inequality and health were ecologic in design, and a number of these studies identified significant associations between income inequality and life expectancy, all-cause and cause-specific mortality, and self-rated health (in the anticipated directions). More recent investigations have applied a multilevel analytic framework and controlled for individual-level SES. Most of the studies supporting an association between income inequality and health have been in the context of the United States, a country with a comparatively high Gini coefficient among developed nations, whereas findings have generally been null in more egalitarian societies such as Japan and Sweden.

Working Conditions

The psychosocial work environment may also play an important role in determining levels of health among individuals. In support of this relation, one classic theoretical model is the *psychological demand-decision latitude model*, which consists of two dimensions: (1) emotional and psychological demands and (2) decision latitude, which corresponds to the degree of control an employee has over work-related tasks. Based on conceptualized interactions between these dimensions (each dichotomized as high or low), a worker may be assigned to one of four quadrants. In the quadrant of high psychological demands and low decision latitude, *job strain* is said to occur. Under these conditions, Robert Karasek hypothesized that the sympatho-adrenal system of the body is excessively activated while the body's ability to repair tissues is reduced, ultimately leading to illness. Job strain has been shown in some studies to predict the development of hypertension and coronary heart disease in both men and women, controlling for one's SES and other lifestyle factors.

A second classic model of the psychosocial work environment was developed by the sociologist Johannes Siegrist and is referred to as the *effort-reward imbalance model*. This model concerns the degree to which workers are rewarded (such as through financial compensation or improved self-esteem) for their efforts. When a high degree of effort is insufficiently met with the degree of reward, emotional stress and the risks of illnesses are hypothesized to increase. For example, in workplaces that offer disproportionately generous salaries and promotions in relation to employees' efforts, employees are expected to have lower levels of stress and better health status. Studies that have followed workers prospectively have found significant associations between effort-reward imbalance and higher risks of blood pressure and coronary heart disease, as well as reduced levels of physical, psychological, and social functioning, controlling for other factors.

Statistical Methods

As a field within the discipline of epidemiology, studies in social epidemiology often apply common statistical methods such as multiple linear regression and logistic regression. Issues of measurement are customary in social epidemiology due to the social constructs of interest, which for the most part cannot be directly observed (e.g., social capital, which is typically measured through multiple survey items on interpersonal trust, reciprocity, and/or associational memberships). In the case of area-level social factors (such as community social capital or neighborhood SES), measures are typically derived by aggregating individual-level measures. Methods such as factor analysis that are customarily applied in other disciplines (e.g., psychology and sociology) are frequently used to help in validating such measures.

When the research aim is to explore associations between contextual factors (such as neighborhood SES and income inequality) and individual-level health behaviors and outcomes, multilevel models aid in promoting validity. Such models account for individual-level observations within the same spatial area being potentially nonindependent and thereby reduce the likelihood of incorrectly concluding there is a true association when it is in fact due to chance (known as a Type I error in statistics). In so doing, applying multilevel methods in social epidemiology can allow for the more valid estimation of *contextual effects* of features of the social environment (such as neighborhood social capital), while controlling for *compositional effects* of spatial areas (such as individual-level SES). These methods can be further extended to more validly assess whether contextual effects vary substantially across subgroups of a population.

—*Daniel Kim*

See also Multilevel Modeling; Social Capital and Health; Socioeconomic Classification

Further Readings

Berkman, L.F., & Glass, T. (2000). Social integration, social networks, social support, and health. In L. F. Berkman & I. Kawachi (Eds.), *Social epidemiology* (pp. 137–173). New York: Oxford University Press.

Kawachi, I., & Berkman, L. F. (2000). Social cohesion, social capital, and health. In L. F. Berkman & I. Kawachi (Eds.), *Social epidemiology* (pp. 174–190). New York: Oxford University Press.

Kawachi, I., Kennedy B. P., & Wilkinson, R. G. (Eds.). (1999). *Income inequality and health: A reader.* New York: New Press.

Kawachi, I., Kim, D., Coutts, A., & Subramanian, S. V. (2004). Commentary: Reconciling the three accounts of social capital. *International Journal of Epidemiology, 33,* 682–690.

Krieger, N. (2001). A glossary for social epidemiology. *Journal of Epidemiology and Community Health, 55,* 693–700.

Theorell, T. (2000). Working conditions and health. In L. F. Berkman & I. Kawachi (Eds.), *Social epidemiology* (pp. 95–117). New York: Oxford University Press.

Williams, D. R. (1999). Race, socioeconomic status and health: The added effects of racism and discrimination. *Annals of the New York Academy of Sciences, 896,* 173–188.

SOCIAL HIERARCHY AND HEALTH

Social organization and population health are inextricably linked. Societies organize their affairs in different ways, and these differences, by means of various pathways, have an effect on the production of health and disease among individuals, as well as between and within communities. Although some of these pathways are not yet fully understood, an ever-mounting body of evidence persuasively supports the contention that the social gradient—the hierarchical organization of society's members along the social ladder, as defined by a number of socioeconomic classifications or representations of social position—is intimately mirrored by a corresponding health gradient. Almost invariably, those who rank lower in the socioeconomic scale have worse health status than those above them in the hierarchy—that is, the higher the social standing, the better the health. Central to the notion of this steadily observed *social gradient in health*—also known as the "status syndrome," the archetype of the relationship between social hierarchy and health—is the generation and persistence of inequalities in health. Current evidence points out the key role of the psychosocial impact of low position in social hierarchy on the generation of both ill health and health inequalities, issues of fundamental concern to both social epidemiology research and practice.

Hierarchy is a prominent ecological aspect of social organization that entails the establishment of a ranking among elements of a group—and hence asymmetrical relationships—based on power, coercion, and access to resources regardless of the needs of others. This hierarchy, which is institutionalized to minimize open conflict, contrasts with social affiliation by friendship, in which reciprocity, mutuality, and solidarity define a social system based on more egalitarian cooperation. Social hierarchy is the human equivalent of the pecking order or dominance hierarchy of nonhuman primates. Even the most egalitarian societies have some hierarchical structure based on distinctions with the result that some people are perceived as having higher social standing than others.

In 1978, a marked social gradient in coronary heart disease was identified along the six occupational classes defined by the British Registrar General's social class scale in the Whitehall study of British civil servants. Since then, even in fairly homogeneous populations, studies have repeatedly found a gradient in health by socioeconomic status: Those at lower socioeconomic positions have worse health status than those above them in the hierarchy. These findings have led researchers to postulate a relationship between position in the social hierarchy and health. Studies of social hierarchies in nonhuman primates have also identified this relationship. Disentangling the relative importance of economic versus pure social hierarchies in humans is, however, challenging due to their degree of overlap.

This profound relationship between social hierarchy and health inequality in human populations has been primarily revealed in studies of income and mortality: The risk of dying follows closely the social gradient defined by the level of income, and poorer societies and poorer population segments within societies have consistently higher mortality rates and lower life expectancy than their less poor counterparts. A solid set of indicators, such as the concentration index and the slope index of inequality, have been used to quantify the degree of inequality in health associated with the social hierarchy defined by a ridit scale (i.e., the succession of relative positions formed with interval midpoints, relative to an identified distribution, of discrete categories with a natural ordering) of income or other variables of socioeconomic status. Early on, the existence of a threshold effect with poverty as well as other egregious measures of material deprivation (such as illiteracy, lack of clean water and sanitation, famine, or even lack of health care access) was demonstrated, above which the association between social hierarchy and health is blurred. Far from denying a relation between hierarchy and health, this evidence suggests that income, and other *absolute* measures of *material* deprivation, may not always be a good proxy of social status and social differentiation and, more important, that nonincome aspects of social rankings operating in specific cultures and communities may overpower single economic measures such as income distribution.

Thus, when material deprivation is severe, a social gradient in mortality could arise from degrees of absolute deprivation. But the effects of social hierarchy in health are not confined to the poor: In rich societies with low levels of material deprivation, the social gradient in health changes the focus from absolute to *relative* deprivation and from material to *psychosocial* deprivation, which relates to a broader approach to social functioning and meeting of human needs. Realizing that social status is a relative—not absolute—concept, scholars have highlighted the significance of relative position for health: It is not what a person has that is important, but what he or she can do with what he or she has. In other words, it is not position in the hierarchy per se that is the culprit of social gradient in health and health inequalities but what position in the hierarchy means for what one can do in a given society. This realization brings the attention to two vital human needs: control over the circumstances in which people live and work and full social participation. The lower individuals are in the social hierarchy, the less likely it is that their fundamental human needs for autonomy and to be integrated into society will be met. This failure, in turn, is a potent cause of ill health in individuals and populations.

A growing body of evidence is being assembled with regard to the paramount importance of autonomy, human freedom to lead a life people have reason to value, and empowerment as determinants of the social gradient in health and socioeconomic inequalities in health. Poor social affiliation and low status carry high population attributable risks. More unequal societies not only suffer more relative deprivation but also tend to have lower rates of trust and of community involvement and social engagement. Interestingly enough, several studies have made the connection between social conditions and biological pathways that plausibly provide the link to violence, cardiovascular conditions, and other diseases. It has been shown that where income inequalities are greater and more people are denied access to the conventional sources of dignity and status in terms of jobs and money, people become increasingly vulnerable to signs of disrespect, shame, and social anxiety, consistently explaining the strong statistical relationship between violence, hierarchy, and inequality.

Likewise, low social position and lack of control are linked to less heart rate variability (i.e., a sign of low sympathetic tone), raised levels of blood cortisol, delayed heart rate recovery after exercise, and low exercise functional capacity (i.e., signs of impaired autonomic activity), all related to activity of the two main biological stress pathways: the sympatho-adreno-medullary axis and the hypothalamic-pituitary-adrenal axis. One plausible mechanism of action of these stress pathways is through an effect on the metabolic syndrome—that is, a cluster of risk factors (including abdominal obesity, atherogenic dyslipidemia, high blood pressure, insulin resistance and prothrombotic and proinflammatory states) that increases the risk of heart diseases and Type II diabetes. Stress at work has been shown to be strongly related to metabolic syndrome, which, in turn, exhibits a clear social gradient, and it is related to those biological stress pathways.

Life contains a series of critical transitions: emotional and material changes in early childhood, moving to successive schools, starting work, leaving home, starting a family, changing jobs, facing retirement, and so on. Each of these changes can affect the ability of individuals to built and maintain social networks, influence their standing on the social ladder, and also impinge on their health by pushing people onto a more or less advantaged path, putting those who have been disadvantaged in the past at the greatest risk in each subsequent transition. The longer people live in stressful economic and social circumstances, the greater the physiological wear and tear they suffer, the greater the social divide, and the less likely they are to enjoy a healthy life.

Health and quality of social relations in a society seem to vary inversely with how pervasive hierarchy is within the society. The most important psychosocial determinant of population health may be the levels of the various forms of social anxiety in the population, which, in turn, are mainly determined by income distribution, early childhood experiences (including intergenerational nongenetically transmitted behaviors), and social networks. More hierarchical, unequal societies may be more differentiated by social rank into relations of dominance and subordination and less able to enjoy more egalitarian and inclusive relations consistent with higher social capital and less class and racial prejudice. In this analysis, far from being an epiphenomenon, social capital may emerge as an important element in the causation of health and illness in the population. The link between health and social capital (and egalitarianism) is emphasized by the epidemiological findings testifying to the importance of social status and social relations—that is, social cohesion as beneficial to societal health.

Social and economic resources shape the social organization and the health of individuals and communities: Different socioeconomic factors could affect health at different times in the life course, operating at different levels of organization and through different causal pathways. Moreover, socioeconomic factors can interact with other social characteristics, such as racial/ethnic group and gender, to produce different health effects and gradients across groups. The existence of wide—and widening—socioeconomic disparities in health shows how extraordinarily sensitive health remains to socioeconomic circumstances and, by consequence, to social hierarchy.

—*Oscar J. Mujica*

See also Determinants of Health Model; Health Disparities; Social Capital and Health; Social Epidemiology; Socioeconomic Classification

Further Readings

Bartley, M. (2004). *Health inequality: An introduction to theories, concepts and methods.* Cambridge, UK: Polity Press.

Krieger, N., Williams, D. R., & Moss, N. E. (1997). Measuring social class in U.S. public health research: Concepts, methodologies, and guidelines. *Annual Review of Public Health, 18,* 341–378.

Marmot, M. (2004). *The status syndrome: How social standing affects our health and longevity.* New York: Henry Holt.

Marmot, M. (2006). Harveian oration: Health in an unequal world. *Lancet, 368,* 2081–2094.

Sapolski, R. M. (2005). The influence of social hierarchy on primate health. *Science, 308,* 648–652.

Wilkinson, R. G. (1999). Health, hierarchy, and social anxiety. *Annals of the New York Academy of Sciences, 896,* 48–63.

Social Marketing

Social marketing is the use of marketing principles and techniques to develop and promote socially beneficial programs, behaviors, and other products. In public health, social marketing has shown great promise as a strategic planning process for developing behavior change interventions and improving service delivery. This entry describes social marketing's distinctive features, steps, and major challenges.

Social Marketing's Distinctive Features

Social marketing is a data-driven strategic planning process that is characterized by its reliance on marketing's conceptual framework to bring about voluntary behavior change. The most distinctive features are a commitment to create satisfying exchanges, the use of the marketing mix to design interventions, segmentation of the target populations, and a data-based consumer orientation.

Satisfying Exchanges

Marketers believe people act largely out of self-interest, searching for ways to optimize the benefits they gain and minimize the costs they pay in their exchanges with others. In commercial transactions, consumers typically exchange money for tangible products or services. In public health, people more often sacrifice comfort, time, and effort for the value gained from adopting a healthy behavior or participating in a program. Social marketing encourages public health practitioners to offer exchanges that satisfy customers' wants as well as their needs.

The Marketing Mix

Marketing also offers public health professionals a set of conceptual tools called the "4 Ps"—product, price, place, and promotion—for planning program interventions. Also, known as the marketing mix, these concepts are carefully considered from the consumers' points of view and used to develop integrated plans that guide all program activities.

The *product* refers to several critical features of an intervention. The actual product refers to the recommended or desired behavior—for example, a protective behavior being promoted, use of a public health program, or abandonment of a risky behavior. The core product refers to the benefits consumers gain from adopting the product. In some cases, tangible commodities, called augmented products, also are involved. For instance, in a program to decrease eye injuries among citrus pickers, the actual product is the use of safety glasses, reduction of daily irritation is the core product or benefit, and specific brands of safety eye wear that are comfortable to wear in Florida's groves are augmented products.

Price refers to monetary and other costs (e.g., embarrassment, hassle) that are exchanged for product benefits. In the eye safety project just described, intangible costs, such as discomfort and loss of productivity when glasses get dirty, were just as significant as the cash outlay to purchase them. Unless costs for public health products are lowered or made acceptable, even appealing offers may be rejected as unaffordable.

Place has several applications: the locations and times consumers perform the desired behavior, the distribution of augmented products and the point at which consumers obtain them, the actual physical location at which services are offered (attractiveness, comfort, and accessibility), and people and organizations that facilitate the exchange process (e.g., refer people to a program or reinforce behavioral recommendations).

Promotion includes a variety of activities intended to affect behavior change. In public health, an integrated set of activities are usually needed. Professional training, service delivery enhancements, community-based activities, and skill building are often combined with communications (e.g., consumer education, advertising, public relations, special events).

Audience Segmentation

Social marketers know that one intervention doesn't fit everyone's needs, so they identify subgroups in a population that respond differentially to marketing tactics (e.g., core benefits offered, spokespersons, information channels). To optimize resource allocation, marketers subdivide groups based on their current behavior (e.g., sedentary vs. moderately active), readiness to change, reasons people have not adopted the desired behavior, and other factors that affect their response to intervention strategies. They also select one or more segments to receive the greatest priority in planning their interventions.

Data-Based Consumer Orientation

Perhaps the most important element of social marketing is its reliance on consumer research to understand and address the respective audience's values, lifestyle, and preferences to make the key marketing decisions that comprise a marketing plan—that is, segments to give greatest priority, benefits to promise, costs to lower, and product placement and promotion requirements. Time and other resources are devoted to audience analysis; formative research; and pretesting of message concepts, prototype materials, and training approaches. Public health managers who use social marketing are constantly assessing target audience responses to all aspects of an intervention from the broad marketing strategy to specific messages and materials.

Steps in the Social Marketing Process

The social marketing process consists of five steps or tasks.

1. *Audience analysis.* The problem is analyzed to determine what is known about its causes and the audiences affected. Situational factors affecting the project are considered and formative research is conducted to understand the issue from the consumers' viewpoints. Of special interest are consumers' perceptions of product benefits, costs, placement, and potential promotional strategies.

2. *Strategy development.* Research findings are used to make key marketing decisions and develop a blueprint or marketing plan to guide program development. The strategy team determines the audience segments to target, the core product to offer, strategies for lowering costs or making them acceptable, places to offer products, partners to support product adoption, and ways to promote the product to select audience segments.

3. *Program development.* Interventions are developed and message concepts, prototype materials, and training and promotional activities are created and tested.

4. *Program implementation.* Social marketers carefully coordinate an integrated set of promotional activities and rely on the marketing plan to guide program implementation.

5. *Program monitoring and evaluation.* All aspects of program interventions are monitored to identify unforeseen problems that may require midcourse revisions to improve their effectiveness.

Social Marketing Applications

During the last 30 years, social marketing has been used in the United States and elsewhere to develop programs to promote family planning, breastfeeding, increased fruit and vegetable consumption, physical activity, immunization, environmental protection, a variety of safety practices, and other healthy behaviors. It also has been used to (re)design and promote programs, such as the food stamp program, the Special Supplemental Nutrition Program for Women, Infants, and Children, Medicaid, and others, with significant success. While its use has increased dramatically, social marketing has yet to realize its potential in public health because of a lack of training and widespread misunderstandings. The most challenging problems limiting its application include the following:

- An overreliance on communications, especially mass media. Many public health professionals still equate social marketing with social advertising and misuse the label to describe campaigns that rely exclusively on mass media messages to bring about change rather than a careful integration of the entire marketing mix.
- A reluctance to invest time and money on consumer research. While marketing research does not always

have to be expensive or complex, it is essential to understand how consumers view the product benefits, costs, placement, and promotion.

- An overreliance on focus groups. Focus groups have many advantages in marketing research, but they can also be misleading if not conducted and analyzed carefully. Like all qualitative data collection methods, the results cannot be verified statistically or used to estimate the prevalence of views within a target population.
- An overreliance on demographic variables to segment audiences and reticence to select segments to target. Many public health professionals try to reach everyone with the same intervention, or if they segment, they do so exclusively with demographic variables.
- Failure to rigorously evaluate social marketing interventions.

Conclusions

Social marketing is widely accepted as a method for promoting healthy behaviors, programs, or policies. It is distinguished from other planning approaches by a commitment to offer satisfying exchanges, use of marketing's conceptual framework, segmentation and careful selection of target audiences, and close attention to consumers' aspirations, preferences, and needs. Although social marketing often uses mass media to communicate with its target audiences, it should not be confused with health communication, social advertising, or educational approaches, which simply create awareness of a behavior's health benefits and/or attempt to persuade people to change through motivational messages. Social marketers use research results to identify the product benefits most attractive to target audience segments, determine what costs will be acceptable and those that must be lowered, identify the best places to offer products, and communicate with consumers and design the best mix of promotional tactics to elicit behavior change.

—*Carol Anne Bryant*

See also Diffusion of Innovations; Health Behavior; Targeting and Tailoring

Further Readings

Donovan, R., & Henley, N. (2003). *Social marketing principles and practice.* Melbourne, Australia: IP Communications.

Grier, S., & Bryant, C. A. (2005). Social marketing in public health. *Annual Reviews in Public Health, 26,* 6.1–6.21.

Kotler, P., Roberto, N., & Lee, N. (2002). *Social marketing: Strategies for changing public behavior.* Thousand Oaks, CA: Sage.

Kotler, P., & Zaltman, G. (1971). Social marketing: An approach to planned social change. *Journal of Marketing, 35,* 3–12.

McKenzie-Mohr, D., & Smith, W. (1999). *Fostering sustainable behavior: An introduction to community-based social marketing.* British Columbia, Canada: New Society.

SOCIOECONOMIC CLASSIFICATION

Socioeconomic classification refers, in broad terms, to the arrangement, categorization, or assignment of individuals of a population (and, by extension, other population-based elements such as families, households, neighborhoods, geopolitical units, etc.) to pre-designated classes, orders, subgroups, or continuous scale or gradient on the basis of perceived common social, societal, and/or economic attributes, characteristics, conditions, relations, or affinities. The goal of any socioeconomic classification is to provide a valid, relevant, and meaningful organization of the population into separate, discrete social classes or, conversely, all along a hierarchical continuum of socioeconomic position. Ample evidence supports the assertion that social and economic resources shape the health of individuals and communities; indeed, socioeconomic status is regarded as a fundamental macro-determinant of population health. Socioeconomic classification is at the core of these considerations, and it can, therefore, critically affect epidemiological and public health research and practice, with direct implications for public health policy.

Social sciences, as well as social epidemiology, consistently recognize that behind any socioeconomic classification there is a multidimensional construct comprising diverse social and economic factors. It is increasingly acknowledged that a fundamental distinction between "social class," "social status," and measures of material living standards is needed to clarify definitions, measures, and interpretations associated with a given socioeconomic classification. This would include distinguishing between *income*, *assets*, and *wealth* (i.e., those based on individual and household ownership of goods), terms frequently used loosely and interchangeably despite their different theoretical foundations.

Social classes—hierarchical distinctions between individuals or groups in societies or cultures—are social groups arising from interdependent economic relationships among people. These relationships are governed by the social structure as expressed in the customs, values, and expectations concerning property distribution, ownership, and labor and their connections to production, distribution, and consumption of goods, services, and information. Hence, social classes are essentially shaped by the relationships and conditions of employment of people in the society and not by the characteristics of individuals. These class relationships are not symmetrical but include the ability of those with access to resources such as capital to economically exploit those who do not have access to those resources.

Unlike social class, *social status* involves the idea of a hierarchy or ranking based on the prestige, honor, and reputation accorded to persons in a society. Societal sources for attribution of status, that is, a relative position in the social ladder, are diverse but chiefly concern access to power, knowledge, and economic resources.

Both social class and social status can be regarded as representations of social position. Yet a growing body of knowledge from research on health inequalities indicates a need to consider a more comprehensive socioeconomic classification that can include class, status, and material asset measures, collectively referred to as *socioeconomic position*. This term is increasingly being used in epidemiology as a generic term that refers to the social and economic factors that influence which positions individuals or groups will hold within the structure of a society. Socioeconomic position is one dimension of social stratification and, as such, is an important mechanism through which societal resources and goods are distributed to and accumulated over time by different groups in the population.

From an analytical standpoint, social class involves categorical (usually nominal as opposed to ordinal), discontinuous variables. Social status, on the other hand, is considered as a continuous variable, although for the purposes of analysis it may be divided into categories using cutpoints or other divisions dependent on the data structure rather than a priori reference points. Characteristics of socioeconomic position pertaining to material resources (such as income, wealth, education attainment, and, by extension, poverty, deprivation, etc.) can be modeled as ordinal or interval categorical variables. Another important implication for data analysis is that, unlike social class or status, socioeconomic position can be measured meaningfully at different levels of organization (such as individual, household, and neighborhood levels), as well as at different points in the lifespan (such as infancy, adolescence, adulthood).

The array of socioeconomic classification schemes and indicators of socioeconomic position includes both individual-level and area-level measures. Among others, there are those based on education; income, poverty, and material and social deprivation; occupation, working life, and exclusion from labor force; house tenure, housing conditions, and household amenities; social class position; proxy indicators; composite measures; and indices of deprivation. Among the best known socioeconomic classifications is the British Registrar General's Social Class (RGSC) scale, used since 1913. This scale, which is based on the occupation of the head of the household, defines six social classes: I, professional; II, managerial; III-NM, skilled nonmanual; III-M, skilled manual; IV, semiskilled manual; and V, unskilled manual. The RGSC scale is said to be based on either general standing in the community or occupational skill, and its categories broadly reflect social prestige, education level, and household income. Despite much criticism for its obvious class and gender biases, as well as for its exclusion of individuals outside the formal paid labor force, this schema has proven to be powerfully predictive of inequalities in morbidity and mortality. Wright class schema or socioeconomic classification is another well-known typology that—based on the contention that the essence of class distinctions can be seen in the tensions of a middle class simultaneously exploiting and being exploited (in terms of ownership, control, and possession of capital, organization, and credential assets)—ultimately distinguishes between four core class categories: wage laborers, petty bourgeois, small employers, and capitalists. Yet other standard socioeconomic classifications include the Erikson and Goldthorpe class schema, the Nam-Powers' occupational status score, the Duncan socioeconomic index, the Cambridge social interaction and stratification scale, the Hollingshead index of social position, the Warner index of status characteristics, and the Townsend deprivation index. These measures and others are discussed in detail in the Further Readings list provided at the end of this entry.

There are many criteria, schemes, and indicators to generate a classification of socioeconomic position; no single measure can be regarded as suitable for all purposes or settings. Ideally, this choice should be informed by consideration of the specific research question and the proposed mechanism linking socioeconomic position to the health outcome. In practice, however, the measures used tend to be driven by what is available or has been previously collected. To reflect on the potential of a given indicator of socioeconomic position to help understand, as opposed merely to describe, health, inequality should be taken as an overarching principle when choosing a socioeconomic classification measure.

—*Oscar J. Mujica*

See also Determinants of Health Model; Health Disparities; Social Capital and Health; Social Epidemiology; Social Hierarchy and Health

Further Readings

Bartley, M. (2004). Measuring socio-economic position. In M. Bartley (Ed.), *Health inequality: An introduction to theories, concepts and methods* (pp. 22–34). Cambridge, UK: Polity Press.

Galobardes, B., Shaw, M., Lawlor, D. A., Davey Smith, G., & Lynch, J. W. (2006). Indicators of socioeconomic position. In J. M. Oakes & J. S. Kaufman (Eds.), *Methods in social epidemiology* (pp. 47–85). San Francisco: Wiley.

Krieger, N., Williams, D. R., & Moss, N. E. (1997). Measuring social class in U.S. public health research: Concepts, methodologies, and guidelines. *Annual Review of Public Health, 18*, 341–378.

Liberatos, P., Link, B. G., & Kelsey, J. L. (1988). The measurement of social class in epidemiology. *Epidemiological Reviews, 10*, 87–121.

Lynch, J., & Kaplan, G. (2000). Socioeconomic position. In L. F. Berkman & I. Kawachi (Eds.), *Social epidemiology* (pp. 13–35). Oxford, UK: Oxford University Press.

SOCIETY FOR EPIDEMIOLOGIC RESEARCH

The mission of the Society for Epidemiologic Research (SER), established in 1968, is to create a forum for sharing the most up-to-date information in epidemiologic research and to keep epidemiologists at the vanguard of scientific developments.

SER is a membership organization governed by a four-member executive committee (president, president-elect, past president, and secretary-treasurer) and a five-member board including one student representative; the executive committee and the board members are elected by the SER membership. SER holds an annual scientific meeting and is one of the sponsors, along with the American College of Epidemiology and the Epidemiology Section of the American Public Health Association, of the North American Congress of Epidemiology, which is held every 5 years (most recently in 2006). In addition, SER sponsors publication of the professional journals *American Journal of Epidemiology* and *Epidemiologic Reviews* and publishes a semiannual newsletter concerning SER activities (available on the SER Web site). The SER office is located in Clearfield, Utah, USA.

The annual meeting of the SER is held in the United States or Canada. The 40th annual meeting was held in Boston, Massachusetts, in June 2007. The 41st annual meeting will be held in Chicago, Illinois, in June 2008. The meeting includes presentation of scientific papers and posters by SER members, round-table discussions, and instructional workshops. The winner of the Abraham Lilienfeld Student Prize, which is awarded annually for the best paper describing research done as a student in an advanced degree program with a concentration in epidemiology, is invited to present his or her research during the plenary session of the annual meeting.

Epidemiologic Reviews is published once a year by Oxford University Press. It publishes review articles focused on a particular theme, which is changed annually: The 2006 issue focused on vaccines and public health, and the 2007 issue focuses on the epidemiology of obesity. The *American Journal of Epidemiology* is published 24 times a year by Oxford University Press and publishes original research articles, reviews, methodology articles, editorials, and letters to the editor. In 2005, the impact factor for *Epidemiologic Reviews* was 4.722, and the impact factor for the *American Journal of Epidemiology* was 5.068, ranking them second and fourth among 99 journals in public, environmental, and occupational health.

—*Sarah Boslaugh*

See also American College of Epidemiology; American Public Health Association; Journals, Epidemiological

Further Readings

Web Sites

American Journal of Epidemiology: http://aje .oxfordjournals.org.
Epidemiologic Reviews: http://epirev.oxfordjournals.org.
Society for Epidemiologic Research: http://www .epiresearch.org.

SPECIFICITY

See SENSITIVITY AND SPECIFICITY

SPIRITUALITY AND HEALTH

Interest in the role of spirituality in health outcomes has increased in recent years in both scientific and lay circles, as evidenced by increases in published articles and in funding for research in this area. This entry provides a brief review of the research on spirituality and health, methodological challenges, and future research directions. This area of research not only has theoretical value but may also lead to applied knowledge relevant to health education and promotion.

Discussions of research in this area should generally begin with a brief definition of concepts, including what is meant by the term *spirituality*. These discussions typically also involve the concept of religion, as the two concepts are often used interchangeably in this literature even though they refer to distinct—yet potentially overlapping—constructs. Although there has been debate over the usage of these terms, *spirituality* is often used to refer to people's experience of what gives them meaning in life, which may include things such as nature or a higher power. The term *religion*, on the other hand, is often used to refer to an organized system of worship involving doctrine, beliefs, and a higher power often but not always referred to as "God." Research in spirituality and health is not as developed as in religion and health, largely due to the difficulty of assessing the construct of spirituality. There has been widespread disagreement on what is meant by spirituality. Although it poses its own set of conceptual challenges, religion is easier to define; as a result, the majority of research on "spirituality and health" has actually focused on a concept more related to religion. Thus, for the purpose of this entry, the term *spirituality/religion* is used, with the recognition that these terms are not interchangeable.

Research Methodology

Early Work

Research in the area of spirituality/religion and health began with large population-based data sets examining the association between single indicators of religion (e.g., church attendance, religious affiliation) and health outcomes such as mortality. Because positive relationships were often found even with these crude indicators, interest in this area increased.

Emergence of Multidimensional Assessment

Researchers began to recognize that the single-item indicators of religion needed much improvement relative to the way that other psychological constructs were being assessed. Multiple-item scales began to be developed, and later came the recognition that religion and spirituality are indeed multidimensional constructs having several dimensions. These dimensions were reflected in instruments assessing dimensions such as public and private religiosity and religious beliefs and behaviors.

Other Methodological Challenges

Measurement was not the only methodological challenge to be overcome in spirituality/religion and health research. Even when positive associations were found between spirituality/religion and a health outcome (and this was not always the case), there were questions as to whether there was another variable, such as health status or age, that was confounding the relationship. Researchers in this area must be aware of the potential for confounding; for example, they must ask whether those who attend church are more likely to experience positive health outcomes for some reason other than their spirituality/religion. These variables must then be assessed and controlled for in research studies, as is being done in some research. But even when the confounding factors are controlled for, a cause-effect relationship cannot be demonstrated without longitudinal studies, and this is difficult to accomplish. Finally, most of the studies in the United States have focused on Christian populations. While

this approach was taken to enhance generalizability by studying relatively large populations, it is inherently limited since it applies only to these populations. Much less is known about those of other faiths such as Buddhists and Muslims.

The Relationship Between Spirituality/Religion and Health

Is there a relationship between spirituality/religion and health? Although this is a complex question beyond the scope of this entry, several large-scale reviews of the literature in this area have concluded that the weight of the evidence for the relationship between spirituality/religion and health is generally, although not always, positive. Some studies have found negative relationships and others found no such relationship, but most do find a modest positive association with outcomes such as health-related behaviors, conditions, and general mortality.

After many studies attempting to answer the question of *whether* there is an association between spirituality/religion and health, the research in this area has generally moved on to ask *why* such an association might exist, for whom, and under what conditions. To address the "why" question, several excellent theoretical articles have proposed mechanisms for the relationship between health and spirituality/religion. These mechanisms include the hypotheses that spiritual/religious individuals experience health benefits because they have more social support, experience more positive affect, have a healthier lifestyle, engage in healthier behaviors, experience more social pressure to avoid unhealthy behaviors (e.g., not smoking in front of fellow church members), or cope better with stress than do less spiritual/religious individuals. Although there are little actual data to support many of these mechanisms to date, the future of the research points to studies that can provide data to support such mediational relationships and build the much needed theory in the area. It is also important, when examining an area such as spirituality/religion and health mediators, to begin this work with qualitative studies before making assumptions about what is certainly a very complex set of relationships. This will help ensure that the quantitative studies are asking the right questions.

Another question is for whom spirituality/religion might have a health benefit. Again, studies have begun to address this question but many more are needed to identify population subgroups that are more or less apt to experience the connection. For example, it may be that particular racial/ethnic groups, those of different age groups, of different denominational affiliations, or of different socioeconomic strata differ in the strength of the spirituality/religion-health connection.

Finally, there is the question of under what conditions spirituality/religion might have a health benefit. It is possible that there may be a positive association for some health outcomes and not others. For example, individuals may view their spiritual/religious beliefs as a basis for avoiding behaviors such as tobacco, drug, or alcohol use but not for adopting health-promoting behaviors such as a healthy diet and physical activity. Additionally, it may be that the association holds only for individuals who have adequate social support systems in place or in other conditions of which researchers are unaware. Again, this is where qualitative methods such as in-depth interviews and focus groups can shed some light on these complex phenomena.

Why Study the Relationship Between Spirituality/Religion and Health?

Besides being a challenging area in terms of measurement and controlling for confounding variables, and an intriguing area in terms of the complexity of the spirituality/religion-health mediators, there is potential applied value in this area of research. For example, when researchers learn more about the nature of the association between spirituality/religion and health, this information can be used to improve the effectiveness of the many church-based health promotion programs that are now being used to better the health of these communities. Additionally, many patients are asking that their spiritual needs be addressed within the context of clinical care. This research may be able to inform how these situations are handled.

Future Research

There are many potential directions for research on the relationship between spirituality/religion and health, including answering the aforementioned questions (why, for whom, and under what conditions this relationship exists). In addition, another promising area of research that has applied value deals with ways to improve effectiveness of church-based health

promotion programs by using a spiritually based approach to health education. Finally, it is important to bring together a multidisciplinary group of scholars to study this area—including theologians, who have not traditionally been included in past research. This is a dynamic area of research that has made significant advances in recent years and still has much opportunity for growth and discovery.

—*Cheryl L. Holt*

See also Cultural Sensitivity; Health Communication; Health Disparities; Locus of Control; Measurement

Further Readings

George, L. K., Larson, D. B., Koenig, H. G., & McCullough, M. E. (2000). Spirituality and health: What we know, what we need to know. *Journal of Social and Clinical Psychology, 19,* 102–116.

Hill, P. C., & Hood, R. W. (1999). *Measures of religiosity.* Birmingham, AL: Religious Education Press.

Holt, C. L., Kyles, A., Wiehagen, T., & Casey, C. M. (2003). Development of a spiritually-based breast cancer educational booklet for African American women. *Cancer Control, 10,* 37–44.

Holt, C. L., Lewellyn, L. A., & Rathweg, M. J. (2005). Exploring religion-health mechanisms among African American parishioners. *Journal of Health Psychology, 10,* 511–527.

Koenig, H. G., McCullough, M. E., & Larson, D. B. (2001). *Handbook of religion and health.* New York: Oxford University Press.

Levin, J. S. (2001). *God, faith, and health: Exploring the spirituality-healing connection.* Hoboken, NJ: Wiley.

Levin, J. S., & Vanderpool, H. Y. (1989). Is religion therapeutically significant for hypertension? *Social Science and Medicine, 29,* 69–78.

SPREADSHEET

Spreadsheets are among the most common types of computer software used by people working in epidemiology and public health. When desktop computers were introduced in the late 1970s, the first "killer app" ("killer application," i.e., the software that everyone wants to have) was the spreadsheet. Visicalc, the first major spreadsheet application, was so useful that it justified the purchase of a computer. For people working in fields such as statistical analysis, scientific research, economics, and finance, the ability to easily manipulate large amounts of numerical data presented an immense advantage over manual methods. The consequent time and cost savings easily paid back the investment in a desktop (or "personal") computer. In fact, spreadsheet software quickly became so popular that it helped establish the notion of the personal computer—a computer used primarily by a single individual and small enough to sit on a desktop, in contradistinction to the mainframe computers that were far more common at the time.

When the IBM PC was introduced in the early 1980s, Lotus 1-2-3 became its killer app. Lotus became the accepted standard for over a decade. Its success was coincidental with the runaway success of the PC. By the 1990s, with the introduction of the visual interface of Microsoft Windows and Apple's Macintosh, Microsoft Excel overtook Lotus 1-2-3 as the market leader and remains the standard to this day. Although there are other choices in spreadsheet software, Excel has a market share of more than 90%. Because Excel is bundled with the dominant word-processing program Microsoft Word in the ubiquitous Microsoft Office package and because many other programs can use Excel data files, it has become the accepted standard.

Spreadsheet software (the name is derived from the spreadsheet used by accountants to record financial information) is a computer program that presents a rectangular matrix of rows and columns to display data (see Figure 1). Each cell can contain numerical or textual data. Columns are defined by letters and rows by numbers. Cells are referenced as the intersection of those two criteria, A1 or D37, for example. In this figure, each row contains the information for one case, in this instance for one patient. Each column represents a variable (gender, date of birth, etc.) for that patient. In database terminology, each row is a record and each column is a field in that record.

Spreadsheets are most commonly used in epidemiology and public health for three purposes:

1. to create, store, and share electronic data files;

2. to perform basic calculations on data; and

3. to visually examine data and create reports, graphs, and charts based on the data in a spreadsheet.

The most common use of spreadsheets in epidemiology is to enter, store, and share electronic data files. Spreadsheets offer several advantages in data entry.

They allow data to be copied and pasted, rearranged, and reused. Spreadsheets also have time-saving features such as the fill function, which will copy formulas and number series to other cells. Features such as sorting and filtering make it easy to look at data in a spreadsheet, and most statistical applications programs can easily import data stored in a spreadsheet. Numbers and text can be entered and displayed in a variety of formats, and columns and rows can be resized vertically and horizontally to accommodate varying lengths of entries.

Figure 1 shows an excerpt of a spreadsheet storing information about a medical study, in standard rectangular file format (in cells A5:D15: Rows 1 to 4 are used for descriptive information and would not be used in statistical analysis). Each row represents information about a single patient, while each column represents a single variable. Row 5 contains labels that can be preserved as variable names when we import these data into a statistical package. Therefore, the first patient (with ID #1) is a female born on May 4, 1956, and whose first office visit was on August 1, 2005; the second patient is a male born on March 15, 1953, and whose first office visit was on September 3, 2005.

Spreadsheets can also be used to process data. They include many built-in functions that automate tasks such as computing the sum of a column of numbers or the number of days between two dates. This allows the user to perform simple data manipulations without using dedicated statistics software such as SAS. Using these functions, epidemiologists can also

	A	B	C	D	E
1	Dr. Lionel Schmerz				
2					
3	Patient Records				
4					
5	Patient_ID	DOB	Gender	1st Visit	
6	1	04-May-56	F	01-Aug-05	
7	2	15-Mar-53	M	03-Sep-05	
8	3	27-Mar-53	M	10-Oct-04	
9	4	17-Jun-90	F	08-May-05	
10	5	20-Dec-63	F	08-Jan-05	
11	6	09-Jun-42	M	09-Jul-04	
12	7	08-Apr-62	F	07-Sep-05	
13	8	17-Mar-59	M	28-Jan-05	
14	9	08-May-62	F	19-Aug-05	
15	10	05-Nov-68	F	08-Dec-05	

Figure 1   A Typical Spreadsheet Where Each Row Contains Data About a Patient

test the results of "what if?" scenarios. For example, if one assumes that 2% of the population per year will become infected with a disease, how many cases will one have in 10 years? What if one assumes 3% or 4%? Using a spreadsheet, one can see the results of these different scenarios immediately.

Spreadsheets provide many options for displaying data: It can be sorted, rows and columns can be hidden, data can be filtered so that only particular cases are displayed, and so on. Database designers often use a spreadsheet to analyze the structure of a data set before incorporating it into another system. Modern spreadsheet software also offers the capability to create graphic representations directly from spreadsheet data, including pie charts, bar graphs, and scatterplots. Charts created from spreadsheets are instantly updated when the underlying data are changed. The resulting charts can be saved in a variety of formats or pasted into Word or PowerPoint files.

As spreadsheet software evolved, the features took on many of the capabilities of relational database software. Using the relational model, data in other spreadsheets can be incorporated into a single file. Data can also be searched, sorted, and extracted by criteria. For example, instead of just displaying the sum of a column of numbers, the software can show subtotals by specified categories of the data, even from other files. Specified data can also be extracted into another file and reused.

—*Daniel Peck*

See also Relational Database

Further Readings

Frye, C. (2004). *Microsoft Office Excel 2003 step by step.* Redmond, WA: Microsoft Press.

Keller, G. (2000). *Applied statistics with Microsoft Excel.* Pacific Grove, CA: Duxbury Press.

Langer, M. (2004). *Excel 2003 for Windows: Visual QuickStart guide.* Berkeley, CA: Peachpit Press.

STATISTICAL AND CLINICAL SIGNIFICANCE

See HYPOTHESIS TESTING

STEM-AND-LEAF PLOT

The stem-and-leaf plot was developed by John Tukey and is used for continuous data during exploratory data analysis. It gives a detailed description of the distribution of the data and gives insight into the nature of the data. It is more informative than a simple tally of the numbers or a histogram because it retains individual data points. Using the information in a stem-and-leaf plot, the mean, median, mode, range, and percentiles can all be determined. In addition, when the stem-and-leaf plot is turned on its side, one is looking at a histogram of the data. From this, one can get an idea of how the data are distributed. For example, whether the data appear to be described by a normal curve or whether they are positively or negatively skewed. It also can point to unusual observations in the data that may be real or a result of reporting errors or data entry errors.

To make a stem-and-leaf plot by hand, the data should be ordered and made into categories or groups. If no logical categories exist for the data, a rough guide for the number of stems to use in the plot is two times the square root of the number of data points. When using a statistical program to create a stem-and-leaf plot, the number of categories is determined by the software. The leaf is generally the last digit of the number, and the stem includes the digits that come before the leaf. For example, if the data are whole numbers ranging from 20 to 75, the categories may be from 20 to 24, from 25 to 29, from 30 to 34, and so on. The stem is the digit in the tens position, valued from 2 to 7, and the leaf is the digit in the ones position, valued from 0 to 9. It is useful, especially when there is a place filler as in the example shown here, to add a key so that it is clear what number one's stem and leaf is portraying. See Table 1 for an illustration of a stem-and-leaf plot. By simply looking at this plot, it can be seen that the mode is 60 (the most frequent value) and the median, boldface in the table, is 59 (21 of the values fall above this number, and 21 of the values fall below this number).

The stem-and-leaf plot can also be used to compare data sets by using a side-by-side stem-and-leaf plot. In this case, the same stems are used for both data sets. The leaves of one data set will be on the right, and the leaves of the other will be on the left. When the leaves are side by side like this, the distributions, data ranges, and where the data points fall can be compared.

The stem-and-leaf plot becomes more difficult to create by hand as the amount of data increases. In addition,

Table 1	Height in Inches in U.S. Children Aged 0 to 17 Years
Stem	*Leaf*
2 *	0
2.	99
3 *	0
3.	556688
4 *	1224
4.	88889
5 *	34
5.	**9**9
6 *	0000001234
6.	55677789
7 *	22

Key: 2 * = 20 to 24, 2. = 25 to 29, and so on.

Source: Data from a random selection of 43 points from Centers for Disease Control and Prevention, National Center for Health Statistics, State and Local Area Integrated Telephone Survey, National Survey of Children's Health, 2003.

with large amounts of data, the benefits of being able to see individual data values decrease. This is the case because it becomes increasingly difficult to determine summary measures, such as the median, which is part of the value of using a stem-and-leaf plot. A histogram or a box-and-whisker plot may be a better option to visually summarize the data when the data set is large.

—*Rebecca Harrington*

See also Box-and-Whisker Plot; Histogram; Measures of Central Tendency; Percentiles; Tukey, John

Further Readings

Tukey, J. (1977). Scratching down numbers (stem-and-leaf). In J. Tukey (Ed.), *Exploratory data analysis* (pp. 1–26). Reading, MA: Addison-Wesley.

STRATIFIED METHODS

Confounding is a major consideration in etiological investigation because it can result in biased estimation of exposure effects. Control of confounding in data analysis is achieved by stratified analysis or by multivariable analysis. (Control of confounding in research design stage is achieved by matching for observational studies and by randomization for experimental studies.) Stratified analysis is accomplished by stratifying the confounding variable into homogeneous categories and evaluating the association within these strata. Multivariable analysis, on the other hand, involves the use of a regression model and allows the researcher to control for all confounders at the same time while looking at the contribution of each risk factor to the outcome variable. Stratified analysis is a necessary preliminary step to performing regression modeling to control for confounding. Unlike regression models, stratified analysis requires few assumptions.

Here is a simple example of how the stratified method works. In comparing mortality statistics for Mexico and the United States in the 1990s, we observe that Mexico's crude death rate is lower than the crude death rate in the United States. Yet Mexico's age-specific death rates are higher than those of the United States for every age categories. The different age distributions of the two populations explain the direction and magnitude of the difference in the crude death rates between the two countries. The crude death rate may be expressed as $\sum_i m_i w_i$, which is a weighted average of the age-specific death rates m_i with age distribution w_i as weights. The population of Mexico is younger. Mexico has relatively more people in the younger age categories and less people in the older age categories than the United States—w_i differs as a function of i between the two countries. There is a strong positive association between age and mortality—m_i is an increasing function of i for both countries. Thus, the existence of the confounding variable age i leads to a lower sum of products of m_i and w_i, the crude death rate for Mexico in the unstratified analysis, whereas a stratified analysis with confounding variable age as the stratification variable provides the true picture—Mexico has higher death rates at every age. Consequently, comparison of directly standardized rates of the two countries will show higher mortality for Mexico.

Generally, epidemiologists consider stratified methods for controlling for confounding to include the following steps:

1. Perform an unstratified analysis by calculating the crude measure of association ignoring the confounding variable (depending on the study design, the measure of association could be risk

difference, rate difference, risk ratio, rate ratio, or odds ratio).

2. Stratify by the confounding variable.

3. Calculate the adjusted overall measure of association.

4. Compare the crude measure with the adjusted measure.

If the crude estimate differs from the adjusted estimate by 10% or more, there is confounding, and the adjusted estimate should then be calculated by stratifying the confounder. If the estimates differ by less than 10%, there is no confounding. If there is confounding, formal significance testing and the calculation of 95% confidence interval may then be carried out to determine the significance of the association between the risk factor and the outcome variable for the different strata.

Analysis of *n*-Way Contingency Tables

Stratified analysis is more rigorously performed using categorical data analysis. To do so, we need to categorize all variables to construct *n*-way contingency tables with *n* equal to or greater than 3. Analysis of such a contingency table is done by computing statistics for measures and tests of association between two variables (usually a risk factor and an outcome variable) for each stratum defined by the third variable (usually the confounding variable) as a stratification variable, as well as computing the adjusted overall measures and tests.

Suppose we are interested in the association between the two variables y and z but we know that a third variable, sex, is a potential confounder. For an unstratified analysis, we would ignore sex and compute an asymptotic chi-square or an exact test statistic to test for the significance of association between y and z (this may be done by using SAS procedure frequency with tables statement tables $y * z$/chisq;). To account for sex as a confounder, we need to perform a stratified analysis adjusting for the stratification variable sex. This is done by analyzing a three-way contingency table with sex defining the strata. We first compute the chi-square test of association for each stratum of sex and then pool the strata to produce the Cochran-Mantel-Haenszel test statistic to conclude on whether or not rows (y) and columns (z) are associated after controlling for the stratification variable sex (the tables statement for SAS

procedure frequency is now changed to tables sex $* y * z$/chisq cmh;). Finally, the Mantel-Haenszel estimate provides the adjusted overall measure of association.

Suppose in the unstratified analysis we found no significant association between y and z. However, in the stratified analysis we found a significant association between y and z among males but not among females and the Cochran-Mantel-Haenszel statistic shows that there is a significant association between y and z. Thus, when we adjust for the effect of sex in these data, there is an association between y and z and the source of association is the male sex. But, if sex is ignored, no association is found.

If stratified analysis has ruled out confounding as a possible explanation for results and association is found to be not statistically significant, there are two possibilities. Either this is a true finding and there is actually no association between the suspected risk factor and the outcome, or the study did not have the power to show the difference even if it exists in the population because of insufficient sample size. In the latter case, another study may need to be conducted to exclude the possibility of confounding.

—*John J. Hsieh*

See also Confounding; Direct Standardization; Life Tables; Matching; Regression

Further Readings

Kleinbaum, D. G., Kupper, L. L., & Morgenstern, H. (1982). *Epidemiologic research: Principles and quantitative methods.* New York: Van Nostrand Reinhold.

Rothman, K. J., & Greenland, S. (1998). *Modern epidemiology.* Philadelphia: Lippincott-Raven.

Silva, I. (1999). *Cancer epidemiology: Principles and methods.* Lyon, France: IARC.

STRESS

Stress is one of the most talked about psychosocial constructs in popular discourse. We invoke the language of stress when we want sympathy, to convey that we feel inundated by demands, responsibility, or worry. The harried young mother in a store, a student at exam time, and the busy corporate executive are all familiar images of the stressed individual. Less prominent in the popular imagination is the stress of the impoverished, the unemployed, those facing discrimination, and outcasts at the margins of society. Stress is central to the study of health disparities because the disadvantaged members of society bear it in disproportion.

In its epidemiological sense, stress is a way to characterize those aspects of experiencing the social and physical environment that influence the well-being of individuals. A variety of definitions have been put forth, but a prevailing theme is that stress results either from socioenvironmental demands that strain the adaptive capacity of the individual or from the absence of means for the individual to obtain desired ends. Stress therefore is not strictly an attribute of the environment but arises from discrepancies between social conditions and characteristics of the individual. Similar to stress in engineering, psychosocial stress can be thought of as a force on a resisting body that flexes within, but may exceed, a normal range. Social stress research differs from engineering in that it treats the capacity to resist as a separate construct, that of coping. Epidemiologists also distinguish stressors from distress: Stressors refer to the environmental stimulus, while distress is the psychological or behavioral response to the stressor. This entry will describe the origin and development of stress concepts, the continuum of stress, stress as a process, and social patterns of stress exposure.

Origin and Development of Stress Concepts

Early-20th-century investigations with laboratory animals suggested that emotion-provoking stimuli produce physiological changes related to the fight or flight response. It was soon recognized that persistent stimuli of this type could produce physical illness. Cases of clinical pathology in humans were noted to follow severe emotional trauma, and eventually, physicians were trained to use a life chart as a diagnostic tool. By the mid-20th century, the general adaptation syndrome was posited as a mechanism by which physical environmental stressors could lead to diseases of adaptation. This led the way for the investigation of psychosocial stimuli as potential stressors, and soon life stresses became accepted risk factors for disease, especially psychosomatic disease. Stress events represented a change in a person's life, and hence the need to adapt. The life event checklist, which typically provided a count of life change events over the preceding 6 months or year, was a standard tool to rate the level of stress in people's lives. By the late 20th century, it was accepted that only undesired change, and not change per se, constituted stress. The field of social epidemiology has generally not pursued the biophysiological mechanisms by which the experience of negative events can produce illness, although some scientists now study the related concepts of allostasis and allostatic load.

Work proceeded in the social sciences on the concept of role-related stress. This emphasized chronic or recurrent conditions rather than "eventful" stress. Stressfulness in the work role, for example, is characterized in terms of task demands, degree of control over the amount or pace of work, danger, and noise. Jobs that are high in demand and low in control represent a particularly stressful work environment. Stress in the marital role may arise from interpersonal conflict, lack of intimacy or reciprocity, or conflict with the demands of other roles. The parent role, as suggested at the beginning of this entry, can bring with it stressful conditions that may be enduring, as living with adolescent turmoil. The absence of roles is another source of social stress: Consider the strains associated with childlessness for those who aspire to parenthood, or the lack of a partner or job.

Stress also results from one's social identity as an immigrant or a minority group member. Newcomers to a society may experience acculturation stress as they adapt to new customs, places, and an unfamiliar language. Intergenerational conflict may arise within immigrant families as parents and their children do not acculturate at the same pace. Visible minority individuals are at risk for exposure to discrimination stress, as are members of other marginalized groups who are defined by age, sexual orientation, or religion. These forms of stress exposure are distinct from life event stress in that they are embedded in the social roles and status characteristics that individuals have and tend to be chronic or recurring.

A Continuum of Stress Exposure

Stress phenomena occur across a spectrum from discrete events to continuous. The most discrete stressors are sudden, unexpected traumatic events such as an automobile accident, natural disaster, or criminal victimization. Somewhat less discrete are events that take some time to conclude—for example, a divorce, serious illness, or going on welfare. Near the middle of the spectrum is the category of daily hassles. While hassles are not major stressors individually, their accumulation from day to day may represent an important stress source. More continuous in nature is the ongoing absence of an expected or desired social role, or non-event. Stressors of this type include joblessness and childlessness. Chronic stress is the most continuous type; examples include living in a dangerous neighborhood, poverty, and living with a disability.

Eventful and chronic stress may be related through a process of stress proliferation. One example is when a worker loses a job because macroeconomic conditions led to the closure of a plant. Soon the loss of the individual's worker role and his or her source of income precipitate a financial crisis and increased conflict in the marital and parent roles—the "event" of job loss has proliferated stressful experience in a whole constellation of life domains. Social roles, and hence role-related stressors, do not occur in isolation.

Sometimes, the stressful meaning of a normally undesirable life event is negated by the context within which it occurs. Consider the separation or divorce of a person whose marital role history had been fraught with disappointment, conflict, and unhappiness—the event in such a case does not demand the kind of adaptation that is a threat to the person's well-being.

Stress as a Social Process

Stress may be viewed as the central means by which the structural arrangements of society create differential health outcomes for the people who occupy different social statuses and roles. Stress theory does not treat stress exposure as a health determinant in isolation: Stress is one element within a process that is closely linked to the social system. The amount of stress experienced is largely determined by an individual's social location. So are the social and personal resources that are available to forestall or cope with stressful events and circumstances as they occur. Stressful experiences may motivate social support (if it is available), which can mitigate their deleterious consequences. Successful resolution of a stressful event, such the loss of a home in a natural disaster, can build confidence that one can cope with future losses. Or it could be devastating to a person who had limited access to coping resources in the first place. Social inequality in the exposure to stress and in the availability of protective factors

amplifies the production and reproduction of health disparities. That is because social structural arrangements are systematically related both to the amount a person is exposed to stress and access to the resources needed to mitigate its ill-health effects.

Stress arises from the social context of people's lives. There is systematic variation in the level of stress and coping resources across social status dimensions. Greater exposure to stress is associated with low education and poverty, unmarried status, minority group membership, and youth. The existence of a gender difference is less clear. Since stress and coping resources are important determinants of health and illness outcomes, stress functions as an epidemiological link between a society's structure and the health outcomes of its members.

—*Donald A. Lloyd*

See also Geographical and Social Influences on Health; Health Disparities; Social Capital and Health; Social Epidemiology; Social Hierarchy and Health

Further Readings

Aneshensel, C. S. (1992). Social stress: Theory and research. *Annual Review of Sociology, 18*, 15–38.

Cohen, S., Kessler, R. C., & Gordon, L. U. (1995). *Measuring stress: A guide for health and social scientists.* New York: Oxford University Press.

Dohrenwend, B. P. (1998). *Adversity, stress, and psychopathology.* New York: Oxford University Press.

Pearlin, L. I., Lieberman, M., Menaghan, E., & Mullan, J. T. (1981). The stress process. *Journal of Health and Social Behavior, 22*, 337–356.

Thoits, P. A. (1995). Stress, coping, and social support processes: Where are we? What next? [Extra issue]. *Journal of Health and Social Behavior*, 53–79.

Turner, R. J., Wheaton, B., & Lloyd, D. A. (1995). The epidemiology of social stress. *American Sociological Review, 60*, 104–125.

STRUCTURAL EQUATION MODELING

The roots of structural equation modeling (SEM) begin with the invention of least squares about 200 years ago, the invention of factor analysis about 100 years ago, the invention of path analysis about 75 years ago, and the invention of simultaneous equation models about 50 years ago. The primary focus with SEM is on testing causal processes inherent in our theories. Before SEM, measurement error was assessed separately and not explicitly included in tests of theory. This separation has been one of the primary obstacles to advancing theory. With SEM, measurement error is estimated and theoretical parameters are adjusted accordingly—that is, it is subtracted from parameter estimates. Thus, SEM is a fundamental advancement in theory construction because it integrates measurement with substantive theory. It is a general statistical methodology, extending correlation, regression, factor analysis, and path analysis.

SEM is sometimes referred to as "latent variable modeling" because it reconstructs relationships between observed variables to infer latent variables. Many variables in epidemiological research are observable and can be measured directly (e.g., weight, pathogens, mortality). However, many variables are also inherently unobservable or *latent*, such as well-being, health, socioeconomic status, addiction, and quality of life. Measuring and interpreting latent variables requires a measurement theory. Latent variables and its respective measurement theory can be tested using an SEM technique called "confirmatory factor analysis." This involves specifying which latent variables are affected by which observed variables and which latent variables are correlated with each other.

SEM also provides a way of systematically examining reliability and validity. Reliability is the consistency of measurement and represents the part of a measure that is free from random error. In SEM, reliability is assessed as the magnitude of the direct relations that all variables except random ones have on an observed variable. This capability of SEM to assess the reliability of each observed variable and simultaneously estimate theoretical and measurement parameters is a fundamental methodological advancement. The potential for distortion in theoretical parameters is high when measurement error is ignored, and the more complicated the model the more important it becomes to take measurement error into account. Validity is the degree of direct structural relations (invariant) between latent and measured variables. SEM offers several ways of assessing validity. Validity differs from reliability because we can have consistent invalid measures. The R^2 value of an observed variable offers a straightforward measure of reliability. This R^2 sets an upper limit for validity because the validity of a measure cannot exceed its reliability.

Major Assumptions

Like other kinds of analyses, SEM is based on a number of assumptions. For example, it assumes that data represent a population. Unlike traditional methods, however, SEM tests models by comparing sample data with the implied population parameters. This is particularly important because the distinction between sample and population parameters has been often ignored in practice. SEM generally assumes that variables are measured at the interval or ratio level, and ordinal variables, if used at all, are truncated versions of interval or ratio variables. Hypothesized relationships are assumed to be linear in their parameters. All variables in a model are assumed to have a multivariate Gaussian or normal distribution. Therefore, careful data screening and cleaning are essential to successfully work with SEM.

SEM shares many assumptions with ordinary least squares regression and factor analysis. For example, the error of endogenous latent variables is uncorrelated with exogenous variables. The error of the endogenous observed variables is uncorrelated with the latent endogenous variables. The error of the exogenous observed variables is uncorrelated with the latent exogenous variables. The error terms of the endogenous latent variables and the observed endogenous and exogenous variables are mutually uncorrelated. This is the result of combining factor analysis and regression in one overall simultaneous estimation.

Steps in SEM

Specification

Models are constructed by defining concepts, clarifying the dimensions of each concept, forming measures of the dimensions, and specifying the expected empirical relationships between the measures and the construct. The accuracy of parameter estimates is partly dependent on the correctness of the theory and partly dependent on the validity of the measurement. There is always more than one model that fits the data, and thinking about these alternative models and testing them helps refine theory. Depicted in Figure 1 is a path diagram—a common way to represent models. The circles represent latent variables, squares represent observed variables, double-headed arrows represent correlations, and single-headed arrows represent causal effects. The one-to-one correspondence between path diagrams and sets of structural equations facilitates communication and clarification of all

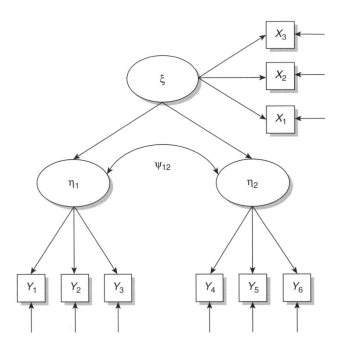

Figure 1   Example of a Path Diagram in SEM

parameters and their interrelationships. Model parameters are fully specified, which means stating a hypothesis for every parameter.

Identification

Models are composed of a set of equations with known and unknown parameters. Identification is the problem of determining whether there is a unique solution for each unknown parameter in the model. It is a mathematical problem involving population parameters, not sample size. A model can fail to be identified even with a large sample. There are a number of rules that if followed ensure identification. The most common is the t rule. The t in the t rule refers to the number of free parameters specified in the model. Specifically, a model is identified if the t value is equal to or smaller than half the number of observed variables multiplied by the number of observed variables plus 1 $[t \leq (1/2)(p)(p+1)]$. The t rule is a necessary but not sufficient condition for identification. Other rules are the scaling rule, three-indicator rule, null-β rule, recursive rule, and rank-and-order rules.

Estimation

SEM estimation procedures use a particular fitting function to minimize the difference between the

population and the sample. Basically, this is a recipe to transform data into an estimate. The data matrix for SEM must be positive definite, a mathematical requirement for the estimation algorithms. Maximum likelihood is the default estimator in most SEM programs. Maximum likelihood is based on the idea that the sample is more likely to have come from a population of one particular set of parameter values than from a population of any other set of values. Maximum likelihood estimation is the vector of values that creates the greatest probability of having obtained the sample in question. This method of estimation is asymptotically unbiased, consistent, and asymptotically efficient, and its distribution asymptotically normal. If the sample is large, no other estimator has a smaller variance. There are two drawbacks with maximum likelihood. First, it assumes a normal distribution of error terms, which is problematic for many measures in the health and social sciences fields. Second, the assumption of multinormality is even more problematic, again because of the extensive use of crude measures.

In choosing estimators, the main choice is between maximum likelihood and weighted least squares. The weighted least squares estimator is used when multivariate normality is lacking and, especially, when some of the variables are ordinal. Although weighted least squares is computationally demanding, it is important to have a large sample size when some variables are ordinal. Other choices in estimators include generalized least squares and unweighted least squares. Maximum likelihood and generalized least squares are very similar. The generalized least squares estimator weights observations to correct for unequal variances or nonzero covariance of the disturbance terms. It is used when variable distributions are heteroscedastic or when there are autocorrelated error terms. An unweighted least square is used with variables that have low reliability. This estimator is less sensitive to measurement error than maximum likelihood or generalized least squares. Research shows estimates from the unweighted least square to be similar in models with and without error, while maximum likelihood estimates without and without errors are very different.

Fitting

After a model is estimated, its fit must be assessed. There are more than 20 different fit measures to assess misfit and goodness of fit. They are based on six different criteria: (1) the discrepancy between the sample covariance matrix and the fitted (population) covariance, (2) accounting for observed variances and covariance, (3) maximizing the fit of a cross-validated model, (4) including a penalty for unnecessarily estimating parameters or creating fewer degrees of freedom, (5) the amount of improvement over a baseline model, and (6) separating the measurement model from the latent variable model.

Most of the existing fit measures are tied directly or indirectly to the chi-square ratio. This chi-square statistic is based on the same general idea as the familiar chi-square comparison between the observed and expected values. The difference is that in SEM our substantive interest or hypothesis is the null hypothesis. In traditional applications, we want to reject the hypothesis of no difference between observed and expected frequencies so that we can accept the alternative hypothesis of a difference. In contrast, with SEM, we want to find no difference between the expected and observed values. Therefore, the smaller the chi-square values the better because this leads to a failure to reject the null hypothesis, which is our substantive interest.

The chi-square statistic assumes that the variables in a model are multivariate normal, that the data are unstandardized (covariance as opposed to correlations matrixes), that sample sizes are at least $N > 100$ and preferably $N > 200$, and that the model holds exactly in the population. This chi-square has been found robust to skew violations but sensitive to Kurtosis violations. The interpretation of chi-square depends on adequate sample sizes. With large samples tiny deviations can lead one to reject the null hypothesis, which again in SEM is of substantive interest.

SEM fit measures are not applicable in exactly identified models. In exactly identified models (when degrees of freedom = 0), the sample variances and covariance always equal the estimates of the population variances and covariance because there is only enough information to calculate one estimate per parameter. A limitation of chi-square is that the closer the model is to being exactly identified, the higher the chi-square value. In other words, chi-square values always decrease when parameters are added to the model. With an overidentified model (degrees of freedom > 0), the overall fit can differ from the fit of different parts of the model. A poor overall fit does not help to detect areas of poor fit. The overall fit statistics also do not tell us how well the independent variables predict the dependent variables.

A good fit does not mean that model is "correct" or "best." Many models fit the same data well. Measurement parameters often outnumber theoretical parameters. Therefore, a "good fit" may reflect the measurement and not the theory. There is considerable discussion about fit measures. The best current advice in evaluating model fit is to seek a nonsignificant chi-square (at least $p > .05$ and preferably .10, .20, or better); an IFI (incremental fit index), RFI (relative fit index), or CFI (comparative fit index) greater than .90; low RMSR (root mean square residual) and RMSEA (root mean square of approximation) values, plus a 90% confidence interval for RMSEA < .08; and a parsimony index that show the proposed model as more parsimonious than alternative models.

Modification

It is not uncommon for models to exhibit a poor fit with the data. There are many potential sources of error, including an improperly specified theory, poor correspondence between the theory and the model, and causal heterogeneity in the sample. Modifications are typically made to poor-fitting models, and most SEM software packages provide modification indices that suggest which changes can improve model fit. However, using these indices in the absence of theory represents one of the main abuses of SEM. It is important that a systematic search for error is conducted and that modifications are based on theory or to generate new theory. A well-fitting respecified model does not represent a test. Respecified models must be tested on new data.

Specialized Techniques

SEM is a highly flexible methodology that allows for many special types of models to be examined. The most common models are those with unidirectional (recursive) causal effects, but SEM also allows for bidirectional (nonrecursive) effects to be tested. Stacked or multiple groups can also be examined, which facilitates interpretation and tests of interaction. Repeated measures designs can be analyzed using an SEM technique called "latent growth curves." This provides a way of examining both linear and nonlinear changes over time. Recent advances in software also provide a way of accounting for hierarchical or nested data structures, including survey weights.

Summary

SEM is a flexible and extensive method for testing theory. These models are best developed on the basis of substantive theory. Hypothesized theoretical relationships imply particular patterns of covariance or correlation. Statistical estimates of the hypothesized covariance indicate, within a margin of error, how well the models fit with data. The development and testing of these models advance theory by allowing latent variables, by including measurement error, by accepting multiple indicators, by accommodating reciprocal causation, and by estimating model parameters simultaneously. Structural equation models subsume factor analysis, multiple regression, and path analysis. The integration of these traditional types of analysis is an important advancement because it makes possible empirical specification of the linkages between imperfectly measured variables and theoretical constructs of interest.

The capabilities, technical features, and applications of SEM are continually expanding. Many of these advances are reported in the journal *Structural Equation Modeling* and communicated on the international and interdisciplinary SEM listserv called SEMNET. This listserv also archives its discussion and provides a forum for offering and receiving advice, which makes it an invaluable resource for epidemiologists and other social scientists learning and using SEM.

—David F. Gillespie and Brian Perron

See also Factor Analysis; Measurement; Regression

Further Readings

De Stavola, B. L., Nitsch, D., Silva, I. D. S., McCormack, V., Hardy, R., Mann, V., et al. (2005). Statistical issues in life course epidemiology. *American Journal of Epidemiology, 163*, 84–96.

Der, G. (2002). Structural equation modelling in epidemiology: Some problems and prospects [Commentary]. *International Journal of Epidemiology, 31*, 1199–1200.

Hoyle, R. H. (Ed.). (1995). *Structural equation modeling.* Thousand Oaks, CA: Sage.

Keller, S. D., Ware, J. E., Jr., Bentler, P. M., Aaronson, N. K., Alonso, J., Apolone, G., et al. (1998). Use of structural equation modeling to test the construct validity of the SF-36 Health Survey in ten countries: Results from the IQOLA project. *Journal of Clinical Epidemiology, 51*, 1179–1188.

Kline, R. B. (2004). *Principles and practice of structural equation modeling* (2nd ed.). New York: Guilford Press.

Schumacker, R. E., & Lomax, R. G. (2004). *A beginner's guide to structural equation modeling* (2nd ed.). Mahwah, NJ: Lawrence Erlbaum.

Singh-Manous, A., Clarke, P., & Marmot, M. (2002). Multiple measures of socio-economic position and psychosocial health: proximal and distal measures. *International Journal* of Epidemiology, *31*, 1192–1199.

STUDY DESIGN

Epidemiologic studies have traditionally been categorized as having "descriptive" or "analytic" designs. Descriptive studies are viewed primarily as hypothesis-generating studies and usually take advantage of routinely collected data to describe the distribution of a disease in a population in terms of the basic descriptors of person, place, and time. Analytic studies are further divided into "observational" and "experimental" study designs and are viewed as approaches suitable for testing specific hypotheses about disease etiology or the efficacy of disease prevention strategies. The main categories of observational studies are the cohort, case-control, nested case-control, case-cohort, case crossover, and cross-sectional designs. The most commonly employed experimental designs used in epidemiologic research include the classic randomized clinical trial and the quasi-experimental nonrandomized study design used to evaluate the effectiveness of population-based disease prevention approaches.

Descriptive Epidemiology

Data Sources

Descriptive epidemiologic studies are designed to determine the distribution of a disease in a population with regard to person, place, and time. The numbers of individuals in the population who are diagnosed with or die from various diseases are obtained from sources such as vital records files, disease registries, and surveys. Death certificates provide information on the underlying cause of death and provide basic socio-demographic data on the decedent such as age, gender, race/ethnicity, marital status, and place of residence at the time of death. Birth certificates are used to study the incidence of various birth outcomes such as low birthweight (LBW) and its relationship to various parental factors such as maternal age. Birth defects registries also exist in some areas and combine data from birth certificates and reports from hospitals, physicians, and genetic testing laboratories.

Cancer registries now exist in all regions of the United States and are used to enumerate the number of total and specific forms of cancer that occur in a defined population over a specified time period. Cancer registries routinely collect information from hospital records and pathology laboratories regarding various clinical factors such as the cancer's anatomic location and histological type, clinical and pathologic stage of the disease, and information on the methods used to diagnosis the cancer. The cancer records also include data on various sociodemographic characteristics such as age, gender, race/ethnicity, marital status, and place of residence at the time of diagnosis. The address listed in the vital record or disease registry report at the time of death, birth, or diagnosis can be coded to the individual's census tract of residence using computer-based matching algorithms. The census tract reports contain data on various measures of socioeconomic status such as income and education for the geographic area in which the individual resided at the time of birth, death, or disease diagnosis. These numerator data are then combined with population denominator data to create disease incidence or death rates by person, place, or time.

Person, Place, and Time

Characteristics of persons include age, gender, race/ethnicity, marital status, and various measures of socioeconomic status such as education and income. Most diseases show distinct patterns of occurrence with regard to these personal characteristics. Breast cancer steadily increases with age until about the age of menopause at which time the age curve flattens. After the menopause, breast cancer incidence again increases with advancing age, albeit at a slower rate. These and other observations have led researchers to consider the possibility that pre- and postmenopausal breast cancer arise from separate etiologic processes. Numerous other examples exist regarding the relationship between disease incidence and mortality and age.

Descriptive epidemiologic studies have also shown that incidence and mortality rates for many diseases vary in relationship to personal characteristics. For example, mortality attributed to hypertension has been shown to occur more frequently among African Americans when compared with whites, while the risk for adult brain tumors is higher in men than women, most likely due to occupational exposures to chemicals.

Disease incidence and mortality patterns may also show distinctive geographic patterns. One of the earliest clues that early infection with hepatitis B virus (HBV) might be related to the development of liver cancer came from observations that countries with a high incidence of liver cancer were the same counties that reported high HBV infection rates. Researchers observed a strong concomitant geographic variation in liver cancer and HBV infection rates around the world. These data led to the development of case-control, cohort, and intervention studies that confirmed a strong association between HBV and liver cancer. The findings from the epidemiologic studies were further supported by strong evidence derived from animal models.

Variations in disease incidence and mortality over time have also provided insights into disease etiology and the effectiveness of intervention programs in a population-based setting. In the mid-1960s, approximately 60% to 65% of white males in the United States were cigarette smokers. Due in large part to the success of public health smoking prevention and cessation programs, the number of American males who currently smoke cigarettes is approximately 20%. An examination of age-adjusted lung cancer death rates for males in the United States between the years 1930 and 2005 show the waxing and waning of the cigarette-induced lung cancer epidemic. Between 1930 and 1980, male lung cancer death rates increased every year at a steady rate. However, by 1980 the success of the smoking prevention and cessation programs began to take effect, and the annual rate of increase in lung cancer mortality began to slow and then level off by 1990. Beginning in 1991, lung caner death rates began to fall for the first time in more than 60 years and have continued to decrease for the past 15 years.

Analytic Epidemiology

Analytic studies are further divided into "observational" and "experimental" designs. Observational studies include cohort, case-control, nested case-control, case-cohort, case crossover, and cross-sectional designs. These types of studies have also been referred to as natural experiments in that they are designed to take advantage of exposure/disease relationships that occur naturally in human populations.

Cohort Studies

The word *cohort* comes from Latin and originally referred to "one of 10 divisions of an ancient Roman legion [and later] a group of individuals having a statistical factor [such] as age or class" in common (*Merriam-Webster Online Dictionary*, www.m-w.com). The epidemiologic cohort represents a study base that is defined according to various characteristics. Figure 1 shows the basic structure of a typical cohort study. Note that baseline medical examinations or reviews of medical records are used to identify individuals who have already been diagnosed with the disease of interest. Since the purpose of the cohort study is to calculate incidence rates among exposed and nonexposed subgroups within the cohort, it is vital to start with a cohort that does not include prevalent cases. Various exposures of interest are collected at baseline through a variety of methods. A cohort study of factors related to heart disease might use questionnaires to collect baseline data on various lifestyle exposures such as diet, physical activity, and tobacco and alcohol use. Serum samples could also be drawn to measure levels of cholesterol, triglycerides, and other biochemical

markers, while anthropometric methods could be used to categorize cohort members based on body fat deposition using measures such as body mass index and skin fold measurements. Since some of these measures may change over time, cohort members would be reexamined and reinterviewed on a periodic basis, perhaps annually. The annual follow-up surveys and clinic visits would also be designed to identify members of the cohort who have been diagnosed or died from heart disease during the past year. To confirm a diagnosis reported by a cohort member during the annual follow-up, every attempt is made to obtain medical records related to the diagnosis. Physicians trained in cardiology would review the available medical records to confirm the diagnosis. The reviewers should be blinded as to the exposure status of the cohort member and use standardized diagnostic criteria in making their decisions. Deaths that occur between annual surveys or clinic visits are obtained from family members or by matching cohort member information against the National Death Index. High-quality cohort studies maintain excellent follow-up rates of 90% or higher and obtain medical records for 98% of patients with a diagnosis of the disease of interest. Maintaining a small loss to

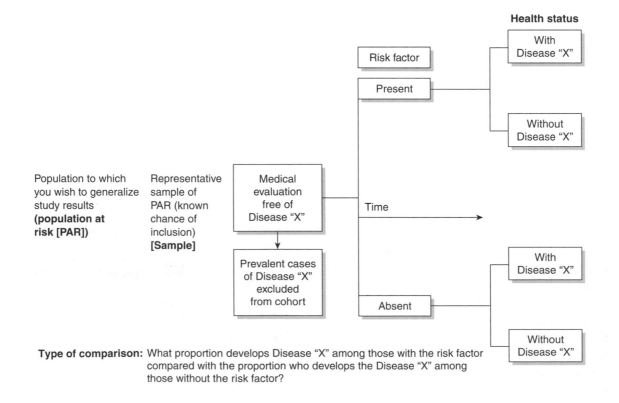

Figure 1   Basic Design of a Cohort Study: Flow Chart

follow-up rate is critical to ensuring that study results are not affected by selection bias where cohort members who are lost to follow-up are different from those who are not lost to follow-up with regard to both exposure and disease status.

Cohorts may be either "static" or "dynamic." In a static cohort study, all cohort members are enrolled at about the same time and are followed for a short period of time, thus minimizing loss to follow-up and the effects of competing causes of death. An example would be a cohort study of maternal factors related to LBW where a cohort of women are all registered in a prenatal clinic during their third month of pregnancy at about the same calendar time and are then followed to term. Let's assume that the exposure of interest is maternal cigarette smoking during the pregnancy and that LBW ($< 2{,}500$ g) serves as the outcome variable. This is a static cohort given that all cohort members are enrolled at the same time and the number of young, healthy mothers who are lost to follow-up or who die during the short 6-month period of the study is likely to be small. The task is to calculate a cumulative incidence of LBW children among smoking and nonsmoking mothers. Dividing the cumulative incidence of LBW among smoking mothers by the cumulative incidence among nonsmoking mothers provides the relative risk of a LBW child among smoking mothers when compared with nonsmoking mothers. The calculations are as follows:

$$\frac{\text{Number of LBW children among smoking mothers}}{\text{Number of smoking mothers initially enrolled}}$$
$$= \frac{30}{1000} = 30 \text{ per } 1000,$$

$$\frac{\text{Number of LBW children among nonsmoking mothers}}{\text{Number of nonsmoking mothers initially enrolled}}$$
$$= \frac{15}{1000} = 15 \text{ per } 1000,$$

Relative risk
$$= \frac{\text{Cumulative incidence in smoking mothers}}{\text{Cumulative incidence in nonsmoking mothers}}$$
$$= \frac{30/1000}{15/1000} = 2.0.$$

If the cohort structure is dynamic, cohort members are enrolled over a longer period of time and the follow-up time is usually measured in years. The long follow-up time leads to more cohort members being lost to follow-up or dying before they develop the disease of interest. These follow-up issues and the staggered enrollment period call for the use of a different approach to calculating disease occurrence among the exposed and nonexposed. This type of design calls for the calculation of an incidence density rate (IDR) where the numerator of the rate is still the number of cohort members diagnosed with the disease of interest, over a specified period of time. On the other hand, since each cohort member will enter and leave the cohort at different times, the investigators need to calculate the person-years of risk (PYR) for each cohort member. The sum of the individual PYR forms the denominator for calculating the IDR. Dividing the IDR among the exposed by the IDR among the nonexposed give us the rate ratio as an estimator of the relative risk.

In a dynamic cohort where the number of cohort members diagnosed with the disease during the follow-up period is small relative to a large number of PYR, the rate ratio is an excellent estimator of the relative risk. The calculations of the IDR and the incidence density rate ratio (IDRR) for a hypothetical cohort study of the risk of developing lung cancer among smokers versus nonsmokers are as follows:

$$\frac{\text{Number of smoking cohort members diagnosed with lung cancer}}{\text{PYR among nonsmoking cohort members}}$$
$$= \frac{60}{5800} = 10.3 \text{ per } 1000 \text{ PYR,}$$

$$\frac{\text{Number of nonsmoking cohort members diagnosed with lung cancer}}{\text{PYR among nonsmoking cohort members}}$$
$$= \frac{15}{10100} = 1.5 \text{ per } 1000 \text{ PYR,}$$

$$\text{IDRR} = \frac{\text{Incidence density rate among smokers}}{\text{Incidence density rate among nonsmokers}}$$
$$= \frac{10.3}{1.5} = 6.9.$$

Case-Control Studies

The basic idea of the case-control design is to select a group of cases (individuals with the disease of interest) and a group of controls (individuals without the disease of interest) and then measure the extent of exposure in the two groups. The basic outline of the case-control design is shown in Figure 2. A more detailed discussion of the issues covered in this section can be found in the series of three articles published by Wacholder et al., which are listed below in the "Further Readings" section. In theory, all case-control studies are embedded within a cohort, although the nature and structure of the underlying cohort is not always easy to discern. Cases and controls may be sampled from either a primary or a secondary study base. A primary study base requires a mechanism for ensuring complete or nearly complete ascertainment of all eligible cases in a defined population and a mechanism for assuring that all non-cases have an equal chance of being selected from the same underlying population that produced the cases. The basic principle is that there is a reciprocal relationship between the case and control selection procedures such that if a case had not been diagnosed with the disease, the individual would have the opportunity to be selected as a control and vice versa. Let us assume that we want to study the relationship between estrogen replacement therapy in postmenopausal women and the risk of developing breast cancer. Let us further assume that we decide to conduct this study in a small country that has a high-quality national cancer registry the existence of which ensures that we can ascertain all or nearly all eligible cases. Furthermore, the country maintains a complete registry of the population from which we can select control women without breast cancer. The use of the case-control design in the presence of these resources would help to ensure that we have satisfied the reciprocity principle and that we are dealing with a primary study base. Access to a primary study base helps reduce the potential for creating selection bias at the design phase by minimizing the chances that cases and controls are selected for inclusion in the study based on the presence or absence of the exposure of interest.

However, these conditions frequently do not exist and investigators are often forced to use a secondary study base to select cases and controls. A common example involves selecting cases from one or more hospitals or medical care practices. The exact nature and structure of the underlying study base that gave rise to the hospitalized cases and controls is not always clear. In addition, the chances of being selected as a case or control depends on the extent to which the case and

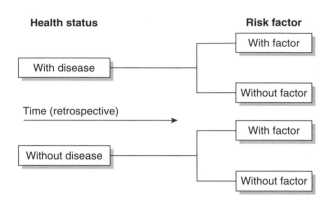

Type of comparison: The prevalence of the risk factor among those with the disease compared with those without

Figure 2   Basic Design of a Case-Control Study: Flow Chart

control diseases usually result in hospitalization and the hospital referral patterns for the case and control diagnoses in the underlying target population. If referral of the case and control diseases to the hospital is based on the presence or absence of the exposure, then there is a clear chance that study findings will be affected by design-based selection bias. Selection bias may also occur in case-control studies when not all eligible controls agree to be interviewed, tested, or examined and exposure information is absent for these nonparticipating study subjects and if the patterns of nonparticipation are related to both disease and exposure status.

The investigator needs to pay careful attention to methods and materials used to confirm the existence of the disease in cases. A standard and well-recognized set of diagnostic criteria should be employed. Diagnoses may be based on information from a variety of sources, including disease registry, hospital, and pathology reports. In some cases, it may be necessary to have an expert panel of pathologists conduct a blinded review of the original biopsy slides to accurately classify the disease, a step that is necessary, for instance, when attempting to classify subtypes of non-Hodgkin's lymphoma.

Another major threat to the internal validity of the case-control study is the difficulty encountered when attempting to assess exposure status retrospectively. The extent to which valid measurement of prior exposure can be obtained depends on the nature of the exposure, the amount of details required, and the length of time that has existed between the interview and the exposure event. Cigarette smoking and alcohol consumption patterns can be assessed with a fair degree of accuracy through the use of structured questionnaires. Other lifestyle behaviors such as diet and physical activity are more difficult to measure. Using similar methods to collect exposure data for cases and controls is vitally important.

Investigators also employ biomarkers of internal dose as a means of determining exposures. Although these biomarkers can be quite useful, the laboratory values may only reflect recent rather than long-term exposures. In addition, the investigator is often forced to use a surrogate biologic source such as sera in place of another tissue source, which may lead to more accurate results but is highly invasive and therefore impractical in a population-based study. The collection of biomarker specimens may also add to respondent burden, increasing the nonresponse rate and thus increasing the potential for selection bias.

Nested Case-Control and Case-Cohort Studies

This variant of the basic case-control study is used to select study subjects from within an established cohort study. Cases are defined as individuals who have been ascertained through the cohort follow-up procedures to have the disease of interest. Controls are selected from among the remaining cohort members who have not developed the disease. One or more control subjects are selected for each case from among the nondiseased cohort members who were at risk at the time the case was diagnosed. This "matching" procedure provides close control over time as a potential confounding variable. If the follow-up rate for cohort members is high, then the cases and controls are derived from the same primary study base and participation rates are a nonissue. The quality of the exposure information is improved because these data are collected closer in time to the actual events. The temporal relationship between the exposure and disease is also assured because the exposure data are collected within the original cohort structure prior to the development of the disease. Nested case-control studies can be especially useful when the exposure measurement involves an expensive laboratory assay. Assume, for example, that we want to assess the relationship between various hormone patterns and breast cancer risk in a cohort of 10,000 women followed for 7 years. While the baseline blood draws might be reasonable to obtain, the cost of 10,000 hormone assays would be prohibitive. Another

approach is to obtain and freeze the baseline serum samples. Once a sufficient number of cases are identified through the cohort follow-up procedures, the investigators can then thaw and test the samples for the much smaller number of cases and controls. The case-cohort and nested case-control studies are similar in design and vary only with respect to the control sampling procedures employed. In the case-cohort study, the controls are selected at random from among all nondiseased cohort members without regard to matching at the design phase by time at risk. Rather, information is collected on time at risk and included as a potential confounding variable at the time of analysis.

Case-Crossover Studies

The selection of an appropriate control group is particularly difficult when attempting to identify risk factors for acute disease outcomes. One example would be a study attempting to determine the events that immediately preceded a sudden nonfatal myocardial infarction. Another example would include a study of events that occurred close in time to an occupational injury. In both examples, the investigators would be hard pressed to select a separate control group to assess these proximal risk factors. The case-crossover design has been developed for these types of situations. In the case-crossover design, the case serves as his or her own control. The basic idea is to determine if a particular exposure occurred close in time to the acute event and how frequently this exposure occurred during a "control" time period. Let us assume a hypothesis that acute nonfatal myocardial infarctions may be triggered by heavy physical exertion just prior to the event. Let us further assume that we know the days and times when the acute nonfatal myocardial infarctions occurred. A key event exposure could be defined as heavy physical exertion occurring within 30 min of the acute nonfatal myocardial infarction. The "control" period could be chosen as the same day and time during the previous week. One approach to the analysis of data from a case-crossover design involves a matched pair design. Using a case as his or her own control also has a number of other advantages, including savings in time and money that result from not having to interview members of a separate control group. Another is that personal characteristics that do not change over time, such as gender and race/ethnicity, are controlled at the design phase. Data on other potential confounders that are more transient by nature need to be collected and included in the analysis.

Cross-Sectional Studies

The cross-sectional study is usually considered to be a hypothesis-generating design. In cross-sectional studies, a population of individuals is cross-classified with regard to a disease and potential risk factors at one point in time. The basic cross-sectional design is shown in Figure 3. Because data on the disease and the exposure are collected at a point in time, this approach cannot provide estimates of disease incidence but instead produces an estimate of disease prevalence with regard to the possible risk factors. In addition, the lack of a time dimension also prohibits the investigator from drawing any firm conclusions regarding the temporal relationship between the disease and the exposures. However, a series of cross-sectional surveys embedded within a community-based intervention study can help to test a hypothesis. Conducting multiple surveys in intervention and comparison communities can help to show that the prevalence of the desired behavioral changes is occurring more readily in the intervention community rather than in the comparison community.

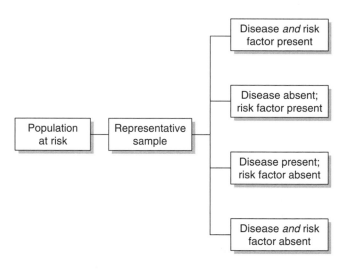

Figure 3   Cross-Sectional Studies: Flow Chart

Experimental and Quasi-Experimental Designs

Randomized Clinical Trials

Randomized trials are conducted to assess the efficacy and safety of a clinical intervention such as surgery, medical devices, and drug therapies. An outline of the basic design is shown in Figure 4. In some instances, a new intervention is tested against an existing form of treatment, such as testing a standard coronary artery metal stent against a new medicated stent. The study could be designed to assess a short-term outcome such as restenosis of the treated artery or long-term effects such as patient survival. In situations where a suitable treatment for the disease does not exist, the investigators might consider testing the new treatment against a "placebo" group, which typically receives no treatment or no effective treatment. Randomized trials are also conducted to assess the efficacy of various disease-screening techniques, the efficacy of natural products such as beta carotene for cancer chemoprevention, or the efficacy of various counseling approaches to effect desired behavioral changes.

The first phase of a randomized clinical trial involves developing inclusion criteria for patients. These criteria include sociodemographic factors such as age and clinical parameters that measure the patient's current health status as related to the disease under study and to other comorbid conditions. Individuals who meet the inclusion criteria are then randomized to either the intervention or comparison group. The randomization helps ensure that the intervention or treatment group and the comparison group will be similar with regard to baseline characteristics (potential confounders) that are strongly associated with the outcome under study. The extent to which randomization has equalized the distribution of potential confounding variables among the intervention and comparison groups can be determined by creating a table that compares the characteristics of the two groups at baseline following randomization.

Where feasible, a procedure called double-blinding is also used. For example, we might want to test the extent to which a new analgesic relieves headache better than buffered aspirin. Given that the outcome "pain relief" is somewhat subjective, the investigator might be concerned that if patients were aware of which drug they received, those treated with the "new" drug might be inclined to report more relief than those who knew they were treated with aspirin. To avoid this potential problem, a double-blind design is used where the patients and their primary care givers are not told whether the patient has been randomized to aspirin or the new drug. In addition, the individuals charged with interviewing the patients about their perceptions of pain relief are also blinded to the patients' treatment assignment. As an aid to maintaining patient blinding,

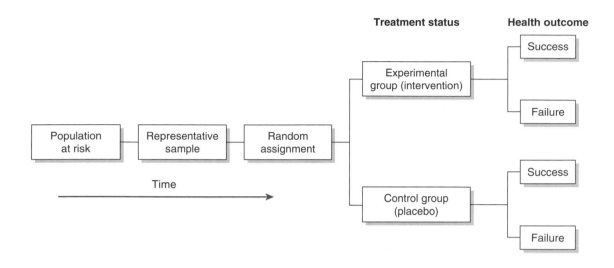

Figure 4   Experimental Design: Flow Chart

aspirin and the new drug would be designed to have the same shape, color, taste, and packaging. It is more difficult but not impossible to implement double-blinding in studies of interventions involving surgical or medical device interventions. In acupuncture treatment, the needles are often inserted using a small plastic tube as a guide. In studies of the potential therapeutic benefits of acupuncture, patients have been randomized to receive either real acupuncture treatments or to a "sham" acupuncture treatment group. The touch of the plastic guide tube on the patient's skin has been used to create a false sense that needles are actually being inserted. The procedures are applied to the patients' back in such a way that the patient is blinded to whether they are receiving the real or sham acupuncture treatment. The individuals charged with assessing the patients' perceptions of pain relief could also be blinded as to which group the patient had been randomized to.

Conduct of randomized trials should involve periodic analysis of the study data to determine if a preset level of statistical significance has been reached that would indicate that the new treatment has been shown to be superior to the old treatment or has more negative side effects than the old treatment. If either of these outcomes is observed, then the trial should be stopped on ethical grounds. These decisions are the main prevue of the safety monitoring board, which works closely with the analysis group to determine on an ongoing basis the observed benefits and risk associated with the new treatment.

Another key issue involves the extent to which patients randomized to the intervention group can be maintained on the intervention, particularly over long periods of time. Patient adherence is affected by the burden imposed by the intervention, including the amount of discomfort or negative side effects caused by the intervention. Adherence to the treatment regimen is measured in a number of ways, such as counting pills or weighing pill bottles at periodic visits to the clinic or through measuring the drug or its metabolites in blood or urine. The number of dropouts from the intervention group needs to be kept as low as possible and measured against the number of patients in the comparison group who adopt the intervention independently of the randomization process. Patients who switch groups during the course of the trial create some interesting issues with regard to data analysis. The most common approach to calculating an outcome measure such as the relative risk or the risk ratio involved has been referred to as the "intent to treat" approach. This approach analyzes the frequency of the outcome in the groups as originally randomized irrespective of whether patients failed to be maintained in their original groups.

Studies involving community-based interventions often involve what is described as a quasi-experimental design. Let us suppose that we are interested in determining if a media-based intervention can increase the number of adults in a population who are screened for hypertension and placed on an appropriate treatment regimen. Since the intervention will be community based, it will not be feasible to randomize individuals to intervention or comparison group. The unit of analysis now becomes the community and not the individual. One approach would be to stratify the communities within a target area according to various sociodemographic characteristics and then randomly assign communities within each stratum to either the intervention group or the comparison group. To measure the impact of the intervention, the investigator could conduct special surveys of the population both prior to and after the intervention has been in operation. These cross-sectional surveys could provide a measure of increased medical surveillance for hypertension over time in both the intervention and comparison communities. Other design and measurement approaches that follow the general quasi-experimental design could, of course, be employed in these community-based studies.

—*Philip C. Nasca*

See also Bias; Causal Diagrams; Causation and Causal Inference; Descriptive and Analytic Epidemiology; Randomization; Sequential Analysis

Further Readings

Journal Articles

Wacholder, S., McLaughlin, J. K., Silverman, D. T., & Mandel, J. (1992). Selection of controls in case-control studies: 1. Principles. *American Journal of Epidemiology*, *135*, 1019–1028.

Wacholder, S., Silverman, D. T., McLaughlin, J. K., & Mandel, J. (1992). Selection of controls in case-control studies: 2. Types of controls. *American Journal of Epidemiology*, *135*, 1029–1041.

Wacholder, S., Silverman, D. T., McLaughlin, J. K., & Mandel, J. (1992). Selection of controls in case-control studies: 3. Design options. *American Journal of Epidemiology*, *135*, 1042–1050.

Introductory Epidemiologic Methods

Aschengrau, A., & Seage, G. R. (2007). Essentials *of epidemiology in public health* (2nd ed.). Boston: Jones & Bartlett.

Bhopal, R. (2002). *Concepts of epidemiology: An integrated introduction to the ideas, theories, principles, and methods of epidemiology.* New York: Oxford University Press.

Friis, R. H., & Sellers, T. (2004). *Epidemiology for public health practice* (3rd ed.). Boston: Jones & Bartlett.

Kleinbaum, D. G., Sullivan, K. M., & Barker, M. D. (2002). *ActivEpi* (CD-ROM and Companion Textbook). New York: Springer.

Koepsell, T. D., & Weiss, N. S. (2003). *Epidemiologic methods: Studying the occurrence of illness.* New York: Oxford University Press.

Merrill, R. M., & Timmreck, T. C. (2006). *Introduction to epidemiology* (4th ed.). Boston: Jones & Bartlett.

Oleckno, W. A. (2002). *Essential epidemiology: Principles and applications.* Long Grove, IL: Waveland Press.

Rothman, K. J. (2002). *Epidemiology: An introduction.* New York: Oxford University Press.

Intermediate to Advanced Epidemiologic Methods

Brownson, R. C., & Petitti, D. B. (2006). *Applied epidemiology: Theory to practice* (2nd ed.). New York: Oxford University Press.

Elwood, J. M. (2007). *Critical appraisal of epidemiological studies and clinical trials.* New York: Oxford University Press.

Rothman, K. J., Greenland, S., & Lash, T. L. (2007). *Modern epidemiology* (3rd ed.). Philadelphia: Lippincott Williams & Wilkins.

Szklo, M., & Nieto, J. (2007). *Epidemiology: Beyond the basics* (2nd ed.). Boston: Jones & Bartlett.

Woodward, M. (2004). *Epidemiology: Study design and data analysis* (2nd ed.). New York: Chapman & Hall.

SUICIDE

The term *suicide* refers to deliberately ending one's own life and may also refer to someone who ends his or her life. Because the actor's intention is part of the definition of suicide, it is often a matter of judgment whether a particular death was due to suicide, was accidental, or was caused by a third party. Studies of suicide are complicated by inconsistent reporting due to the fact that different religions and cultures judge the act of suicide differently. In ambiguous cases, a death may be classified as suicide in a society for which that is a morally defensible choice and classified as accidental in a society in which suicide is considered shameful and in which consequences such as the inability to be buried among one's ancestors may follow. In addition, legal or practical considerations such as difficulty in collecting on a life insurance policy after the insured person has committed suicide may also influence whether a death is classified as suicide or not. It is even more difficult to get an accurate estimation of the number of people who attempted suicide and did not die: If they do not seek medical treatment, they will not be counted; and if they do seek treatment, there is no guarantee that attempted suicide will be recorded as a cause.

Suicide in the United States

According to the Centers for Disease Control and Prevention, in the United States in 2001, 30,622 people died by suicide and about nine times that number were hospitalized or treated in emergency departments for attempted suicide. Suicide rates in the United States are highest in the spring and lowest in the winter, contrary to popular belief, and rates are higher in the western states as opposed to the eastern and Midwestern states. Women are about three times more likely than men to report attempting suicide in their lifetime, but men are four times more likely to die from suicide. Suicide rates are highest among Caucasians, followed by Native Americans and Alaska Natives.

Although rates of suicide among young people have declined in recent years, it is the third leading cause of death among people aged 15 to 24 years. In this age group, suicide rates are highest among Native Americans and Alaskan Natives and about six times as high for males as for females. Suicide rates increase with age and are highest among those aged 65 years and older; the male/female ratio of suicides in this age group is similar to that among persons aged 15 to 24 years.

A number of risk factors have been identified for suicide. Personal history factors associated with increased suicide risk include previous suicide attempts, a history of mental disorders, a history of alcohol and substance abuse, a family history of child abuse, and a family history of suicide. Concurrent medical and psychological risk factors include impulsive or aggressive tendencies, feelings of hopelessness or isolation, and physical illness. Other risk factors include lack of access to mental health care, recent traumatic events, access to lethal methods of suicide such as firearms, and local epidemics of suicide. Protective factors include access to medical and psychological care, family and community support, maintaining ongoing relationships with medical and mental health care providers, and personal skills in problem solving and conflict resolution.

Suicide in a Global Context

Statistics concerning suicide and related topics must be interpreted with even greater care when comparing

rates across countries or estimating the global incidence of suicide, because the cultural and reporting issues discussed previously are that much greater when dealing with information from different countries with widely varying cultural attitudes and reporting systems. In addition, when making global comparisons over time, researchers must consider that the estimates for different years may not include data from the same set of countries.

The World Health Organization reports that in 2000 approximately 1 million people died from suicide, a mortality rate of 16 per 100,000. Suicide rates have increased by 60% worldwide over the last 45 years. Traditionally, suicide rates have been highest among elderly males, but they have been increasing among young people; in 1950, most cases of suicide (60%) were older than 45 years, while in 2000, the majority of cases (55%) were among people aged 5 to 44 years. Suicide rates for individual countries, as reported by the World Health Organization, are generally higher for men than for women and show considerable range: For some countries, the rate is less than 1.0 per 100,000 while some of the highest rates are for men in countries of the erstwhile Soviet Union, including Lithuania (74.3 per 100,000), the Russian Federation (69.3 per 100,000), Belarus (63.3 per 100,000), Kazakhstan (50.2 per 100,000), Estonia (47.7 per 100,000), and Ukraine (46.7 per 100,000). Reported suicide rates for women are highest in Asian and Eastern European countries and Cuba, including Sri Lanka (16.8 per 100,000), China (14.8 per 100,000), Lithuania (13.9 per 100,000), Japan (12.8 per 100,000), Cuba (12.0 per 100,000), the Russian Federation (11.9 per 100,000), and the Republic of Korea (11.2 per 100,000).

Physician-Assisted Suicide

Physician-assisted suicide or physician-assisted dying refers to a practice in which a doctor provides a means, such as an injection or prescription drugs, intended to hasten the death of a patient on the request of that patient. It is part of the larger category of *euthanasia*, a term formed by the Greek words for "good" and "death," which is sometimes translated as "the good death" or "the merciful death." Usage of the term *euthanasia* differs, and some include within this category the involuntary killing of people who have not requested to die and the hastening of death through the withdrawal of life-support systems. Physician-assisted suicide is a controversial topic because of the ethical issues involved, the problems of protecting vulnerable people from abuses, and the association of euthanasia with the Nazi regime in Germany and similar historical abuses. Laws regarding physician-assisted suicide are constantly changing, but as of 2006 some form of physician-assisted suicide was legal in several European countries, including Switzerland, the Netherlands, and Belgium. Within the United States, in 2006 only Oregon had legislation allowing physician-assisted suicide.

—Sarah Boslaugh

See also Ethics in Health Care; Eugenics; Psychiatric Epidemiology; Violence as a Public Health Issue

Further Readings

Anderson, R. M., & Smith, B. L. (2003). Deaths: Leading causes for 2001. *National Vital Statistics Report, 52,* 1–86.

Jamison, K. R. (1999). *Night falls fast: Understanding suicide.* New York: Vintage Books.

National Center for Injury Prevention and Control. (n.d.). *Suicide: Fact sheet.* Retrieved November 24, 2006, from http://www.cdc.gov/ncipc/factsheets/suifacts.htm.

Oregon Department of Human Services. (n.d.). *FAQs about the Death with Dignity Act.* Retrieved November 24, 2006, from http://www.oregon.gov/DHS/ph/pas/faqs.shtml.

SURGEON GENERAL, U.S.

The term *Surgeon General* is used in the United States to denote the supervising medical officer of the Public Health Commissioned Corps within the U.S. Department of Health and Human Services. The term is also applicable when referring to the senior medical officer within the U.S. Army and Air Force. Foreign governments also have equivalent positions but do not make use of this particular title.

The position of U.S. Surgeon General was created as a result of the reorganization and recognition of the Marine Hospital Service, a group of hospitals originally constructed to provide health services at key sea and river ports to merchant marines. Expansion of the military and growth in the science of public health led to the need for a national hospital system with centralized administration. The newly reconstructed Marine Hospital system was overseen by a Supervising Surgeon from 1871 to 1872, a Supervising Surgeon General from 1873 to 1901, and a Surgeon General from 1902 to date. Dr. John Woodworth was appointed the first Supervising Surgeon of the U.S. Marine Hospital Service, predecessor of today's U.S. Public Health Service, and Walter Wyman (1891–1911) was the first surgeon to hold the title of Surgeon General.

The U.S. Surgeon General oversees more than 6,000 members of the Public Health Commissioned Corps, holds the rank of Admiral of the Commissioned Corps, and ex officio is the spokesperson on matters of national public health. The U.S. Surgeon General conducts duties under the direction of the Assistant Secretary for Health and the Secretary of Health and Human Services. The Office of the Surgeon General is part of the office of Public Health and Science, Office of the Secretary, U.S. Department of Health and Human Services.

The U.S. Surgeon General is appointed to a 4-year term. This appointment is made after a recommendation from the President of the United States and the endorsement of the U.S. Senate. Official duties of this office are the following:

- Oversee the Commissioned Corps, a diverse collection of health professionals considered experts in public health.
- Provide leadership and direct response to public health matters, current and long term, and provide direction in matters of emergency preparedness and response.
- Establish, protect, and represent a commitment to national health through education and endorsement of empirically supported disease prevention and health promotion programs for the nation.
- Carry out communicative, advisory, analytical, and evaluative roles in matters of domestic and international scientific health policy with both governmental and nongovernmental agencies.
- Ensure quality in existing and planned public health practice throughout the professions by establishing research priorities and appropriate standards.
- Participate in various traditional and statutory federal boards, governing entities, and nongovernmental health organizations such as Board of Regents of the Uniformed Services University of the Health Sciences, the National Library of Medicine, the Armed Forces Institute of Pathology, the Association of Military Surgeons of the United States, and the American Medical Association.

—Floyd Hutchison

See also Governmental Role in Public Health; U.S. Public Health Service

Web Sites

U.S. Department of Health and Human Services, Office of the Surgeon General: http://www.surgeongeneral.gov.

SURVEY RESEARCH METHODS

See SAMPLING TECHNIQUES

SURVIVAL ANALYSIS

Survival analysis is a collection of methods for the analysis of data that involve the time to occurrence of some event and, more generally, to multiple durations between occurrences of events. Apart from their extensive use in studies of survival times in clinical and health-related studies, these methods have found application in several other fields, including industrial engineering (e.g., reliability studies and analyses of equipment failure times), demography (e.g., analyses of time intervals between successive child births), sociology (e.g., studies of recidivism, duration of marriages), and labor economics (e.g., analysis of spells of unemployment, duration of strikes). The terms *duration analysis*, *event-history analysis*, *failure-time analysis*, *reliability analysis*, and *transition analysis* refer essentially to the same group of techniques, although the emphases in certain modeling aspects could differ across disciplines.

The time to event T is a positive random variable with distribution function $F(t) = P[T \leq t], t \geq 0$. In biostatistics and epidemiology, it is more common to use the survivorship function or survival function $S(t) = 1 - F(t)$. Thus, $S(t)$ is the probability of being free of events at time t. In clinical studies, where T is the time of death of a patient, one refers to T as the *survival time* and $S(t)$ as the *probability of survival beyond t*. Since time and duration must have an origin, the specific context determines an appropriate starting point from which T is measured. For example, consider a clinical trial of competing treatments in which patients entering the study are randomized to treatment conditions. The time origin is the time of randomization or initiation of treatment, and T is the time until the primary endpoint (e.g., death) is reached.

Censoring

In clinical studies, patients enter the study at different points in time. For example, a 5-year study might be planned with a 2-year recruitment phase in which patients enter randomly. Patient follow-up begins at entry and ends at death (or some terminal endpoint) if observed before the end of year 5. The survival time T is then known. If the terminal event is not reached by the end of study, T is not observed but we know that $T > U$, where U is the follow-up time from entry to the end of study. The survival times of these patients are censored, and U is called the *censoring time*. Censoring would also occur if a patient died from causes unrelated to the endpoint under study or withdrew from the study for reasons not related to the endpoint. Such patients are lost to follow-up.

The type of censoring described above is called *right censoring*. If the true event time T was not observed but is known to be less than or equal to V, we have a case of *left censoring*. If all that is known about T is that it lies between two observed times U and V $(U > V)$, we say it is *interval censored*. For example, when periodic observations are made for the time to seroconversion in patients exposed to the human immunodeficiency virus, if seroconversion is observed, the time of conversion lies in the interval between the previous negative assessment and the first positive assessment. Right censoring occurs if seroconversion is not observed by the end of study, while left censoring is the case if the patient tests positive at the very first assessment.

Hazard Function

A useful concept in survival analysis is the hazard function h, defined mathematically by $h(t) = \lim_{\Delta t \to 0} P[T < t + \Delta t | t \geq t] / \Delta t$. The quantity $h(t)$ is not a probability. However, because $h(t)\Delta t \approx P[T < t + \Delta t | T \geq t]$, we can safely interpret $h(t)\Delta t$ as the conditional probability that the event in question occurs before $t + \Delta t$, given that it has not occurred before t. For this reason, $h(t)$ has been referred to as the *instantaneous risk* of the event happening at time t.

If the distribution of T is continuous, $h(t) = -d(\log S(t))/dt$. Then, $S(t) = \exp(-H(t))$ and $H(t) = \int_0^t h(u)\, du$ is the cumulative hazard function. (The relationship between S and H is more subtle when the distribution T is not continuous.) Other useful concepts in survival analysis are

Mean survival time	$\mu = E(T) = \int_0^\infty S(t) dt$
Mean survival restricted to time L	$\mu_L = E(\min(T, L)) = \int_0^\infty S(t) dt$
Percentiles of survival distribution	$t_p = \inf\{t > 0 : S(t) \leq 1 - p\}$, $0 < p < 1$
Mean residual life at time t	$r(t) = E(T - t\|T > t)$ $= \int_0^\infty S(u) du / S(t)$

Just as the H determines S, there is a unique relationship between r and S given by

$$S(t) = \frac{r(0)}{r(t)} \exp\left(-\int_0^t \frac{du}{r(u)}\right).$$

Because survival data are often quite skewed with long right tails, the restricted mean survival μ_L or the median survival time $t_{0.5}$ are generally preferred as summary statistics.

Parametric Distributions

Some common distributions for an event time T used in survival analysis are given below. The parameters α and λ have different interpretations, and $\alpha > 0$ and $\lambda > 0$.

1. *Exponential distribution:* $h(t) = \lambda, H(t) = \lambda,\ S(t) = \exp(-\lambda t)$, and $E(T) = \lambda^{-1}$.

2. *Weibull distribution:* $h(t) = \lambda t^{\alpha - 1},\ H(t) = (\lambda t)^\alpha,\ S(t) = \exp(-(\lambda t)^\alpha)$, and $E(T) = \lambda^{-1}\Gamma(1 + \alpha^{-1})$, where Γ is the gamma function.

3. *Log-normal distribution:* Here, $\log T$ has a normal distribution with mean μ and standard deviation σ. Then,

$$S(t) = 1 - \Phi\left(\frac{\log t - \mu}{\sigma}\right),$$

$$h(t) = \frac{1}{\sigma t} \frac{\phi\left(\frac{\log t - \mu}{\sigma}\right)}{\left[1 - \Phi\left(\frac{\log t - \mu}{\sigma}\right)\right]},$$

and $E(T) = \exp(\mu + 1/2\sigma^2)$, where ϕ and Φ are, respectively, the standard normal density and cumulative distribution functions.

4. *Log-logistic distribution:*

$$h(t) = \frac{\lambda^\alpha \alpha t^{\alpha - 1}}{1 + (\lambda t)^\alpha},$$

$$H(t) = \log(1 + (\lambda t)^\alpha),$$

$$S(t) = \frac{1}{1 + (\lambda t)^\alpha},$$

and $E(T) = \lambda^{-1}\Gamma(1 + \alpha^{-1})\Gamma(1 - \alpha^{-1})$, if $\alpha > 1$, where Γ is the gamma function.

5. *Pareto distribution:*

$$h(t) = \frac{\lambda \alpha}{1 + \lambda t},$$

$$H(t) = \alpha \log(1 + \lambda t),$$

$$S(t) = \frac{1}{(1 + \lambda t)^\alpha},$$

$$E(T) = \lambda^{-1}(\alpha - 1)^{-1},\ \alpha > 1.$$

These distributions provide considerable flexibility in fitting a parametric distribution to survival data. For example, the Weibull distribution with $\alpha > 1$ has increasing hazard function, with $\alpha < 1$ the hazard function is decreasing, and with $\alpha = 1$ the hazard is constant. This last case results in the exponential distribution. For the log-logistic distribution with $\alpha \leq 1$, the hazard is decreasing. With $\alpha > 1$, the hazard is increasing up to time $\lambda^{-1}(\alpha - 1)^{1/\alpha}$ and then decreases.

Generally, survival data exhibit skewness. To mitigate this, one might consider a log transformation. A general class of distributions in the location-scale family is specified by $\log T = \mu + \sigma \varepsilon$, where the constants μ and σ are called, respectively, the *location* and *scale* parameters. By specifying a distribution for the random variable εs, one induces a distribution on T. Clearly, the log-normal distribution is in this class. The Weibull distribution also belongs to this class where ε has a standard extreme value distribution $P[\varepsilon > y] = \exp(-e^y)$, $-\infty < y < \infty$, with $\sigma = \alpha^{-1}$, $\mu = -\log\lambda$. The log-logistic distribution is in this class with ε having a standard logistic distribution,

$P[\varepsilon > y] = 1/(1 + e^y)$, $-\infty < y < \infty$, with $\sigma = \alpha^{-1}$, $\mu = -\log\lambda$. However, the Pareto distribution does not belong to the location-scale family.

The location-scale family of survival distributions may also be expressed as $T = e^\mu T_0^\sigma$, with $\log T_0 = \varepsilon$. The survival distribution of T takes the form $S(t) = P[T_0 > (te^{-\mu})^{1/\sigma}] = S_0((te^{-\mu})^{1/\sigma})$, where S_0 denotes the survival distribution of T_0. Therefore, $S(t)$ is obtained from S_0 by either accelerating or decelerating the time. For example, if $\sigma = 1$ and $\mu < 0$, the time is accelerated. Distributions in the location-scale family are also called *accelerated failure time* (AFT) distributions.

Modeling Survival Data

Survival data obtained from a sample of patients often exhibit variation that sometimes can be explained by incorporating patient characteristics in survival models. For each patient, the observable data consist of the survival time T or the follow-up time U and a vector $\mathbf{x} = (x_1, x_2, \ldots, x_p)$ of p covariates. For example, in clinical studies these covariates included indicator variables for treatment group; patient demographic variables such as age, race/ethnicity, level of educational attainment, and so on; and clinical variables such as comorbidities, laboratory assessments, and so on.

In longitudinal studies, some of these covariates might be assessed at several time points throughout the study making them dependent on time. The observed time is $X = \min(T, U)$ and an indicator δ of whether $X = T$ or $X = U$. The observable data on n patients are $\{(X_i, \delta_i, \mathbf{x}_i) : 1 \leq i \leq n\}$ with the subscript i indexing the patient. We generally assume that observations across patients are independent, and survival times are independent of the censoring times, given the covariates, which for now we assume are also fixed (i.e., are independent of time). The independence of T and U is important. A patient who is still at risk at time t, meaning that $X \geq t$ does not provide more information on survival than a patient with $T \geq t$. Censoring is therefore noninformative: It does not remove patients under study because they are at a higher or lower risk of death.

In the location-scale family of distributions, $\log T = \mu + \sigma\varepsilon$, we can incorporate covariate effects by modeling μ in the linear form $\mu = \mathbf{x}'\beta = \beta_0 + x_1\beta_1 + \cdots + x_p\beta_p$ with an intercept β_0. Additional patient heterogeneity could be accommodated by modeling the scale parameter σ, usually on the log scale as

$\log\sigma = \mathbf{z}'\gamma$, where $\mathbf{z}$ is a subset of $\mathbf{x}$. The underlying model for our survival data looks like the familiar linear regression model, $Y_i \equiv \log T_i = \mathbf{x}_i'\beta + \sigma\varepsilon_i$, except that $E(\varepsilon_i|\mathbf{x}_i)$ is not necessarily zero, although it is a constant. Furthermore, we will not have complete observations on Y_i since some patients will have censored survival times. For inference, we must maintain the assumption of a parametric distribution for ε that is independent of $\mathbf{x}$. Because of this assumption and that of noninformative censoring, estimation of all regression parameters can be accomplished via maximum likelihood estimation using the censored sample $\{(X_i, \delta_i, \mathbf{x}_i) : 1 \leq i \leq n\}$. Standard tests such as the Wald test and the likelihood ratio test could be used to assess the statistical significance of components of (β, γ). In the interest of parsimony, one might choose to retain only significant covariate effects in the model.

An easy interpretation of the β coefficients is directly from $E(\log T|\mathbf{x}) = \mathbf{x}'\beta + (\varepsilon)$. For example, consider a placebo-controlled treatment study with a single treated group. Patients are randomized to treatment ($x_1 = 1$) or placebo ($x_1 = 0$). If σ is constant, the effect of treatment (vs. placebo) is $\beta_1 = E(\log T|x_1 = 1) - E(\log T|x_1 = 0)$. The aforementioned maximum likelihood estimation allows one to test the hypothesis of no treatment effect—namely, $H_0 : \beta_1 = 0$. If our model has additional covariates, $\mathbf{x}^* = (x_2, \ldots, x_p)$, that have no interactions with the treatment indicator x_1, then β_1 is called the adjusted effect of treatment because $\beta_1 = E(\log T|x_1 = 1, \mathbf{x}^*) - E(\log T_1 = 0, \mathbf{x}^*)$—that is, the treatment effect keeping all other covariates $\mathbf{x}^*$ held fixed in the treated and placebo groups. For a continuous covariate x_1 (e.g., age), the interpretation of β_1 is the partial effect—the effect of one unit increase in x_1 on the expected log survival, holding all other covariates fixed (and assuming no interactions with x_1).

The effect of a covariate on any summary measure, such as the survival function, mean survival time $E(T|\mathbf{x})$, or the median survival time (or other percentiles), may be used to provide comparisons on the original untransformed scale. For example, suppose the underlying survival distribution is Weibull and we want to assess the effect of treatment on mean survival time. From $E(T|\mathbf{x}) = \exp(\mathbf{x}'\beta + \log\Gamma(\sigma + 1))$, we get $E(T|x_1 = 1, \mathbf{x}^*)/E(T|x_1 = 0, \mathbf{x}^*) = \exp(\beta_1)$; that is, $\exp(\beta_1)$ is the adjusted effect of treatment, relative to placebo, on mean survival. This interpretation carries over to all the previously mentioned location-scale models. Similarly, a common structure applies to the percentiles of the survival distributions in location-scale models. The upper $100p$th percentile t_p of the survival distribution is given by $t_p = \exp(\mathbf{x}'\beta + \sigma z_p)$, where z_p is the corresponding percentile of the distribution of ε. For example, in the log-normal distribution the median survival is $t_{0.5} = \exp(\mathbf{x}'\beta)$ and therefore in the aforementioned scenario we obtain an entirely equivalent interpretation of $\exp(\beta_1)$ as the adjusted effect of treatment relative to placebo, on median survival time. It is worthy of note that these structural similarities do not carry over to the survival function $S(t|\mathbf{x}) = S_0((te^{-\mathbf{x}'\beta})^{1/\sigma})$, which has very different functional forms for different survival distributions.

Nonparametric Methods

In the absence of a plausible parametric assumption for the survival distribution, its estimation may be based on the relationship $S(t) = \exp(-H(t))$. For right-censored survival data $\{(X_i, \delta_i, \mathbf{x}_i) : 1 \le i \le n\}$, we define two basic quantities: $N(t)$ is the number of events observed up to time t, and $Y(t)$ is the number of patients at risk of the event just prior to time t. While $N(t)$ is a step function that increases only at event times and remains constant between event times, $Y(t)$ decreases just after event and censoring times. Hence, $\Delta N(t)/Y(t)$ is the proportion of patients with events at t among those who are at risk and not censored just prior to t. This provides an estimator $\hat{S}(t) = \exp(-\hat{H}(t))$, where $\hat{H}(t) = \sum_{u \le t} \Delta N(u)/Y(u)$. These are called the Nelson-Aalen estimators. Because $Y(t) = 0$ if t is larger than the largest observed time (called $X_{(n)}$) in the sample, whether it is an event or censoring time, we cannot define these estimators for $t > X_{(n)}$. Generally, the Nelson-Aalen estimator $\hat{S}(t)$ is close to the Kaplan-Meier estimator $\tilde{S}(t)$ given by $\tilde{S}(t) = \prod_{u \le t}(1 - \Delta N(u)/Y(u))$. If $X_{(n)}$ is an event time, then $\tilde{S}(t) = 0$ for $t \ge X_{(n)}$. If not, $\tilde{S}(t)$ is left undefined for $t > X_{(n)}$.

The two estimators $\hat{S}(t)$ and $\tilde{S}(t)$ have equivalent large-sample properties. The fact that they are consistent and asymptotically normal estimators of $S(t)$ allows one to compute pointwise confidence intervals for $S(t)$. For example, a $100(1-\alpha)\%$ confidence interval for $S(t)$ has approximate confidence limits given by $\tilde{S}(t) \pm z_{1-\alpha/2}\tilde{\sigma}(t)$, where

$$\sigma^2(t) = \{\tilde{S}^2(t)\} \sum_{u \le t} \frac{\Delta N(u)}{Y(u)(Y(u) - \Delta N(u))}$$

is an estimate of the large sample variance of $\tilde{S}(t)$. However, better approximations may be obtained by first computing a confidence interval for a transformed $S(t)$, such as $\log[S(t)]$ or $\log[t\log S(t)]$, and then retransforming back to the original scale.

Another innovation is to compute a simultaneous confidence band for $S(t)$ over the interval $t_L \le t \le t_U$, where t_L and t_U are appropriately specified time points. Practically, these points should be between the smallest and largest failure times in the observed sample. A simultaneous confidence band will preserve the confidence level $1 - \alpha$ by deriving statistics $\hat{L}(t)$ and $\hat{U}(t)$ such that the interval $[\hat{L}(t), \hat{U}(t)]$ contains $S(t)$ for all $t_L \le t \le t_U$ with probability $1 - \alpha$—that is, $P[[\hat{L}(t), \hat{U}(t)]\ S(t), t_L \le t \le t_U] = 1 - \alpha$. In contrast, a pointwise confidence interval will only guarantee $P[[\hat{L}(t), \hat{U}(t)]\ S(t)] = 1 - \alpha$ for each t. When confidence intervals for the survival function are desired at several time points, using a simultaneous band is recommended.

Semiparametric Models

Many applications require comparison of survival across groups after controlling for other covariates that might have influence on survival. For parametric models within the location-scale family, we have seen how comparisons can be made after the estimation of regression parameters via maximum likelihood estimation. A widely used model is the proportional hazards model (PHM) in which the hazard function $h(t|\mathbf{x})$ is given by $h(t|\mathbf{x}) = h_0(t)\exp(\mathbf{x}'\beta)$, where $h_0(t)$ is a baseline hazard function that is left completely unspecified. Because this part of the model is nonparametric, the term *semiparametric* is used. The model was introduced by D. R. Cox in 1972 and has since received unprecedented attention. Because inference is often focused on the parameter β, Cox suggested an approach to its estimation by using a partial likelihood function that is independent of h_0. After the estimation of βs, we can estimate the cumulative hazard $H(t|\mathbf{x}_0) = H_0(t)\exp(\mathbf{x}_0'\beta)$ and the survival function $S(t|\mathbf{x}_0) = \exp(-H(t|\mathbf{x}_0))$ at a specified covariate profile $\mathbf{x}_0$.

The PHM and AFT models are distinct. In fact, the Weibull distribution is the only member of both classes. For the Weibull, $h(t|\mathbf{x}) = \alpha t^{\alpha-1}\lambda_0^\alpha(t)\exp(-\alpha\mathbf{x}'\beta)$, where $h_0(t) = \alpha t^{\alpha-1}$. The two parameterizations differ slightly.

To interpret the PHM model, consider once again a treatment study of survival with a single treated group ($x_1 = 1$) and a placebo group ($x_1 = 0$). Because $h_0(t)$ is arbitrary, there is no need for an intercept parameter. The hazard at time t in the treated group is $h(t|x_1 = 1) = h_0(t) \exp(\beta_1)$, whereas in the placebo group it is $h(t|x_1 = 0) = h_0(t)$ that provides an interpretation for $h_0(t)$. Therefore, the relative hazard (treated vs. placebo) is $h(t|x_1 = 1)/h(t|x_1 = 0) = \exp(\beta_1)$. When $\beta_1 > 0$, the treated group has at each time t a higher probability of the event (e.g., death) than the placebo group. When $\beta_1 < 0$, this is reversed. Indeed, $S(t|x_1 = 1) = \{S(t|x_1 = 0)\}^{\exp(\beta_1)}, t > 0$, and so the two survival functions are ordered. With additional covariates, $\mathbf{x}^* = (x_2, \ldots, x_p)$, which have no interactions with x_1, $\exp(\beta_1)$ is the adjusted relative hazard for treated versus placebo when $\mathbf{x}^*$ is held fixed in both groups. Similarly, for a continuous covariate the interpretation of $\exp(\beta_1)$ is the relative hazard for a unit increase in x_1 while holding all other covariates fixed (and assuming no interactions with x_1).

In multicenter studies where survival data are collected from different sites, it is appropriate to consider a stratified PHM in which the hazard in site j is specified by $h_j(t|\mathbf{x}) = h_{j0}(t) \exp(\mathbf{x}'\beta)$, that is, we incorporate a separate baseline hazard for each site (stratum). Stratification could also be considered if the standard proportion hazard assumption might seem inapplicable. For example, instead of using age within the covariate mix $\mathbf{x}$ we could form age strata, and within each age stratum, the proportional hazards assumption applies to all other covariates under consideration.

Another extension of the PHM is to incorporate time-dependent covariates. This is often necessary in longitudinal studies with periodic measurements of important factors related to survival. The time-dependent model is $h(t|\mathbf{x}(t)) = h_0(t) \exp(\mathbf{x}'(t)\beta)$, where $\mathbf{x}(t)$ denotes the cumulative covariate history up to time t. Although the regression parameter β can still be estimated using the partial likelihood function, inference on the survival function will require some assumptions on the relationship between the stochastic development of $\{\mathbf{x}(t) : t \geq 0\}$ and the event time T. To retain the expression $S(t|\mathbf{x}(t)) = \exp(-\int_0^t h(u|\mathbf{x}(u)) \, du)$, strict exogeneity of $\{\mathbf{x}(t) : t \geq 0\}$ with respect to T is sufficient. This means $P[\mathbf{x}(t + \Delta t)|T \geq t + \Delta t, \mathbf{x}(t)] = P[\mathbf{x}(t + \Delta t)|\mathbf{x}(t)]$, that is, given $\mathbf{x}(t)$, future values of the covariates are not influenced by future values of T. Time-fixed covariates are obviously strictly exogenous. A patient's age at any time t is independent of the event $T \geq t$ and is therefore strictly exogenous. There are other types of time-dependent covariates for which

inference on the relative hazard parameter β is still valid. However, for more general considerations we need to model jointly the covariate process $\{\mathbf{x}(t) : t \geq 0\}$ and event time T.

Other Extensions

Several important developments that extend the basic survival analytic technique have arisen to support applications in many fields. One important extension is to multistate models and multiple failure times. The finite-state Markov process in continuous time is ideally suited to consider transitions from one state to another. The concepts of hazard functions are replaced by intensity functions and survival probabilities by transition probabilities. For example, in follow-up studies in cancer patients, we might consider periods of remission (State 0) and relapse (State 1) before death (State 2). A simple three-state model examines the impact of covariates on the transitions $0 \rightarrow 1$, $1 \rightarrow 0$, $0 \rightarrow 2$, and $1 \rightarrow 2$ by modeling the intensities $\alpha_{jk}(t|\mathbf{x}) = \alpha_{jk0}(t) \exp(\mathbf{x}'_{jk}\beta)$ just like in a proportional hazard model. Here, α_{jk} is the transition intensity for $j \rightarrow k$. The interpretation of these intensities is as follows: from entry into State j, $\alpha_{jj} = \sum_{k \neq j} \alpha_{jk}$ is the hazard function for the duration in state j; given that exit from state j occurs at time t, the exit state k is selected with probability α_{jk}/α_{jj}.

The survival model is a special case of a multistate model with just two states, alive and dead. A competing risks model has one origination state (alive, State 0) and several destination states (States $k = 1, \ldots, K$) corresponding to causes of death. The intensities α_{0k} are the cause-specific hazard functions, and $\alpha_{00} = \sum_k \alpha_{0k}$ is the overall hazard for survival.

Multiple failure times arise when an individual can potentially experience several events or when there is a natural clustering of event times of units within a cluster (e.g., failure times of animals within litters, survival times of zygotic twins). Often, this situation can also be cast in the framework of a multistate model if interest lies in modeling only the intensities of each event type and not on the multivariate joint distribution of the event times. Other important developments in survival analysis include Bayesian survival analysis and frailty models.

—Joseph C. Gardiner and Zhehui Luo

See also Censored Data; Cox Model; Hazard Rate; Kaplan-Meier Method

Further Readings

Andersen, P. K., Borgan, O., Gill, R. D., & Keiding, N. (1993). *Statistical models based on counting processes.* New York: Springer-Verlag.

Box-Steffensmeier, J. M., & Jones, B. S. (2004). *Event history modeling—A guide for social scientists.* Cambridge, UK: Cambridge University Press.

Collett, D. (2003). *Modelling survival data for medical research* (2nd ed.). London: Chapman & Hall.

Cox, D. R., & Oakes, D. (1984). *Analysis of survival data.* London: Chapman & Hall.

Elandt-Johnson, R. C., & Johnson, N. L. (1980). *Survival models and data analysis.* New York: Wiley.

Fleming, T. R., & Harrington, D. P. (1991). *Counting processes and survival analysis.* New York: Wiley.

Heckman, J. J., & Singer, B. (Eds.). (1985). *Longitudinal analysis of labor market data.* Cambridge, UK: Cambridge University Press.

Hosmer, D. W., & Lemeshow, S. (1999). *Applied survival analysis: Regression modeling of time to event data.* New York: Wiley.

Hougaard, P. (2000). *Analysis of multivariate survival data.* New York: Springer-Verlag.

Ibrahim, J. G., Chen, M.-H., & Sinha, D. (2001). *Bayesian survival analysis.* New York: Springer-Verlag.

Kalbfleisch, J. D., & Prentice, R. L. (1980). *The statistical analysis of failure time data.* New York: Wiley.

Klein, J. P., & Moeschberger, M. L. (1997). *Survival analysis: Techniques for censored and truncated data.* New York: Springer-Verlag.

Lancaster, T. (1990). *The econometric analysis of transition data.* Cambridge, UK: Cambridge University Press.

Lawless, J. F. (1982). *Statistical models and methods for lifetime data.* New York: Wiley.

Lee, E. T. (1992). *Statistical methods for survival data analysis.* New York: Wiley.

Marubini, E., & Valsecchi, M. G. (1995). *Analysing survival data from clinical trials and observational studies.* New York: Wiley.

Nelson, W. (1982). *Applied lifetime data analysis.* New York: Wiley.

Thernau, T. M., & Grambsch, P. M. (2000). *Modeling survival data: Extending the Cox model.* New York: Springer-Verlag.

SYNDEMICS

A syndemics model of health and illness focuses attention on the multiple interconnections that occur between copresent diseases and other health-related problems in a population as well as within individual sufferers at both the biological and social levels.

This orientation, which developed initially within medical anthropology and diffused to epidemiology and public health, emerged in response to the dominant biomedical conceptualization of diseases as distinct entities in nature, separate from other diseases, and independent of the social contexts in which they are found. While isolating diseases, assigning them unique labels (e.g., AIDS, TB), and narrowly focusing on their immediate causes and expressions laid the foundation for the development of modern pharmaceutical and other biomedical approaches to sickness, it has become increasingly clear that diseases and other health conditions (e.g., nutritional status) interact synergistically in various and consequential ways and that the social conditions of disease sufferers are critical to understanding the impact of such conditions on the health of both individuals and groups. A syndemics approach examines disease concentrations (i.e., multiple diseases affecting individuals and groups), the pathways through which they interact biologically within individual bodies and within populations and thereby multiplying their overall disease burden, and the ways in which social environments, especially conditions of social inequality and injustice, contribute to disease clustering and interaction.

Disease Interactions

Interest in a syndemics approach has been driven by growing evidence of significant interactions among comorbid diseases. One such interaction has been found, for example, between type 2 diabetes mellitus and various infections, such as hepatitis C viral infection. Several factors are known to contribute to the onset of type 2 diabetes, including diet, obesity, and aging. The role of infection, however, is only beginning to be understood. Already, it is known that risk for serious infections of various kinds increases significantly with poor diabetes control, but appreciation of more complex relationships between infection and type 2 diabetes is now emerging as well. The Third National Health and Nutritional Examination Survey (NHANES III) found that the frequency of type 2 diabetes increases among people who have been infected with the hepatitis C virus. Similarly, several health reports note that diabetes is present in as many as 37% of those who are critically ill with severe acute respiratory syndrome.

The nature of interaction among diseases may vary and need not require direct physical interaction to produce new or amplified health consequences (e.g., as in AIDS, changes in biochemistry, or damage to organ systems caused by one pathogenic agent may facilitate the spread or impact of another agent). Direct interaction, however, including gene mixing among different types of pathogenic agents, has also been described, such as the molecular in vivo integration of the avian leukosis virus and Markek's disease virus (MDV) in domestic fowl. Both these cancer-causing viruses are known to infect the same poultry flock, the same chicken, and even the same anatomic cell. In coinfected cells, the retroviral DNA of the avian leukosis virus can integrate into the MDV genome, producing altered biological properties compared with the parental MDV. In studies of human populations, a lethal synergism has been identified between influenza virus and pneumococcus, a likely cause of excess mortality from secondary bacterial pneumonia during influenza epidemics. It is disease interactions of this sort that are a central biological component in syndemics. Syndemic theory seeks to draw attention to and provide a framework for the analysis of these interactions.

Social Origins of Syndemics

Beyond disease clustering and interaction, the term *syndemic* also points to the importance of social conditions in disease concentrations, interactions, and outcomes. In syndemics, the interaction of diseases or other health-related problems commonly occurs because of adverse social conditions (e.g., poverty, stigmatization, oppressive social relationships, health care disparities) that put socially devalued and subjugated groups at heightened risk for disease or limit access to timely and effective care. With reference to tuberculosis, for example, it is impossible to understand its persistence in poor countries as well as its recent resurgence among the poor in industrialized countries without assessing how social forces, such as political violence and racism, come to be embodied and expressed as individual pathology.

Identified Syndemics

Various syndemics (although not always labeled as such) have been described in the literature, including the SAVA syndemic (substance abuse, violence, and AIDS); the hookworm, malaria, and HIV/AIDS syndemic; the Chagas disease, rheumatic heart disease, and congestive heart failure syndemic; the asthma and infectious disease syndemic; the malnutrition and depression syndemic; the mental illness and HIV/AIDS syndemic; and the sexually transmitted diseases syndemic. Additional syndemics are being identified around the world as public health officials, researchers, and service providers begin to focus on the connections among diseases and the social context factors that foster disease interactions.

Syndemic Research

Several lines of future syndemics inquiry have been described. First, there is a need for studies that examine the processes by which syndemics emerge, including the specific sets of health and social conditions that foster the occurrence of multiple epidemics in a population and how syndemics function to produce specific kinds of health outcomes in populations. Second, there is a need to better understand processes of interaction between specific diseases with each other and with health-related factors such as malnutrition, structural violence, discrimination, stigmatization, and toxic environmental exposure that reflect oppressive social relationships. Finally, there is a need for a better understanding of how the public health systems and communities can best respond to and limit the health consequences of syndemics. Systems are needed to monitor the emergence of syndemics and to allow "early-bird" medical and public health responses designed to lessen their impact. Systematic ethno-epidemiological surveillance with populations subject to multiple social stressors must be one component of such a monitoring system. Current efforts by researchers at the Centers for Disease Control to expand the discussion of syndemics in public health discourse is an important step in the development of a funded research agenda that addresses these research needs. Given the nature of syndemics, this research requires a biocultural/social approach that attends to both clinical and social processes.

—*Merrill Singer*

See also Comorbidity; Geographical and Social Influence on Health; Global Burden of Disease Project; Health Disparities; Medical Anthropology

Further Readings

Freudenberg, N., Fahs, M., Galea, S., & Greenberg, A. (2006). The impact of New York City's 1975 fiscal crisis on the tuberculosis, HIV, and homicide syndemic. *American Journal of Public Health, 96*, 424–434.

Singer, M. (1996). A dose of drugs, a touch of violence, a case of AIDS: Conceptualizing the SAVA syndemic. *Free Inquiry in Creative Sociology, 24*, 99–110.

Singer, M., & Clair, S. (2003). Syndemics and public health: Reconceptualizing disease in bio-social context. *Medical Anthropology Quarterly, 17*, 423–441.

Singer, M., Erickson, P., Badiane, L., Diaz, R., Ortiz, D., Abraham, T., et al. (2006). Syndemics, sex and the city: Understanding sexually transmitted disease in social and cultural context. *Social Science and Medicine, 63*, 2010–2021.

Stall, R., Mills, T., Williamson, J., & Hart, T. (2003). Association of co-occurring psychosocial health problems and increased vulnerability to HIV/AIDS among urban men who have sex with men. *American Journal of Public Health, 93*, 939–942.

SYNERGISM

See EFFECT MODIFICATION AND INTERACTION

T

TARGETING AND TAILORING

Information and communication are important and powerful tools for helping enhance population health. Generally speaking, health information that is carefully designed for a specific group or individual is more effective in capturing attention and motivating changes in health-related attitudes and behaviors than information designed for a generalized audience or with no particular audience in mind. The two most common types of health information customized for specific audiences are *targeted* and *tailored* communication.

Both targeted and tailored health communication are audience-centered approaches driven by a careful analysis of intended recipients. Both approaches use what is learned from this analysis to customize health messages, sources of information, and channels of information delivery to maximize the reach and effectiveness of a health communication to a particular audience. In targeted communication, the unit of audience analysis and customization is a particular *group*, while in tailored communication the unit of audience analysis and customization is one specific *individual*. Thus, these approaches are often referred to as "group targeted" and "individually tailored" health communication.

Targeted Health Communication

The rationale for group-targeted health communication is summarized in three key assumptions: (1) there is diversity among the members of any large population with respect to the determinants of a given health decision or behavior and also among the characteristics that affect exposure and attention to, processing of, and influence of health messages; (2) for any health-related behavior, homogeneous population subgroups can be defined based on shared patterns of these determinants and characteristics; and (3) different health communication strategies are needed to effectively reach different population subgroups. In health communication terminology, these population subgroups are called *audience segments.*

The concept of audience segmentation has its roots in marketing and advertising consumer products and services and is now widely accepted as a best practice in health communication. Historically, audience segmentation in public health has been driven by findings from disease surveillance and epidemiological studies that identified population subgroups with elevated risk or burden of disease. Because of the limited types of data typically collected in these surveillance and research activities, the resulting audience segments were often fairly unsophisticated, relying on only demographic variables (e.g., teenagers, African Americans), health status indicators (e.g., pregnancy, blood pressure), broad behavioral categories (e.g., smokers, men having sex with men), or sometimes simple combinations of the three (e.g., pregnant teenage girls who smoke). Boslaugh, Kreuter, Nicholson, and Naleid (2005) showed that simple segmentation strategies such as those relying on demographic variables alone provided little improvement over no segmentation at all in understanding physical activity behavior. Thus, while epidemiological data such as these are invaluable for identifying population subgroups with great need for risk reduction, they are of little use in helping health communication planners and developers make critical decisions about effective message design or selection of interpersonal and media channels to reach members of those subgroups.

More sophisticated, multivariable approaches to audience analysis and segmentation consider demographic, psychographic, geographic, health status and behavioral characteristics, and the dynamic interplay among them. For example, Vladutiu, Nansel, Weaver, Jacobsen, and Kreuter (2006) observed that parents' beliefs and behaviors related to child injury prevention varied significantly based on whether or not they were first-time parents and by the age of their oldest child. In short, beliefs about the effectiveness of injury-prevention measures and perceptions of how important injury prevention was to others in their lives were related to injury prevention behaviors among parents of preschool children, but not among parents of infants and toddlers. Attitudes about injury prevention (i.e., "injuries are normal part of childhood," "injuries can't be prevented") predicted injury-prevention behaviors for first-time parents but not parents of multiple children. Thus, rather than promoting injury prevention by delivering the same information to all parents, these findings suggest that it may be more effective to segment the population of parents into multiple subgroups, for example, those with only one child versus those with two or more children. For parents with only one child, targeted communications would focus on changing specific beliefs that may undermine child injury-prevention behaviors.

Although one could conceivably identify hundreds of population subgroups or audience segments for any behavior of interest, some segments will be higher priorities than others for receiving targeted communication. When the level of need or health risk is equal, audience segments that are larger in size, easily identifiable in the population, and accessible through existing channels are generally more promising as prospects for population health improvement through targeted communication.

Tailored Health Communication

While targeted health communication seeks to reach a given population subgroup, tailored health communication is designed to reach one specific person. To customize health information in this way, data from or about an individual are gathered and processed to determine what messages will be needed to address one's unique needs, then these messages are assembled in a predesigned template for delivery to the individual. This process of assessing behaviors and key determinants of behavior change for different individuals, matching messages to those determinants, and providing tailored feedback to the individual is usually automated using a computer database application. In a typical tailoring program, a patient in a primary care setting might answer questions about his or her dietary behaviors and beliefs on a paper form or computer kiosk while in the waiting room. One's answers would be processed using a set of computerized algorithms that identify not only potential problem areas in one's diet, but also beliefs and skills that would affect one's motivation or ability to make dietary changes. Using this information, the computer program would then select from a large library of messages only those that were appropriate given one's answers on the assessment. These messages would then be printed in a magazine or newsletter for the person or shown as on-screen feedback.

Findings from individual studies and a growing number of literature reviews indicate that tailored communication is more effective than nontailored communication for capturing attention, increasing motivational readiness to change a behavior, and stimulating behavioral action. Tailoring effects have been found for a wide range of behaviors (e.g., diet, physical activity, smoking cessation, immunization, cancer screening, injury prevention), in diverse populations, and across many settings (e.g., health care, worksites, online). Tailored health communication has also taken many forms, including calendars, magazines, birthday cards, and children's storybooks. Most tailoring to date has been based on individuals' responses to questions assessing behaviors (e.g., fruits and vegetables consumed per day, injury-prevention devices used) and/or determinants of behavior change derived from theories of health behavior change (e.g., readiness to change, perceived benefits and barriers). While health information in any medium—audio, video, Internet—can be tailored to individual recipients, the evidence base for tailoring effects comes almost exclusively from tailored print communication.

Why does tailored health communication have these effects? One explanation is that recipients of tailored health information perceived it as personally relevant. The theories of information processing propose that individuals are more motivated to thoughtfully consider messages when they perceive them to be personally relevant. In a randomized trial, Kreuter, Bull,

Clark, and Oswald (1999) showed that participants exposed to tailored weight loss materials engaged in significantly more cognitive processing of the information than those exposed to two different types of nontailored weight loss materials. Webb, Simmons, and Brandon (2005) suggest that the mere *expectation* of customized communication (i.e., telling people they will receive information made just for them) may be sufficient to stimulate tailoring-like effects. In a study of what they call "placebo tailoring," smokers were randomly assigned to receive one of three booklets that shared identical smoking-related content but varied in degrees of ostensible tailoring. As the amount of apparent tailoring increased, so too did the favorability of smokers' responses to the booklets, although no differences in actual behavior change were observed.

Because the cost and time involved in developing tailored health communication programs can exceed that required for less customized forms of communication, it should be undertaken only in situations when it has distinct advantages over other approaches. Perhaps obviously, tailoring health messages would be unnecessary and even wasteful if a single message was equally effective for all or most members of a larger group (i.e., as in *targeted* communication). However, if members of that same group vary significantly on behavioral determinants of some outcome of interest, the added effort to tailor messages for each individual might be justified. Similarly, because individual-level data are required to tailor messages, this approach should only be considered when there is a feasible way to obtain data from (i.e., through an assessment) or about (i.e., through an existing database) individual members of the intended audience. To date, no studies have directly compared effects or cost-effectiveness of targeted with tailored communication. However, for practical purposes, it is probably less important to identify one superior approach than it is to determine how the two can be used in concert to help achieve public health objectives.

—*Matthew W. Kreuter and Nancy L. Weaver*

See also Health Behavior; Health Communication

Further Readings

Boslaugh, S. E., Kreuter, M. W., Nicholson, R. A., & Naleid, K. (2005). Comparing demographic, health status, and psychosocial strategies of audience segmentation to promote physical activity. *Health Education Research, 20*(4), 430–438.

Kreuter, M. W., Bull, F. C., Clark, E. M., & Oswald, D. L. (1999). Understanding how people process health information: A comparison of tailored and untailored weight loss materials. *Health Psychology, 18*(5), 487–494.

Kreuter, M. W., Strecher, V. J., & Glasman, B. (1999). One size does not fit all: The case for tailoring print materials. *Annals of Behavioral Medicine, 21*(4), 1–9.

Kreuter, M. W., & Wray, R. J. (2003). Tailored and targeted health communication: Strategies for enhancing information relevance. *American Journal of Health Behavior, 27*(Suppl. 3), S227–S232.

Slater, M. D. (1996). Theory and method in health audience segmentation. *Journal of Health Communication, 1*, 267–283.

Vladutiu, C. J., Nansel, T. R., Weaver, N. L., Jacobsen, H. A., & Kreuter, M. W. (2006). Differential strength of association of child injury prevention attitudes and beliefs on practices: A case for audience segmentation. *Injury Prevention, 12*, 35–40.

Webb, M. S., Simmons, N., & Brandon, T. H. (2005). Tailored interventions for motivating smoking cessation: Using placebo-tailoring to examine the influence of expectancies and personalization. *Health Psychology, 24*(2), 179–188.

TARGET POPULATION

The terms *statistical population, population of interest, universe*, and simply *population* are often used interchangeably when referring to a target population. What they have in common is that they define a group of people or other units that are the focus of a study and to whom the results are intended to generalize. The term *population* derives from the origins of statistics being used to describe human populations. However, a population may be people (such as the population of smokers), objects (such as hospital records), events (such as deaths or births), or measurements on or of the people, objects, or events (such as ages of smokers or occurrence of births).

A group may be defined as a population due either to an inherent characteristic of the group itself (such as residence in a particular city) or to a particular characteristic of interest to the researcher (such as having a particular health condition). A population may be very large (such as the population of the United States, estimated at more than 300 million in 2007) or very small (such as the population of patients with progeria, of whom only 42 were known in the world as of 2006).

If a target population consists of people, objects, or events, then it is the set of sampling units about which investigators would like to draw conclusions or the set of all the members of the group under consideration. This population is the entire set of units to which findings of the survey are to be generalized. If the population consists of measurements taken on people, objects, or events, then, ideally, it is the set of all measurements that a researcher would like to have in answering a scientific question. These data are all possible or all hypothetically possible observations of those measurements.

In a statistical study, the researcher must define the population being studied. Typically, defining the target population is easy: It is all subjects possessing the common characteristics that are being studied. However, often for practical reasons the researcher must also define a study population, meaning the actual population of people from whom the sample will be drawn. For instance, if a researcher working in Ohio is interested in the effects of smoking on systolic blood pressure in adults aged 18 to 65 years, this would be the target population (sometimes called the "theoretical population"), while for practical reasons, the study population from whom the sample would be drawn might be all people between the ages of 18 and 65 years on January 1, 2007, residing within Greene County, Ohio. Additionally, each set of measurements that might be drawn on these individuals may be considered a population, so we could speak of the population of systolic blood pressure measurements or the population of smoking status indicators (whether each individual smokes) for adults aged 18 to 65 years in Greene County, Ohio.

It is important to note that whether a data set is considered a population or a sample depends on the context in which the data are to be viewed. In the previous example, if the researcher is interested in generalizing the study to all adults within southwestern Ohio, then the set of data for all adults in Greene County would be a sample. However, if the researcher is interested only in studying the relationship of smoking and blood pressure within Greene County, then that same set of data would constitute the population. Additionally, the population "adults aged 18 to 65 years in Greene County" could be used to draw a sample for study: If the results are intended to generalize all adults in southwestern Ohio (or the entire

United States), this would be a study population; if a sample was drawn with the intent of generalizing only the adults of Greene County, it would be the target population.

The researcher must be careful when defining the population to ensure that the appropriate sampling units are included in the sampling frame to avoid exclusion bias. In the smoking and blood pressure example, the ideal sampling frame would be a list of all adults between the ages of 18 and 65 on January 1, 2007, who reside in Greene County, Ohio; this ideal sampling frame is simply a list of all the members of the target population. If there is a difference between the target population and the study population, then the list of the people who will actually be sampled is called a "notional sampling frame." The sampling units (or sampling elements) are the individual entities that are the focus of the study; in this example, these are the individual adults who meet these criteria. A sample is a subset of those adults from which observations are actually obtained and from which conclusions about the target population will be drawn. Of course, in practice such lists frequently do not exist or are incomplete, and other methods must be used to define and sample the study population.

Some other examples of studies and their populations include the following: (1) If researchers want to conduct a survey to estimate the number of people living in California who have never visited a dentist, the population consists of all people living in California, and each person is a sampling unit; (2) if researchers want to determine the number of hospital discharges during a given year that left against medical advice, then each hospital discharge is a sampling unit, and all discharges during the year are the population; and (3) if researchers want to know the number of people living in Montana who had scarlet fever in 2006, then the population is all residents of Montana in 2006, and each person is a sampling unit.

—*Stacie Ezelle Taylor*

See also Bias; Convenience Sample; Probability Sample; Sampling Techniques; Study Design

Further Readings

Hassard, T. H. (1991). *Understanding biostatistics.* St. Louis, MO: Mosby-Year Book.

Levy, P. S., & Lemeshow, S. (1999). *Sampling of populations: Methods and applications* (3rd ed.). New York: Wiley.

TERATOGEN

Teratology is the study of the effects of exposures during pregnancy on a developing fetus. These exposures, known as teratogens, can be quite varied and include agents such as medications, illicit drugs, infectious diseases, maternal metabolic states, and occupational and environmental exposures. A teratogen can cause a spontaneous loss of pregnancy or structural and/or functional disability in a child. It has been estimated that 5% to 10% of birth defects are due to an exposure during pregnancy.

The following are the five characteristics of a teratogen. The first characteristic is that the occurrence of the birth defect or pattern of birth defects is higher in the population exposed to the teratogen as compared with the general population. Since 3% to 5% of all newborns have a birth defect, the number of malformed infants must exceed that of the background risk. More specifically, the occurrence of the exact malformation or pattern of malformations must be increased. The second characteristic is that an animal model should duplicate the effect seen in humans. Animal models serve as a good system for "red flagging" an agent but can never be used to directly determine effects from human exposure or the magnitude of any potential risk. The third characteristic is that a dose-response relationship has been established; the greater the exposure, the more severe the phenotypic effect. A corresponding concept is that of a threshold effect; effects are only seen above a specific exposure level. The fourth characteristic is that there should be a plausible biologic explanation for the mechanism of action. The fifth characteristic asserts that a genetic susceptibility increases the chance of an adverse outcome from the exposure. This area of pharmacogenetics holds great promise for advancing our understanding of human teratology and the provision of individualized risk assessments.

Using the above principles, it is possible to develop a risk assessment for an individual exposed pregnancy. Several pieces of information, including the timing of the exposure, the dose of the agent, and family medical and pregnancy history information, are critical. A review of the available literature is essential. Scientific data concerning outcomes of exposed pregnancies are often conflicting, difficult to locate, and hard to interpret. Much of the data are in the form of case reports, animal studies, and retrospective reviews. To provide complete information, it may be necessary to consult various resources. It is important to appreciate the risk-benefit ratio regarding a particular agent to provide an individualized risk assessment on which pregnancy management may be based.

Despite scientific advances in clinical teratology, exposures prior to and during pregnancy still cause great anxiety and misunderstanding among both the public and health care professionals. Teratology Information Services (TIS) are comprehensive, multidisciplinary resources that provide information on prenatal exposures to health care providers and the public. The national consortium of individuals providing these services is the Organization of Teratology Information Specialists. An individual TIS has three components: service (toll-free, confidential phone consultations), education (to health care providers and the public), and research (national and international studies on specific agents).

—*Dee Quinn*

See also Birth Defects; Environmental and Occupational Epidemiology; Maternal and Child Health

Further Readings

Briggs, G. B., Freeman, R. K., & Yaffe, S. J. (2005). *Drugs in pregnancy and lactation: A reference guide to fetal and neonatal risk* (7th ed.). Philadelphia: Lippincott Williams & Wilkins.

Web Sites

Clinical Teratology Web: A resource guide for clinicians: http://depts.washington.edu/ ~ terisweb.
Organization of Teratology Information Specialists, which provides further information on the individual programs, research projects, and fact sheets: http://www.otispregnancy.org.
Reprotox: An information system on environmental hazards to human reproduction and development: http://www.reprotox.org.

TERRORISM

See WAR

Thalidomide

Thalidomide is a pharmaceutical product that was synthesized in West Germany in 1953 and sold as an antinausea drug and sleep aid under a number of different brand names beginning in 1957. Because it was believed to be nontoxic and to have no side effects, it was widely prescribed to pregnant women for relief of morning sickness and insomnia. However, thalidomide proved to be anything but nontoxic; more than 10,000 women who took the drug during pregnancy gave birth to children with severe birth defects. The best-known sign of prenatal thalidomide exposure was phocomelia (misshapen limbs), but children exposed to thalidomide before birth (commonly referred to as "thalidomide babies") suffered many other birth defects, including missing limbs, cleft palate, spinal cord defects, missing or abnormal external ears, and abnormalities of the heart, kidneys, genitals, and digestive system. Some women who took thalidomide also reported abnormal symptoms, including peripheral neuropathy. Thalidomide was removed from the market in most countries in 1961, and the events surrounding its approval and release are considered perhaps the worst case of insufficient pharmacological oversight in the modern world. In particular, thalidomide had not been tested on humans at the time of its release, and its pharmacological effects were poorly understood.

Thalidomide was never approved by the Food and Drug Administration (FDA) for sale in the United States, so the impact of the drug was much less in this country than in Europe and other countries. However, the experience of seeing thousands of "thalidomide babies" born in countries where the drug had been approved for general sale led to strengthening of several protections in the U.S. drug approval process. The major changes were incorporated in the Kefauver-Harris Amendment, passed in 1962, which required that new pharmaceutical products had to be demonstrated as both safe and effective and required that adverse reactions to prescription drugs be reported to the FDA.

Although thalidomide should not be taken by pregnant women, it has legitimate medical uses and is used in some countries to treat serious conditions such as cancer, leprosy, and AIDS. Because of thalidomide's history, any use of the drug today is controversial and some medical professionals believe that the drug should be banned entirely, while others feel that it is the best available drug to treat certain specific conditions.

One primary medical use of thalidomide today is in the treatment of leprosy, in particular to treat the symptoms of erythema nodosum leprosum. Thalidomide is also used in some cancer therapies and has become a common treatment for multiple myeloma. Thalidomide is also used to treat AIDS patients, in particular to fight mouth ulcers and wasting syndrome. Theoretically, the therapeutic use of thalidomide is carefully supervised and monitored; in practice, however, the risk of improper use remains (e.g., a thalidomide baby was born in Brazil in 1995), and this potential harm must be weighed against the benefits achieved by wider use of this drug.

—*Sarah Boslaugh*

See also Birth Defects; Teratogen

Further Readings

Franks, M. E., Macpherson, G. R., & Figg, W. D. (2004). Thalidomide. *Lancet, 363*(9423), 1802–1811.

Pannikar, V. (2006). *The return of thalidomide: New uses and renewed concerns.* Retrieved August 8, 2007, from http://www.who.int/lep/research/Thalidomide.pdf.

Stephen, T. D., & Rock, B. (2001). *Dark remedy: The impact of thalidomide and its revival as a vital medicine.* New York: Perseus.

Theory of Planned Behavior

An extension of the theory of reasoned action, the theory of planned behavior (TPB) is today one of the most popular models for explaining, predicting, and changing human social behavior. It has been applied to study a number of health behaviors, including exercise, smoking, drug use, and compliance with medical regimens. According to the TPB, human behavior is guided by three kinds of considerations:

1. Beliefs about the likely outcomes of the behavior and the evaluations of these outcomes (*behavioral beliefs*); in their aggregate, these beliefs produce a positive or negative attitude toward the behavior.

2. Beliefs about the normative expectations of important others and motivation to comply with these

expectations (*normative beliefs*) that result in perceived social pressure or a subjective norm.

3. Beliefs about the presence of various internal and external factors and the perceived power of these factors to facilitate or impede performance of the behavior (*control beliefs*). Collectively, control beliefs give rise to a sense of self-efficacy or perceived behavioral control.

Attitudes toward the behavior, subjective norms, and perceived behavioral control jointly lead to the formation of a behavioral intention. The relative weight or importance of each of these determinants of intention can vary from behavior to behavior and from population to population. However, as a general rule, the more favorable the attitude and subjective norm, and the greater the perceived control, the stronger the person's intention to perform the behavior in question. Finally, given a sufficient degree of actual control over the behavior, people are expected to carry out their intentions when the opportunity arises. Intention is thus assumed to be the immediate antecedent of behavior. However, because many behaviors pose difficulties of execution, the TPB stipulates that degree of control moderates the effect of intention on behavior: Intentions are expected to result in corresponding behavior to the extent that the individual has volitional control over performance of the behavior.

Beliefs serve a crucial function in the TPB; they represent the information people have about the behavior, and it is this information that ultimately guides their behavioral decisions. According to the TPB, human social behavior is reasoned or planned in the sense that people take into account the behavior's likely consequences, the normative expectations of important social referents, and factors that may facilitate or impede performance. Although the beliefs people hold may be unfounded or biased, their attitudes, subjective norms, and perceptions of behavioral control are thought to follow reasonably from their readily accessible beliefs, to produce a corresponding behavioral intention, and finally to result in behavior that is consistent with the overall tenor of the beliefs. However, this should not be taken to imply deliberate, effortful retrieval of information and construction of intention prior to every behavior. After a person has at least minimal experience with a behavior, his or her attitude, subjective norm, and perceived behavioral control are assumed

to be available automatically and to spontaneously produce a behavioral intention.

In sum, the behavioral, normative, and control beliefs that are readily accessible in memory serve as the fundamental explanatory constructs in the TPB. Examination of accessible beliefs provides substantive information about the considerations that guide people's behavior and can thus also serve as the basis for interventions designed to change behavior.

Empirical Support

The TPB has been used to predict and explain a myriad of social behaviors, including investment decisions, dropping out of high school, blood donation, driving violations, recycling, class attendance, voting in elections, extramarital affairs, antinuclear activism, playing basketball, choice of travel mode, and a host of other activities related to protection of the environment, crime, recreation, education, politics, religion, and virtually any imaginable area of human endeavor. Its most intense application, however, has been in the health domain, where it has been used to predict and explain varied behaviors such as drinking, smoking, drug use, exercising, dental care, fat consumption, breast self-examination, condom use, weight loss, infant sugar intake, getting medical checkups, using dental floss, and compliance with medical regimens.

The results of these investigations have, by and large, confirmed the theory's structure and predictive validity. Armitage and Conner (2001) found, in a meta-analytic review of 185 data sets, that the theory accounted on average for 39% of the variance in intentions, with all three predictors—attitude toward the behavior, subjective norm, and perceived behavioral control—making independent contributions to the prediction. Similarly, intentions and perceptions of behavioral control were found to explain 27% of the behavioral variance. Godin and Kok (1996), in a meta-analysis of 76 studies in the health domain related to addiction, clinical screening, driving, eating, exercising, AIDS, and oral hygiene, found that the TPB was shown to explain, on average, 41% of the variance in intentions and 34% of the variance in behavior.

Sufficiency

Investigators have suggested a number of additional variables that might be incorporated into the theory to improve prediction of intentions and behavior. Among the proposed additions are expectation, desire, and need; affect and anticipated regret; personal or moral norm; descriptive norm; self-identity; and past behavior and habit. Some of these proposed additions can be viewed as expansions of the theory's existing components. Thus, it is possible to subsume expectation, desire, and need to perform the behavior under intention; anticipated regret and other expected affective consequences of a behavior arguably are a proper part of attitude toward the behavior; and descriptive norms perhaps contribute to perceived social pressure—that is, subjective norm.

Other proposed factors, such as self-identity and moral norms, are conceptually distinct from the original constructs in the TPB, and some studies have shown that these factors can make an independent contribution to the prediction of intentions and actions. Perhaps of greatest concern because it touches on the theory's reasoned action assumption is the suggestion that, with repeated performance, behavior habituates and is no longer controlled by intentions but, instead, by critical stimulus cues. However, evidence for the role of habit in the context of the TPB is weak; intentions are found to predict behavior well even for frequently performed behaviors that would be expected to habituate.

From Intention to Behavior

For the TPB to afford accurate prediction, intentions measured at a certain point in time must not change prior to enactment of the behavior. Empirical evidence strongly supports this expectation, showing that the intention-behavior relation declines with instability in intentions over time. Even when intentions are stable, however, people do not always act on their intentions. The concern about lack of correspondence between intentions and actions can be traced to LaPiere's classic 1934 study in which ready acceptance of a Chinese couple in hotels, motels, and restaurants contrasted sharply with stated intentions not to accept "members of the Chinese race" in these same establishments. Similar discrepancies have been revealed in investigations of health behavior where it has been found that between 25% and 50% of participants fail to carry out their stated intentions to perform behaviors such as using condoms regularly, undergoing cancer screening, or exercising. A variety of factors may be responsible for observed failures of effective

self-regulation, yet a simple intervention can do much to reduce the gap between intended and actual behavior. When individuals are asked to formulate a specific plan—an implementation intention—indicating when, where, and how they will carry out the intended action, the correspondence between intended and actual behavior increases dramatically. For example, Sheeran and Orbell (2000) found that asking participants who planned to undergo a cervical cancer screening to form a specific implementation intention increased participation from 69% to 92%.

Behavioral Interventions

Given its predictive validity, the TPB can serve as a conceptual framework for interventions designed to influence intentions and behavior. Thus far, only a relatively small number of investigators have attempted to apply the theory in this fashion. The results of these attempts have been very encouraging. For example, Brubaker and Fowler (1990) developed an intervention designed to increase testicular self-examination (TSE) among high school students based on the TPB-addressed beliefs about the outcomes of TSE. This theory-based intervention was found to be considerably more successful than merely providing information about testicular cancer and TSE or a general health message. The theory-based intervention had a significantly greater impact on attitudes toward TSE, the factor directly attacked in the intervention, it was more effective in raising intentions to perform TSE, and it produced a 42% rate of compliance over a 4-week period, compared with 23% and 6% compliance rates in the other two intervention conditions, respectively. The theory has also been applied in interventions designed to promote vegetable and fruit consumption, smoking cessation, safer sex, physical exercise, and a host of other, mostly health-related behaviors; these applications are reviewed by Hardeman et al. in 2002.

—*Icek Ajzen*

See also Health Behavior; Health Belief Model; Intervention Studies; Self-Efficacy

Further Readings

Ajzen, I. (1991). The theory of planned behavior. *Organizational Behavior and Human Decision Processes, 50,* 179–211.

Ajzen, I. (2005). *Attitudes, personality, and behavior* (2nd ed.). Maidenhead, UK: Open University Press.

Armitage, C. J., & Conner, M. (2001). Efficacy of the theory of planned behavior: A meta-analytic review. *British Journal of Social Psychology, 40*, 471–499.

Brubaker, R. G., & Fowler, C. (1990). Encouraging college males to perform testicular self-examination: Evaluation of a persuasive message based on the revised theory of reasoned action. *Journal of Applied Social Psychology, 20*, 1411–1422.

Godin, G., & Kok, G. (1996). The theory of planned behavior: A review of its applications to health-related behaviors. *American Journal of Health Promotion, 11*, 87–98.

Hardeman, W., Johnston, M., Johnston, D. W., Bonetti, D., Wareham, N. J., & Kinmonth, A. L. (2002). Application of the theory of planned behaviour in behaviour change interventions: A systematic review. *Psychology and Health, 17*, 123–158.

LaPiere, R. T. (1934). Attitudes vs. actions. *Social Forces, 13*, 230–237.

Sheeran, P., & Orbell, S. (2000). Using implementation intentions to increase attendance for cervical cancer screening. *Health Psychology, 19*, 283–289.

TIME SERIES

Time series are time-ordered observations or measurements. A time series can consist of elements equally spaced in time—for example, annual birth counts in a city during four decades—or measurements collected at irregular periods, for example, a person's weight on consecutive visits to a doctor's office. Time plots, that is, graphical representations of time series, are very useful to provide a general view that often allows us to visualize two basic elements of time series: short-term changes and long-term or secular trends.

Time series are often used in epidemiology and public health as descriptive tools. For instance, time plots of life expectancy at birth in Armenia, Georgia, and Ukraine during the years 1970 to 2003 (see Figure 1) reveal relatively stagnant health conditions before the 1990s in these three countries of the former USSR, as well as a substantial deterioration of health

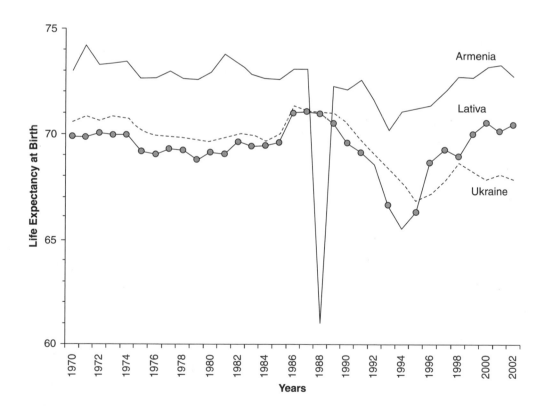

Figure 1   Life Expectancy at Birth (Years) in Three Countries Formerly Part of the USSR

Source: Created by the author using data from the European Health for All database (HFA-DB).

in the early to mid-1990s, after the breakdown of the USSR. The sharp trough in 1988 in Armenian life expectancy reflects the impact of the Spivak region earthquake that killed tens of thousands of people, including many children.

In describing a time series in mathematical terms, the observation or measurement is considered a variable, indicated for instance by y_t, where the subscript t indicates time. It is customary to set $t = 0$ for the first observation in the series, so that the entire expanded series will be represented by y_0, y_1, y_2, $y_3, \ldots, y_m$ for a series containing $m + 1$ elements. The element for time k in this series will be therefore y_k, with $k > 0$ and $k < m$.

In some cases, time series are well described by a mathematical model that can be exponential, logistic, linear (a straight line), and so on. They often reveal recurring patterns, for instance seasonal ones, associated with different seasons of the year. A series of monthly deaths due to respiratory disorders during several consecutive years will show a yearly peak in winter and a yearly trough in summer. Other patterns may be periodic but not seasonal; for instance, among

Jews in Israel, deaths are more frequent on Sundays. Still other patterns are recurrent but are acyclical, that is, not periodical; for instance, in market economies, the unemployment rate reveals successive peaks (recessions) and troughs (periods of economic expansion) that make up what has come to be called the "business cycle" (Figure 2), which is not a "cycle" in the ideal sense because it occurs at irregular intervals.

In most time series, there is strong first-order autocorrelation, which means that consecutive values are highly correlated. That is, the value y_k is usually not very far from its neighbors, y_{k-1} and y_{k+1}. This is the basis for *interpolation* and *extrapolation*, the two techniques used to estimate an unknown value of a time series variable. A missing value inside a time series can be estimated by *interpolation*, which usually implies an averaging of the values in the neighborhood of the missing one. For instance, if the value for Year 8 in a series of annual values was unobserved, it can be estimated as an average of the observed values for years 6, 7, 9, and 10. In general, the error in the estimation through interpolation will

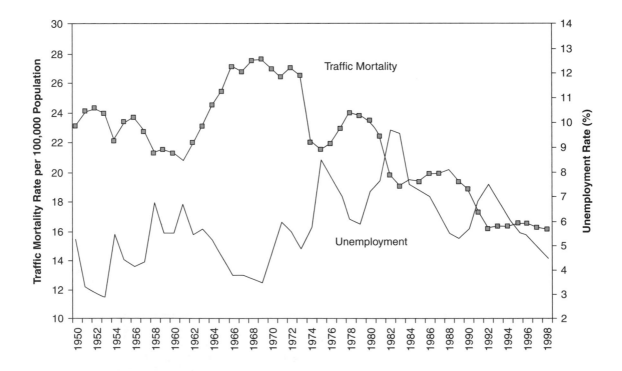

Figure 2   Traffic Mortality and Unemployment in the United States, 1950–1999

Source: Created by the author using data in the U.S. Bureau of the Census "Historical Statistics of the United States" and the National Health for Health Statistics "Vital Statistics of the United States." Available in several online and printed sources.

be smaller than the error in estimating through extrapolation, which implies estimating an unobserved value out of the time range of the time series, usually in the future. (Backward extrapolation to the past is also possible, though usually uninteresting.) *Forecasting* is a term used for predicting the value of a variable at a later time than the last one observed. When a causal model involving the major determinants of the variable to be predicted is not available, forecasting is done through more or less sophisticated techniques of extrapolation. For instance, if the suicide rates during the past 5 years in a nation were, respectively, 12.7, 13.4, 12.9, 12.2, and 13.1 per million, using a somewhat rough extrapolation we might forecast that the suicide rate next year will probably be around 12 or 13 per million. This conclusion, as any other forecast, has a large uncertainty associated with it, because time series may have sudden upturns or downturns that cannot be predicted. Obviously, the uncertainty grows exponentially as the future we try to forecast becomes more distant. The formal techniques of forecasting imply fitting a mathematical model (linear, exponential, etc.) to the observed data, then computing the expected value in the future with that mathematical model. The *a*utoregressive *i*ntegrated *m*oving *a*verage models or ARIMA models, often used in forecasting (frequently referred to as the Box-Jenkins models or methodology), have been sometimes applied in biomedical sciences and epidemiology, but they constitute a quite specialized field of statistics. Like ARIMA models, spectral analysis is another specialized technique in the field of time series analysis.

Establishing causal relations between time series variables is not straightforward. While high absolute values of the correlations between variables observed in cross-sectional studies may be suggestive of causal associations, high correlations between two time series are very common and prove nothing. For instance, in many advanced countries the proportion of persons below 15 years of age in the population, the annual volume of typewriting machines sold, and the percentage of adult women not having paid work secularly dropped during the past half century. Therefore, the correlation between any two annual series of these three variables will be very high, but this does not suggest any causal relationship at all between them. To investigate causal relations between time series, the series must be *stationary*. A stationary series is one consisting of values oscillating over and

above a constant mean for the whole period. Thus, a stationary series is one that has no trend. The series with trends have to be detrended or "prewhitened" if we are looking for causal associations. *Differencing* and *filtering* with a smoothing tool are common methods of detrending. For differencing a series, the differences between successive elements of the series are computed, so that the original series $y_0, y_1, y_2, \ldots, y_m$ is transformed into the series $z_0, z_1, z_2, \ldots, z_{m-1}$, where $z_0 = y_1 - y_0$, $z_1 = y_2 - y_1$, and $z_{m-1} = y_m = y_{m-1}$. The differenced series will be one unit shorter than the original one. The transformation of a variable y_t into its rate of change $r_t = (y_t - y_{t-1})/y_{t-1}$ is a variety of the procedure of differencing. Detrending a series through *filtering* involves computing a smooth trend line, and then the detrended series is computed by subtracting the values of the filtered series from the values of the original series. There are many filtering procedures or "filters," the most commonly used are moving averages (moving means), moving medians, and combinations of both, such as the T4253H smoother provided by SPSS. The Hodrick-Prescott filter is another popular tool for detrending. Since in time series analysis it is common to work with transformed values, the term *in levels* is often used to refer to the original observations (say, the annual rate of infant mortality), while "in differences" refers to their changes from one observation period to the next (the absolute change in infant mortality) and "in rate of change" refers to its period-to-period percent change (the year-to-year relative change in the infant mortality rate).

High absolute values of the cross-correlation of two stationary time series imply a strong comovement and, possibly, a causal connection, with one series causing the other or both being caused by a third variable. The graphs showing parallel movements in two series (with peaks in one coinciding with peaks in the other, and troughs in one coinciding with troughs in the other) are evidences of comovement and highly suggestive of some direct causal connection. The same is true when graphs show mirroring movements (with peaks in one series coinciding with troughs in the other, and vice versa). For example, mirroring time plots of unemployment and mortality due to traffic injuries (Figure 2) are highly suggestive of traffic deaths increasing during periods of accelerated economic activity, when unemployment diminishes, and dropping during recessions, when unemployment is high.

Panel regression methods are often useful to analyze relationships between time series variables.

—*José A. Tapia Granados*

See also Causation and Causal Inference; Data Transformation; Panel Data; Pearson's Correlation Coefficient; Regression

Further Readings

Diggle, P. J. (2000). *Time series: A biostatistical introduction.* Oxford, UK: Clarendon Press.

Dominici, F., Peng, R. D., Bell, M. L., Pham, L., McDermott, A., Zeger, S. L., et al. (2006). Fine particulate air pollution and hospital admission for cardiovascular and respiratory diseases. *Journal of American Medical Association, 295*(2), 1127–1134.

Pope, C. A., III, & Schwartz, J. (1996). Time series for the analysis of pulmonary health data. *American Journal of Respiratory Care Medicine, 154,* 5229–5233.

Tapia Granados, J. A. (2005). Increasing mortality during the expansions of the US economy, 1900–1996. *International Journal of Epidemiology, 34,* 1194–1202.

Warner, R. M. (1998). *Spectral analysis of time-series data.* New York: Guilford Press.

Zeger, S. L., Irizarry, R., & Peng, R. D. (2006). On time series analysis of public health and biomedical data. *Annual Review of Public Health, 27,* 57–79.

Web Sites

The European Health for All database (HFA-DB), compiled by the Regional Office for Europe of the World Health Organization: http://www.euro.who.int/hfadb.

TOBACCO

The term *tobacco* refers to plants of the genus *Nicotiana*, which may be consumed in various ways. Because cigarette smoking is the predominant method of tobacco consumption in the United States, in public health the term *tobacco use* is often used as a synonym for *cigarette smoking* without consideration of the different modes of tobacco consumption and differing health risks posed by them. This entry describes the health risks associated with cigarette smoking, other tobacco smoking, and environmental tobacco smoke (ETS) and contrasts these to the effect of nicotine in itself and to the use of smokeless tobacco (ST). It also explores the importance of tobacco research in the

history of epidemiology and the potential of epidemiological studies in reducing the health impacts of smoking.

Tobacco is native to the Americas, where it was cultivated by indigenous populations from about 4000 BCE and used in smoked and smokeless forms, largely for ceremonial purposes. Less than 100 years after its discovery by European explorers around AD 1500, tobacco was being used throughout the world, a testimony to the powerful psychoactive properties it delivers to human brains. Cigarette smoking started to become popular only around 1900 with the introduction of efficient mass production and wide distribution of cigarettes during the 20th century's two world wars made it the dominant form of tobacco use globally.

Ochsner and DeBakey recognized a link between smoking and lung cancer as early as 1939. Schairer and Schöniger (1943) published one of the first epidemiologic studies of this relationship, in German, during World War II (it was not widely distributed or indexed at the time, but was resurrected in English in 2001). But it was not until the studies of cigarette smoking and lung cancer by Doll and Hill (1950), Wynder and Graham (1950), and others a half century ago that the dangers of smoking were clearly established. While difficult to imagine today, the medical community that then dominated public health was sufficiently conservative that these results were not immediately accepted despite previous evidence. These early studies of the relationship between smoking and health risks also played an important role in establishing the merits of observational epidemiologic studies.

Today, it is well established that regular moderate or heavy cigarette smoking (and to a lesser extent, smoking of tobacco in other forms) causes well-known morbidity and mortality risks, with total attributable risk far exceeding that from any other voluntary exposure in wealthy countries. Cigarette smoke also creates an environmental exposure, labeled "second-hand smoke" or "environmental tobacco smoke" (ETS). Because smoking has been so prevalent for so long and causes high relative risks for many diseases, and because it offers little opportunity for experimental intervention, smoking stands as a near-perfect demonstration of what can be done with observational epidemiology (though perhaps also as a rarely attainable archetype).

In contrast, nicotine, the primary reason people smoke or otherwise use tobacco, is a relatively benign mild stimulant, similar to caffeine. Nicotine causes transient changes in cardiovascular physiology, as do many mild stimulants that might cause a small risk of cardiovascular disease. There is general agreement that nicotine is addictive for many people (the term *addictive* is not well-defined, but nicotine consumption fits most proposed definitions, at least for a portion of the population). But nicotine by itself does not appear to cause a substantial risk of any life-threatening disease; the epidemiologic evidence on nicotine in the absence of smoking is sufficiently limited that it is impossible to distinguish small risks from zero risk. Although not extensively studied, research suggests that nicotine may have psychological and neurological health benefits, protecting against Parkinson's disease and possibly dementia, and providing acute relief from schizophrenia and other psychological morbidities.

Substantial research shows that the use of modern ST products is associated with very small health risks, similar to those from nicotine alone. There has been little research on the health effects of very light smoking or long-term pharmaceutical nicotine use, in part because it is difficult to find populations with such long-term usage patterns (not interrupted by periods of heavier smoking), and in part because most tobacco and nicotine research funding is driven by a prohibitionist agenda, and so there is limited support for quantifying these practices' presumably modest health effects.

Cigarette smoking probably remains the most researched exposure in epidemiology. However, the set of exposures related to tobacco also generate a great deal of advocacy and rhetoric, often making it a challenge to sort out the epidemiology from the politics. Epidemiology related to tobacco suffers from publication bias against studies that show no increased risk (which is particularly relevant to harm reduction and to ST), from overinterpretation of results of a few favored studies, and from a "ratchet effect," where any association found in one study is treated as established, regardless of what other evidence shows. For example, many studies of ETS have shown very small or undetectable health effects for all but extreme exposure levels, but these studies are widely ignored, or even vilified, in the popular discourse. Similarly, a few studies have found positive associations of ST use and oral or pancreatic cancer, but most studies have not; nevertheless, these positive associations are discussed as if they are indisputably established.

Perhaps these problems are no worse than in other subject matter areas, but they pose a potentially greater threat to epidemiology as an honest science because of the high stakes and high profile of tobacco issues, and are less excusable given the overwhelming amount of epidemiologic evidence that exists.

The greatest confusion comes from treating exposures to tobacco as homogeneous, despite the very different pathways and different levels of health risk. Using the term *tobacco* is particularly misleading when referring only to the health effects of smoking, since the major health impact is from inhaling smoke, which is quite unhealthy no matter what is burning; thus, emphasizing the plant rather than using the term *smoking* confuses people about the cause of the health effects.

Cigarette Smoking

Smoking prevalence peaked at about 50% in most Western countries, reaching a maximum in the 1950s and 1960s in most male populations, though often continuing to rise among women. But the health risks of smoking, highlighted in reports from the Royal College of Physicians (the United Kingdom, 1962) and the United States Surgeon General (1964), and in thousands of studies since, resulted in a steady decline over about two decades, to the prevalences in the 20-some percent range (similar for men and women) found in most Western countries today. However, despite near-universal knowledge of the health risks and aggressive antismoking advocacy and policies in many places, the rate of the decline has slowed or stopped over the past several decades. National average prevalence has dropped substantially less than 20% only in Sweden, where ST use has largely replaced smoking. Outside the West, prevalence is increasing in many countries; male prevalence remains more than 50% in many countries in Eastern Europe, the former Soviet Union, Africa, and Asia, while prevalence among women varies from negligible to quite high.

Since the lung cancer link was established, smoking has been shown to cause other cancer mortality and an even greater absolute risk of fatal cardiovascular disease. Popular claims attribute about one fifth of all current mortality in wealthy countries to smoking or in excess of 150 deaths per 100,000 person years. Extrapolations of present worldwide trends predict dramatically increasing smoking-attributable mortality in the future, predominantly in developing countries.

It should be noted that some of the most widely cited statistics about tobacco and health are produced primarily by antitobacco advocates using proprietary data and methods, and thus cannot be validated. For example, estimates of smoking-attributable deaths released by the U.S. Centers for Disease Control and Prevention (CDC) are based on relative risks derived from the American Cancer Society's (ACS) Second Cancer Prevention Study (CPS-II). Nearly everyone has heard of the CDC estimate of about 400,000 annual smoking-attributable deaths in the United States. But few realize that this and other findings from the CDC relating to health consequences of tobacco use, the basis of tobacco policies at all levels of American government, are based on data and analyses that are kept secret from investigators outside the CDC or ACS.

However, few would doubt that the true mortality from smoking is at least half of what is usually claimed, so there is no serious question that among behavioral health exposures, smoking is among the most important at the individual and social levels. In the world's healthier countries, it has a greater impact on mortality and morbidity than any other behavioral exposure. Smoking is often called the greatest or most important preventable source of disease; while such phrasing belongs to advocacy rhetoric and is scientifically meaningless (most notably, it strains the definition of "preventable" to apply it to an exposure that remains very prevalent despite massive efforts to eliminate it), the epidemiologic evidence makes clear that if we could substantially reduce the rate of smoking, it would result in greater health improvement in wealthy countries than any other change imaginable within the bounds of current technology and budgets.

By exposing the lungs, airway, and mouth to concentrated combustion products, smoking causes a still-increasing majority of the world's lung cancer. In Western men, smoking is estimated to cause as much as 90% of lung cancer and 75% of the oral, pharyngeal, esophageal, and laryngeal cancers; attributable risk for women, historically lower due to a lag in smoking uptake in the 20th century, is largely equivalent today. Smoking has also been convincingly linked to cancers of the stomach, pancreas, and urinary bladder, as well as leukemia. It is sometimes also linked to cancers of the breast and colon, but these associations are less well established. Smoking is responsible for reversing what otherwise would have been a steep decline in overall cancer mortality in Western countries during the latter half of the 20th century.

The relative risks for cardiovascular diseases are much lower than those for the sentinel cancers, but because of the greater baseline risk, the absolute total risk is higher. In the West, smoking is estimated to cause about 40% of coronary heart disease and stroke deaths in people below 65 years of age and more than 50% of deaths from aortic aneurysms. In addition, smoking is considered the proximate cause of about 20% of pneumonia and influenza deaths and about 80% of deaths related to bronchitis, emphysema, and chronic airway obstruction.

Other Tobacco Smoking

Smoking of tobacco in various types of pipes and cigars is an exposure similar to smoking cigarettes, though many (but not all) smokers of these products have lower consumption and do not draw smoke into the lungs, both of which result in lower risks. Because of the great heterogeneity of usage patterns, it is difficult to generalize about these exposures. But epidemiologic studies generally show these exposures, as practiced in the West, to cause substantially less risk than regular cigarette smoking on average, though the total risk of serious disease associated with their use is still high compared with almost every other common voluntary exposure.

Environmental Tobacco Smoke

There is fierce debate about the magnitude of the health risk to nonsmokers from ETS exposure. ETS has been linked to various acute changes in respiratory and cardiovascular physiology, but the epidemiologic evidence is only suggestive of a small risk of lung cancer and cardiovascular disease after concentrated long-term exposure such as that experienced by the nonsmoking spouses of smokers or by people who work in very smoky environments. Popular claims attribute that about 2 deaths per 100,000 person years to ETS in wealthy countries, with claimed relative risks for lung cancer and heart disease as high as about 1.3, but these numbers come from antismoking advocates and selective citation of the research, and are not widely accepted by nonadvocates. For example, the scientific literature contains competing summary analyses of studies of ETS and cardiovascular disease, with a widely cited study written by employees of an antitobacco advocacy group finding a relative risk in excess of 1.2, while a recent study of that literature produces a summary estimate of approximately 1.05. While it stands to reason that ETS creates some of the same risks as active smoking (since it involves exposure to the same chemicals that harm smokers, via the same pathway, albeit in much lower doses), the absolute risk appears to be lower than what can be accurately measured by available epidemiologic methods.

Smokeless Tobacco

Since most of the health risk from smoking comes not from the tobacco plant, but from inhaling concentrated smoke, oral use of modern Western ST products (e.g., snuff dipping) has little in common with smoking other than nicotine absorption. This exposure has become popular in Sweden and Norway, and seems to be gaining popularity in parts of North America, due in part to the low health risks and to availability of modern products that can be used invisibly and without spitting, in contrast to traditional chewing tobacco.

The epidemiologic evidence does not definitively demonstrate an association between ST use and any life-threatening disease. There is a widespread misunderstanding, among both health professionals and the general population, that ST use creates substantial risk of oral cancer, but this is based on erroneous conclusions from early research. Extensive modern epidemiology has consistently shown that ST use causes very little or no risk of oral cancer (clearly much less than the substantial risk of oral cancer from smoking) or of any other life-threatening disease.

In contrast to studies of smoking, epidemiologic studies of ST use face considerable challenges because the prevalence of ST use in Western countries is very low (e.g., no more than 5% among adult men and well under 1% among women in the United States), the diseases putatively linked to ST use (such as oral cancer) are rare, and the relative risks, even among long-term users, are very low. Despite these challenges, there has been sufficient epidemiologic research on the subject, most usefully from the past 15 years, to conclude that Western ST use causes only a tiny fraction of the total mortality risk of smoking; calculated estimates put it at 1% to 2% and clearly less than 5%. A recent meta-analysis of epidemiologic studies of ST use and oral cancer found that the use of modern American and Swedish products (moist snuff and chewing tobacco) was associated with undetectably low risks for cancers of the oral cavity and other upper respiratory sites (relative risks ranging from 0.6 to 1.7); older studies of American dry snuff showed substantially elevated risk (relative risks ranging from 4 to 13), with the contrast due to an unknown combination of the archaic products causing measurable risk and improved study methods (e.g., better control for smoking).

ST use in South Asia and Africa may cause substantially greater disease risks. The products used are quite different from Western ST, because they use different manufacturing processes and typically include other ingredients that have their own psychoactive and health effects (indeed, sometimes these products do not even contain tobacco, but are classified in analyses as being tobacco products). The epidemiology suggests that these products are associated with a substantially increased risk of oral cancer, with relative risks for this disease similar to or higher than those from smoking. Since oral cancer is much more common outside the West, this represents a greater absolute risk than it would in the West. Little is known about other mortality risks from these products, though there is no reason to doubt that total risk is greater than that from Western ST, but still only a small fraction of that from smoking.

Epidemiology and Reducing the Health Impacts of Smoking

Beyond showing that smoking is unhealthy, epidemiologic research also contributes to identifying predictors of smoking behavior, assessing smoking cessation interventions (generally finding them to provide very little or no benefit), and measuring the effects of antismoking regulations. Important unanswered epidemiologic questions with practical implications for health policy include the health effects of very low levels of smoking (in the range of one cigarette per day), the nature of the benefits of nicotine for some users and its effect on their quality of life, and whether smokers derive important benefits from smoking apart from the nicotine.

Epidemiologic research has revealed the potential of tobacco harm reduction (the substitution of less harmful sources of nicotine for smoking) as an important public health intervention. The effectiveness of traditional antismoking efforts has plateaued in the Western world. But since other products (particularly ST, which has similar pharmacokinetics to smoking) contain the nicotine that smokers seek, and those products have been shown to cause very little of the health risk associated with smoking, encouraging smokers to switch products is a promising intervention. Swedish men substantially replaced smoking with ST use over the past several decades, and descriptive epidemiology confirmed that the predicted reduction in disease occurred. Swedish women and Norwegians are making a similar substitution, and the approach is increasingly considered a promising option in North America and elsewhere.

—*Carl V. Phillips and Brad Rodu*

See also Cancer; Doll, Richard; Harm Reduction; Health Behavior; Hill, Austin Bradford; Observational Studies

Further Readings

Doll, W. R., & Hill, A. B. (1950). Smoking and carcinoma of the lung: Preliminary report. *British Medical Journal, 2,* 739–748.

Doll, R., & Hill, A. B. (1956). Lung cancer and other causes of death in relation to smoking: A second report on the mortality of British doctors. *British Medical Journal, 2,* 1071–1081.

Gately, I. (2001). *Tobacco: A cultural history of how an exotic plant seduced civilization.* New York: Grove Press.

Office of the Surgeon General. (2004). *The health consequences of smoking: A report of the Surgeon General.* Atlanta, GA: National Center for Chronic Disease Prevention and Health Promotion.

Ochsner, A., & DeBakey, M. (1939). Primary pulmonary malignancy: Treatement by total pneumonectomy. Analysis of 79 collected cases and presentation of 7 personal cases. *Surgery, Gynecology & Obstetrics, 68,* 435–451.

Phillips, C. V., Rabiu, D., & Rodu, B. (2006). Calculating the comparative mortality risk from smokeless tobacco versus smoking. *American Journal of Epidemiology, 163,* S189. Retrieved August 8, 2007, from http://www.tobaccoharmreduction.org/calculating.htm.

Phillips, C. V., Rodu, B., & the Alberta Smokeless Tobacco Education & Research Group, University of Alberta. (2006). *Frequently asked questions about tobacco harm reduction.* Retrieved August 8, 2007, from http://www.tobaccoharmreduction.org/faq/menu.htm.

Rodu, B., & Godshall, W. T. (2006). Tobacco harm reduction: An alternative cessation strategy for inveterate smokers. *Harm Reduction Journal, 3,* 37.

Royal College of Physicians of London. (1962). *Smoking and health: Summary and report of the Royal College of Physicians of London on smoking in relation to cancer of the lung and other diseases.* Toronto, Ontario, Canada: McClelland & Stewart.

Schairer, E., & Schöniger, E. (1943). Lungenkrebs und Tabakverbrauch [Lung cancer and tobacco consumption]. *Zeitschrift für Krebsforschung, 34,* 261–269. (Republished in English: *International Journal of Epidemiology* (2001), *30,* 24–27)

Surgeon General's Advisory Committee on Smoking and Health. (1964). *Smoking and health: Report of the advisory committee to the Surgeon General of the Public Health Service.* Washington, DC: U.S. Department of Health, Education, and Welfare, Public Health Service.

Wynder, E. L., & Graham, E. A. (1950). Tobacco smoking as a possible etiologic factor in bronchiogenic carcinoma: A study of 684 proved cases. *Journal of the American Medical Association, 143,* 329–336.

TOXIC SHOCK SYNDROME

Toxic shock syndrome (TSS) is a rare but potentially fatal disease caused by toxins produced by two types of bacteria. It is most commonly associated with tampon use but has also been linked to the use of contraceptive diaphragms, wound infections, complications following surgery, and infection resulting from childbirth or abortion.

TSS is caused by the release of toxins from the strains of bacteria, *Staphylococcus aureus,* and less commonly, *Streptococcus pyogenes.* Infections caused by the latter strain are called streptococcal toxic shock-like syndrome (STSS), and although it is a similar syndrome to TSS, it is not identical. The median incubation period of infection of TSS is approximately 2 days.

Symptoms of TSS infection can develop very suddenly and typically include fever, nausea, diarrhea, vomiting, and muscle aches. A sunburn-like rash on the palms and the soles is typically present during the acute phase and peels within a few weeks. More serious complications include hypotension and sometimes even multiorgan failure. Infection is subsequently diagnosed with tests that may include blood and urine tests. On confirmation of diagnosis, treatment typically involves the administration of antibiotics, and in general, the patient recovers in approximately 7 to 10 days. In more serious cases, treatment may include hospitalization and administration of intravenous fluids.

TSS was first described in 1978 in the United States in an outbreak of seven young children. However, it became more commonly known in 1980 as a result of an epidemic associated with the prolonged use of highly absorbent tampons in menstruating, healthy, young women. This association was due to the efficiency of superabsorbent tampons in absorbing magnesium, low levels of which are associated with increased production of TSS-associated toxin, TSS Toxin 1. After this initial epidemic, TSS became a nationally reportable disease in the United States in 1980.

Following this epidemic, the number of cases of TSS has declined significantly. Influencing factors might include changes that were made in tampon production that led to a decrease in tampon absorbency, greater knowledge of TSS among women and physicians, and the standardized labeling required by the U.S. Food and Drug Administration. Specifically, superabsorbent tampons were removed from the market after the outbreak in 1980. In 1979, before these tampons were removed from the market, menstrual TSS accounted for approximately 90% of all cases. By 1996, it accounted for approximately half of all cases. The annual incidence rate when the last surveillance was done in 1986 was approximately 1 per 100,000 women. It is fatal in about 5% of all cases.

An additional change in the epidemiology of TSS since this time is the relative increase in the proportion of nonmenstrual cases, particularly those reported following surgical procedures. This could be due to an increase in outpatient procedures and therefore increased opportunity for infection. Preventive efforts focus on patient education about early signs and symptoms and risk factors for TSS.

—Kate Bassil

See also Food and Drug Administration; Notifiable Disease; Women's Health Issues

Further Readings

Hajjeh, R. A., Reingold, A., Weil, A., Shutt, K., Schuchat, A., & Perkins, B. A. (1999). Toxic shock syndrome in the United States: Surveillance update, 1979–1996. *Emerging Infectious Diseases, 5*(6), 807–810.

TRANSTHEORETICAL MODEL

The transtheoretical model (TTM) was developed by James Prochaska and Carlo DiClemente around 1980 to explain how people change in psychotherapy. The model was soon adapted to describe behavior change with respect to addictions, especially smoking cessation. In the past 10 years, the model has been applied across a wide range of behaviors important to public health, including diet, exercise, sun exposure, alcohol and drug abuse, mammography screening, condom use, stress management, weight control, diabetes self-management, and many more. First conceptualized primarily as a model of self-change, the model was elaborated to include how people change with professional help and has now become one of the most widely used frameworks for the development and dissemination of public health interventions.

The basic premise of the TTM is that behavior change occurs in a series of *stages of change* and that at each stage different strategies or *processes of change* are best suited to help individuals change behavior. The model is frequently referred to as the stages of change model; however, that name overlooks several important additional constructs that are integral to the change process, including several intervening or intermediate outcome variables: *decisional balance* (the pros and cons of change) and *self-efficacy* (confidence in the ability to change and temptations to engage in unhealthy behaviors across challenging situations). Together with the stages and processes of change, these constructs provide a multidimensional view of how people change.

Stages of Change

The stages of change serve as the central organizing construct of the TTM, describing change as a process instead of a singular event. Five ordered categories of readiness to change have been defined: precontemplation, contemplation, preparation, action, and maintenance.

Precontemplation

Individuals in the precontemplation stage do not intend to change in the next 6 months. People in this stage may think that their unhealthy behavior is not a real or serious problem for many reasons. They may avoid thinking, reading, or talking about their behavior, and may seem resistant, defensive, and unmotivated.

Contemplation

In the contemplation stage, individuals admit that their behavior is a problem and they are seriously considering change within the next 6 months. They acknowledge the benefits of change but are keenly aware of the costs, resulting in ambivalence. These individuals often delay acting on their intentions and may remain in this stage for a long time ("chronic contemplation").

Preparation

Individuals in the preparation stage intend to change behavior in the next 30 days. They have a specific plan of action that includes small steps forward, such as smoking fewer cigarettes, quitting smoking for 24 hr, enrolling in an online program, or talking to a health professional. Often, they have made recent short-term attempts to change behavior.

Action

Individuals in the action stage must meet a specific and well-established behavioral criterion, such as quitting smoking (rather than cutting down), or eating five or more daily servings of fruits and vegetables (rather than eating more in one serving). Ideally, the criterion reflects expert consensus on how much change is necessary to promote health or reduce disease risk. The action stage lasts for 6 months, since this includes the period of greatest relapse risk.

Maintenance

Maintenance is defined as 6 months of successful action. The goals for this stage are to consolidate the gains achieved during action so as to continue to prevent relapse. While relapse risk diminishes during maintenance, it does not disappear. For some individuals and for some behaviors, maintenance may be a lifelong struggle.

Generally, individuals need to complete the tasks and consolidate the gains of one stage before they are ready to progress to the next. Progress through the stages is not usually linear, but more likely to be cyclical. Individuals reaching action or maintenance may lapse and recycle to an earlier stage. Once included as a distinct stage in the model, relapse is viewed as an event that initiates recycling through the stages. Most relapses do not result in regression all the way back to precontemplation since many of the gains made before the relapse remain, thus facilitating subsequent action attempts. The TTM views relapse as providing opportunities to learn from previous mistakes, to weed out unsuccessful change strategies, and to try new approaches.

Processes of Change

The processes of change are cognitive, affective, and behavioral strategies that individuals use to progress through the stages of change. Ten basic processes have been found consistently across most health behaviors (several additional processes have been identified as important for a more limited set of behaviors). These processes are organized into two higher-order processes. The experiential processes incorporate cognitive and affective aspects of change, and the behavioral processes include more observable change strategies. The experiential processes include *consciousness raising* (increasing awareness and understanding of the behavior), *dramatic relief* (experiencing feelings of personal susceptibility related to the behavior), *environmental reevaluation* (affective and cognitive understanding of how the behavior affects the psychosocial environment), *self-reevaluation* (cognitive/affective understanding of personal values and self-image with respect to behavior), and *social liberation* (awareness of social norms and support for alternative, healthier choices). The behavioral processes include *contingency (reinforcement) management* (rewarding oneself or being rewarded by others for making healthy changes), *counterconditioning* (substitution of alternative healthier behaviors for unhealthy ones), *helping relationships* (accepting and using others' support), *self-liberation* (choosing and committing to change), and *stimulus control* (removal of cues for unhealthy behaviors, addition of cues for healthy alternatives, avoiding challenging situations, and seeking supportive environments).

Decisional Balance: Pros and Cons of Change

Part of the decision to move from one stage to the next is based on the relative evaluation of the pros and cons of changing behavior. The pros are positive aspects or advantages of change, and the cons are negative aspects or disadvantages of change. The comparative weight of the pros and cons varies depending on the individual's stage of change. This relationship between the stages of change and decisional balance has been found to be remarkably consistent across a wide range of health behaviors.

Self-Efficacy: Confidence and Temptation

Adapted from cognitive-social learning theory, in the TTM self-efficacy is operationalized as how confident individuals are that they will engage in the new healthy behavior and how tempted they would be to engage in the unhealthy behavior across a range of challenging situations. Both constructs assess multidimensional situational determinants of relapse. Confidence and temptation typically show small relationships to stage of change from precontemplation to preparation, followed by strong and nearly linear increases and decreases from preparation to maintenance, respectively. Both constructs serve as good indicators of relapse risk for individuals in later stages.

Integration of TTM Constructs

TTM constructs are integrally related providing an important foundation for intervention. Transitions between stages are mediated by the use of distinct subsets of change processes and are associated with substantial changes in decision making, self-efficacy, intention, and ultimately, behavior. Individuals in the earlier stages of change tend to use experiential processes of change and report relatively low confidence and fairly high temptation, as well as overvaluing the cons of change relative to the pros. Individuals in the later stages tend to use behavioral processes, report more confidence in their ability to change and relatively less temptation to slip into unhealthy behaviors, and evaluate the pros of change more highly than the cons. These interrelationships are vital to the development of effective interventions. When treatment programs ignore or mismatch processes to stages, recruitment, retention, and behavior change efforts are likely to suffer. Stage-tailored intervention programs accelerate progress through the stages. An important advantage of this approach is that stage-tailored interventions are relevant not just to those select individuals who may be ready to change but also to the full population who may be neither prepared nor motivated to change. The TTM intervention approach, including effective treatment for individuals at all stages of readiness to change, can greatly increase the population impact of programs, by effectively increasing recruitment, retention, reach, and efficacy.

—Joseph S. Rossi and Colleen A. Redding

See also Health Belief Model; Self-Efficacy; Social-Cognitive Theory; Targeting and Tailoring; Theory of Planned Behavior

Further Readings

Prochaska, J. O. (2004). Population treatment for addictions. *Current Directions in Psychological Science, 13*, 242–246.

Prochaska, J. O., Redding, C. A., & Evers, K. (2002). The transtheoretical model and stages of change. In K. Glanz, B. K. Rimer, & F. M. Lewis (Eds.), *Health behavior and health education: Theory, research, and practice* (3rd ed., pp. 99–120). San Francisco: Jossey-Bass.

Prochaska, J. O., & Velicer, W. F. (1997). The transtheoretical model of health behavior change. *American Journal of Health Promotion, 12*, 38–48.

Prochaska, J. O., Velicer, W. F., Rossi, J. S., Goldstein, M. G., Marcus, B. H., Rakowski, W., et al. (1994). Stages of change and decisional balance for 12 problem behaviors. *Health Psychology, 13*, 39–46.

TUBERCULOSIS

Tuberculosis (TB) is a contagious disease caused by the bacilli *Mycobacterium tuberculosis*, which usually attacks the lungs but can also attack the brain, spine, and other parts of the body. TB was once the leading cause of death in the United States but is much less deadly today due to the development of drugs and combination therapies to treat it; however, the development of drug-resistant strains of TB is cause for concern. Worldwide, TB remains a major cause of morbidity and mortality, particularly in Africa and South East Asia.

TB is spread primarily through the air, when a person with active TB puts the bacilli in the air through coughing or sneezing and other people breathe in the bacilli. When a person breathes in TB, the bacilli may settle in the lungs and from there can move to other parts of the body. TB is not a highly contagious disease, and in fact only 20% to 30% of people exposed to TB bacilli become infected. Infection is most common among people who have daily or frequent contact with a person with active TB, such as a family member or coworker. The symptoms of active TB include persistent cough, coughing up blood, weakness and fatigue, weight loss, chills, fever, and night sweats.

The most common test for TB is a skin test that involves inserting a small amount of fluid under the skin of the forearm; after 2 or 3 days the skin test is "read" by a health care worker to determine if it is positive or negative. A positive skin test generally indicates exposure to TB, but does not mean that the person has active TB. In fact, most people who test positive for TB have only an inactive or latent infection, meaning that they are not currently sick but that the TB bacilli are present in their body, so they are at heightened risk of developing TB later in their lives. Persons with latent TB have no symptoms and cannot spread the disease to others. Risk factors for developing active TB include age (babies and young children are at greater risk), gender (males are more at risk during infancy and after 45 years of age, women in adolescence and early adulthood), occupational exposure to silicosis, and stress. Any condition that weakens the immune system also places a person with latent TB at risk: Today a common cause of diminished immunity is infection with HIV, and the combination of the two diseases has worsened the global TB burden. Persons with latent TB infection are often advised to take medication to prevent the latent infection from becoming active, and persons known to have weakened immune systems are sometimes treated prophylactially if they have frequent contact with someone known to have active TB.

Active TB is usually treated with a combination of drugs, the most common of which include streptomycin, isoniazid, rifampin, ethambutol, thiacetazone, and pyrazinamide. In most cases, a course of treatment must be continued for at least 6 months to kill all the TB bacilli in a person's body. However, because the person often feels better with only a few weeks of treatment, he or she may cease to take medications on schedule, therefore risking the chance of becoming ill again and also of breeding drug-resistant strains of TB. Directly observed therapy, in which a TB patient takes medications in the presence of a health care worker, has become common for at least initial TB treatment and is recommended by both the Centers for Disease Control and Prevention (CDC) and the WHO.

History

TB is an ancient disease: It was known to the ancient Greeks as *phthisis* and to the Romans as *tabes*, and evidence of TB has been detected in Egyptian mummies and remains of Neolithic man in Germany, France, Italy, and Denmark. It was established in Western Europe and the Mediterranean states by AD 100, but became a major health concern with the mass population migrations to cities beginning in the 17th century: The crowded city environment created excellent conditions for spreading the disease. In the United States, TB arrived with *the Mayflower* and was well established in the colonies by the 1700s. TB was largely unknown in Africa until the early 1900s, when it was spread by European colonists. Robert Koch identified the *Mycobacterium tuberculosis* in 1882 and received the Nobel Prize in 1905 in recognition of this discovery.

Early treatment of TB involved rest, exercise, dietary changes, bloodletting, and sometimes a change of climate (such as moving to the mountains or the seaside), none of which may have had any effect on the disease. In the late 1850s, sanatorium treatment became popular, and TB patients were often sent to live in institutions built in mountainous or rural areas solely for that purpose, a practice that may not have helped the patients (beyond what could have been gained by normal bed rest in any climate) but did decrease the probability of their spreading the disease to others. The first effective treatment developed for TB was streptomycin, introduced in 1946. However, streptomycin-resistant strains appeared within months of its introduction. Other early drugs demonstrated to be effective against TB were sulfanilamide, isoniazid, and para-aminosalicylic acid. The success of pharmacological treatment of TB led many in the medical community to believe that the disease was a thing of the past, at least in the industrialized world.

Neglect of TB control programs, coupled with emergence of HIV, led to resurgence in TB rates in the 1980s, both in the industrialized world and in developing countries. The WHO in 1993 declared TB to be a global health emergency, which led to increased efforts toward TB control. Particularly in developing countries, the high prevalence of latent TB infection, high prevalence of HIV infection, and the emergence of drug-resistant strains of TB make the disease particularly difficult to control.

A vaccine for TB was developed in 1921 by Albert Calmette and Camille Guerin; their vaccine, known as BCG (Bacille Calmette Guerin), was first put into common use in France in 1924. Vaccination became common in Europe, until the "Lübeck Disaster" of 1930 in which a number of children were accidentally vaccinated with virulent tubercle bacilli and many died. After World War II, use of the BCG vaccine was reinstated in Europe and today is a standard vaccine in the WHO Expanded Programme on Immunization and is used in most countries in the world but is not recommended by the CDC for use in the United States except under very limited conditions. The BCG vaccine has variable effectiveness in different populations and on average probably prevents about half of infections. A BCG-vaccinated individual will be positive for a skin test while the vaccine is still effective. Therefore, its use complicates the identification of individuals with latent or newly acquired disease in low-risk areas such as the United States.

Incidence, Prevalence, and Mortality

The WHO collects and reports data on global TB annually: Reporting is voluntary but nearly all countries in the world participate. The WHO estimates that one third of the world's population, approximately 1.9 billion people, is infected with TB. It is the 8th leading cause of death in the world and caused approximately 1.8 million deaths in 2003, more than any infectious disease other than HIV. Most TB cases occur in the developing world, where it causes 25% of adult preventable deaths.

The WHO annual TB reports are presented by geographic region, which somewhat confuses the picture because some regions include countries with both high and low incidence. Africa has the highest annual incidence (new cases) rate, with 345 cases per 100,000 people, followed by South East Asia (including India, Pakistan, Bangladesh, Nepal, the Maldives, Thailand, Indonesia, Timor-Leste, Myanmar, and North Korea) with 190 cases per 100,000. The WHO estimates that 60% to 70% of adults in the African and South East Asian regions are infected with latent TB. The incidence of TB is lowest in Europe and the Americas, with 50/100,000 and 43/100,000 cases, respectively, although there is wide variation by country within these regions.

In the United States, data on TB have been collected by the CDC, in cooperation with state and local health departments, since 1953. In 2005, 14,097 cases of TB were reported, for a case rate of 4.8/100,000. Asians (25.7/100,000) had the highest case rate among ethnic groups, and the rate was much higher for foreign-born (21.9/100,000) than for U.S.-born

(2.5/100,000) persons. Approximately, 1.0% of the U.S. cases were of primary multidrug-resistant TB.

—*Sarah Boslaugh*

See also Epidemiology in Developing Countries; Public Health Surveillance; World Health Organization

Further Readings

Centers for Disease Control and Prevention. (2005). *Questions and answers about TB*. Atlanta, GA: Author. Retrieved December 13, 2006, from http://www.cdc.gov/nchstp/tb/default.htm.

Coberly, J. S., & Chaisson, R. E. (2007). Tuberculosis. In K. E. Nelson & C. F. M. Williams (Eds.), *Infectious disease epidemiology: Theory and practice* (2nd ed., pp. 653–697). Sudbury, MA: Jones & Bartlett.

National Center for HIV, STD and TB Prevention: Division of Tuberculosis Elimination. (2006). *Reported tuberculosis in the United States, 2005*. Atlanta, GA: Centers for Disease Control and Prevention. Retrieved December 13, 2006, from http://www.cdc.gov/nchstp/tb/surv/surv2005/default.htm.

World Health Organization. (2006). *Global tuberculosis control: Surveillance, planning, financing*. Geneva, Switzerland: Author. Retrieved December 13, 2006, from http://www.who.int/tb/publications/global%5Freport/2006/pdf/full%5Freport.pdf.

World Health Organization. (2006). *Tuberculosis* (Fact Sheet No. 104). Geneva, Switzerland: Author. Retrieved December 13, 2006, from http://www.who.int/mediacentre/factsheets/fs104/en.

TUKEY, JOHN
(1915–2000)

John W. Tukey was a mathematician and statistician responsible for many innovations in data analysis. He was born in New Bedford, Massachusetts, and educated at home until he entered Brown University in 1933. After earning degrees in chemistry at Brown, Tukey entered Princeton University in 1937 to continue his study of chemistry. He began attending lectures in the Department of Mathematics, and, in 1939, received a Ph.D. in mathematics at Princeton. He remained there for the rest of his career as Professor of Mathematics, and later, he served as the founding chairman of the Department of Statistics. For most of his career, Tukey also held positions at AT&T's Bell Laboratories, where he worked on projects such as the Nike missile system, the methods for estimating the depth of earthquakes, and the development of an index for the literature on statistics. He retired from both Princeton and Bell Laboratories in 1985.

Tukey served as a consultant for many clients, including the U.S. government. During World War II, he joined Princeton's Fire Control Research Office, where he worked on issues related to artillery fire control. Later, he applied his expertise in solving time-series problems to the issue of distinguishing nuclear explosions from earthquakes. As a consultant for Merck, he worked on statistical methods for clinical trials, drug safety, and health economics. His education-related consulting included work for the Educational Testing Service and on the development of the National Assessment of Educational Progress.

In 1950, Tukey was a member of an American Statistical Association committee that criticized, in a balanced report, the methodology used in Alfred C. Kinsey's research on sexuality. From 1960 until 1980, he worked for NBC on the development of methods for rapidly analyzing incoming election-night data. Later, he argued in favor of using statistical procedures to adjust U.S. Census enumerations.

Tukey was a proponent of exploratory data analysis (EDA), a data-driven approach that he thought provided a much-needed complement to inferential, model-driven, confirmatory data analysis methods. EDA emphasizes visual examination of data and the use of simple paper-and-pencil tools such as box-and-whisker and stem-and-leaf plots, both of which were developed by Tukey for quickly describing the shape, central tendency, and variability of a data set. These methods remain in use today and have been incorporated into most statistical software programs.

Tukey's work on the problem of controlling error rates when performing multiple comparisons using a single data set resulted in the development of his "honestly significant difference" test. His creation of the "jackknife" procedure for estimating uncertainty in a statistic whose distribution violates parametric assumptions is one widely recognized product of his work on the issue of statistical robustness. With this method, the variability of a statistic is estimated by successively excluding different subsets of data from computations. Because he viewed this procedure as a tool that is suitable for many tasks but ideal for none, Tukey coined the term *jackknife*. Other widely known terms first used by Tukey include *bit* (for

binary digit), *software*, *data analysis*, and the acronym "ANOVA" (to refer to analysis of variance).

—Scott M. Bilder

See also Box-and-Whisker Plot; Robust Statistics; Stem-and-Leaf Plot

Further Readings

Brillinger, D. R. (2002). John W. Tukey: His life and professional contributions. *Annals of Statistics, 30(6),* 1535–1575.

TUSKEGEE STUDY

The Tuskegee Study of untreated syphilis in the African American male was conducted between 1932 and 1972. It was the longest nontherapeutic study conducted on humans in the history of medicine. When the numerous breaches of ethical behavior by researchers conducting the Tuskegee Study became known, public outcry was so great that the protection of the rights of participants in medical research were made a priority through legislation and administration.

The Tuskegee Study, conducted by the U.S. Public Health Service, included 616 participants (412 infected with syphilis and 204 controls). The study participants were low-income African American males in Macon County, Alabama, a poor community with a high prevalence of the disease. The purpose of the study was to assess the course of untreated syphilis in African American males and to compare it with that noted in the Oslo, Norway, Study (1929), a retrospective study of untreated primary and secondary syphilis in whites, which was conducted at a time when minimal treatment and no cure was available for syphilis. Other purposes of the Tuskegee Study included raising the public's consciousness of the problem of syphilis, maintaining the momentum of public health work in the area by sustaining cooperative arrangements among state and local governments and the Tuskegee Institute medical personnel, and standardization and developing invention of serologic tests for syphilis.

The researchers involved in the Tuskegee Study believed it represented high-quality research and published various articles on its findings; the idea that the study was unethical on any level was not considered.

Although the researchers may have had good intentions, multiple ethical violations occurred, including (1) there was no informed consent of participants, even though in 1914 the U.S. Supreme Court ruled that every adult human being of sound mind has the right to determine what is to be done with his or her own body; (2) participants were denied treatment of their disease (arsenic and bismuth were available as a treatment for syphilis at the initiation of the study, and penicillin became available as a cure for syphilis during the 1940s); (3) participants were not informed of their illness; (4) participants were not educated as to how their illness was transmitted; and (5) participants were not informed of the risks of participating in the study.

The Tuskegee Study has also been criticized as being the first to address potential biological and genetic differences as rationale for the differences in syphilis among blacks and whites rather than addressing differences in social class, environment, education level, cultural differences, and access to health care. The ramifications of the study are still apparent today with mistrust of the medical and research fields by minorities in America.

The study has been credited by some for its attempt to be culturally sensitive in its approaches to recruitment and retention of research subjects in the midst of unethical practices. Eunice Rivers, an African American nurse, was the liaison for the Public Health Service physicians and the subjects. Eunice Rivers also provided transportation to subjects along with organizing and tracking them for physical examinations.

As a result of the Tuskegee Study, the National Research Act of 1974 was passed by the U.S. Congress. The act led to the creation of the National Commission for the Protection of Human Subjects in Biomedical and Behavioral Research. In 1978, the Commission released *The Belmont Report: Ethical Principles and Guidelines for the Protection of Human Subjects*. The report recommended three principles that should guide research on human subjects: beneficence, personal respect, and justice. Beneficence is the performance of actions or behaviors that actively do good or that actively protect from harm. The principle of beneficence requires protection of research participants and mandates specific safeguards to minimize risks that might occur to subjects. It requires that benefits to participants, research investigators, scientific disciplines, and society at large be maximized. The second principle, respect for persons, requires acknowledgment of the research subject's right to autonomy and informing the subject of his or her rights and protection of those with diminished autonomy. The requirements of personal respect involve specific policies to ensure that research subjects are protected from the following: (1) involvement in a study without knowledge or consent, (2) coercion of subjects to participate in studies, (3) invasion of privacy, (4) unfairness and lack of consideration, (5) nondisclosure of the true nature of the study, and (6) deception. Finally, the principle of justice requires fairness in the distribution of the burdens and the benefits of research. Researchers should make every attempt to involve subjects who are most likely to benefit from the research findings in any application. The Belmont principles were also developed to prevent exploitation of vulnerable populations because of race, ethnicity, gender, disability, age, or social class.

The National Research Act also mandated the installation of an institutional review board (IRB) at all research institutions receiving federal funding. The IRB was initially introduced in the 1960s to ensure that adequate measures are taken to secure informed consent in experimental studies. The role of the IRB is to determine if the proposed selection of patients is equitable and to protect the rights and welfare of human subjects.

—*Keneshia Bryant*

See also Ethics in Health Care; Ethics in Human Subjects Research; Health Disparities; Institutional Review Board; Sexually Transmitted Diseases

Further Readings

Cassell, E. (2000). The principles of the Belmont Report revisited: How have respect for persons, beneficence and justice been applied to clinical medicine? *Hastings Center Report, 30*(4), 12–21.

Corbie-Smith, G. (1999). The continuing legacy of the Tuskegee syphilis study: Considerations for clinical investigation. *American Journal of Medical Science, 317*(1), 5–8.

Jones, J. (1993). *Bad blood: The Tuskegee syphilis experiment*. New York: Free Press.

Sales, B., & Folkman, S. (2000). *Ethics in research with human participants*. Washington, DC: American Psychological Association.

White, R. (2000). Unraveling the Tuskegee study of untreated syphilis. *Archives of Internal Medicine, 160*(5), 585–598.

TWIN STUDIES

Twin studies have been instrumental in building our knowledge of the etiology of common disorders because they provide a mechanism for estimating the relative magnitude of genetic and environmental contributions to disease. Monozygotic (identical) twins share 100% of their genes, and dizygotic (fraternal) twins share on average 50% of their genetic material—the same as in any pair of full siblings. By combining information from monozygotic (MZ) and dizygotic (DZ) twin pairs, an index of heritability can be calculated in the form of a ratio of MZ to DZ twin correlations for a given disorder. Since DZ twins are the same age (unlike other sibling pairs), differences observed between members of DZ twin pairs cannot be attributed to age or cohort differences. A higher correlation among MZ versus DZ twins therefore suggests a genetic contribution to the disorder.

Origins and Assumptions of the Twin Model

The identification of familial clustering of a disorder is only the starting point for investigating its heritability. Because parents provide both genes and environment to offspring, attributions of genetic versus environmental causes of disease cannot be properly made in a traditional parent-offspring study. Studies of twins reared apart allow for a clear distinction to be drawn between genetic and environmental factors in the etiology of disorders. Variability in outcomes between individuals with the same genes in two different environments are attributed to factors that distinguish the two environments. However, the relatively unusual circumstances under which twins are separated at birth need to be considered in interpreting findings (including their possible relationship to parenting behaviors and/or heritable traits). Even more important, the rarity of twins being reared apart creates significant obstacles in the acquisition of samples that are sufficiently large to detect differences between affected and unaffected individuals, especially in the study of relatively uncommon diseases.

Studies of twins reared together do not suffer from the above limitations and, although distinguished from single births by shorter gestational periods, disadvantages associated with twin status do not appear to persist beyond 5 years of age. The prevalence or risk factors for numerous adult health conditions, including psychiatric disorders, do not differ between twins and singletons, making findings from twin studies generalizable to the larger population.

The twin method is based on the premise that the environments of etiologic relevance to the trait being studied do not differ significantly between DZ and MZ twins. The equal environments assumption (EEA) is critical in the interpretation of findings from twin studies because it is the basis on which distinctions between MZ and DZ similarity in a given trait are attributed to genetic rather than environmental sources. It has been argued that MZ twins experience environmental conditions that differ from those of DZ twins in that MZ twins are treated more similarly by parents and other individuals in their social environments and that they typically spend more time together and enjoy a closer emotional bond. Whereas critics of the twin method have argued that these apparent violations of the EEA invalidate findings from twin studies, twin researchers have argued for testing the assumption in a number of ways, including measuring the relationship between environmental similarity and outcomes under study and, in cases in which parents are misinformed about zygosity of twins, comparing the impact of actual versus perceived zygosity on twin resemblance. Little evidence of violations of the EEA has been produced, but twin researchers continue to promote rigorous testing and adjustments for violations when they are found.

A Brief History of Twin Studies

Francis Galton is credited with being the first to recognize the utility of twin methodology in establishing heritability of a trait or disorder. In his 1875 paper "The History of Twins," he described twins as affording a means for evaluating the effects of nature versus nurture and acknowledged that there are two kinds of twins, one in which both twins are derived from a single ovum (MZ) and a second in which twins develop from two separate ova (DZ). It was not until the 1920s, however, that the idea of comparing MZ and DZ concordance rates was proposed as a method for assessing heritability. In 1924, both dermatologist

Herman Siemens's study examining melanocytic naevi (moles) and psychologist Curtis Merriman's study on cognitive abilities described comparisons between identical and nonidentical twin similarity to determine the heritability of the traits under investigation, marking these as the first true twin studies. An article published by John Jinks and David Fulker in 1970 signified another major development in the history of twin studies, as it argued for the application of a biometrical genetic approach to the study of human behavior and proposed a framework for testing hypotheses in genetically informed designs.

Partitioning Variance in Twin Models

The goal in using twin methodology is to estimate the proportion of variance in a given phenotype (the detectable outward manifestation of a genotype) attributable to each of three sources: genetic factors, shared environment, and unique environment. Genetic variance, represented by "a" in the twin path model (see Figure 1), refers to the combined effect of all additive genetic factors that contribute to variability in the phenotype, which in the case of complex traits generally means multiple genes. Covariance between a1 and a2 is 1.0 for MZ twins and 0.5 for DZ twins, as MZ twins are genetically identical and DZ twins share on average half of their genes. Shared environment is denoted as "c" in the model and by definition has a covariance of 1.0 in both MZ and DZ twins, as it represents environmental factors common to both members of the twin pair. Unique variance ("e") refers to variance that is not attributable either to genetic factors or to environmental factors common to both twins and is by definition unshared between twin pairs of either zygosity. Using the above nomenclature, variance of a given phenotype is denoted as a2 + c2 + e2. The covariance between MZ twins is represented as a2 + c2 and the covariance between DZ twins as (0.5)a2 + c2.

Computer programs such as Mx and LISREL have been created to build more complex models that take into account additional factors that affect variance estimations, but simple comparisons between correlations of MZ versus DZ twins provide broad indicators of the proportion of variance in a phenotype attributable to genetic and environmental sources. Genetic influence is suggested by higher correlations between MZ than DZ twins, as it is the greater genetic similarity between MZ twins that distinguish them from DZ

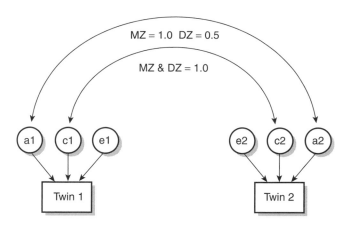

Figure 1   Partitioning Variance in Twin Models

twins. Shared environmental influence is indicated by DZ twin correlations exceeding half of MZ twin correlations. That is, if DZ twins are more alike than would be expected if similarities were based entirely on genetic factors, the implication is that influences in the shared environment are playing a role in the development of the phenotype. Unique environmental influences are approximated by subtracting the MZ twin correlation for the phenotype (which encompasses both genetic and shared environmental influences on MZ twins) from 1, the total variance.

Extensions of the Twin Model and Future Directions

One major limitation of traditional twin methodology is that genetic effects are confounded with gene-environment interactions and genotype-environment correlations. Inflated estimates of genetic contributions to disorders can result from failure to control for variability in genetically controlled sensitivity to environmental factors associated with the phenotype (e.g., responsiveness to stress and depression). Similarly, as individuals with certain genotypes are more likely to seek out particular environments or to evoke differential responses from the environment, environmental exposures cannot be assumed to be randomly distributed in the population. Individuals with (heritable) antisocial traits, for example, are more likely to associate with deviant peers—a known environmental risk factor for developing substance use disorders. Assortative mating or nonrandom choice of sexual partners (and coparents of offspring) based on similarities that have a genetic basis can also influence patterns of family resemblance.

Data from spouses and additional family members, collected in twin-family studies, can be informative in assigning genetic and environmental sources of variance to the disorder of interest. Another approach designed to address gene-environment correlations and interactions is the offspring of twins model, in which offspring of twins are characterized as high versus low environmental risk and high versus low genetic risk based on the twin parent's status in combination with the parent's cotwin's status on the phenotype. For example, an individual whose father is not depressed but whose father's cotwin meets depression criteria would be considered at high genetic and low environmental risk for depression. Gene-environment effects may also be addressed in part by determining whether estimates of heritability vary according to a specified environmental exposure.

Finally, in addition to its continued utility in evaluating genetic and environmental sources of variance in disease, the twin method has the potential to contribute significantly to the identification of specific genes that impact the development of various disorders. Using DZ twins in linkage studies can increase power because they provide built-in controls for family environment and age. Association studies similarly benefit from the use of twins through their provision of ethnically matched controls as well as the means for estimating genetic variance attributable to a given polymorphism.

—*Carolyn E. Sartor*

See also Gene-Environment Interaction; Genetic Epidemiology; Genotype; Phenotype

Further Readings

Boomsma, D., Busjahn, A., & Peltonen, L. (2002). Classical twin studies and beyond. *Nature Reviews Genetics, 3*, 872–882.

Kendler, K. S. (1993). Twin studies of psychiatric illness. Current status and future directions. *Archives of General Psychiatry, 50*, 905–915.

MacGregor, A. J., Snieder, H., Schork, N. J., & Spector, T. D. (2000). Twins: Novel uses to study complex traits and genetic diseases. *Trends in Genetics, 16*, 131–134.

Martin, N., Boomsma, D., & Machin, G. (1997). A twin-pronged attack on complex traits. *Nature Genetics, 17*, 387–392.

Neale, M. C., & Maes, H. H. M. (1992). *Methodology for genetic studies of twins and families.* Dordrecht, The Netherlands: Kluwer Academic.

TYPE I AND TYPE II ERRORS

Type I and Type II errors are two types of errors that may result when making inferences from results calculated on a study sample to the population from which the sample was drawn. They refer to discrepancies between the acceptance or rejection of a null hypothesis, based on sample data, as compared with the acceptance or rejection that reflects the true nature of the population data. Both types of error are inherent in inferential statistics, but they can be minimized through study design and other techniques.

Type I Error

The probability of a Type I error, also known as alpha (α), is the probability of concluding that a difference exists between groups when in truth it does not. Another way to state this is that alpha represents the probability of rejecting the null hypothesis when it should have been accepted. Alpha is commonly referred to as the significance level of a test or, in other words, the level at or below which the null hypothesis is rejected. It is often set at 0.05 which, although arbitrary, has a long history that originated with R. A. Fisher in the 1920s. The alpha level is used as a guideline to make decisions about the p value that is calculated from the data during statistical analysis: Most typically, if the p value is at or below the alpha level, the results of the analysis are considered significantly different from what would have been expected by chance. The p value is also commonly referred to as the significance level and is often considered analogous to the alpha level, but this is a misuse of the terms. There is an important difference between alpha and p value: Alpha is set by the researcher at a certain level before data are collected or analyzed, while the p value is specific to the results of a particular data analysis. For instance, a researcher might state that he or she would use an alpha level of 0.05 for a particular analysis. This means two things: First, that he or she accepts the fact that if his or her analysis was repeated an infinite number of times with samples of equal size drawn from the same population, 5% of the time the analysis will return significant results when it should not (a Type I error) and that results with p values of 0.05 or less will be considered significant—that is, not due to chance. The p value calculated for a particular experiment can be any number between 0 and 1: In this example, a p value of 0.02 would be considered significant while a p value of 0.8 would not be.

As an example of a Type I error, consider the case of two normally distributed populations whose true means are equal. If an infinite number of samples are drawn from those populations, the means of the samples will not always be equal, and sometimes will be quite discrepant. Because in most cases we do not know the true population means, we use statistics to estimate how likely the differences in the means found in our samples are, if the population means were truly the same. In doing this, we accept that in some percentage of the cases, we will make the wrong decision, and conclude that the population means are different when they are truly the same: The probability of making this incorrect decision is Type I error or alpha.

Type II Error

The probability of a Type II error is known as beta (β). Beta is the probability of concluding that no difference exists between groups when in truth it does exist. As with alpha, we accept that there is some probability of drawing incorrect conclusions merely by chance: Often, the probability is set at 20%.

The complement of beta (i.e., $1 - \beta$) is known as statistical power, and describes the probability of detecting a difference between sample groups when a difference of specified size truly exists in the population. The commonly accepted power level is 80%, corresponding to a beta of 20%, meaning that if a true difference at least as large as we specify truly exists in the population from which our samples are drawn, over an infinite number of trials, we will detect that difference 80% of the time. If the power of a study is low, it may not be able to detect important differences that may truly exist, thereby missing potentially important associations.

Importance of Type I and Type II Errors

Type I and Type II errors are generally thought of in the context of hypothesis testing. In hypothesis testing, the null hypothesis (H_0) is often that there is no difference between groups while the alternative hypothesis (H_a) is that there is a difference between groups. Type I and Type II errors are the two types of errors that may occur when making a decision based on the study sample as to whether the null hypothesis or the alternative hypothesis is true. The 2×2 table shown below (Table 1) illustrates when a Type I or Type II error occurs in the context of hypothesis testing. These errors are important concepts in epidemiology because they allow for the conceptualization of how likely study results are to reflect the truth. From them, guidelines can be set as to what is an acceptable amount of uncertainty to tolerate in the sample to make an inference to the truth in the population and gives an idea of how likely the data are to be able to detect a true difference.

The probability of a Type I error, alpha, and the complement of the probability of a Type II error, power, are used in the calculation of sample size. Prior to beginning a study, it is necessary to decide on the levels of error that are acceptable and from this, determine the sample size that corresponds to the chosen levels of error. As stated previously, although the common alpha and power level are 0.05 and 0.80, respectively, sometimes researchers choose different levels. Their choice depends in part on the relative importance of making a Type I or Type II error, because there is a trade-off between the alpha and power levels: When the alpha level is set lower, the beta necessarily becomes higher and vice versa. Figure 1 demonstrates why this trade-off occurs. Figure 1a shows a scenario where, using a one-sided test and specifying the alternative hypothesis as the average amount by which males are taller than females, or delta (Δ), the alpha is set at 0.05, and the beta is 0.20. When the alpha level is changed to 0.10, keeping all

Table 1   Hypothesis Testing and Errors

	H_0 Is True	H_0 Is Not True
Accept H_0	Correct	Type II error
Reject H_0	Type I error	Correct

other factors (i.e., sample size) the same, the beta necessarily lowers to 0.12 as seen in Figure 1b. This happens because the amount of overlap between the two curves is predetermined by the values given to the null and alternative hypotheses. Increasing the alpha level shifts the cutoff to the left, thereby decreasing the size of beta (and increasing power).

Generally, beta is set much higher than alpha because some consider it to be a less serious error to make, though there is controversy in this statement. Deducing that no difference exists between groups when it does seems a less harmful mistake because it may lead to lack of action on the part of scientists (i.e., not implementing an efficacious intervention or drug treatment). On the other hand, deducing that there is a difference when there really is not may lead to inappropriate action and could lead to harmful side effects that do not bring with it the expected benefits. The debate, however, comes about with the realization that lack of action is not always less harmful and, therefore, the levels at which the alpha and beta are set depend on the potential costs or benefits that may result from a Type I or Type II error.

The concepts of Type I and Type II errors also pertain to instances where the outcome measure is a categorical variable, not continuous. The principle is the same although statistics appropriate to categorical data are used to estimate effect size, such as chi-square or odds ratio (OR), rather than a statistic such as mean difference between groups. An example using the OR is demonstrated in Figure 2, which also demonstrates the influence of sample size on Type I and Type II errors. Let us assume the real effect is

$OR = 1.5$ in the population and the alpha level is set at 0.05. The larger study sample has a smaller confidence interval (CI) range and is able to detect the difference between the experiment and the control groups at the set alpha level (0.05); whereas a smaller study sample fails to do so because the CI includes $OR = 1$ (H_0). In other words, the analysis based on the smaller study sample resulted in a Type II error, failing to detect a true difference, which could also be stated as failing to reject the null hypothesis when it should have been rejected.

In general, increasing the study sample size decreases the probability of making a Type II error without having to increase the alpha level. This is, in part, because increasing the sample size decreases sample variance and increases statistical power. Along the same line, when the sample size is very large, there is a high likelihood of finding statistically significant differences between study groups; however, the differences are not necessarily clinically significant.

In epidemiology, there has been some discussion as to the ethicality of conducting a study that has a high probability of Type II error, even if the likelihood of a Type I error is low. The issue arises because study participants are asked to take on risks by being in a study that they wouldn't take on otherwise, such as the use of experimental drugs or potential breaches to confidentiality, and many researchers consider it unethical to expose them to those risks unless the study has a high probability of finding differences if they truly exist. In a well-designed study with proper methodology, human subjects' protections, and ample power, the risks taken on by

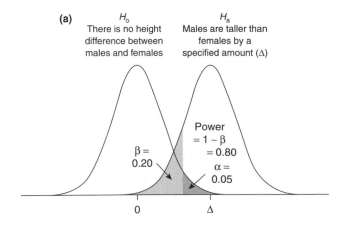
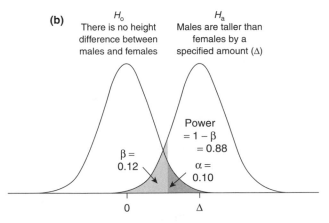

Figure 1   Type I and Type II Error Trade-Off

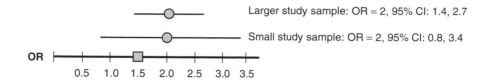

Figure 2   Type I and Type II Errors for Categorical Variables

participants are outweighed by the potential benefits to society that come with scientific findings. However, in a study with low power, the risks may not be outweighed by the potential benefits to society because of the lesser probability that a true difference will be detected. Grant applications and institutional review board proposals often require a power analysis for this reason, and further require that researchers demonstrate that they will be able to attract sufficient study subjects to give them adequate power.

—Rebecca Harrington and Li-Ching Lee

See also Hypothesis Testing; Multiple Comparison Procedures; *p* Value; Sample Size Calculations and Statistical Power; Significance Testing

Further Readings

Gordis, L. (2004). Randomized trials: Some further issues. In *Epidemiology* (3rd ed., pp. 130–146). Philadelphia: W. B. Saunders.

Rosner, B. (2000). Hypothesis testing: One-sample inference. In *Fundamentals of biostatistics* (5th ed., pp. 211–271). Pacific Grove, CA: Duxbury Press.

Rothman, J. R., & Greenland, S. (1998). Approaches to statistical analysis. In J. R. Rothman & S. Greenland (Eds.), *Modern epidemiology* (2nd ed., pp. 181–199). Philadelphia: Lippincott-Raven.

Clemson University. (2001). Type I and type II errors: Making mistakes in the justice system. *Amazing applications of probability and statistics*. Retrieved August 12, 2006, from http://intuitor.com/statistics/T1T2Errors.html.

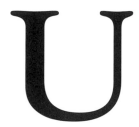

UNITED NATIONS CHILDREN'S FUND

The United Nations Children's Fund (UNICEF) is a United Nations program focused on the rights of children. UNICEF is headquartered in New York City and is primarily funded by governments and charitable donations.

History

Originally dubbed the United Nations International Children's Emergency Fund, UNICEF was founded in December 1945 to provide food, clothing, and health care to impoverished children in Europe after World War II. In 1950, UNICEF's mandate was expanded to address the needs of children and women in all developing countries, becoming a permanent program of the United Nations in 1953. UNICEF was awarded the Nobel Peace Prize in 1965. In 1989, the General Assembly of the United Nations adopted the Convention on the Rights of the Child, a set of standards ensuring human rights of children aged 18 years and younger. This framework serves as the basis for UNICEF's work.

Priorities

Working in 191 countries, UNICEF currently has five focus areas: child survival and development; provision of basic, compulsory education for all boys and girls; HIV/AIDS prevention for children; protection of children from violence and exploitation; and public policy. The child survival program centers on using evidence-based, high-impact interventions to lower the number of preventable maternal, newborn, and child deaths. The education program is based on the principles of human rights and gender equality, with the philosophy that education is a means to ending poverty and disease. In fighting HIV/AIDS, UNICEF has set out to reduce the number of new infections in children, particularly among infants and young adults. In addition, the program focuses on providing support to orphans and families affected by HIV/AIDS. The child protection focus area advocates for the development of a protective environment for children, free from the threats of violence, abuse, and exploitation. Finally, the public policy focus area uses data analysis to clarify the pathways by which policy affects the well-being of women and children in developing countries.

The Millennium Development Goals

In 2000, the world's leaders met at a summit to address the eradication of poverty, resulting in eight Millennium Development Goals with a target date of 2015. Six of the eight goals have an intrinsic link to children: eradicate poverty and hunger; achieve universal education; promote gender equality and empower women; reduce child mortality; improve maternal health; and combat HIV/AIDS, malaria, and other diseases. UNICEF's work in the five focus areas directly relates to these goals. UNICEF indicators are used as measures of progress toward a number of goals.

—Anu Manchikanti

See also Child and Adolescent Health; Health, Definitions of; Maternal and Child Health Epidemiology

Web Sites

UNICEF: http://www.unicef.org.

UNIT OF ANALYSIS

In a statistical model, the unit of analysis is the entity about which inference is being made. For example, in a clinical study, an investigator must decide if inference is to be made with regard to individual patient outcomes or with regard to the physicians treating the patients. If the former, then the unit of analysis is the patient, and the resulting odds ratios or relative risks (or other statistics) would be interpreted as reflecting changes in patient risk or differences in patient characteristics. Similarly, it may be desirable to make inference regarding the treating physicians, each of whom may have treated multiple patients. In this case, statistical methods should be chosen so as to address questions related to the physician.

In most instances, the selection of the unit of analysis is straight-forward. In a cross-sectional survey of patients in the emergency department waiting room, the unit of analysis would be the survey respondent, the patient. In a randomized clinical trial of the effectiveness of a new medication treatment, the unit of analysis would again be the individual patient.

Proper identification of the unit of analysis is critical. Failure to do so may result in biased or invalid results. In a clinical study of 100 patients treated by 5 different doctors, if the unit of analysis is the patient, we end up ignoring the fact that patients treated by one doctor will have certain characteristics in common compared with patients treated by another doctor. That is, a doctor is likely to approach different patients in a roughly similar way. Ignoring this "clustering" by physician, or selecting analytic techniques that do not take this into account will yield incorrect estimates of variance, leading to erroneous confidence intervals or p values.

If we are interested in making inference with regard to the treating physicians, patient outcome measures can be summarized with means or proportions within treating physician. The analyses of these types of data require different statistical tests and have a different interpretation than if the patient was the unit of analysis. Analyses that take into consideration effects at these different levels (e.g., patient and physician) are often referred to as "multilevel" or "hierarchical" models.

—Annette L. Adams

See also Confidence Interval; Inferential and Descriptive Statistics; Multilevel Modeling; Point Estimate; Predictive and Associative Models

Further Readings

Divine, G. W., Brown, J. T., & Frazier, L. M. (1992). The unit of analysis error in studies about physicians' patient care behavior. *Journal of General Internal Medicine*, 7(6), 623–629.

Pollack, B. N. (1998). Hierarchical linear modeling and the "unit of analysis" problem: A solution for analyzing responses of intact group members. *Group Dynamics: Theory, Research, and Practice*, 2(4), 299–312.

Raudenbush, S. W., & Bryk, A. S. (2002). *Hierarchical linear models: Applications and data analysis methods* (2nd ed.). Thousand Oaks, CA: Sage.

URBAN HEALTH ISSUES

Demographic trends suggest that there is an urgent need to consider the health of urban populations. Cities are becoming the predominant mode of living for the world's population. According to the United Nations, approximately 29% of the world's population lived in urban areas in 1950. By 2000, 47% lived in urban areas, and the United Nations projects that approximately 61% of the world's population will live in cities by 2030. Overall, the world's urban population is expected to grow from 2.86 billion in 2000 to 4.94 billion in 2030. As the world's urban population grows, so does the number of urban centers. The number of cities with populations of 500,000 or more grew from 447 in 1975 to 804 in 2000. In 1975, there were four megacities with populations of 10 million or more worldwide; by 2000, there were 18, and 22 are projected by 2015. Most cities are in middle- to low-income countries; in 2000, middle- to low-income countries contained 72% of the world's cities.

Epidemiology can play a central role in studying both health and disease in the urban context and how urban characteristics may influence the health of populations. Characteristics of the urban environment that may shape population health include features of the social and physical environment and features of the urban resource infrastructure. Features of the social and physical environment and the urban resource infrastructure in turn are shaped by municipal, national, and global forces and trends.

Defining Urban Areas

One of the key challenges that faces epidemiologic inquiry about health in cities and how city characteristics influence health is that there is little consensus about the definition of *urban* and what constitutes a city. The U.S. Bureau of the Census defines an urbanized area by specifying a minimum population (50,000 people) and a particular minimum population density (1,000 people per square mile). The Census Bureau thus provides a dichotomy whereby territory, population, and housing units within specific size and density parameters are designated as urban and those that are outside those parameters are nonurban. However, there are inherent limitations to these definitions; urban areas exist in contrast to rural or simply in contrast to nonurban areas. In the 21st century, only a few cities, such as Las Vegas, exist in extreme isolation where what is not defined as city is rural. Most cities (e.g., New York City, London, Bangkok) are actually far-reaching densely populated areas, containing periurban and suburban areas, which continue relatively uninterrupted for miles beyond the municipal city boundaries and the city center. To accommodate varying conceptions of what constitutes an urban area, alternative definitions have been developed. They vary in how they define rates of disease, risk, and protective behaviors.

The definition of *urban* also varies widely between countries. Among 228 countries for which the United Nations had data in 2000, almost half (100) include size and density as criteria, 96 include administrative definitions of *urban* (e.g., living in the capital city), 33 include functional characteristics (e.g., economic activity, available services), 24 have no definition of urban, and 12 define all (e.g., Anguilla, Bermuda, the Cayman Islands, Gibraltar, the Holy See, Hong Kong, Monaco, Nauru, Singapore) or none (e.g., Pitcairn Island, Tokelau, and Wallis and Futuna Islands) of their population as urban. Official statistics (e.g., United Nations statistics detailed above) rely on country-specific designations and, as such, vary widely. In specific instances, definitions of *urban* in adjacent countries vary tremendously (e.g., Cambodia vs. Vietnam). Furthermore, definitions of *urban* have evolved in different ways in different countries. Therefore, global statistics are subject to country-level differences in the definition of *urban* that may be based on population density or specific urban features (e.g., proportion of agricultural workers, municipal services).

Urban "Exposure" As a Determinant of Health

It may be heuristically and methodologically useful to conceptualize urban exposure in two main ways: urbanization and the urban environment. Epidemiologic inquiry can be guided by an understanding of how these different facets of urban exposure may influence population health.

Urbanization refers to the change in size, density, and heterogeneity of cities and provides a perspective for public health planning. Factors such as population mobility, segregation, and industrialization frequently accompany urbanization. More simply stated, urbanization is the process that involves the emergence and growth of cities. Thus, the process of urbanization does not depend on definition of *urban* per se but rather on the dynamics of agglomeration of individuals. Although the pace of urbanization is independent of the base size of the population, the population size and density of surrounding areas may shape the pace of urbanization. For example, urbanization may include the establishment (or destruction) of new buildings or neighborhoods, development (or removal) of transportation routes and the in-migration and out-migration of people, and changing racial/ethnic composition of cities.

How the dynamics of urbanization affect health can be considered with examples. An influx of impoverished peoples to a city (e.g., immigration driven by food or work shortages in nonurban or other urban areas) in search of jobs and services may tax available infrastructure, including transportation, housing, food, water, sewage, jobs, and health care. Overtaxed sanitary systems may directly lead to rapid spread of disease, as has been the case many times in North America during the past century and as continues to be the case in the developing world today. Also, the population strain on available jobs may result in devaluation of hourly wage rates, higher unemployment, and changing socioeconomic status for persons previously living in a given city. This lowering of socioeconomic status can result in more limited access to health care and may lead to poorer health. Therefore, characteristics of urbanization—including the intensity, rate, and duration of such changes as well as the response to these changes—may have health effects on urban residents. Common mechanisms may exist through which urbanization affects health independent of the size of the city in question.

The *urban context or environment* can be defined as the specific characteristics or features of cities that influence health within a particular city. It is helpful to think of the urban environment as involving three distinct concepts: the social environment, the physical environment, and the urban resource infrastructure. The social urban environment comprises contextual factors that include social norms and attitudes, disadvantage (e.g., neighborhood socioeconomic status), and social capital (e.g., social trust, social institutions). The urban physical environment refers to the built environment, pollution, access to green space, transportation systems, and the geological and climatic conditions of the area that the city occupies. Features of the urban resource infrastructure that influence health may include factors such as the availability of health and social services and municipal institutions (e.g., law enforcement). Features of the social and physical environment and infrastructural resources are all, in turn, shaped by municipal, national, and global forces and trends.

Studies of Health in Urban Populations

Three study designs—urban versus rural studies, interurban studies, and intra-urban studies—have been principally employed to consider both the health of urban populations and how characteristics of cities may influence the health of urban residents. Each has strengths and weaknesses, and these methods may lend themselves to addressing different questions. A multiplicity of methods, including qualitative and quantitative methods, may be employed within each of these designs.

Urban Versus Rural Studies

Urban versus rural studies typically contrast urban areas with rural areas in the same country or consider morbidity and mortality in urban versus nonurban areas. Essentially, these studies seek to determine whether morbidity and mortality due to a specific health outcome is different in specific urban areas as compared with specific nonurban areas.

Urban versus rural (or nonurban) comparisons are useful in drawing attention to particular health outcomes that may be more or less prevalent in urban areas and merit further investigation to examine the specific features of the urban (or rural) environment that are associated with that outcome. Recognizing that urban-rural comparisons are too blunt, more recent work has refined distinctions such as urban core, urban adjacent, urban nonadjacent, and rural. However, such studies are limited in their ability to identify what those factors may be and the pathways through which they affect the health of urban dwellers. Features of cities change over time, and some factors may not be conserved between cities (e.g., racial/ethnic distribution). Thus, it is not surprising that different urban-rural comparisons have provided conflicting evidence about the relative burden of disease in urban and nonurban areas. At best, these studies reveal gross estimates of the magnitude and scope of health measures in broad areas by geographical areas typically defined by size and population density.

Interurban Studies

Interurban studies typically compare health outcomes between two or more urban areas between or within countries. Such studies can simply identify differences between cities or can examine specific features of cities that influence health. Examples of the former are numerous. For example, Vermeiren, Schwab-Stone, Deboutte, Leckman, and Ruchkin (2003) have compared mental health outcomes among adolescents in New Haven (United States), Arkhangelsk (Russia), and Antwerp (Belgium), providing insights into the cross-cultural, cross-urban similarities and differences in antisocial behavior, depression, substance use, and suicide. A study of Puerto Rican injection drug users in New York City (United States) and Bayamóa (Puerto Rico) revealed several differences between the two ethnically similar populations; injection drug users in Puerto Rico injected more frequently and had higher rates of needle sharing as compared with their New York counterparts. The authors pointed to similarities in drug purity and differences in the onset of the crack epidemic as city-level factors that influenced injector risk behaviors. When using the city as the unit of analytic interest, one implicitly assumes that city-level exposures are equally important for all residents. Studying differences in drug use risk behaviors among two cities does not permit analysis of differences in behaviors within cities because of location of residence, intra-urban variability in barriers to safer behaviors, or variations in access to key services (e.g., drug treatment, needle exchange) provided to different urban residents. However, interurban studies such as the examples mentioned here can help guide municipal and state policymakers when making decisions on service provision throughout a city.

Intra-Urban Studies

Intra-urban studies typically compare health outcomes within cities and are being widely used to investigate specific features of the urban environment. These studies often focus on neighborhoods, specific geographic areas within a city that are generally administrative groupings (e.g., census tracts in Canada, subareas or suburbs in South Africa). However, it is important to note that administrative groupings may not represent residents' perceptions of their neighborhoods.

Intra-urban studies may contribute important insights into the relations between specific urban features and health outcomes. However, it may be difficult to generalize from one city to another. For instance, the relation between collective efficacy and violence may be modified by different levels of policing or differential access to illicit substances within a given city. Furthermore, it is important to consider that neighborhood residence is a function of geographical location and other types of social ties that are facilitated or necessitated by the urban environment.

Defining and Quantifying Urban Exposures

When considering a complex and broad exposure such as urbanization or the urban environment, epidemiologic inquiry may fruitfully be guided by considering the elements of urban areas that mechanistically may shape the health of urban populations. It may be useful to consider how the social environment, the physical environment, and the urban resource infrastructure may influence population health.

Social Environment

The urban social environment includes features such as social norms and attitudes, social capital, and income distribution. This list is by no means exhaustive; the further readings provide a more comprehensive look at the urban social environment.

Social norms are patterns of behaviors that are considered accepted and expected by a given society. From the perspective of urban health, the multiple levels of societal and cultural norms are important considerations when thinking about the behavior of urban dwellers. Persons within the urban environment may be influenced by the social norms of their local, geographically defined community, with its unique physical and social structures and cultural characteristics. However, communities may not be limited to one geographic location. Persons in urban areas may also be influenced by the norms operating within the broader urban community.

Social cohesion is typically defined as the connectedness among groups and includes both the presence of strong intra-group bonds and the absence of intra-group conflict. Social capital, a related construct, is thought to provide resources for collective action. Both may be particularly important in densely populated urban areas, where social interaction shapes daily living. There is evidence that the absence of social capital is associated with negative health outcomes such as increases in mortality, poor self-rated perception of health, higher crime rates, and violence.

Income inequality is the relative distribution of income within a city or neighborhood and is typically operationalized with the Gini coefficient. Income inequality is thought to operate through material and psychosocial pathways to shape population health independently of absolute income. Income inequality has been associated with several health outcomes, including self-rated health, cardiovascular mortality, and consequences of illicit drug use. Additionally, emerging work suggests that intra-urban neighborhood income inequality is associated with adverse health outcomes.

Physical Environment

The urban physical environment refers to the built environment (e.g., green space, housing stock, transportation networks), pollution, noise, traffic congestion, and the geological and climate conditions of the area the city occupies. The built environment includes all human-made aspects of cities, including housing, transportation networks, and public amenities. Recent studies have suggested that poor quality of built environments is associated with depression, drug overdose, and physical activity. Green space (e.g., parks, esplanades, community gardens) has the potential to significantly contribute to the health of urban dwellers. Living in areas with walkable green spaces has been associated with increased longevity among elderly urban residents in Japan, independent of their age, sex, marital status, baseline functional status, and socioeconomic status.

Urban transportation systems include mass transit systems (i.e., subways, light rail, buses) as well as streets and roads. Urban transportation systems are key in the economic livelihoods of city residents as well as cities as a whole. On the other hand, there are significant health considerations for mass transit and roadways, including security and violence, noise, and exposure to pollutants. These exposures are relevant not only for transit workers but also for transit riders.

Pollution is one of the well-studied aspects of the urban physical environment. Urban dwellers are exposed to both outdoor and indoor pollutants that include heavy metals, asbestos, and a variety of volatile hydrocarbons. For example, one study conducted by Ruchirawat et al. (2005) in Bangkok (Thailand) reported high levels of benzene and polycyclic aromatic hydrocarbons among street vendors and school children sampled from traffic-congested areas as compared with monks and nuns sampled from nearby temples.

Urban Resource Infrastructure

The urban resource infrastructure can have both positive and negative effects on health. The urban infrastructure may include more explicit health-related resources such as health and social services as well as municipal structures (e.g., law enforcement), which are shaped by national and international policies (e.g., legislation and cross-border agreements).

The relation between availability of health and social services and urban living is complicated and varies between and within cities and countries. In wealthy countries, cities are often characterized by a catalog of health and social services. Even the poorest urban neighborhood often has dozens of social agencies, both government and nongovernmental, each with a distinct mission and providing different services. Many of the health successes in urban areas in the past two decades, including reductions in HIV transmission, teen pregnancy rates, tuberculosis, and childhood lead poisoning, have depended in part on the efforts of these groups. For example, social and health services may be more available in cities than in nonurban areas, contributing to better health and well-being among urban residents. Despite wider availability of social and health services in cities, many cities experience remarkable disparities in wealth between relatively proximate neighborhoods. This variance is often associated with disparities in the availability and quality of care. Low-income urban residents face significant obstacles in finding health care both in wealthy and less wealthy countries.

Municipal, National, and Global Forces and Trends

Municipal, national, and global forces and trends can shape the more proximal determinants of the health of urban populations. For example, legislation and governmental policies can have substantial influence on the health of urban dwellers. Historically, municipal regulations regarding sanitation in the 19th and 20th centuries facilitated vast improvements in population health and led to the formation of national groups dedicated to improving population health such as the American Public Health Association. A contemporary example of the power of legislation to influence health has been ongoing in New York State since the early 1970s. In 1973, the New York State Legislature, with the encouragement of then Governor Nelson Rockefeller, enacted some of the most stringent state drug laws in the United States. Characterized by mandatory minimum sentences, the Rockefeller Drug Laws have led to the incarceration of more than 100,000 drug users since their implementation. Those incarcerated under the Rockefeller Drug Laws overwhelmingly are New York City residents (78%) and Black or Hispanic (94%). Ernest Drucker (2002) estimated the potential years of life lost as a result of the Rockefeller Drug Laws to be equivalent to 8,667 deaths.

Regional and global trends can affect not only urban living but also the rate and process of urbanization or deurbanization. Changes in immigration policies or policy enforcement can affect urban dwellers in a variety of ways, including, but not limited to, changes in access to key health and social services for some subpopulations, changes in community policing practices, and changes in social cohesion and levels of discrimination. Terrorist attacks in urban centers (e.g., Baghdad, Jerusalem, London, Madrid, and New York City) are associated not only with morbidity and mortality among those directly affected by the event but also with significant psychological distress for other residents of the cities. Armed conflicts have resulted in mass displacement of individuals, some of whom have fled cities for other cities, regions or countries, or camps for displaced individuals (e.g., Darfur).

Future Research

Global demographic trends suggest that urban living has become normative, and there is an urgent need to consider how urban living may influence the health of populations. Epidemiologists may fruitfully be engaged in studying how urban characteristics—including features of the social and physical environment and features of the urban resource infrastructure—can influence health and disease in the urban context. The study of urban health requires a multidisciplinary perspective that can consider different types of studies, including inter- and intra-urban studies and urban-rural comparisons. Epidemiologists' work in the area can complement the work of public health practitioners, urban planners, as well as social, behavioral, clinical, and environmental health scientists in conjunction with the active participation of community residents and civic, business, and political leaders.

*—Sandro Galea, Danielle C. Ompad,
and David Vlahov*

See also Epidemiology in Developing Countries; Governmental Role in Public Health; Multilevel Modeling; Urban Sprawl; Violence as a Public Health Issue

Further Readings

Berkman, L. F., & Kawachi, I. (2000). *Social epidemiology.* New York: Oxford University Press.

Bourgois, P. I. (2003). *In search of respect: Selling crack in el barrio* (2nd ed.). New York: Cambridge University Press.

Colon, H. M., Robles, R. R., Deren, S., Sahai, H., Finlinson, H. A., Andia, J., et al. (2001). Between-city variation in frequency of injection among Puerto Rican injection drug users: East Harlem, New York, and Bayamon, Puerto Rico. *Journal of Acquired Immune Deficiency Syndromes, 27*(4), 405–413.

Drucker, E. (2002) Population impact of mass incarceration under New York's Rockefeller drug laws: An analysis of years of life lost. *Journal of Urban Health: Bulletin of the New York Academy of Medicine, 79*(3), 434–435.

Friedman, S. R., Cooper, H. L., Tempalski, B., Keem, M., Friedman, R., Flom, P. L., et al. (2006). Relationships of deterrence and law enforcement to drug-related harms among drug injectors in US metropolitan areas. *AIDS (London, England), 20*(1), 93–99.

Galea, S., Ahern, J., Rudenstine, S., Wallace, Z., & Vlahov, D. (2005). Urban built environment and depression: A multilevel analysis. *Journal of Epidemiology and Community Health, 59*(10), 822–827.

Galea, S., Ahern, J., Vlahov, D., Coffin, P. O., Fuller, C., Leon, A. C., et al. (2003). Income distribution and risk of fatal drug overdose in New York City neighborhoods. *Drug and Alcohol Dependence, 70*(2), 139–148.

Galea, S., & Schulz, A. (2006). Methodological considerations in the study of urban health: How do we best assess how cities affect health? In N. Freudenberg, S. Galea, & D. Vlahov (Eds.), *Cities and the health of the public.* Nashville, TN: Vanderbilt University Press.

Galea, S., & Vlahov, D. (2005). Urban health: Evidence, challenges, and directions. *Annual Review of Public Health, 26,* 341–365.

Ruchirawat, M., Navasumrit, P., Settachan, D., Tuntaviroon, J., Buthbumrung, N., & Sharma, S. (2005). Measurement of genotoxic air pollutant exposures in street vendors and school children in and near Bangkok. *Toxicology and Applied Pharmacology, 206*(2), 207–214.

Sampson, R. J., Raudenbush, S. W., & Earls, F. (1997). Neighborhoods and violent crime: A multilevel study of collective efficacy. *Science, 277*(5328), 918–924.

Semenza, J. C. (2005). Building health cities: A focus on interventions. In S. Galea & D. Vlahov (Eds.), *Handbook of urban health: Populations, methods, and practice.* New York: Springer.

Subramanian, S. V., Delgado, I., Jadue, L., Vega, J., & Kawachi, I. (2003). Income inequality and health: Multilevel analysis of Chilean communities. *Journal of Epidemiology and Community Health, 57*(11), 844–848.

Takano, T., Nakamura, K., & Watanabe, M. (2002). Urban residential environments and senior citizens' longevity in megacity areas: The importance of walkable green spaces. *Journal of Epidemiology and Community Health, 56*(12), 913–918.

Vermeiren, R., Schwab-Stone, M., Deboutte, D., Leckman, P. E., & Ruchkin, V. (2003). Violence exposure and substance use in adolescents: Findings from three countries. *Pediatrics, 111*(3), 535–540.

Whyte, W. F. (1943). *Streetcorner society: The social structure of an Italian slum.* Chicago: University of Chicago Press.

URBAN SPRAWL

Sprawl is a single-use, low-density, disconnected approach to community design. By separating places where people live, work, and play and limiting direct connections between these activities, sprawl most often renders driving as the only rational travel option. Distances are often too vast, and walking is most often difficult, if not dangerous, in sprawl. Urban sprawl is associated with several adverse health outcomes, including less walking and overall physical activity, increased sedentary time, exposure to air pollution from automobiles, and increased rates of obesity.

Sprawl is one extreme of a continuum of approaches to land development and transportation investment that collectively determine the urban form of an area, which in turn influences the behavior of the residents—for instance, by making it easier or more difficult to include walking in their daily routines. Urban forms range from sprawl that is auto-dependent all the way to smart growth or new urbanist design, which is arguably pedestrian and transit supportive at the expense of reduced auto access. Therefore, sprawl is one of many typologies of urban form along a continuum of auto to pedestrian and transit orientation.

There are several ways in which sprawl has been measured. Typical metrics of urban form includes measures of both the proximity between complementary land uses (residential, shopping, work, entertainment) and the connectivity or directness of travel between locations dedicated to these uses. Proximity is based on the compactness or density and the intermixing of land uses. Another element used to describe urban forms is the design of street networks, which may range from a connected grid to a disconnected cul-de-sac sprawl-type environment. Other measures include the presence of a continuous pedestrian or bike network, crosswalks that are safe and well demarcated, and the placement or setback of development from the edge of a street. These microscale or site-level measures have been less studied but create the character of a place. For instance, an extremely different environment emerges based on whether shops are next to the street or set behind a *parking lagoon* (large parking lot), a term coined by Howard Kunstler who authored *The Geography of Nowhere* (1993).

Sprawl is a highly regulated and metered approach to developing land and to investing in transportation, but at a scale that is too vast for the pedestrian: A sprawl environment is designed for movement at 40 miles per hour and is therefore boring to the walker, since walking is relatively static at 3 miles per hour. Sprawl may be better understood in contrast with its opposite, walkability. Where sprawl describes an auto-dependent environment, walkability defines those elements of an environment that support active forms of travel (walking and biking) and public transit and reduce car dependence. A voluminous body of literature has emerged in recent years on the health and environmental benefits of walkability. Research has extended the relationship between urban form (sprawl vs. walkable) and associated travel patterns to vehicle-based air pollution, physical activity, and prevalence of obesity.

There is general agreement at this point that as one moves away from sprawl and toward the walkability end of the urban form continuum, per capita vehicle use, greenhouse gas and air pollutants, and obesity prevalence decline, while walking and physical activity levels increase. More recently, studies are showing significant associations between sprawl, climate change, and per capita energy consumption due to increased auto dependence. It is arguable that this line of reasoning looks at only a part of the relationship between sprawl and climate change. Studies should also evaluate differences in per capita home-based energy consumption due to larger spaces and lack of shared energy sources for heating and cooling in sprawling single family environments—in contrast to the sharing of energy sources that is inherent in multifamily housing.

Taken collectively, sprawl is a resource and energy consumptive development pattern and requires more energy; more land; more roads, sewer, water, and other services; and more time to move about from place to place. One study in Atlanta, Georgia, showed that residents of sprawling environments drove 30% more during the week and 40% more on the weekend than those in more walkable areas of that region. Another report from this same study known as SMARTRAQ showed that households in the most sprawling areas of the Atlanta region consume an average of 1,048 gallons of gas and spend $2,600 per year (assuming two cars per household and $2.50/gallon). Those living in the most walkable areas of the region consumed 262 fewer gallons of gas a year and spend $640 less per year on average. These estimates are conservative. Going from a two- to a one-car household is more feasible in more walkable areas; moreover, inevitable spikes in energy costs can rapidly increase the gap between transportation costs and the expense of heating and cooling a typical home in urban sprawl versus one in a more walkable setting.

Increased awareness of looming natural resource limitations relative to increased population, aging baby boomers, and changing household demographics, and a renewed interest in urban living renders sprawl's future uncertain. Studies are beginning to show that a significant proportion of those who live in sprawl would in fact prefer to be in more walkable environments but that there is an undersupply of homes in walkable neighborhoods, given the patterns of construction and development in the past half century, which produced most new homes in sprawling environments.

Many argue that while there is an association, there is only limited evidence of a causal connection between sprawl and travel patterns, obesity, and the environment (see Special Report 282 from the Transportation Research Board and Institute of Medicine, 2005). This argument rests on the premise that people's behavior is a function of their preferences and predisposition for specific types of travel choices and neighborhood environments. Research to date has most often not disentangled the effect of these preferences versus that of community design on travel, health, and environmental outcomes. More recently, a new body of research is emerging that compares people with similar preferences who are located in different types of urban environments. At least two studies now show that regardless of preferences, exposure to different types of environments (sprawling or walkable) results in different amounts of driving, and that those preferring walkable environments also walk significantly more and have a lower prevalence of obesity when they are located in a walkable environment.

Why do people continue to build and dwell in sprawling urban environments? Over the past several hundred years, people have wanted to have more living space. Also, urban environments created an environment that was ideal for the transmission of disease, leading to people's desire to live in less densely populated areas. Psychological factors may also be at work; some suggest that sprawl offers *defensible space*, a term coined by Oscar Newman as a form of development that does not require dealing with unknown people and where one knows who does and does not belong in their domain. Therefore, living in a sprawling environment has been a rational choice for many. However, the costs of sprawl are now becoming clear, including the costs in terms of health due to increased pollution from automobiles, as well as the barriers to physical activity presented by this form of development.

—*Lawrence Frank*

See also Geographical and Social Influences on Health; Obesity; Physical Activity and Health; Pollution

Further Readings

Frank, L. D., Saelens, B., Powell, K. E., & Chapman, J. (in press). Stepping towards causation: Do built environments or individual preferences explain walking, driving, and obesity? *Social Science and Medicine*.

Frank, L. D., Sallis, J. F., Conway, T., Chapman, J., Saelens, B., & Bachman, W. (2006). Many pathways from land use to health: Walkability associations with active transportation, body mass index, and air quality. *Journal of the American Planning Association, 72*(1), 75–87.

Frumkin, H., Frank, L. D., & Jackson, R. (2004). *The public health impacts of sprawl.* Washington, DC: Island Press.

Kunstler, H. (1993). *The geography of nowhere: The rise and decline of America's man-made landscape.* New York: Simon & Schuster.

Newman, O. (1996). *Creating defensible space.* Washington, DC: U.S. Department of Housing and Urban Development.

Rees, W., & Wackernagel, M. (1996). *Our ecological footprint: Reducing human impact on the earth.* Philadelphia: New Society.

SMARTRAQ final summary report: New data for new era. Goldberg, D., McCann, B., Frank, L., Chapman, J., & Kavage, S. (2007, January). The Active Transportation Collaboratory, University of British Columbia. Retrieved March 22, 2007, from http://www.act-trans.ubc.ca.

SMARTRAQ full final technical report: Integrating travel behavior and urban form data to address transportation and air quality problems in Atlanta. Chapman, J., & Frank, L. (April 2004). Active Transportation Collaboratory, University of British Columbia. Retrieved March 22, 2007, from http://www.act-trans.ubc.ca.

Transportation Research Board & Institute of Medicine. (2005). *Does the built environment influence physical activity? Examining the evidence* (TRB Special Report 282). Washington, DC: Transportation Research Board.

U.S. PUBLIC HEALTH SERVICE

As part of the U.S. Department of Health and Human Services, the U.S. Public Health Service (PHS) works both to investigate the causes of disease and to combat epidemics. It traces its origins to an Act signed by President John Adams in 1798. This Act created the Marine Hospital Service, a network of hospitals intended to serve the nation's merchant marines. In 1873, a "Supervising Surgeon General" was named to oversee the Service, and in 1889, the Commissioned Corps, a uniformed and mobile division of medical officers, was created.

During the late 19th century, the growth of trade, travel, and immigration networks led the Service to expand its mission to include protecting the health of *all* Americans. To reflect this change, the Marine Hospital Service was renamed the Public Health and Marine Hospital Service in 1902. Ten years later, in 1912, the name was shortened to the Public Health Service.

Under this new name, the PHS was given clear legislative authority "to investigate the diseases of man and [the] conditions influencing the propagation and spread" of these diseases in 1912. All types of illness, regardless of their cause, now fell under the purview of the PHS.

However, even before this name change, commissioned officers had advocated the use of aggressive and innovative means to investigate and combat diseases as they emerged. As part of this initiative, the Marine Hospital Service launched the *Bulletin of the Public Health* (later renamed *The Public Health Reports*) in 1878. This weekly report tracked epidemics both within and outside the United States. Throughout the past 125 years, this publication, along with *Mortality and Morbidity Weekly Report*, has provided PHS officers with the latest information on disease outbreaks, enabling them to chart an epidemic as it develops.

With the advent of the 20th century, the PHS began to use increasingly sophisticated techniques to track and fight diseases. In 1906, for example, the PHS initiated and implemented an epidemiological investigation into a typhoid epidemic centered in Washington, D.C. Covering a four-state area, this was one of the most comprehensive epidemiological investigations implemented by a public health agency. The investigation—and the corresponding eradication of the epidemic—provided the nation's legislators with a dramatic and very local demonstration of the power of epidemiological investigations both to prevent and arrest epidemics. In the wake of this success, PHS officer Wade Hampton Frost developed and implemented an innovative epidemiological investigation of the 1918 to 1919 influenza pandemic.

Building on these successes, the PHS launched a program to eradicate malaria within the United States during World War II. Based in Atlanta, the Malaria Control in War Areas program (MCWA) gradually expanded to include the control of other communicable diseases such as yellow fever, typhus, and dengue. In 1946, the MCWA adopted a new name, the Communicable Disease Center (CDC) and became a permanent component of the PHS. The CDC received its current designation as the Centers for Disease Control and Prevention in 1992.

Although the CDC has not been the only PHS agency to investigate the "conditions influencing the propagation and spread" of disease both within and outside the United States, it has consistently been at the forefront of this aspect of the PHS mission. In 1951, the creation of the Epidemic Intelligence Service (EIS) at the CDC provided a blueprint for training medical officers in epidemiology. EIS officers, then and now, received a brief but intensive training in epidemiology and statistics followed by an assignment with a public health unit associated with the PHS or a state or local public health department. These EIS officers are on permanent call and can be dispatched quickly to investigate a disease outbreak.

Today, the PHS continues its work through its eight operating divisions: the Centers for Disease Control (CDC), the National Institutes of Health (NIH), the Indian Health Service (IHS), the Food and Drug Administration (FDA), Substance Abuse and Mental Health Services Administration (SAMHSA), the Health Resources and Services Administration (HRSA), Agency for Healthcare Research and Quality, and the Agency for Toxic Substances and Disease Registry.

—*Alexandra M. Lord*

See also Centers for Disease Control and Prevention; Frost, Wade Hampton; Governmental Role in Public Health; Surgeon General, U.S.

Further Readings

Mullan, F. (1989). *Plagues and politics: The story of the United States public health service*. New York: Basic Books.

Web Sites

Office of the Public Health Service Historian: http://lhncbc.nlm.nih.gov/apdb/phsHistory.

V

VACCINATION

Vaccination is the process of producing immunity against a disease by exposing individuals to weakened, dead, or closely related (but relatively harmless) versions of the pathogen that causes this disease. With the advent of widespread vaccination within populations, rates of vaccine-preventable diseases have dropped dramatically, leading to significant decreases in both morbidity and mortality. Through vaccination, for example, smallpox has been completely eradicated and other diseases, such as polio and measles, are in the process of becoming eliminated. In spite of these successes, however, vaccination is not without controversy. Concerns over possible adverse effects have caused individuals in many areas of the world to question the benefit of vaccines.

Credit for the development of vaccination is given to Edward Jenner, an 18th century English physician. In 1796, Jenner successfully vaccinated an 8-year-old boy against smallpox by exposing him to the related, but much less virulent, cowpox virus. Since Jenner's initial success, many more vaccines have been developed to combat a variety of diseases, including measles, polio, diphtheria, rabies, pertussis, and the flu. Vaccines continue to be developed today to combat diseases, such as HIV and malaria, as well as infections, such as human papillomavirus (HPV) that can cause certain types of cancer.

The central idea behind vaccination is that exposure to weakened or dead microbes, parts of these microbes, inactivated toxins, or, like Jenner's smallpox vaccine, closely related but relatively harmless pathogens, can cause an immune response within individuals that can prevent subsequent infection. More specifically, when a person is vaccinated, he or she is exposed to a version of a pathogen that has been altered so that it does not produce disease, but so that it still contains antigens, or the parts of the pathogen that stimulate the immune system to respond. The B lymphocytes in an individual's blood then detect these antigens in the vaccine and react as if the real infectious organism was invading the body. During this process, the B lymphocytes clone themselves producing two types of cells: plasma cells and memory B cells.

The plasma cells produce antibodies that attach to and inactivate the pathogen. This response is known as the primary immune response; it can take up to 14 days for this process to reach maximum efficiency. Over time, the antibodies gradually disappear, but the memory B cells remain. If an individual is exposed to the disease-causing pathogen again, these dormant memory cells are able to trigger a secondary immune response. This occurs as memory B cells multiply quickly and develop into plasma cells, producing antibodies that in turn attach to and inactivate the invading pathogen. Unlike the primary response, this secondary response usually takes only hours to reach maximum efficiency. It is through this process that vaccination is able to protect individuals from disease.

Vaccination is also beneficial at the population level. When a sufficient number of individuals in a population are immune to a disease, as would occur if a large proportion of a population was vaccinated, herd immunity is achieved. This means that if there is random mixing of individuals within the population then the pathogen cannot be spread through the population. Herd immunity acts by breaking the transmission of infection or lessening the chances of susceptible individuals coming in contact with a person who is infectious. Herd immunity is important because it provides a measure of protection to individuals who are not personally immune to the disease—for instance, individuals who could not receive vaccines due to age or underlying medical conditions or individuals who received vaccines but remain susceptible. It is herd immunity that made the smallpox eradication campaign possible, and it is herd immunity that prevents the spread of diseases such as polio and measles today.

In spite of these benefits to individuals and populations, vaccination itself is not without risk. Common reactions to vaccines include redness and soreness around the vaccination site. More severe adverse reactions are also possible for some vaccinates; these include vomiting, high fevers, seizures, brain damage, and even death, although such reactions are fairly rare. The most serious adverse reactions, for example, occur in less than one case out of a million for most vaccines.

In addition to these known adverse effects of vaccination, claims have also been made that vaccination is responsible for adverse health conditions, such as autism, speech disorders, and heart conditions. While none of these claims is well accepted in the scientific community, they have had a significant impact on individuals' perceptions about the safety of vaccines. Combined with the fact that most individuals have never personally experienced, or seen someone experience, many of the vaccine-preventable diseases in their lifetime, the focus of concern for many people has shifted from the negative effects of the diseases to the possible negative effects of the vaccines themselves. This complacency about vaccine-preventable diseases, combined with concerns over the effects of vaccination, has led to decreasing levels of vaccination coverage in many areas of the world.

Not vaccinating has two general results. Individually, people who are not vaccinated against a disease are at greater risk of contracting this disease than individuals who are vaccinated. At a population level, if vaccination rates are allowed to drop far enough, a loss of herd immunity will result. When herd immunity is not maintained, disease outbreaks occur, and the costs to society in terms of loss of work, medical care,

disability, and even loss of life can be high. Such situations have already occurred in Japan, England, and the Russian Federation, where, after concerns about the pertussis vaccine led to significant decreases in the number of vaccinated children, outbreaks involving thousands of children and resulting in hundreds of deaths occurred.

—*Emily K. Brunson*

See also Disease Eradication; Herd Immunity; Jenner, Edward; Pasteur, Louis; Polio; Smallpox

Further Readings

Feikin, D. R., Lezotte, D. C., Hamman, R. F., Salmon, D. A., Chen, R. T., & Hoffman, R. E. (2000). Individual and community risks of measles and pertussis associated with personal exemptions to immunization. *Journal of the American Medical Association, 284,* 3145–3150.
Gangarosa, E. J., Galazka, A. M., Wolfe, C. R., Phillips, L. M., Gangarosa, R. E., Miller, E., et al. (1998). Impact of anti-vaccine movements on pertussis control: The untold story. *Lancet, 351,* 356–361.
May, T., & Silverman, R. D. (2003). "Clustering of exemptions" as a collective action threat to herd immunity. *Vaccine, 21,* 1048–1051.
Salmon, D. A., Teret, S. P., MacIntyre, C. R., Salisbury, D., & Halsey, N. A. (2006). Compulsory vaccination and conscientious or philosophical exemptions: Past, present and future. *Lancet, 367,* 436–442.

VALIDITY

Validity refers to the extent to which something does what it is intended to do. From this broad perspective, validity equally applies to an object designed to perform certain tasks, to a program targeted to certain goals, or to an instrument intended to measure a given concept or construct. Therefore, it is not limited to the problem of measurement, although it is in this context that we will use it throughout this entry. The concept of validity applies to all measurement situations, but is particularly crucial to social epidemiology, where most research work has to deal with constructs that have to be operationalized. This entry contains a brief review of the concept with emphasis on its empirical and theoretical implications.

The constructs are variables that cannot be directly observed or measured. Quality of life, motivation, satisfaction, and socioeconomic status are typical examples of constructs. Whenever a construct has to be operationalized, that is, defined in terms of concrete data that can be gathered or behaviors that can be observed, one is inevitably confronted with the problem of validity. Measuring a construct by means of an instrument, such as a questionnaire, always poses a problem of validity; for instance, we may try to measure someone's quality of life by asking him or her a series of questions about limitations, pain, and so on, but we must bear in mind that the answers to these questions are not a direct measure of their quality of life but at best an approximation of it. Another frequent example of a validity problem is statistical inference, where we have to estimate some parameters of a finite or infinite population by examining a sample of it. A sample is valid if it adequately reproduces the characteristics of the population that we want to study. Valid samples are usually said to be representative.

An instrument used to measure a construct can be a single indicator (e.g., income as a measurement of socioeconomic status) or can consist of a set of items (e.g., questionnaires designed to measure quality of life). Validity can be assessed on two grounds: theoretical and empirical.

The theoretical validation of an instrument implies a thorough examination of its contents with the purpose of verifying whether it reflects the meaning we have attached to the construct it is intended to measure. On the other hand, the empirical validation entails a careful testing of the properties that should correspond in practice to that meaning. Accordingly, two main dimensions are involved in the process of validation: the ontological and the methodological dimensions.

To theoretically verify that an instrument reflects the meaning of the construct, we must explicitly state what the construct is or what it means for us. We thereby assume an ontological position that is in practice equivalent to making a contextual definition. For instance, an instrument designed to measure quality of life can be validated neither on theoretical nor on practical grounds if we have not previously defined what quality of life is, or what it means for us. Obviously, the definition may vary from one context to another. For example, it may not be the same when applied to patients with cancer as when applied to healthy people, and it may also differ from one cultural setting to another. People with different views of quality of life will surely not agree on the pertinence of an instrument designed to measure it.

Normally, the processes of creating and validating an instrument are parallel. We do not wait for an instrument to be in its final version to validate it. Rather, we build an instrument by validating portions of it, that is, by discarding some of its items, modifying others, and adding new items to it.

Types of Validity

Validity can be subclassified in two conceptually distinct aspects, content validity and criterion validity. Content validity is assessed on theoretical grounds. Criterion validity has to be tested empirically. Other types of validity include convergent validity, discriminant validity, and predictive validity.

Content Validity

Content validity refers to the capacity of adequately reflecting the essence of the construct in the indicators, items, or observable variables we have chosen as components of our instrument. When we make a choice regarding the number and identity of the dimensions underlying satisfaction, academic performance, professional aptitudes, or quality of life, the pertinence of our choice is closely connected with content validity. The questions or other measures of the construct must address those dimensions, while someone with a different theoretical conception of the same construct could object to the inclusion of an indicator or could suggest the addition of some others.

An important component of content validity is called face validity and can be conceived of as the first step in the assessment of content validity. An instrument has face validity or is valid prima facie if it looks valid at a first nonexpert inspection, meaning that a nonexpert in the field would agree that the instrument measures the construct it is intended to measure.

Criterion Validity

An instrument can be theoretically valid if it contains all and only the relevant components of the construct, and yet it may fail to meet one or more of the practical requirements that are required to create a valid measurement of the construct it is intended to measure. For this reason, instruments have to be tested for criterion validity. For example, if a metric for quality of life is sensitive to different stages in the evolution of disease and correlates highly with external factors associated with health and well-being, then it fulfills two criteria of validity.

Let us take, for instance, the construct satisfaction that is crucial in health systems assessment. Choosing the indicators that fully represent and exhaust our notion of satisfaction is typically a problem of content validity. Showing that those indicators are associated with outcomes or processes related to satisfaction, and that they are sensitive to positively effective interventions, is part of what we have to prove for criterion validity.

Convergent and Discriminant Validity

These two criteria work closely together. To establish convergent validity, we need to show that measures of similar constructs are in fact related to each other. On the other hand, if measures of constructs that are theoretically not related to each other are proved to be in fact not related to each other, that is evidence for discriminant validity. A common way to estimate the degree to which any two measures are related to each other is to use the correlation coefficient. Correlations between theoretically similar measures should be high, while correlations between theoretically dissimilar measures should be low. There are no fixed rules to say when a correlation is high and when it is low, but in construct validation we always want our convergent correlations to be higher than the discriminant correlations.

Often, convergent and discriminant validity are tested as part of a single inferential act, for instance, through the administration of a questionnaire containing items to be used to assess both types of validity, so that we can judge the relative values of discriminant and convergent correlations. For example, a group of items that are intended to measure the functional capacity component of the quality of life in people 65 years or more should have higher correlations with each other than with items intended to measure the psychological component of quality of life, and these, in turn, should be more highly correlated among themselves than with items that measure other dimensions.

Predictive Validity

Assessing predictive validity requires examining the relationship of events occurring at different points in time. There are two possible interpretations of predictive validity. One is related to the property of being sensitive to changes over time. For instance, an instrument intended to measure a person's quality of life should reflect changes in his or her health condition over time. For instance, if they are known to have suffered a major illness or injury, this should be reflected by changes in their quality of life score as measured by that instrument. To take another example, a set of indicators designed to assess the quality of a health delivery system should reflect the improvement experienced by the system after interventions that are known to be effective and the deterioration of the system after the ocurrence of events that are known to affect its quality. The same principle is in use when a measure is validated by administering it to groups that are expected to score differently: The evidence for validity is established if the instrument distinguishes between groups that can be theoretically expected to be different. For instance, populations that do not benefit from certain quality health services should show lower levels of satisfaction than populations that do benefit from those services, and an instrument that purports to measure satisfaction is expected to show different levels when applied to those subpopulations. For similar reasons, if the type of surgery is actually relevant with respect to self-perception of quality of life in breast cancer, women who were operated on with conservative surgery should perform better when the instrument used to measure quality of life is applied to them, than those who were operated on with radical surgery.

Another meaning of predictive validity is that a measure is correlated with some event that occurs at a later date. Such an instrument, measure, or model has predictive validity if there is good coincidence between prediction and outcome. For instance, scores on an examination may be used to select students for medical training. If the scores correlate highly with their grades or success in training, this is evidence of the predictive validity of the examination.

—Jorge Bacallao Gallestey

See also EuroQoL EQ-5D Questionnaire; Measurement; Quality of Life, Quantification of; Quality of Well-Being Scale (QWB); SF-36® Health Survey

Further Readings

Foster, S. L., & Cone, J. D. (1995). Validity issues in clinical assessment. *Psychological Assessment, 7,* 248–260.

Guion, R. M., & Cranny, C. J. (1982). A note on concurrent and predictive ability design: A critical re-analysis. *Journal of Applied Psychology*, *74*, 1337–1349.

Kenny, D. A. (1995). The multitrait-multimethod matrix: Design, analysis and conceptual issues. In P. E. Shrout & S. T. Fiske (Eds.), *Personality research, methods and theory: A festschrift honoring Donald W. Fiske* (pp. 111–124). Hillsdale, NJ: Erlbaum.

Schmitt, N., & Landy, F. J. (1993). The concept of validity. In N. Schmitt & W. C. Borman (Eds.), *Personnel selection in organizations* (pp. 275–309). San Francisco: Jossey-Bass.

Smith, G. T. (2005). On construct validity: Issues of method and measurement. *Psychological Assessment*, *17*, 396–408.

Smith, G. T., Fischer, S., & Fister, S. M. (2003). Incremental validity principles in test construction. *Psychological Assessment*, *15*, 467–477.

Vector-Borne Disease

Vector-borne diseases are caused by infectious agents such as bacteria, viruses, or parasites that are transmitted to humans by vectors. In most instances, vectors are bloodsucking invertebrates, usually arthropods such as ticks, mosquitoes, or flies, although vertebrates, including rodents, raccoons, and dogs, can also be vectors of human disease. Infectious agents are most often transmitted by the bite, sting, or touch of a vector, although ingesting or handling the feces of an infected animal can also result in disease transmission. Vector-borne diseases are most common in tropical and subtropical regions where optimal temperatures and moisture levels promote the reproduction of arthropods, especially mosquitoes. Diseases such as malaria, dengue fever, sleeping sickness, and encephalitis have occurred and, in some instances, are still present at endemic or epidemic levels. Reemergence of vector-borne disease is a constant concern due to the rapid rate at which they are capable of spreading. These diseases have played a large role in integrating public health agencies, research, and relief and assistance to areas that are troubled by vector-borne pathogens.

Vector-Borne Disease Transmission

There are two main types of pathogen transmission by vectors, known as internal transmission (sometimes called mechanical transmission) and external transmission. Internal transmission means that a pathogen is carried inside a vector. This can occur as biological transmission, in which the pathogen passes through a necessary stage in its life cycle inside the vector host, which it could not do inside a different host organism. An example of a pathogen that experiences biological transmission is *Plasmodium,* the infectious pathogen that causes malaria. Internal transmission may also occur as harborage transmission, in which the pathogen remains in the same form and life stage inside the vector as when initially entering the vector. The plague bacterium, *Yersinia pestis*, is a harborage transmission pathogen because it does not change morphologically when inside fleas, the common vectors that transmit plague. External transmission occurs when a pathogen is carried on the body surface of the vector. When it lands on a human, the vector passively transmits the pathogen to its new host. An example of a pathogen that is transmitted by external transmission is *Shigella*, which is carried on the legs of flies.

Vector-Borne Pathogens

The list of vector-borne pathogens is long and despite improvements in insect control, understanding of disease, and sanitary conditions of large populations of humans, many of these pathogens are still endemic or epidemic in some parts of the world today. Malaria has beleaguered humans for centuries if not millennia; however, the causative agent *Plasmodium* wasn't identified until 1880 by French army surgeon Charles Louis Alphonse Laveran. There are multiple species of *Plasmodium* that cause malaria, some more infectious than others, with *Plasmodium falciparum* being the most common in occurrence. When a female mosquito bites a human, *Plasmodium* sporozoites are transmitted into the bloodstream, introducing the pathogen to its new, human host. The sporozoites travel through the blood to the liver where they enter cells, mature into schizonts, undergo asexual reproduction, and cause the liver cell to rupture, releasing hundreds of merozoites. Some species of *Plasmodium* will lay dormant in the liver for long periods of time (sometimes years) before maturing and rupturing cells, whereas others will cause liver cell rupture within 2 weeks of initial infection. Merozoites released into the blood enter red blood cells where they rapidly reproduce, causing cell rupture and release of *Plasmodium* that may be in different life-cycle stages. Some may be immature trophozoites that will enter new red blood cells, mature into schizonts, and lead to the release of merozoites, resulting in a continuous proliferation of *Plasmodium* within the human host, sometimes resulting in a chronic case of malaria. Other *Plasmodium* that are released from rupturing blood cells are gametocytes in the sexual stage that cause sporogonic development in mosquitoes. It is these gametocytes that the female mosquito ingests in her bloodmeal from humans, allowing the life cycle of *Plasmodium* to continue. This period of development typically occurs in mosquitoes of the genus *Anopheles*. During this time, gametocytes (male and female) begin the sporogonic stage in the mosquito's stomach, leading to the production of sporozoites that migrate to the mosquito's salivary glands, facilitating their transfer to a human host when the mosquito ingests another bloodmeal. This stage of the *Plasmodium* life cycle highly depends on temperature in that it requires a minimum temperature to be initiated and will stop if temperature becomes too high. Moisture levels also greatly influence the success of pathogen replication. This temperature and moisture dependence is reflected in the greater occurrence of malaria in tropical and subtropical climates that encourage optimal mosquito body temperature and life span and provide sufficient moisture for mosquito breeding, allowing the pathogen to flourish.

Viruses known as flaviviruses that are typically spread by ticks and mosquitoes cause several vector-borne diseases. Among these are West Nile virus, dengue fever, yellow fever, Japanese encephalitis, and Saint Louis encephalitis. In the case of West Nile, the virus is transmitted to a mosquito when it bites an infected animal, usually a bird, which serves as the pathogen reservoir because it develops immunity to the virus. Multiple species of mosquitoes can transmit the disease to humans and horses, although the primary life cycle of the virus only requires interaction between reservoir hosts and mosquitoes; humans and other mammals are considered incidental hosts. Yellow fever virus is another flavivirus of which there exist two types: Jungle yellow fever, which is transmitted to monkeys by infected mosquitoes and rarely infects humans, and urban yellow fever, which is transmitted to humans by infected *Aedes aegypti* mosquitoes. Yellow fever is endemic in areas of Africa and South America where *A. aegypti* mosquitoes thrive in the warm, moist environments.

Often, the virus will lay dormant during the dry season inside < 1% of the population of female mosquitoes. With the onset of the rainy season, the virus travels to the salivary glands of the mosquito and is transmitted to humans when the mosquito bites and feeds on a bloodmeal. Yellow fever virus has experienced a significant reemergence since the 1980s likely due to reduced mosquito control and lack of vaccination in large populations in susceptible areas.

Tick-borne pathogens are of great concern in North America where they cause Lyme disease, Rocky Mountain spotted fever, tularemia, and others. The tick *Ixodes scapularis* is the vector of Lyme disease, which is endemic in certain areas even though only an estimated 2% to 3% of people bitten by *Ixodes* ticks develop the disease. The bacterium *Borrelia burgdorferi* infects tick larvae when they feed on infected animals, such as mice, and establishes itself in the tick as the tick grows and matures. The ticks then transmit the bacteria to animals or humans when they feed. Two species of ticks, *Dermacentor variabilis* and *D. andersoni*, are responsible for transmission of *Rickettsia rickettsii*, the bacterial pathogen that causes Rocky Mountain spotted fever. This disease occurs in North, Central, and South America and is named for the characteristic rash that develops in the late stages of infection. The ticks are both the natural host and reservoir host of *R. rickettsii*, which survives by living inside the cells of the host organism. There are several ways that the bacteria can be passed on through generations of ticks, including infection of eggs by females and through spermatozoa passed by males to females. The bacteria are transmitted to humans by infected tick saliva passed into the bloodstream when the tick bites and feeds on a human. It often takes a few hours before *R. rickettsii* successfully reaches the human bloodstream.

An example of a vector-borne disease transmitted by a vertebrate animal is hantavirus pulmonary syndrome. In 1993, multiple incidences of acute respiratory syndrome occurred in the southwestern United States (specifically, "the four corners" area where Arizona, New Mexico, Colorado, and Utah meet). Researchers quickly identified the cause as a particular type of hantavirus, which they named Sin Nombre virus (SNV). The virus was traced to the deer mouse, *Peromyscus maniculatus*, that was present in unusually high numbers that year due to heavy rainfall that increased rodent food supplies and, consequently, breeding. The SNV is present in the urine, feces, and saliva of infected mice and is transmitted to humans when the virus particles that linger in the air near where the mice have been are inhaled. Humans may also become infected when handling contaminated mice or items that have been within proximity of the infected mice. Rodents are the only animals that can transmit hantaviruses to humans, which cannot be transmitted from human to human. While hantaviruses are not new, the outbreak served as evidence of their destructive capabilities as nearly half of those who were infected lost their lives.

Prevention and Treatment

Most vector-borne diseases can be prevented by following careful sanitation measures and controlling insect populations with insecticides or biological control methods. Some vaccines are available, such as the vaccines against yellow fever and plague; however, many vector-borne diseases are not treated until severe symptoms have developed. Reasons for this may include ambiguity of symptoms, such as the early stages of Rocky Mountain spotted fever or malaria, which are generally vague, or lack of resources (including insecticides and drugs), such as in poorly developed countries where many of these diseases are prevalent. Some drugs are effective in minimizing disease severity or eliminating disease symptoms. However, most treatment can only stabilize persons with severe disease, such as in the case with hantavirus pulmonary syndrome in which antiviral drugs tend to be ineffective, and the use of a respirator is the best option for providing some relief for affected people. There appears to be greater promise in finding ways to control or eliminate vectors of disease, but unfortunately in countries with few resources even this is difficult because of the unpredictability of vector status from year to year. Informing people about vectors and vector-borne diseases in the areas where they live is of great importance and seems to be the most successful way of preventing disease outbreaks available today.

—*Kara E. Rogers*

See also Epidemiology in Developing Countries; Insect-Borne Disease; Malaria; Yellow Fever

Further Readings

Marquardt, W. H. (Ed.). (2004). *Biology of disease vectors* (2nd ed.). New York: Academic Press.
Service, M. W. (Ed.). (2002). *The encyclopedia of arthropod-transmitted infections*. Cambridge, MA: CABI.
Thomas, J. C., & Weber, D. J. (Eds.). (2001). *Epidemiologic methods for the study of infectious diseases*. New York: Oxford University Press.
World Health Organization. (1997). *Vector control*. Geneva, Switzerland: Author.

Vehicle-Related Injuries

Injuries from motor vehicle crashes represent a significant public health issue throughout the world. Recent figures compiled by the World Health Organization estimate that 1.2 million people are killed in road traffic crashes each year. Presently, injuries from road traffic crashes rank as the 11th leading cause of death worldwide. This figure is expected to rise exponentially, by up to 83%, over the next two decades as more vehicles are bought and used in the developing world, with major increases forecast for India and China.

The epidemiology of injuries from motor vehicle crashes were eloquently framed by William Haddon more than 50 years ago in the context of the Haddon Matrix. The Haddon Matrix is a model for understanding the dynamics of events related to crash injury. It is drawn by outlining the issues that lead to, occur during, and follow a crash. Important issues that describe injuries in these three crash phases include human, vehicle, and environmental factors. The Haddon Matrix has been expanded in recent years to also incorporate a sociobehavioral component as an additional issue.

The advent of the Haddon Matrix brought about an enhanced understanding of the multiple factors that underlie crashes and their outcomes. The findings from research over the past 50 years have identified a number of risk factors related to vehicle injuries. These include issues related to gender, age, behavior, education, vehicular safety and safety devices, vehicle and road user relationships, road type, climate, emergency response time, and trauma care availability, among others. Today, varied research and prevention programs are underway to reduce the burden related to motor vehicle crashes, including programs from multiple disciplines, such as epidemiology, engineering, medicine, behavior science, transportation planning, and government.

High-Risk Groups for Motor Vehicle Injury

Several common risk markers have been observed for road traffic crash injury around the world. The major risk groups include younger and older drivers and passengers, persons under the influence of alcohol, aggressive and distracted drivers, motorcycle operators and passengers, and vulnerable road users, primarily pedestrians. While the magnitude of difference in risk of injury may differ for these groups between countries, the general observation that individuals within these groups have a higher injury risk is remarkably consistent. Thus, most present-day research and prevention agendas focus on these risk groups in their road traffic injury prevention efforts.

Young Drivers

Young drivers are often the risk group with the highest reported crash and injury rates. In the United States, the crash rates of young drivers (15 to 20 years of age) are 2 to 3 times higher than drivers of all other ages, except for the elderly. Many issues in young drivers contribute to the higher risks observed. A common factor cited is inexperience with the performance tasks related to driving. The increased crash rate is most pronounced among younger drivers in situations requiring higher performance such as driving in limited visibility and driving at higher speeds. Other factors cited as contributors to higher risks in young drivers are immaturity and higher levels of risk-taking behaviors, particularly alcohol intake. Risks are also borne by the passengers in vehicles driven by younger operators. Most passengers are also between 15 and 20 years of age. Both factors contribute to the fact that injuries from motor vehicle crashes are generally the leading cause of death for persons below 35 years of age in developed regions and a significant cause of death for this age group in the developing regions of the world as well.

Older Drivers and Pedestrians

Older road users are particularly vulnerable to motor vehicle crash injury. Older drivers in developed countries have higher crash rates than all but the youngest drivers. Pedestrian injury is also much higher in persons above 70 years of age. The limitations in physical functioning and performance are the most common factors thought to contribute to this risk. Several reports, for example, note declining visual acuity and peripheral perception in older drivers and link these factors to higher crash frequency. Older drivers also appear to be overly involved in crashes involving turns against traffic, suggesting that lower levels of perception and action and reaction times may contribute to crashes in this group. Older persons are also more vulnerable because their threshold for injury is lower due to declines in muscle mass and bone strength. Injuries in crashes that might have been survivable by younger persons often lead to fatalities in the elderly.

Alcohol Impairment

It is well-known that alcohol is a major contributor to vehicle-related injury globally. Alcohol impairs judgment and delays reaction times in individuals, in general, and is more pronounced with increasing levels of blood alcohol concentration. A motor vehicle crash is considered to be alcohol related in most countries if a driver or pedestrian involved in the crash has a blood alcohol level above the legal limit. In most countries, this limit is between 0.05 and 0.08 g/dl or a blood alcohol level reached by most people consuming one to two drinks in a short period of time. While the frequency of drinking alcohol and driving varies by country, alcohol is generally involved in more than 40% of all fatal motor vehicle crashes. Alcohol involvement in crashes is more pronounced among younger drivers (15 to 34 years of age) and males. Crashes involving alcohol are higher at night (compared with day) and more frequent on the weekend. In the United States, more than one-half of impaired drivers involved in fatal crashes had blood alcohol levels at twice the legal limit or higher. Repeat offending with respect to driving while drinking is common. In the United States, impaired drivers in fatal crashes were 9 times more likely to have a prior conviction for driving under the influence of alcohol compared with drivers with a zero blood alcohol concentration level.

Aggressive Driving

Aggressive driving is emerging as a significant issue in motor vehicle safety. The definition of aggressive driving varies by the context and road culture of an area. In some cultures, for example, aggressive driving may be perceived as the norm. Many believe that they know aggressive driving when they see it, but the classification of aggressive driving behavior differs between individuals. In many locations, authorities consider aggressive driving to be driving that endangers other persons or property. It typically involves multiple violations or moving vehicle traffic offenses. Common traffic offenses under this scenario include speeding, red light running, failing to allow proper distance between vehicles (tailgating), and failure to yield to other vehicles.

Speeding, alone, does not constitute aggressive driving, but it is a major contributor to motor vehicle crashes and injuries. As injuries are characterized by energy transfer and the body's ability to withstand this transfer, the general rule is that the faster you drive, the greater the likelihood of injury, and of greater severity of injuries. According to the World Health Organization's 2004 report on road traffic injury prevention, an increase in speed of 1 km/hr can result in a 3% higher risk of a crash involving injury and a 4% to 5% increase in risk of a fatal crash. Thus, controlling vehicle speed can help reduce the occurrence of a crash and also the development of injuries when a crash occurs. Speeding may be defined as either exceeding the posted speed limit or driving too fast for road conditions. The data compiled by the World Health Organization indicate that speeding is a factor in about 30% of fatal crashes in developed countries. Alcohol impairment is correlated with speeding, with speeding being more frequently involved in fatal crashes where the driver was impaired. Fatal crashes in which speeding was a factor are also more common among males, younger drivers (15 to 34 years of age), at night, and on rural roads.

Distractions While Driving

Recent research indicates that distractions while driving are frequent contributors to motor vehicle crashes and injuries. The 100-car study recorded the driving experiences of 100 cars over a 1-year period of time and assessed driver behavior with computer and video recordings. Eighty-two crashes were observed in this time, although most were minor. Driver inattention to the driving task was found to be a major issue in crashes. Inattention was noted in 78% of all crashes. Driver inattention in

these events was due to the use of a wireless device (cell phone), internal distractions, driver conversations with passengers, and personal hygiene undertaken by the driver. This work is important because many in the highway safety discipline believe that the majority of crashes are related to driver behavior. Interventions to affect driver behavior, then, may provide the greatest success in the future for the prevention of vehicle-related injury. This work, and others, begins to highlight potential areas where interventions might best be placed.

Motorcycles

Lower in cost than automobiles, motorcycles are the primary forms of road vehicle in low-income countries, and they are common in high-income countries as well. Motorcycle riders and operators, though, are vulnerable road users. Limited protection places motorcycle users at greater risk of injury when they are involved in collisions with other vehicles and objects. According to the National Highway Traffic Safety Administration in the United States, "per vehicle mile, motorcyclists are about 34 times more likely than passenger car occupants to die in a traffic crash" (National Center for Statistics and Analysis, 2006, p. 3). One factor for the high vehicle-related injury burden in developing countries is the mix of vehicles on roads, because motorcyclists are vulnerable in crashes with larger vehicles. Motorcycle involvement in crashes varies globally in proportion to the number of motorcycles on the road. In high-income countries, motorcyclists crash fatally with other vehicles about 50% of the time. One aspect behind this frequency is likely to be the limited visibility or lack of awareness of motorcyclists by larger vehicle operators. An age relationship to fatal motorcycle crashes exists, with younger riders at a heightened risk. However, several recent reports also note a high frequency of fatalities in riders above 40 years of age and some link among these riders to higher engine size cycles. In developed countries, most fatalities also involve males and riders operating under the influence of alcohol.

Pedestrians

Pedestrians are the most vulnerable of all road users. A pedestrian is a person on the road who is not in or on a vehicle (motorized or nonmotorized). Injuries to pedestrians occur primarily from mishaps with other motorized vehicles on the road. The World Health Organization data indicate that pedestrians account for a large proportion of road traffic deaths in low- and middle-income countries, particularly in East and South Asia, and at much higher frequencies than found in high-income countries. Older individuals (above 70 years of age) have the highest rates of pedestrian injury of any age group. About one third of pedestrians involved in fatal events are impaired with alcohol.

Prevention Strategies

The high frequency of road traffic injury has drawn a great deal of attention with respect to preventive interventions. Prevention has been a part of the highway safety discipline for several decades now, and success in reducing motor vehicle fatalities has been recognized as one of the top 10 public health achievements in the 20th century. Unique strategies have been employed to reduce the burden of vehicle-related injury. Most center on passive approaches to design safer vehicles and legislation of safety through traffic codes and laws. A few approaches target high-risk individuals and their behavior in an active attempt to change behavior that is detrimental to transportation safety.

Seat Belts and Car Seats

Seat belts are one of the most effective means to reduce motor vehicle injury and are currently estimated to save more lives than any other preventive strategy. The reports find that three-point safety belts (a lap and shoulder belt attached to the vehicle at the hip) reduce the risk of death in front seat occupants of passenger vehicles by 45% to 61% compared with unrestrained individuals. The largest benefit of seat belts appears for frontal impact, rollover, and rear impact crashes. A seat belt, though, is only effective if it is worn. Large differences exist in the use of restraints around the world, with young male drivers in most locations being the least likely group to wear seat belts. The majority of individuals involved in fatal crashes are also not wearing restraints. Current efforts are underway to increase occupant restraint use. Legislation or laws to require the use of seat belts by occupants in motor vehicles represent the most widely applied approach at this time. Studies indicate that primary seat belt laws (where an individual can

be cited by the police simply for not wearing a belt) are more effective in increasing restraint use compared with secondary seat belt laws (where an individual can only be cited for not wearing a belt if they have committed another traffic offense) or no law.

Additional efforts are underway to increase the use of child safety seats, although these efforts are largely focused in high-income countries. Child seats for infants and toddlers can reduce fatality risk by 71% and 54%, respectively. In some areas, booster seats for young children are also required. Booster seats work by placing the child higher in the seat and in a position where the seat belt in the vehicle can be properly deployed. Laws mandating child restraints have been shown to be effective in increasing their use.

Air Bags

Air bags are another safety feature that are a part of most new vehicles today. Air bags work by placing a barrier between the vehicle occupant and the vehicle. The barrier helps dissipate the energy transfer involved in the crash and thereby reduces injury frequency. Over the past 20 years, an estimated 20,000 lives have been saved by air bags in the United States. Air bags combined with three-point seat belts offer the best protection to vehicle occupants. Air bags, though, carry an injury risk of children seated in child safety seats, and children in these seats should not be placed in front seats with air bags. Deployment of the air bag with a rear facing safety seat has led to injury to the child.

Graduated Driver's License

A recent prevention measure focused on young drivers is the graduated driver's license (GDL). A GDL has the intended purpose of controlling the exposure of young drivers to difficult driving situations and increasing the experience level of drivers. There is no standard GDL program, but common features include a permit stage where teenage drivers must be accompanied by an adult for the purpose of getting practice in the driving process. This is usually followed by a provisional license stage, where the driver cannot operate a vehicle late at night and there are restrictions on the number of teenage passengers that can be in the vehicle. A large study has recently found that the most restrictive GDL programs are associated with a 38% reduction in fatal crashes and a 40% reduction in injury crashes. Any type of program also was beneficial, with 11% and 19% reductions in fatal and injury crashes, respectively.

Helmets

Helmets for motorcycle and pedal cycle users are another effective injury prevention measure. Helmets are worn on the head to protect the individual from serious head injury. They are estimated to prevent fatal injuries to motorcyclists by 37%. Helmets, though, are only effective if they are worn. Helmet use rates, unfortunately, are low in many parts of the world. Factors cited in the low use of helmets include few or no laws requiring helmet use and limited enforcement efforts for existing laws. Areas with a law requiring helmet use have markedly higher rate of use than areas without such laws. Recently, arguments have also been against helmet laws with claims that helmet laws hinder civil rights or that helmets hinder hearing or are too hot for some climates.

Law Enforcement

Law enforcement is an important discipline in highway safety. Strenuous and high visibility enforcement of existing traffic safety laws increases compliance and saves lives. Common programs of law enforcement in highway safety focus on efforts to reduce speeding and driving under the influence of alcohol and increase the use of seat belts and helmets.

Conclusion

Our knowledge of vehicle-related injuries and the factors underlying them has expanded tremendously over the past 50 years. Today, it is possible to predict the frequency of crash and injury with precision and, as such, it is possible to view the majority of crashes as largely preventable. Reductions in most high-income countries in motor vehicle fatalities and injuries have been brought about through a multidisciplinary approach to safety. Engineering, law enforcement, public health, medical, and planning strategies can work to significantly reduce injury. Low- and middle-income countries, though, continue to face a large burden related to motor vehicle injuries. This burden is expected to increase over the next 20 years. Strategies exist to lower the burden of injury from motor vehicles in all parts of the world. The implementation of these strategies, raising awareness of the issue, and enforcing existing laws remain the

challenge ahead. These changes and changes in our cultural way of thinking regarding the acceptability of motor vehicle injury will be necessary to improve highway safety.

—*Thomas Songer*

See also Alcohol Use; Governmental Role in Public Health; Injury Epidemiology; Prevention: Primary, Secondary, and Tertiary

Further Readings

Baker, S. P., Chen, L. H., & Li, G. (2007). *Nationwide review of graduated driver licensing.* Washington, DC: AAA Foundation for Traffic Safety. Retrieved April 9, 2007, from http://www.aaafoundation.org/pdf/NationwideReviewOfGDL.pdf.

National Center for Statistics and Analysis. (2006). *Motorcycles, traffic safety facts, 2005 data* (DOT Publication No. DOT-HS-810–620). Washington, DC: National Highway Traffic Safety Administration. Retrieved July 26, 2007, from http://www-nrd.nhtsa.dot.gov/pdf/nrd-30/NCSA/TSF2005/2005TSF/810_620/810620.htm.

Neale, V. L., Dingus, T. A., Klauer, S. G., Sudweeks, J., & Goodman, M. (2005). *An overview of the 100-car naturalistic study and findings* (Paper No. 05–0400). Washington, DC: National Highway Traffic Safety Administration. Retrieved April 9, 2007, from http://www-nrd.nhtsa.dot.gov/pdf/nrd-12/100Car_ESV05summary.pdf.

Peden, M., Scurfield, R., Sleet, D., Mohan, D., Hyder, A. A., Jarawan, E., et al. (Eds.). (2004). World report on road traffic injury prevention. Geneva, Switzerland: World Health Organization.

Traffic Safety Facts 2005. (2005). Various reports on high risk groups and prevention strategies. Washington, DC: National Highway Traffic Safety Administration. Retrieved July 26, 2007, from http://www-nrd.nhtsa.dot.gov/pdf/nrd-30/NCSA/TSFAnn/TSF2005.pdf.

VETERINARY EPIDEMIOLOGY

Veterinary epidemiology is a specialized area within veterinary medicine that was historically termed epizootiology until the mid-1990s. Like human epidemiology, it involves identifying risk factors for diseases, characterizing outbreaks, quantifying incidence and prevalence, describing the natural history of disease, developing disease control and prevention programs, and assessing the effectiveness of these programs. Veterinary epidemiologists participate in these activities in both human and animal populations when disease agents are zoonotic (infectious and capable of spreading between animals and people), although the potential impacts of environmental agents (such as pesticides) on animal and human health and the challenges of cancer and of chronic diseases are also topics for investigation. Veterinarians are trained in medicines of all species, including primates, and so are often involved in identifying disease risks to humans after being alerted to health issues in animals. This can be used in health surveillance, with animals acting as sentinels of human health concerns. One classic example was the use of canaries to detect toxic gases in coal mines.

The concept of "one medicine" was described and expanded by visionary veterinary epidemiologist Calvin Schwabe in the 1980s and refers to the common basis of veterinary and human medical knowledge that can be applied to diseases affecting all species. The value of veterinarians and veterinary epidemiologists in active participation in global health research activities has been recognized fairly recently. As in human epidemiology, a primary goal of veterinary epidemiology is prevention of disease rather than treatment.

From ancient times, it has been important to identify patterns of disease in herds and groups of animals used for human consumption (milk, meat, fiber, and eggs) and activities (transportation and farming), and veterinary medicine had its foundations in the treatment of large animal diseases that have financial and survival consequences. As urban centers increased and smaller animals joined human households as companions, veterinarians have expanded their services to include cats, dogs, mice, rats, ferrets, rabbits, birds, and other creatures small enough to coexist in these smaller spaces. Because veterinarians have been trained to identify and treat diseases in groups or herds, they are well suited for and often "automatically" engaged in epidemiology and, by extension, public health. While veterinary epidemiology has focused on herd health, that is, on disease patterns in large groups of cattle and other farmed animals, the same principles of recognition and control of infectious diseases hold true in large groups of small animals, such as in catteries, breeding kennels, and animal shelters, as well as in veterinary hospitals, where nosocomial (hospital-based) infections are also of concern.

Veterinary epidemiology uses the same tools as human epidemiology, including observational studies, cross-sectional and longitudinal studies, case-control studies, prospective studies, and experimental and field trials of vaccines, diagnostic procedures, medicines, and treatment protocols. Case reports and case series are often reported by veterinarians engaged in clinical practice. Veterinary epidemiologic research often involves methodologic issues, such as sampling techniques for herds and wildlife populations, and appropriate statistical applications to analyze complex data sets such as capture/recapture data. In survey-based studies, veterinary epidemiologists rely nearly exclusively on proxy respondents, such as owners or farmers, for observations and accurate histories of the animals in their care. Observational studies of animal diseases often depend on recruitment of producers (farmers) and owners of small animals contacted through advertisements in publications of trade associations and breed clubs, or through veterinarians to their clients. An area of considerable study is the determination of test characteristics (sensitivity and specificity) for rapid, portable diagnostics used to screen animal populations for common diseases for which "gold standard" testing is too expensive to be used on individual animals. Geographical information system software has been employed to track distributions of herds or disease vectors, the appearance of new disease cases over time (such as of avian influenza), and changes in vegetation (food and shelter habitat for desirable and parasite species) due to weather patterns. Modeling of disease reservoirs and agent transmission has been used to predict outbreaks; other models have been used to show how population sizes may change through implementation of oral contraceptive baiting schemes. As in human epidemiology, a concern in disease reporting is correct identification of denominators, which poses a greater challenge than in human epidemiology because no systematic census exists for wildlife or companion animals.

Financial resources are considerably less for research in veterinary epidemiology compared with epidemiologic studies of humans, especially for the study of small animal diseases, because there has not been the same investment in animal health infrastructure as there is in human medicine. As a consequence, few veterinary epidemiologists have been able to study risk factors for commonly diagnosed animal diseases, particularly of small animals. However, some of these diseases share similarities with human diseases, and thus, these small animals may provide insight into human health. Examples are prostate cancer and feline immunodeficiency virus infection. Dogs can spontaneously develop prostate cancer and are therefore a model for understanding this common human health problem. Cows, monkeys, and cats have species-specific retroviruses that result in immunodeficiency. The feline immunodeficiency virus is a model for the human immunodeficiency virus, and cats have been studied in an effort to develop vaccines effective in stopping the spread of this worldwide human health problem. A very common disease of older cats is hyperthyroidism, which is similar to one form of human hyperthyroidism. In this case, the human disease has served as a model for the identification of risk factors for disease in cats.

Data Sources for Veterinary Epidemiologic Research

While epidemiologic studies of humans have numerous sources of data for investigation and quantifying disease impacts in the human population, including cancer registries, vital statistics records, occupational registries, and hospital records, similar data sources either do not exist or are not readily available for veterinary epidemiologic research. Internationally, the Office International des Epizooties (OIE), also called the World Organization for Animal Health, maintains reports of notifiable diseases that cross species (including zoonotic diseases), such as anthrax, and species-specific diseases, such as African swine fever. A subset of the OIE-listed "multiple species diseases" are on the Centers for Disease Control and Prevention (CDC) Category A or Category B lists of bioterrorism agents or diseases. Because numerous pathogens on these CDC lists are zoonotic, including anthrax and plague, veterinarians work with public health agencies to prepare for and respond to disease outbreaks that affect several species. The Food and Agriculture Organization of the United Nations has been engaged in numerous programs to control livestock diseases, to protect food safety, and to reduce poverty in developing countries, and by extension, all countries.

Veterinary epidemiologists have been somewhat limited in the availability of active surveillance tools for the study of diseases beyond those of consequence to large animal production (diseases that affect meat, milk, and egg production as well as reproduction,

food safety issues, including bacterial diseases such as *Salmonella* spp. and *Listeria* spp., and patterns of antibiotic resistance). The U.S. Department of Agriculture (USDA), Animal and Plant Health Inspection Service (APHIS), and Centers for Epidemiology and Animal Health (CEAH) provide information about animal health issues, emerging diseases, and market conditions, and coordinate animal disease information for international agencies, including the OIE. Within CEAH, the National Center for Animal Health Surveillance includes programs to conduct studies of animal health, and to monitor, integrate, and analyze large animal health data from state and federal agencies to safeguard the food supply and to communicate disease status to agribusiness industries and backyard farmers.

One database tool for veterinary epidemiologists outside government agencies is the Veterinary Medical Database (VMDB), established in 1964 through a grant from the National Cancer Institute. The VMDB receives veterinary medical records for cows, horses, sheep, goats, pigs, birds, dogs, and cats from participating veterinary school hospitals in the United States and Canada. Not all veterinary schools have provided records continuously to the VMDB since its creation, and limitations include the potential for wide disparity in reporting of diagnoses, because standards for animal disease reporting are relatively recent. In spite of limitations, the VMDB has until recently provided the only generally available database of animal diseases, particularly of small animals.

In 2002, the National Companion Animal Surveillance System at Purdue University was established for near-real time syndromic surveillance of signs and symptoms of disease in small animals that could provide alerts of potential outbreaks of zoonotic disease of suspicious origin. This system analyzes records of a nationwide chain of small animal veterinary clinics that are uploaded daily to centralized hubs to evaluate practice methods. The database has been used to identify geographic patterns in the distribution of serovars (strains) of *Leptospira* spp. infections in dogs and potentially in humans (since this is a zoonotic disease) and to examine patterns of vaccine reactions in dogs. These and future studies will benefit from the large number of records made possible by this nationwide primary veterinary care reporting to find patterns in otherwise rare events. The VMDB has also been used in this way, but depends on records from the few veterinary school hospitals (third-tier referrals), and with time lapses and potentially inconsistent reporting, many more common or rare diseases may not be identified or reported for study.

Training and Employment as a Veterinary Epidemiologist

Most veterinarians engaged in epidemiology have obtained advanced training beyond veterinary school in specialized graduate programs, either at veterinary schools or schools of public health. Program participants are often international, and the focus of research is generally on large animal diseases of economic consequence, such as bluetongue (a vector-borne viral disease of sheep, goats, cattle, and other species), foot-and-mouth disease (a viral disease impacting milk production in cattle, sheep, goats, and pigs), and Newcastle disease (a viral disease in chickens and other bird species). Research results include descriptions of geographic ranges of vectors of disease agents (such as flies, mosquitoes, fleas, and ticks), weather-related disease risks, and management and demographic risk factors.

Veterinary epidemiologists work in government agencies (county, state, national, and international), including the CDC and its Epidemic Intelligence Service, the USDA's Food Safety and Inspection Service and APHIS, and the Center for Veterinary Medicine within the Food and Drug Administration of the U.S. Department of Health and Human Services, in academia at veterinary and medical schools and at schools of public health, and in private industry and consulting. Veterinary epidemiologists at the CDC have studied waterborne disease outbreaks as well as injuries from second-hand smoking. Veterinarians in state government have been instrumental in identifying and tracing the sources of monkeypox in Indiana and the Midwest and rabies in California. Veterinarians with epidemiologic training make up a small cadre within the uniformed Public Health Service.

While many veterinary epidemiologists concentrate on large animal disease recognition and prevention, some veterinary epidemiologists have focused on small animal issues, including diseases of dogs such as bladder cancer, prostate cancer, and breed-specific diseases, and of cats such as hyperthyroidism and *Bartonella* spp. (the zoonotic agents responsible for cat scratch disease), as well as upper respiratory diseases of cats and dogs in animal shelters and their

prevention with vaccines. Others have looked at the interface between human society and animals: hoarding of companion animals, injuries to owners of companion animals as well as the social and exercise benefits of dog ownership, reasons for shelter relinquishment of dogs and cats, infectious disease prevalence among feral cats, and risk factors for human failures to evacuate in disasters such as fires or floods. Veterinary epidemiologists also work at the interface between wildlife, domestic animal, and human populations to study disease transmission patterns and potential zoonotic risks. Examples include chronic wasting disease in wild and potentially farmed deer and elk (a disease similar to bovine spongiform encephalopathy (mad cow disease), severe acute respiratory syndrome in humans and wildlife sold in markets, raccoon roundworms and larval migrans disease, rabies in bats and companion animals, tuberculosis in cattle and humans, and avian influenza in migratory and farmed bird populations.

Organizations of veterinary epidemiologists include the Association for Veterinary Epidemiology and Preventive Medicine (formerly the Association of Teachers of Veterinary Public Health and Preventive Medicine), the International Symposium for Veterinary Epidemiology and Economics, the Canadian Association of Veterinary Epidemiology and Preventive Medicine, and the European-based Society for Veterinary Epidemiology and Preventive Medicine. Other groups include the National Association of State Public Health Veterinarians and the Veterinary Public Health special interest group within the American Public Health Association. Board certification in veterinary preventive medicine is available through the American College of Veterinary Preventive Medicine, with an additional subspecialization available in Epidemiology, and may be valuable for veterinarians in government agencies or large human medical institutions.

—Charlotte H. Edinboro

See also Foodborne Diseases; Public Health Surveillance; Zoonotic Disease

Further Readings

Dohoo, I., Martin, W., & Stryhn, H. (2004). *Veterinary epidemiologic research*. Charlottetown, Prince Edward Island, Canada: AVC.

Hugh-Jones, M. E., Hubbert, W. T., & Hagstad, H. V. (2000). *Zooneses: Recognition, control, and prevention.* Ames: Iowa State University Press.

Martin, W. S., Meek, A. H., & Willeberg, P. (1987). *Veterinary epidemiology: Principles and methods.* Ames: Iowa State University Press.

Salman, M. D. (Ed.). (2003). *Animal disease surveillance and survey systems: Methods and applications.* Ames: Iowa State University Press.

Schwabe, C. W. (1984). *Veterinary medicine and human health* (3rd ed.). Baltimore: Williams & Wilkins.

Slater, M. R. (2002). *Veterinary epidemiology (practical veterinarian).* Oxford, UK: Butterworth-Heinemann.

Smith, R. D. (2005). *Veterinary clinical epidemiology* (3rd ed.). Boca Raton, FL: CRC Press.

Thursfield, M. (2005). *Veterinary epidemiology* (3rd ed.). Oxford, UK: Blackwell Science.

VIOLENCE AS A PUBLIC HEALTH ISSUE

In 1996, the 49th World Health Assembly declared violence to be a leading worldwide public health problem. The World Health Organization (WHO) defines violence as

> the intentional use of physical force or power, threatened or actual, against oneself, another person, or against a group or community, that either results in or has a high likelihood of resulting in injury, death, psychological harm, maldevelopment or deprivation. (WHO, 2002, p. 5)

This entry describes the types of violence, its consequences, and its prevalence worldwide. It also examines characteristics of interpersonal violence as experienced by women, the elderly, and children and adolescents. Although violence as a criminal act remains primarily within the purview of judicial system, public health interventions can reduce the incidence of violence and its impact. A scientific approach to understanding the underlying causes of violence and risk factors is necessary to devise effective prevention programs and protecting health. Such an understanding can provide a basis for public health interventions that can reduce the incidence of violence and its impact.

Types of Violence

Violent acts include physical attacks, sexual abuse, psychological threat, and deprivation or neglect. Violence is categorized into three broad categories according to characteristics of the perpetrators: self-directed violence, interpersonal violence, and collective violence. Suicidal behavior and self-abuse are self-directed violence. Intimate partner violence, child abuse within a family, and violence between unrelated individuals are examples of interpersonal violence. Collective violence refers to that committed by larger groups of individuals (terrorist activities, insurgency, gang and mob violence) or by states (war).

Consequences of Violence

There are serious consequences of violence for individuals, families, communities, health care systems, and countries. Globally, violence is a major cause of death for people aged 15 to 44 years, and the economic and social costs of violence are substantial. More than 1.6 million people worldwide died as a result of self-inflicted, interpersonal, or collective violence in 2000, for an overall age-adjusted rate of 28.8 per 100,000 population. Nearly, half of these 1.6 million violence-related deaths were suicides, almost one third were homicides, and about one fifth were war-related. Among low- and middle-income countries, self-inflicted injuries and violence accounted for 8.9% of deaths. Suicide was the third leading cause of death for women in the age group 15 to 44 years.

Interpersonal Violence

Women, children, and elderly people are the major victims of interpersonal violence.

Violence Toward Women

Physical abuse by an intimate partner is the most common form of violence that women experience. It is estimated that between 10% and 52% of women experience some form of violence at the hands of their husband or male partner. Intimate partner violence, often referred to as domestic violence, includes the range of sexually, psychologically, and physically coercive acts used against adult and adolescent women by current or former male intimate partners without their consent.

A WHO multicountry study conducted in 2001 found that the lifetime prevalence of physical or sexual domestic violence varied widely, from 6% to as high as 71% across the countries studied. There is growing recognition of the pronounced burden that violence against women exacts on their reproductive and overall health. Using a disability-adjusted life years approach, a World Bank study estimated that physical and sexual violence jointly account for 5% to 16% of healthy years of life lost by women of reproductive age in developing countries, ranking with obstructed labor, HIV, and cancer as causes of disability among women. Abused women are more likely to report gynecological morbidity, sexual problems, pelvic inflammatory disease, HIV, STD, urinary tract infections, and substance abuse. Studies found strong association between domestic violence and depressive disorders.

A substantial proportion of women experiencing physical violence also experience sexual abuse. In Mexico and the United States, studies estimate that 40% to 52% of women experiencing physical violence by an intimate partner have also been sexually coerced by that partner. Both physical and sexual domestic violence have been shown to be significantly associated with an increased risk of unintended pregnancy, short interpregnancy intervals, and lower contraceptive use, including condom use.

Effects of Violence During Pregnancy

Studies have shown that domestic violence does not abate during pregnancy and may possibly even be aggravated during this period. Violence is a major cause of death for pregnant and postpartum women in the United States, but still remains underreported. The percentage of women reporting domestic violence at the hands of their husband or intimate partner during pregnancy has varied between 0.9% and 20.1% in different studies. Deleterious maternal health correlates of abuse during pregnancy include depression, premature labor, injury, kidney infections, and antepartum hemorrhage. Homicide by partners, the most extreme form of abuse during pregnancy, has been identified as an important cause of maternal mortality in several countries.

Violence during pregnancy not only adversely affects the health of women but also affects birth outcomes. The adverse consequences of violence during pregnancy on birth outcomes such as low birthweight and prematurity have been extensively studied. Research has also shown that violence during pregnancy increases perinatal and infant mortality. The pathways through which domestic violence may lead to elevated risks of early childhood mortality are not fully understood. One possible pathway is through the direct effects of blunt physical trauma and resultant fetal death or subsequent adverse pregnancy outcome. A second potential pathway is through elevated maternal stress levels and poor nutrition, both associated with low birthweight or preterm delivery, well-known risk factors for adverse early childhood mortality outcomes. A third mechanism through which domestic violence may contribute to elevated risks of childhood mortality is through its deterrent effect on women's use of preventive or curative health services during pregnancy or delivery, or postnatally.

Risk Factors

Alcohol abuse is an important risk factor for interpersonal violence. Community-level cultural and contextual variables are also important determinants of intimate partner violence across cultures. Women's status, including personal autonomy, economic opportunity, political power, and the ability to participate in women's group activities, affects the risk of violence. Intergenerational exposure to domestic violence—witnessing family violence as a child—has shown to be one of the few consistent predictors with the risk of being a perpetrator (men) or victim (women) of domestic violence.

Elder Abuse

It is estimated that 4% to 6% of older people (above 65 years of age) experience violence, either at home or at institutional facilities (nursing homes, residential care, hospitals, and day care facilities). It is generally agreed that abuse of older people is either an act of direct abuse or of neglect and that it may be either intentional or unintentional. The abuse may be of a physical nature, it may be psychological (involving emotional or verbal aggression), or it may involve financial or other material maltreatment.

Children and Adolescents as Victims of Violence

Children are subjected to both physical and sexual abuse. The term battered child syndrome drew attention to the problems of physical abuse in young children in the late 1980s. In 1999, the WHO Consultation on Child Abuse Prevention defined violence to children as follows:

Child abuse or maltreatment constitutes all forms of physical and/or emotional ill-treatment, sexual abuse, neglect or negligent treatment or commercial or other exploitation, resulting in actual or potential harm to the child's health, survival, development or dignity in the context of a relationship of responsibility, trust or power. (WHO, 2002, p. 59)

According to the World Health Organization, there were an estimated 57,000 deaths attributed to homicide among children below 15 years of age in 2000. Global estimates of child homicide suggest that infants and very young children are at greatest risk, with rates for the 0- to 4-year-old age group more than double those of 5- to 14-year-olds. The highest homicide rates for children below 5 years of age are found in the WHO African Region—17.9 per 100,000 for boys and 12.7 per 100,000 for girls.

Often, children are neglected by the parents and caregiver. There are many forms of child neglect, including failure to seek appropriate health care, noncompliance with health care recommendations, and deprivation of food. Abandonment, inadequate parental supervision, exposure to poor living conditions and hygiene, and lack of schooling may also be forms of child neglect. Parent's negligence to the exposure of children to drugs and alcohol remains a major public health concern.

There are serious adverse health consequences for child abuse. Abused children not only experience severe form of physical injuries, but also develop reproductive health problems, psychological and behavioral problems, including alcohol and drug habits, risk taking, antisocial and suicidal behaviors. They are more likely to experience unwanted pregnancy, STDs, poor academic performance, and drop out from the school.

Homicide and nonfatal injuries are the major causes of premature deaths and disability among youths. In 2000, an estimated 199,000 youth homicides (9.2 per 100,000 population) occurred globally. In other words, an average of 565 children, adolescents, and young adults between 10 and 29 years of age die each day as a result of interpersonal violence. Among all the homicide cases, three fourths are male victims and youth violence is the underlying factor.

—*Saifuddin Ahmed*

See also Child Abuse; Intimate Partner Violence; War

Further Readings

Robertson, L. S. (1992). *Injury epidemiology.* New York: Oxford University Press.

Rosenberg, M. L., Butchart, A., Narasimhan, V., Waters, H., & Marshall, M. S. (2006). *Interpersonal violence.* In D. T. Jamison, J. G. Breman, A. R. Measham, G. Alleyne, M. Claeson, D. B. Evans, et al. (Eds.), *Disease control priorities in developing countries* (2nd ed., pp. 755–770). New York: Oxford University Press.

Winett, L. B. (1998). Constructing violence as a public health problem. *Public Health Reports, 113*(6), 498–507.

World Health Organization, WHO Consultation. (1996). *Violence against women.* Geneva, Switzerland: Author.

World Health Organization. (2001). *Putting women first: Ethical and safety recommendations for research on domestic violence against women.* Geneva, Switzerland: Author.

World Health Organization. (2002). *World report on violence and health.* Geneva, Switzerland: Author.

World Health Organization. (2002). *Guide to United Nations resources and activities for the prevention of interpersonal violence.* Geneva, Switzerland: Author.

VITAMIN DEFICIENCY DISEASES

Vitamins are required in the diet for human consumption. Compounds that are known collectively as vitamins are either insufficiently produced in the body or are not synthesized at all and yet are essential to normal body functions. In general, the concentrations of vitamins stored within the body vary. Some vitamins (such as A and B12) remain in the body in sufficient quantity such that a person may not develop a deficiency for months or years despite low dietary intake. However, other vitamin deficiencies may develop within a matter of weeks. Deficiencies of vitamins (and minerals) may be caused by, and may result in, a variety of diseases. This entry discusses the principal vitamin deficiencies and highlights important contributing factors and treatment regimens. Although the discussion of trace mineral deficiencies is beyond the scope of this entry, additional information and further readings on the topic are presented at the end of this section.

Water-Soluble Vitamins

These vitamins are soluble in water and generally cannot be stored within the body for an extended period of time. Vitamins that are naturally water soluble must be constantly replenished through diet intake; otherwise, a deficiency of one or more of these vitamins can result.

Thiamine (B1)

Thiamine converts to a coenzyme in its active form, catalyzing the conversion of amino acids and the metabolism of carbohydrates. Primary food sources of thiamine include pork, beans, and other legumes, nuts, beef, and whole grains. Deficiency is primarily a result of poor dietary intake; however, in developed countries, thiamine deficiency more often results from chronic illness (e.g., cancer) or alcoholism.

A person in the early stages of thiamine deficiency will show symptoms of irritability and poor food intake. The full manifestation of thiamine deficiency is known as beriberi, and is characterized by muscle weakness and wasting, an enlarged heart (cardiomyopathy), pain in the legs and hands (peripheral neuropathy), weakness of one or more eye muscles (opthalmoplegia) and possible swelling of the extremities (edema). If the deficiency arises as a result of chronic alcoholism, the person may also experience central nervous dysfunction that may include loss of balance and psychosis.

The diagnosis of thiamine deficiency is confirmed by functional enzymatic assay. Treatment consists of intravenous or oral thiamine supplementation.

Riboflavin (B2)

Riboflavin is essential as a contributing factor in carbohydrate, fat, and protein metabolism. The most important sources of this vitamin are dairy products and whole grains. Other foods containing riboflavin include broccoli, legumes, eggs, fish, and other meats. Deficiency usually results from lack of dietary intake, and those who follow particularly strict diets (e.g., vegetarians and vegans) are at particular risk if they do not ensure adequate intake of vegetable sources of riboflavin.

The clinical manifestations of riboflavin deficiency include red or purple coloration of the tongue, cracking of the skin around the corners of the mouth, and dandruff. Additional indications of deficiency may include anemia, irritability, or other personality changes.

The diagnosis of riboflavin deficiency can be confirmed with laboratory testing of the blood or urine. Lab diagnostic tools are commonly used, because the clinical symptoms are nonspecific and similar to other vitamin deficiencies. Riboflavin deficiency is treated with supplementation of riboflavin.

Niacin (B3)

This vitamin catalyzes DNA repair and calcium transport reactions. The most common sources of niacin include protein-rich foods: dairy, meat, eggs, and beans. Another food source includes enriched flour, and daily intake of niacin in the United States usually exceeds FDA recommended guidelines. Deficiency results from poor dietary intake and is typically found among people who subsist on corn-based diets (as in parts of China, India, and Africa). Similar to thiamine deficiency, niacin deficiency in developed countries often is seen in chronic alcoholics. Niacin deficiency also occurs in people with congenital malabsorption or a chronic disease such as carcinoid syndrome, where niacin is insufficiently produced from its amino acid derivative.

Deficiency of niacin results in the clinical disease known as pellagra. This constellation of symptoms is manifested by a characteristic rash, a bright red tongue, diarrhea, disorientation, and possible memory loss. Severe niacin deficiency can result in death. The factors that may contribute to a niacin deficiency include alcoholism, pyridoxine (vitamin B6) deficiency, or riboflavin deficiency.

Diagnosis of this deficiency is usually based on clinical assessment, and treatment consists of oral niacin supplements.

Pyridoxine (B6)

Vitamin B6 is an essential cofactor for amino acid metabolism. It is also involved in the metabolism of certain other vitamins, including niacin. This vitamin is available in all food groups, but it is found in highest concentration in meats, whole grains, nuts, and legumes. Deficiency is usually due to alcoholism or use of specific medications for treatment of a chronic condition. The medications that can cause B6 deficiency include isoniazid (used for treating tuberculosis), L-dopa (used for the treatment of Parkinson's disease), and penicillamine (for patients with rheumatoid arthritis or Wilson's disease). It is rare that a person is born with a congenital disorder that would require B6 supplementation, but examples of such conditions include sideroblastic anemia and cystathionine beta-synthase deficiency.

Vitamin B6 deficiency results in symptoms similar to those seen in other B vitamin deficiencies, in particular, skin changes such as dandruff and cracking of the skin. Additionally, severe deficiency can affect the nervous system, resulting in pain, seizures, and confusion. Anemia also may be associated with this vitamin deficiency.

Diagnosis of B6 deficiency is confirmed by measuring low levels of pyridoxal phosphate in the blood. Treatment consists of B6 supplementation.

Folate

Folate, also known as folic acid, is the coenzyme for metabolism of amino and nucleic acids and is essential in cell DNA synthesis. Folate is also involved in embryogenesis, and recent studies have shown that increased folate intake to be associated with a reduced risk of neural tube defects in the newborn. The primary sources of folate include raw vegetables and fruits. In addition, grain products sold in the United States are now enriched with folate. Deficiency commonly results from malnutrition but tends to manifest itself clinically only after several months of poor dietary intake. Those with folate deficiency are often severely undernourished and include persons suffering from chronic alcoholism, narcotic addiction, chronic hemolytic anemia, or intestinal malabsorption. Additionally, certain prescription drugs (sulfasalazine, pyrimethamine) can cause folate deficiency.

Clinical findings in folate deficiency include megaloblastic anemia (red blood cells are larger than normal), inflammation of the tongue, depression, diarrhea, and cracking at the edges of the mouth. In contrast to cobalamin deficiency, no neurological symptoms occur as a result of a deficiency in folate. Children born to women with folate deficiency have an increased risk of spinal cord malformations, including spina bifida.

Diagnosis of folate deficiency is based on the finding of sufficiently large blood cells (cell volume > 100 fl) on blood smear. Treatment usually consists of oral folic acid supplements. Women in their first 6 weeks of pregnancy, as well as women of child-bearing age, are recommended to supplement their diet with a multivitamin containing folate to reduce the risk of neural tube defects in the newborn.

Cobalamin (B12)

Vitamin B12, also known as cobalamin, catalyzes the reaction that forms methionine, which is a key factor in the metabolism of folate. Cobalamin can only be found in animal products: either meat or dairy foods. Deficiency is often the result of malabsorption due to chronic illness, such as pernicious anemia or disease of the small intestine. Deficiency can also be the result of poor dietary intake and can be seen in people taking certain prescription drugs or who are strict vegetarians.

Features of cobalamin deficiency include megaloblastic anemia (similar to folate deficiency), inflamed tongue, weight loss, and diarrhea. In addition, deficiency of cobalamin can eventually cause peripheral nerve degeneration resulting in numbness, pain, muscle weakness and imbalance. Some of these findings may be permanent if the deficiency is not treated immediately.

Diagnosis of cobalamin deficiency is based on characteristic red blood cell changes similar to those seen in folate deficiency. These laboratory findings are used in combination with clinical symptomatology. Cobalamin deficiency can also occur without the characteristic anemia and is quite common in elderly persons. Treatment of the deficiency includes cobalamin supplementation and treatment of the underlying disorder.

Vitamin C

Vitamin C, also known as ascorbic acid, functions as an antioxidant and facilitates several biochemical reactions, including iron absorption and norepinephrine synthesis. It also plays a role in maintaining connective tissue and is important in several enzyme systems, including the mixed-function oxidase system. Vitamin C is found in leafy vegetables, citrus fruits, and tomatoes. Deficiency usually results from poor dietary intake, although in developed countries, deficiency is usually seen in alcoholics and in those who consume less than 10 mg of vitamin C per day (the elderly or those with very low incomes).

The constellation of symptoms that result from vitamin C deficiency is known as scurvy. Symptoms include poor wound healing, bleeding gums, extensive bruising, and additional internal bleeding. Deficiency in children is often associated with reduced bone growth.

Diagnosis of vitamin C deficiency is based primarily on clinical assessment and is confirmed by low levels of white blood cells in the blood. Oral vitamin C supplementation is the usual treatment for deficiency.

Fat-Soluble Vitamins

These vitamins are soluble in lipids (fat) and are stored within the tissues of the body. Generally, once these vitamins are stored, they tend to remain in the body. However, if a person has too little fat intake, or they are unable to absorb fat adequately, those fat-soluble vitamins will also be poorly absorbed, leading to a vitamin deficiency.

Vitamin A

Vitamin A and its active metabolites are essential for normal vision, growth, and cell specialization. Food sources of vitamin A include fish, liver, brightly colored fruits, and green leafy vegetables. Children in particular are susceptible to deficiency, because sufficient levels of vitamin A are not supplied through either cow's or breast milk. The particular areas that have high levels of vitamin A deficiency include Southern Asia, South America, and parts of Africa. In developed nations, factors that contribute to deficiency include alcoholism, malnutrition, malabsorption syndromes, and infection. Additionally, patients taking mineral oil, neomycin, or cholestyramine are at risk of deficiency, because these medications interfere with vitamin A absorption.

Clinical manifestations of vitamin A deficiency include night blindness, impaired development, increased susceptibility to infection (as a result of immune dysfunction), and skin lesions. Children with vitamin A deficiency are at particular risk of death due to measles, diarrhea, and respiratory infection.

Diagnosis of vitamin A deficiency is confirmed with measurement of retinol levels in the blood. Treatment consists of vitamin A supplementation, and for those persons with night blindness, this can be given in the form of an intramuscular injection or in the form of oral supplements.

Vitamin D

Vitamin D is a combination of two active metabolites that act to maintain adequate levels of calcium and phosphorus in the blood. The principal sources of vitamin D are actually nondietary, as it can be produced within the skin during sun exposure. In response to ultraviolet radiation, precursor chemicals within the skin are cleaved into vitamin D. As a result, vitamin D is classified as a hormone rather than a vitamin. There are, however, dietary sources of vitamin D, including fish oil and fortified dairy and cereal products. Deficiency may be caused by a number of things: poor dietary intake, malabsorption, impaired production within the skin, the use of specific drugs (barbiturates, phenytoin, isoniazid, or rifampin), liver disease, kidney disease, or congenital disorders.

Vitamin D deficiency has several clinical manifestations. In young children, deficiency causes a characteristic retardation of bone growth known as rickets that results in lack of bone mineralization and is distinguished by bowed legs, scoliosis, and deformities of the chest wall. In developed countries, rickets due to vitamin D deficiency is quite rare, although rickets can occur as a result of several other diseases and disorders. In adults, deficiency of vitamin D is known as osteomalacia. This condition is often the result of poor dietary intake and is the result of impaired mineralization of bone. Small fractures in the scapula, pelvis, and femur are common in adults with this condition. In both children and adults, weakness of the upper arm and thigh muscles are characteristic.

Diagnosis of vitamin D deficiency can be done by assessing patient symptoms in combination with radiology and laboratory findings. Supplementation with vitamin D, in combination with calcium, is recommended to prevent vitamin D deficiency. Treatment of clinical deficiency varies based on the underlying disorder.

Vitamin E

Vitamin E is important as an antioxidant and also serves to regulate several enzyme pathways that inhibit blood clotting. This vitamin is actually a family of eight different vitamins; alpha-tocopherol is the most important type in humans. The important food sources of vitamin E include olive oil, sunflower and safflower oils, and wheat germ. Additional sources include meats, grains, nuts, leafy vegetables, and some fruits. Deficiency of vitamin E as a result of poor dietary intake does not exist; however, severe and prolonged malabsorption can result in deficiency. Additionally, those with cystic fibrosis or a congenital disorder are also susceptible to vitamin E deficiency.

This deficiency is characterized by a variety of signs and symptoms. Hemolytic anemia, muscle wasting, and retinal disease are some of the manifestations.

Severe deficiency can also cause degeneration of specific neural pathways, resulting in uncoordinated walking and loss of vibration and position sense in the lower limbs.

Diagnosis is based primarily on knowledge of the condition underlying the deficiency, since poor dietary intake does not cause deficiency. Treatment consists of oral supplementation with alpha-tocopherol.

Vitamin K

This vitamin is essential in the formation of blood clots. Primary food sources include green leafy vegetables, but vitamin K can also be found in meats and dairy products. Deficiency is often the result of an underlying disease; however, newborns are also susceptible because they lack fat stores at birth and receive only a minimal amount of vitamin K through breast milk. In adults, deficiency is seen in patients with poor fat absorption (i.e., diseases of the small intestine), liver disease, alcoholism, or using particular antibiotics.

Symptoms of deficiency are manifested by widespread bleeding. Severe deficiency can result in intracranial hemorrhage, intestinal bleeding, and poor wound healing.

Diagnosis of this vitamin deficiency is confirmed with an elevated prothrombin time, one of two laboratory tests that measure blood clot formation. For adults, treatment consists of oral vitamin K supplementation. Newborns are given an injection of vitamin K at birth as standard prophylaxis against deficiency.

—*Ashby Wolfe*

See also Alcohol Use; Birth Defects; Cancer; Child and Adolescent Health; Eating Disorders; Malnutrition, Measurement of; Pellagra

Further Readings

Babior, B. M., & Bunn, H. F. (2005). Megaloblastic anemias. In D. L. Kasper, E. Braunwald, A. S. Fauci, S. L. Hauser, D. L. Longo, & J. L. Jameson (Eds.), *Harrison's principles of internal medicine* (pp. 601–607). New York: McGraw-Hill.

Fairfield, K. M., & Fletcher, R. H. (2002). Vitamins for chronic disease prevention in adults: Scientific review. *Journal of the American Medical Association, 287*(23), 3116–3126.

Institute of Medicine. (1999). *Dietary reference intakes for calcium, phosphorous, magnesium, vitamin D and flouride.* Washington, DC: National Academies Press.

Institute of Medicine. (2000). *Dietary reference intakes for thiamin, riboflavin, niacin, vitamin B6, folate, vitamin B12, pantothenic acid, biotin and choline.* Washington, DC: National Academies Press.

Institute of Medicine. (2000). *Dietary reference intakes for vitamin C, vitamin E, selenium and carotenoids.* Washington, DC: National Academies Press.

Institute of Medicine. (2001). *Dietary reference intakes for vitamin A, vitamin K, arsenic, boron, chromium, copper, iodine, iron, manganese, molybdenum, nickel, silicon, vanadium and zinc.* Washington, DC: National Academies Press.

Office of Dietary Supplements, National Institutes of Health. (2005). *Vitamin and mineral supplement fact sheets.* Bethesda, MD: Author. Retrieved July 30, 2006, from http://ods.od.nih.gov/Health_Information/ Vitamin_and_Mineral_Supplement_Fact_sheets.aspx.

Russell, R. M. (2005). *Vitamin and trace mineral deficiency and excess.* In D. L. Kasper, E. Braunwald, A. S. Fauci, S. L. Hauser, D. L. Longo, & J. L. Jameson (Eds.), *Harrison's principles of internal medicine* (pp. 403–411). New York: McGraw-Hill.

VOLUNTEER EFFECT

The volunteer effect is a form of selection bias, sometimes referred to as self-selection or volunteer bias. This phenomenon is based on the idea that individuals who volunteer to participate in epidemiological studies are different in some way from the target population that they have originated from. The result of this effect is that the resulting measure between exposure and disease is distorted.

The selection of the study population is a critical part of any epidemiological study. One of the methods of selecting individuals is to recruit volunteer participants from the target population. However, the main risk in this method is that this subset of the population differs in some way from the general population. It has been suggested that individuals who volunteer to participate in epidemiological studies are often healthier than the general population, and it is their interest in health that motivates them to participate in such studies. As a result, healthier individuals who may be more knowledgeable about health in general will be overrepresented in the study population. A consequence of this is that the measure of effect could be distorted, and the results cannot be generalized to the larger population. An example of this was seen in the Iowa Women's Health Study that investigated the relationship between mortality and cancer in women. When participants and nonparticipants were compared, it was found that there was a higher proportion of smokers in the nonparticipant group. This group also had a greater occurrence of smoking-related cancers. A similar situation is seen in studies examining treatment interventions and alcoholism. Often, individuals who volunteer for these studies have a different baseline level of alcoholism severity than those who do not volunteer.

Participants who volunteer may not actually be healthier than the target population, but it could be that they are interested in a study because they have a family history of the disease in question and are actually more at risk of the disease than the general population. This is another form of the volunteer effect. For example, a study investigating a potential intervention on the subsequent development of breast cancer that recruits women may actually find little effect simply because the volunteer participants are at a higher risk of developing breast cancer anyway.

Individuals who volunteer to participate in studies may also differ from the general population by education, gender, socioeconomic status, and other demographic characteristics. The result of this is that it can limit the generalizability of results to the general population. In situations where the possibility of volunteer bias is a concern, random sampling methods can be used to recruit study participants and therefore minimize the volunteer effect.

—*Kate Bassil*

See also Bias; Participation Rate; Sampling Techniques; Target Population; Validity

Further Readings

Rychtarik, R. G., McGillicuddy, N. B., Connors, G. J., & Whitney, R. B. (1998). Participant selection biases in randomized clinical trial of alcoholism treatment settings and intensities. *Alcoholism: Clinical and Experimental Research, 22*(5), 969–973.

Stohmetz, D. B., Alterman, A. I., & Walter, D. (1990). Subject selection bias in alcoholics volunteering for a treatment study. *Alcoholism: Clinical and Experimental Research, 14*(5), 736–738.

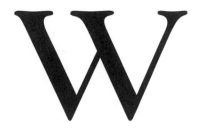

WAR

War is generally defined as armed conflict conducted by nation-states. The term is also used to denote armed action by a group within a nation against governmental or occupying forces; such armed actions are often termed *civil wars*, *wars of liberation*, or *revolutionary wars*. This entry examines the physical and psychological impact of war, terrorism, and other forms of armed violence, and the role that epidemiology can play in understanding and preventing violence.

War accounts for more death and disability than many major diseases. War destroys families, communities, and sometimes entire nations and cultures. War siphons limited resources away from health and other human services and damages the infrastructure that supports health. War violates human rights. The mindset of war—that violence is the best way to resolve conflicts—contributes to domestic violence, street crime, and other kinds of violence. War damages the environment.

An estimated 191 million people died during wars in the 20th century, more than half of whom were civilians. The exact figures are unknowable because of poor recordkeeping during wartime. Over the course of the 20th century, an increasing percentage of people killed in war were civilians; in some wars in the 1990s, possibly 90% of the people killed were noncombatant civilians. Most of them were caught in the crossfire of opposing armies or were members of civilian populations specifically targeted during war.

During most years of the past decade, there were approximately 20 wars, mainly civil wars that were infrequently reported by the news media in the United States. For example, more than 3.8 million people died in the civil war in the Democratic Republic of Congo during the past several years. As another example, more than 30 years of civil war in Ethiopia led to the deaths of 1 million people, about half of whom were civilians.

Several of these civil wars have been considered to be genocidal. In the Iraq War, which began in 2003, more than 2,500 U.S., British, and other Coalition troops had been killed as of March 2006, and more than 16,000 were wounded. An unknown number of Iraqi civilians have died as a result of the war; estimates range to more than 650,000, based on a cluster sample survey of Iraqi households that was performed in September 2006.

Many people survive wars only to be physically scarred for life. Millions of survivors are chronically disabled from injuries sustained during wars or the immediate aftermath of wars. Landmines are a particular threat; in Cambodia, for example, approximately 1 in 250 people is an amputee as a result of a landmine explosion. Approximately one third of the soldiers who survived the civil war in Ethiopia were injured or disabled; at least 40,000 had lost one or more limbs.

Millions more are psychologically impaired from wars, during which they have been physically or sexually assaulted, have been forced to serve as soldiers against their will, witnessed the death of family members, or experienced the destruction of their communities or entire nations. Psychological trauma may be demonstrated in disturbed and antisocial behavior, such as aggression toward others, including family members. Many military personnel suffer from post-traumatic stress disorder (PTSD) after military service.

Rape has been used as a weapon in many wars. In acts of humiliation and revenge, soldiers have raped female family members of their enemies. For example, at least 10,000 women were raped by military personnel during the war in the 1990s in Bosnia and Herzegovina. The social chaos brought about by war also creates conditions permitting sexual violence.

Children are particularly vulnerable during and after wars. Many die as a result of malnutrition, disease, or military attacks. Many are physically or psychologically injured. Many are forced to become soldiers or sexual slaves to military personnel. Their health suffers in many other ways as well, as reflected by increased infant and young-child mortality rates and decreased rates of immunization coverage.

The infrastructure that supports social well-being and health is destroyed during many wars, so that many civilians do not have access to adequate and safe food, water, medical care, and/or public health services. For example, during the Persian Gulf War in 1991 and the years of economic sanctions that followed, the United Nations Children's Fund (UNICEF) estimated that at least 350,000 more children than expected died, with most of these deaths due to inadequate nutrition, contaminated water, and shortages of medicines. Many of these deaths were indirectly related to destruction of the infrastructure of civilian society, including health care facilities, electricity-generating plants, food-supply systems, water-treatment and sanitation facilities, and transportation and communication systems. The Iraq War has further damaged this health-supporting infrastructure.

In addition, many civilians during wartime flee to other countries as refugees or become internally displaced persons within their own countries, where it may be difficult for them to maintain their health and safety. Refugees and internally displaced persons are vulnerable to malnutrition, infectious diseases, injuries, and criminal and military attacks. Many of the 35 million refugees and internally displaced persons in the world were forced to leave their homes because of war or the threat of war.

War and the preparation for war divert huge amounts of resources from health and human services and other productive societal endeavors. This is true for many countries, including the United States, which ranks first among nations in military expenditures and arms exports, but 38th in infant mortality rate and

45th in life expectancy. In some less developed countries, national governments annually spend $10 to $20 per capita annually on military expenditures, but only $1 per capita on all health-related expenditures. The same types of distorted priorities also exist in more developed, or industrialized, countries.

War often creates a cycle of violence, increasing domestic and community violence in the countries engaged in war. War teaches people that violence is an acceptable method for settling conflicts. Children growing up in environments in which violence is an established way of settling conflicts often choose violence to settle conflicts in their own lives. Teenage gangs mirror the activity of military forces. Returning military servicemen commit acts of violence against others, including their wives or girlfriends.

War and the preparation for war have profound impacts on the environment. Specific examples include the following:

- destruction of mangrove forests in Vietnam by the defoliant Agent Orange or by bombs, with the resultant bomb craters filling with stagnant water and becoming breeding sites for mosquitoes that spread malaria and other diseases;
- destruction of human environments by aerial carpet bombing of major cities in Europe and Japan during World War II; and
- ignition of more than 600 oil well fires in Kuwait by retreating Iraqi troops in 1991.

Less obvious are other environmental impacts of war and the preparation for war, such as the huge amounts of nonrenewable fossil fuels used by the military before and during wars, and the environmental hazards of toxic and radioactive wastes, which can contaminate air, soil, and both surface water and groundwater.

In the early 21st century, new geopolitical, tactical, and technological issues concerning war are arising that have an impact on health and health services. These include use of new weapons, use of "suicide-bombers," use of drone (unmanned) aircraft and high-altitude bombers, and newly adopted United States policies on "preemptive" wars and on "usable" nuclear weapons. An example of the introduction of new weaponry has been the use of shell casings hardened with depleted uranium (DU), a toxic and radioactive material employed for its density and ability to ignite on impact. DU has been used by the United States in the Persian Gulf War, the wars in the Balkans and Afghanistan, and (also by the United Kingdom) in the Iraq War. An estimated 300 metric tons of DU remain in Iraq, Kuwait, and Saudi Arabia. Because of the lack of data on the number of troops and civilians exposed, the levels of exposure, and the short-term and long-term consequences, epidemiological studies of the health impact have been fragmented and inadequate.

Terrorism

Closely related to war are forms of armed violence, often termed *terrorism*, in which individuals or groups, often clandestine, use politically motivated violence or the threat of violence, especially against civilians, with the intent to instill fear. These individuals or groups may be seen as "resistance fighters" or "freedom fighters" by those who support their actions or as "terrorists" by those who oppose them. Nation-states generally refuse to consider as "terrorism" their own governmental military actions that target civilians with the intent to instill fear.

Although there is much discussion about the possibility of chemical, biological, radiological, and nuclear weapons being used in terrorist attacks, the vast majority of terrorist attacks have used conventional weapons, mainly explosives. Since the 9/11 attacks in the United States and the transmittal of anthrax bacteria through the U.S. mail shortly thereafter, the U.S. government has conducted what it terms a *war on terror*. This has led to the restriction of civil liberties of U.S. citizens and the arrest, detention without charges, and violation of the human rights of noncombatant citizens of other countries whom the U.S. government has suspected of being "terrorists" or having "terrorist" ties. The United States has given much attention and devoted many human and financial resources to terrorism preparedness since 2001, often at the cost of reducing attention and resources for major public health problems, such as tobacco, alcohol, and other forms of substance abuse; gun-related deaths and injuries; and HIV/AIDS, cardiovascular disease and cancer.

The Roles of Epidemiology

Epidemiology has an important role in documenting and understanding the adverse health effects of war, terrorism, and other forms of armed violence, and thereby helping to prevent these effects. Epidemiologic surveillance, research, and analysis can, for example, help document and describe the morbidity and mortality due to the direct and indirect effects of war. Epidemiology can also elucidate the adverse health effects of a variety of chemical, biological, physical, and psychosocial exposures that occur during war among both combatants and noncombatants. It can also help us better understand the long-term physical, psychological, and social consequences of war. Epidemiologists have responsibilities not only to perform this type of surveillance, research, and analysis but also to share their findings with the scientific community and the general public. The results of, and conclusions drawn from, epidemiologic surveillance and research on war, terrorism, and other forms of armed violence are useful for developing and implementing policies to prevent armed violence and its adverse health consequences and for better providing for needs of those adversely affected.

—Victor W. Sidel and Barry S. Levy

See also Bioterrorism; Firearms; Genocide; Immigrant and Refugee Health Issues; Post-Traumatic Stress Disorder; Violence

Further Readings

Austin, J. E., & Bruch, C. E. (Eds.). (2000). *The environmental consequences of war*. Cambridge, UK: Cambridge University Press.

Cukier, W., & Sidel, V. W. (2006). *The global gun epidemic: From Saturday night specials to AK-47s*. Portsmouth, NH: Praeger Security International.

Levy, B. S., & Sidel, V. W. (Eds.). (2008). *War and public health* (2nd ed.). New York: Oxford University Press.

Levy, B. S., & Sidel, V. W. (Eds.). (2003). *Terrorism and public health: A balanced approach to strengthening systems and protecting people*. New York: Oxford University Press.

Levy, B. S., & Sidel, V. W. (Eds.). (2006). *Social injustice and public health*. New York: Oxford University Press.

Power, S. A. (2002). *A problem from hell: America and the age of genocide*. New York: Basic Books.

Sidel, M. (2004). *More secure, less free? Antiterrorism policy and civil liberties after September 11*. Ann Arbor: University of Michigan Press.

Stockholm International Peace Research Institute. (2006). *SIPRI yearbook 2006: Armaments, disarmament and international security*. Oxford, UK: Oxford University Press.

Taipale, I., Makela, P. H., Juva, K., Taipale, V., Kolesnikov, S., Mutalik, R., et al. (Eds.). (2002). *War or health? A reader*. London: Zed Books.

WATERBORNE DISEASES

In the mid-1800s, physician John Snow recommended removal of the handle from a water pump in a London neighborhood, ending an outbreak of cholera that had killed more than 500 people in a 10-day period. In the past 150 years, much progress has been made in understanding and preventing the transmission of infectious waterborne diseases. Even so, waterborne pathogens continue to be transmitted to humans via recreational water contact and contaminated drinking water supplies throughout the world, resulting in morbidity and mortality that is preventable. Infections that result from contact with waterborne pathogens can result in either endemic or epidemic disease. Most waterborne diseases are endemic in a population—there is some baseline level of disease that occurs normally in a population. An epidemic is defined when cases occur in excess of the normal occurrence for that population.

The Centers for Disease Control and Prevention (CDC) estimates that each year infectious waterborne diseases account for approximately 2 billion episodes of diarrhea leading to an estimated 1 million deaths worldwide. Most of these diarrheal deaths occur among children in developing countries, but the elderly and immunocompromised populations are also at an increased risk for waterborne infections. Table 1 lists the primary agents of infectious waterborne disease worldwide. These bacteria, viruses, and protozoa typically cause gastrointestinal symptoms, although some may cause a variety of other health effects, including neurological disorders (e.g., primary amoebic meningoencephalitis caused by *Naegleria fowleri*) and respiratory illness (e.g., pneumonia caused by *Legionella* species.

The CDC reports biennial estimates of waterborne outbreaks attributed to bacteria, viruses, and protozoa in the United States. In 2001 and 2002, 31 drinking water outbreaks were reported in 19 states, resulting in 1,020 cases of illness. Sixty-five recreational water outbreaks were reported by 23 states, resulting in 2,536 cases of illness. The number of cases from recreational and drinking water outbreaks for selected pathogens is shown in Table 2. Endemic waterborne disease is more difficult to quantify, but the 1996 Amendments to the Safe Drinking Water Act mandated that the U.S. Environmental Protection Agency (EPA) and the CDC jointly develop a national estimate of waterborne disease occurrence in the United States. Preliminary estimates by the EPA indicate that of all cases of acute gastrointestinal illness occurring in the U.S. population served by community water systems, approximately 8.5% may be attributed to their drinking water ($\sim$ 16.4 million cases per year).

Waterborne Disease Surveillance Systems

Public health surveillance systems are critical for detection and control of waterborne diseases. In many developed countries, governmental systems are in place requiring laboratories, hospitals, and clinicians to report certain diseases to a central agency. In the United States,

Table 1   Primary Agents of Infectious Waterborne Diseases

Bacteria	Viruses	Protozoa
Campylobacter jejuni	Hepatitis A	Balantidium coli
Escherichia coli	Norwalk virus	Cryptosporidium species
Francisella tularensis	Rotavirus	Cyclospora cayetanensis
Legionella species		Entamoeba histolytica
Leptospira species		Giardia species
Mycobacterium species		Naegleria fowleri
Salmonella typhi		
Shigella species		
Vibrio cholerae		

Source: Heymann (2004).

Table 2   Two-Year Case Counts for Primary Agents Associated With Selected Infectious Waterborne Disease Outbreaks in the United States 2001–2002

	U.S. Reported Cases*	
Pathogen	Recreational Water	Drinking Water
Bacteria		
Campylobacter jejuni	–	25
Escherichia coli	78	2
Legionella species	68	80
Shigella species	78	–
Viruses		
Norwalk virus	146	727
Protozoa		
Cryptosporidium species	1474	10
Giardia species	2	18
Naegleria fowleri	8	2
Unknown	145	117

Sources: Blackburn et al. (2004) and Yoder et al. (2004).
* Does not include infectious waterborne outbreaks due to *Pseudomonas aeruginosa*, *Bacillus species*, *Staphylococcus species*, or Avian schistomsomes.

individual states require different "notifiable diseases" to be reported to public health officials, which are later compiled in the National Notifiable Diseases Surveillance System (NNDSS) by the CDC and the Council of State and Territorial Epidemiologists (CSTE). These notifiable diseases include a variety of bioterrorism-related conditions, as well as many potential waterborne diseases, such as cryptosporidiosis, giardiasis, and legionellosis. These types of data can provide some insight into endemic disease, but reporting requirements are not limited to waterborne infections. For example, giardiasis may be transmitted by contaminated water or food, or it may be sexually transmitted. The NNDSS is an example of a passive surveillance system since these data are voluntarily reported to the CDC by state, territorial, and local public health agencies.

In contrast to passive surveillance, active surveillance relies on solicitation of disease reports from laboratories, hospitals, and clinicians (e.g., the CDC's FoodNet Program). Active surveillance overcomes the problem of underreporting by health care providers and can be specifically tailored to identify secondary complications associated with infections. Syndromic surveillance is a specific type of surveillance that may be useful in detecting waterborne disease outbreaks. Syndromic surveillance involves the systematic gathering of population behavior and health data, such as antidiarrheal sales or emergency room visits, to identify anomalous trends. Syndromic surveillance may increase timely detection of outbreaks before laboratory or clinically confirmed diagnostic information is available, but empirical evidence of the efficacy of syndromic surveillance to mitigate the effects of waterborne disease outbreaks through earlier detection and response is lacking.

In the United States, epidemics may be identified through the Waterborne Diseases Outbreak Surveillance System (WBDOSS)—a database of drinking and recreational water outbreaks maintained by the CDC, the EPA and the CSTE. The ability of the WBDOSS to accurately capture the disease burden associated with waterborne outbreaks may be limited due to the difficulty of outbreak detection and inherent limitations of passive surveillance system data. These limitations include the following:

- Waterborne infectious disease often manifests as gastroenteritis or other self-limiting illnesses with mild symptoms; therefore, only a small proportion of cases may seek medical attention.
- Waterborne outbreaks that result in mild symptoms, have low attack rates, or are not caused by an easily identifiable etiologic agent may go unrecognized because the medical community never has an opportunity to make a formal diagnosis.
- The ability to detect waterborne outbreaks depends on the capacity of local public health agencies and laboratories to identify cases of illness and link these in a timely manner to a common source of exposure or to an etiologic agent.
- Water service system type, source water type, and size of the population served by the contaminated water system may affect the likelihood that an outbreak is attributed to a waterborne source.

Prevention of Waterborne Diseases

Drinking water sources are vulnerable to contamination from point and nonpoint sources. Point sources, such as improperly treated sewage discharged to a water source, can lead directly to infectious waterborne disease transmission. Nonpoint sources, such as agricultural or urban runoff, can introduce pathogens to surface waters or to groundwater under the influence of surface water.

Prevention of waterborne disease transmission in public drinking water systems can be accomplished in several ways, including (1) watershed management and protection of source waters, (2) use of treatment techniques intended to remove or inactivate pathogens prior to distribution, (3) presence of residual disinfectant and implementation of routine pipe flushing programs to prevent growth of disease-causing organisms in the water distribution system, and/or (4) implementation of measures to prevent cross-connections between wastewater and drinking water in the distribution system. Often, a combination of actions is employed to help ensure multiple barriers of protection of water supplies. If monitoring results suggest contamination of drinking water, actions can be taken to prevent waterborne spread. These include issuing of "boil water" advisories, implementing additional treatment, or ceasing use of the water source.

In recreational waters, disease transmission can be prevented by careful monitoring and sanitation practices. In public swimming pools and spas, practices that prevent transmission of disease include (1) maintenance and monitoring of disinfectant and pH levels, (2) policies to require showers prior to entering the pool or spa, and (3) measures to prevent accidental fecal release. Prevention of accidental fecal release is especially important at facilities that serve young children; measures such as implementation of bathroom breaks as part of the pool schedule and providing separate pools for young children are effective at reducing fecal-oral transmission. In the United States, states and local jurisdictions enforce environmental health laws governing sanitation practices for pools, spas, and other recreational waters. In marine and fresh recreational waters, eliminating potential sources of pathogens such as wastewater discharge near public beaches is an important step to help reduce recreational waterborne infections. Water monitoring and beach closure postings are also essential for reducing potential exposure to pathogens.

Routine monitoring is another effective measure employed to ensure that drinking and recreational water is safe to use. In the United States, regulations require monitoring for biological, chemical, and radiological parameters in public drinking water supplies. Routine monitoring for both drinking and recreational

waters usually includes tests for coliform bacteria, which are used to indicate the possibility of fecal contamination that could spread waterborne diseases. Additional monitoring and treatment requirements for more specific pathogens, such as *Cryptosporidium* and *Giardia*, are required for drinking waters with surface water sources in the United States. In recreational waters, monitoring for specific pathogens is expensive and may require specialized equipment not readily available, so indicator bacteria such as total coliform, *Escherichia coli*, and *Enterococci* are typically used as surrogates for the pathogenic organisms that might be present. One drawback to the use of indicators is that they may not always be well correlated with specific pathogen occurrence or risk of illnesses. An additional disadvantage of current pathogen testing methods (i.e., bacteria, viruses, and protozoa) is that these tests require 24 hr or more to generate results, so there is a lag in time between when exposure is potentially occurring and when any preventative actions may be initiated. These problems are likely to diminish as rapid testing methods and new indicators are developed and become more widely available.

—*June M. Weintraub and J. Michael Wright*

See also Centers for Disease Control and Prevention; Notifiable Disease; Outbreak Investigation; Public Health Surveillance; Snow, John

Further Readings

Berger, M., Shiau, R., & Weintraub, J. M. (2006). Review of syndromic surveillance: Implications for waterborne disease detection. *Journal of Epidemiology and Community Health, 60,* 543–550.

Blackburn, B. G., Craun, G. F., Yoder, J. S., Hill, V., Calderon, R. L., Chen, N., et al. (2004). Surveillance for waterborne-disease outbreaks associated with drinking water: United States, 2001–2002. *Morbidity and Mortality Weekly Report Surveillance Summaries, 53,* 23–45.

Centers for Disease Control and Prevention. (2006, June). 12 Steps for prevention of recreational water illnesses (RWIs). Retrieved August 11, 2006, from http://www.cdc.gov/healthyswimming/twelvesteps.htm.

Fewtrell, L., & Colford, J. M., Jr. (2005). Water, sanitation and hygiene in developing countries: Interventions and diarrhoea—a review. *Water Science and Technology, 52,* 133–142.

Gerba, C. P., Hunter, P. R., Jagals, P., & Peralta, G. L. (Eds.). (2006). Estimating disease risks associated with drinking water microbial exposures. *Journal of Water and*

Health, *4*(Suppl. 2), 1–2. Retrieved July 27, 2007, from http://www.epa.gov/nheerl/articles/2006/waterborne_disease.html.

Heymann, D. L. (Ed.). (2004). *Control of communicable diseases manual* (18th ed.). Washington, DC: American Public Health Association.

U.S. Environment Protection Agency. (1986). *Ambient water quality criteria for bacteria: 1986*. EPA440/5-84-002. Washington, DC: Office of Water Regulations and Standards Division.

Wade, T. J., Calderon, R. L., Sams, E., Beach, M., Brenner, K. P., Williams, A. H., et al. (2006). Rapidly measured indicators of recreational water quality are predictive of swimming-associated gastrointestinal illness. *Environmental Health Perspectives*, *114*, 24–28.

Wade, T. J., Pai, N., Eisenberg, J. N., & Colford, J. M., Jr. (2003). Do U.S. Environmental Protection Agency water quality guidelines for recreational waters prevent gastrointestinal illness? A systematic review and meta-analysis. *Environmental Health Perspectives*, *111*, 1102–1109.

Wheeler, J. G., Sethi, D., Cowden, J. M., Wall, P. G., Rodrigues, L. C., Tomkins, D. S., et al. (1999). Study of infectious intestinal disease in England: Rates in the community, presenting to general practice, and reported to national surveillance. *British Medical Journal*, *318*, 1046–1050.

Yoder, J. S., Blackburn, B. G., Craun, G. F., Hill, V., Levy, D. A., Chen, N., et al. (2004). Surveillance for waterborne-disease outbreaks associated with recreational water: United States, 2001–2002. *Morbidity and Mortality Weekly Report Surveillance Summaries*, *53*, 1–22.

WOMEN'S HEALTH ISSUES

Women constitute 51% of the U.S. and 50% of the world's population. The familiar paradox of women's health, that women live longer than men but have poorer health throughout their lives, continues to be true. In most developed countries, women live about 6.5 years longer than men, on average. Women's mortality advantage has been reduced somewhat in recent years, reflecting decreased heart disease and cancer death rates among men, but not women. Women's morbidity and mortality are influenced by a variety of conditions that preferentially affect them, as noted below.

Women's health is a broad topic that has gained recognition as a discipline. Multiple definitions have been proposed with more recent definitions focusing on the variety of factors that influence a woman's health during her life span. For example, the National Academy on Women's Health Medical Education defines women's health as devoted to facilitating the preservation of wellness and prevention of illness in women; it includes screening, diagnosis, and management of conditions that are unique to women, are more common in women, are more serious in women, or have manifestations, risk factors, or interventions that are different in women. As a discipline, women's health also recognizes (a) the importance of the study of gender differences; (b) multidisciplinary team approaches; (c) the values and knowledge of women and their own experience of health and illness; (d) the diversity of women's health needs over the life cycle and how these needs reflect differences in race, class, ethnicity, culture, sexual preference, and levels of education and access to medical care; and (e) the empowerment of women to be informed participants in their own health care.

One issue for women's health research, reporting, and interpretation is the conflation of the terms sex and gender. Sex is a biological phenomenon, whereas gender is a social construction resulting from culturally shaped norms and expectations for behavior. Biological differences may not be taken into account because they are regarded as a product of cultural influences; on the other hand, differences in the socialization of women are sometimes not taken into account in the exploration of sex differences. Thus, the conflation of sex and gender is problematic and may obscure questions such as whether women experience pain differently than men—a sex difference—or have been trained to seek care more frequently—a gender difference. Nonspecific use of the terms *sex* and *gender* has had an impact on the equitable treatment of women in biomedical research and clinical medicine and on how sex differences have been conceived, studied, and addressed in biomedicine.

Not long ago, women were routinely excluded from large-scale clinical trials. For instance, most trials for the prevention of heart disease studied middle-aged males and excluded women because of a complex and sometimes conflicting set of assumptions. On the one hand, women's hearts were assumed to be the same as men's; therefore, it was unnecessary to include both sexes in the trial. On the other hand, women were assumed to be sufficiently different from men (because of hormonal and reproductive factors, for instance) to justify their exclusion from trials. This paradoxical attitude toward sex difference in clinical trials persists today and highlights the complexities of addressing sex differences in health. Human subject guidelines, and the National Institutes of Health grant requirements, have mandated women's inclusion in clinical trials and research, yet the question remains as to how similarities and differences between men and women will be conceived, studied, and compared. The way research questions are posed will dictate the answers investigators obtain and will have implications for women's treatment and overall health. For instance, it is well recognized that woman are diagnosed with depression in greater numbers than are men. Is this difference a sex difference (Are women at higher risk of depression by virtue of being women?), a gendered difference (Are women more likely to seek care for depression than men?), or is it something else (Are doctors more likely to diagnose depression in women than in men?)? Precision of language and thought demands that we focus on the ways we measure and report differences between men and women and allows us to specify what these differences mean for biomedical research and ultimately for patients care.

In epidemiology, the subject of women's health is frequently organized by life course, by anatomical feature, or by chronic/infectious states. This entry incorporates and supplements these schemas by considering women's health issues by life stage, by anatomy, and by social origin, focusing primarily on the experience of women in the United States.

Women's Health Issues: By Life Stage

Adolescence and Menarche

Adolescence is a period of tremendous change in women's lives, resulting in physical and sexual maturation. The rate at which maturation occurs depends on ethnicity, nutritional status, and physical activity. According to the National Survey of Family Growth (1988), median age at menarche for American women in 1988 was 12.5 years. Health issues of greatest concern during adolescence include development through puberty; menarche, or first menstrual bleeding; menstrual disorders; premenstrual syndrome; and adolescent pregnancy.

Reproductive Years

Women's reproductive years span the time from puberty to menopause, usually characterized as from 15 to 44 years. Hormones are clearly connected with health during the reproductive years and fluctuate cyclically, except during pregnancy and lactation. During the reproductive period of a woman's life, the health issues of greatest concern include the following: sexual dysfunction; fecundability, or ability to conceive; contraception; abortion, both induced and spontaneous; pregnancy; labor and delivery; infertility; assisted reproductive technology; adverse birth outcomes, such as preterm birth, low birthweight, small for gestational age, and birth defects; myoma and leiomyomata (benign tumors of the uterine muscle, also known as uterine fibroids); abnormal uterine bleeding; pelvic pain; pelvic floor relaxation; and endometriosis (which results from endometrial cells growing outside the uterus).

Perimenopause, Menopause, and Postmenopause

The most frequently used definition of menopause comes from the World Health Organization and defines menopause as the permanent cessation of menstruation resulting from the loss of ovarian follicular activity. Perimenopause, or climacteric, includes the period prior to menopause when endocrinological, clinical, and biological changes associated with menopause are occurring. Postmenopause is defined as the period after menopause and begins 12 months after spontaneous amenorrhea. Health tends to decline as women age, so many of the health issues we identify as chronic health conditions become of concern during this period of life. Most of these will be considered in the following section on anatomy. One health decision directly associated with reproductive senescence is whether to take hormone replacement therapy (HRT). HRT has been implicated as both beneficial and harmful to the health and quality of life for menopausal and postmenopausal women. Definitive information from randomized controlled trials is forthcoming.

Elderly and Frail Elderly Years

Almost 60% of people above the age of 65 years in 1999 were women. Although older women face many risks related to chronic disease as they age, most are healthy well into their later years. In 1994, 75% of women aged between 65 and 74 rated their health as good to excellent. The presence of chronic conditions increases with age. Nearly half of women aged 75 or older reported activity limitations resulting from chronic conditions. Two nonchronic health conditions faced by women in older age are sensory impairment (age-related loss of vision, hearing, and chemical senses such as taste and smell) and Alzheimer's disease, which is a degenerative disease of the brain, associated with the development of abnormal tissues and protein deposits in the cerebral cortex and characterized by confusion, disorientation, memory failure, speech disturbances, and the progressive loss of mental capacity.

Women's Health Issues: By Anatomy

Another organizational schema for discussing women's health issues is by anatomical feature. Men and women share the bulk of their anatomy, but the extent to which these anatomical structures operate, age, and degenerate identically is unknown. Most of the conditions grouped by anatomy are chronic in nature and will subsequently be more prevalent in older ages than among younger women.

Bone and Musculoskeletal Disorders

Two bone/skeletal disorders of particular concern for women's health are osteoporosis and osteoarthritis. Osteoporosis is a disease of bone in which the bone mineral density (BMD) is reduced, bone micro-architecture is disrupted, and the noncollagenous proteins in bone is altered, resulting in increased propensity to fracture. Arthritis is a group of conditions where there is damage caused to the joints of the body; it is the leading cause of disability among women above the age of 65 years.

Cancer

In the United States, cancer is the second leading cause of death for both men and women. Although there are more than 40 forms of cancer, six sites accounted for more than 60% of all deaths due to cancer among American women: breast, lung, colorectal, cervical, uterine, and ovarian. Cancer rates have been relatively stable among white women but have increased among nonwhites. Endogenous hormones, such as estrogen, have been implicated in the growth and development of several of these cancers (breast, cervical, uterine, and ovarian).

Cardiovascular Disease (CVD)

CVD is the leading cause of death among women, including young women. Age-specific CVD death rates lag about 10 years behind those for men. Until 1990, there was little information on women and heart disease because women were excluded from almost all major CVD randomized trials. It is unclear what role women's hormones, including those taken via hormone replacement therapy, play in protecting women against CVD.

Digestive Diseases

Gastrointestinal disorders represent some of the most poorly understood conditions in the female body. Many share a constellation of symptoms that currently have little structural or biochemical explanation. Despite the lack of clear diagnostic and physiologic understanding, digestive diseases have significant impacts on women's health. Relevant gastrointestinal issues for women's health include irritable bowel syndrome, characterized by abdominal pain or discomfort associated with a change in bowel function; gallstone disease (the formation of stones in the gallbladder or bile ducts); peptic ulcer disease, which refers to a discrete mucosal defect in the portions of the gastrointestinal tract exposed to acid and pepsin secretion; dyspepsia or stomach pain; aerophagia (swallowing too much air and the resultant belching), rumination (regurgitation of previously consumed food); functional constipation; functional diarrhea; and functional abdominal pain.

Immunity and Autoimmune Diseases

Diseases of the immune system demonstrate sex differences in incidence, natural history, and disease severity. These differences are illustrated in the cytokines measured, the degree of immune responsiveness, and the presence of sex hormones. Furthermore, the degree of immune responsiveness differs between men and women. The common theme connecting autoimmune disorders is the presence of an autoimmune response based on genetic risk factors that interact with environmental triggers. These triggers might be exposure to infection, chemicals, physical stress, or other unknown exposures. Immune and autoimmune diseases that affect women's health include asthma; allergic diseases; multiple sclerosis, a disease that affects the central nervous system in which the protective myelin around nerve fibers is lost, leaving scar tissue called sclerosis; rheumatoid arthritis; thyroid diseases; systemic lupus erythematosus (a chronic, inflammatory autoimmune disease that targets various organs); and Sjögren's syndrome, a chronic disease in which white blood cells attack the moisture-producing glands, including the mouth, eyes, and organs.

Oral Health

Changing hormonal levels over the life course, particularly during puberty, menses, and menopause, have been implicated in frequency of cold sores, gingivitis during puberty, dry mouth, taste changes, increased risk of gum disease, and bone weakness around menopause. Oral health issues of particular concern for women's health include periodontal disease and temporomandibular disorders, a variety of disorders that causes pain and tenderness in the temporomandibular joint.

Urologic and Kidney Conditions

Urinary incontinence, the inability to hold urine until arriving at a toilet, is often temporary and always results from an underlying medical condition. Women experience incontinence twice as often as men. Pregnancy and childbirth, menopause, and the structure of the female urinary tract account for this difference. Another urologic condition is interstitial cystitis, which is a long-lasting condition also known as painful bladder syndrome or frequency-urgency-dysuria syndrome, which results from the wall of the bladder becoming inflamed or irritated. This irritation affects the amount of urine the bladder can hold and causes scarring, stiffening, and bleeding in the bladder. Diabetes is the most important of the kidney conditions facing women's health. The overall age-adjusted prevalence of physician-diagnosed diabetes is the same in women and in men (5.2% vs. 5.3%), but its sequelae, including kidney disease and end-stage renal disease, are serious. Diabetes is the seventh leading cause of death in the United States.

Other Conditions

A number of poorly understood conditions adversely affect women's health in the United States, including migraines, fibromyalgia, and chronic fatigue syndrome.

Migraine headache is a severe pain felt on one side, and sometimes both sides, of the head, and lasting from a few hours up to 2 days. Migraines may be accompanied by nausea, vomiting, and light sensitivity. Migraines are more common in women than in men and are most common in women between the ages of 35 and 45. Hormones have been implicated in migraine prevalence; more than half of women with migraine report having them right before, during, or after their period.

Fibromyalgia, formerly known as fibrositis, is a chronic condition causing pain, stiffness, and tenderness of the muscles, tendons, and joints. Fibromyalgia is also characterized by restless sleep, awakening feeling tired, fatigue, anxiety, depression, and disturbances in bowel function. Its cause is currently unknown. Fibromyalgia affects predominantly women between the ages of 35 and 55.

Chronic fatigue syndrome (CFS) is an illness characterized by profound disabling fatigue lasting at least 6 months accompanied by symptoms of sleep disturbance, musculoskeletal pain, and neurocognitive impairment. A unifying etiology for CFS is yet to emerge. More women than men are diagnosed with CFS, but it is unclear if this differential results from women seeking care for CFS more frequently than men or some underlying predilection.

Neuroscience and Women's Health

In addition to the health issues noted above, the ways in which neuroscience intersects women's health, for example, sex differences in cognition, sex differences in drug behavior, sex differences in manifestations of brain disorders, sex differences in sensory perception and pain, sex differences in balance and the vestibular system, and so on, will remain an important area for improving understanding of women's health.

Women's Health Issues: Social Origin

Many issues that affect women's health result from the intersection of women and social interactions or social structure.

Sexually Transmitted Diseases

In the United States from 1973 to 1992, more than 150,000 women died of causes related to sexually transmitted diseases (STDs), including human immunodeficiency virus (HIV). Women bear a rate and burden of STD that is disproportionate compared with men. Much of this overrepresentation can be attributed to increased biological and behavioral susceptibility. As women age, the female ecology becomes less susceptible to colonization by STD-causing agents, but among all women, adolescents are at particularly high risk for STDs. STDs of particular concern for women's health include chlamydia, gonococcal infection, syphilis, genital herpes, human papilloma virus (HPV, which causes genital warts and is associated with the development of cervical and other genital tract squamous precancerous lesions and cancers), HIV/acquired immunodeficiency syndrome (AIDS), and pelvic inflammatory disease (PID, a general term that describes clinically suspected infection with resultant inflammation of the female upper reproductive tract, including the fallopian tubes, ovaries, and uterine lining).

Mental Health Issues

Men and women differ in the prevalence and severity of mental illness, but the validity of this finding is undermined by mental illness diagnosis (based largely on subjective symptoms), gender-based behavioral training (women more likely to seek help), and physician assumptions (physicians may expect to see more mental disorders among women). The mental health picture is further complicated by hormonal effects on brain function, brain maturation, and pharmacological response. Despite the limited information on mental health issue etiology, ascertainment, diagnosis, and treatment, multiple mental health issues affect women's health, including the following: depression, gender and mood disorders, anxiety disorders, post-traumatic stress disorder (PTSD), eating disorders and body image concerns (including anorexia, bulimia, overweight, obesity), and addictive disorders (tobacco, alcohol, and other drug abuse). As currently understood, many of these mental health issues preferentially influence women's health.

Violence

Research indicates that women experience many forms of violence, and both physical and psychological violence can occur from perpetrators who are strangers, acquaintances, family members, or partners. In 1995, the National Crime Victimization Survey, conducted by the U.S. Department of Justice, estimated that approximately 4% of women in the United States reported experiences of violent crime during the past year. The estimated number of incidents perpetrated against women is more than 4.7 million, and in 1994, women were raped at a rate of 4.6 per 1,000 women. Violence has long-reaching effects, including both mental and physical health consequences.

Global Issues in Women's Health

Women living outside the United States, particularly those living in nondeveloping and developing countries, are faced with many of the same health issues as women living in the United States, but some have different concerns as well. Three areas that are of particular concern for women living outside the United States are high maternal morbidity and mortality associated with childbearing, female genital mutilation/circumcision, and HIV/AIDS.

It is important to note that women's health issues are differentially distributed; not all issues affect all women equally. In the United States and elsewhere, social hierarchies exist that contribute to significant disparities between racial groups, particularly between white and nonwhite women. In addition, the health needs of lesbians are barely understood and ill appreciated by the health care and research community. Health disparities arise from differential exposure, diagnosis, and treatment, and virtually all women's health issues can be considered through a health disparities framework.

—*Lynne C. Messer*

See also Chronic Disease Epidemiology; Health Disparities; Life Course Approach; Maternal and Child Health Epidemiology

Further Readings

Boston Women's Health Book Collective. (2005). *Our bodies, ourselves for the new century*. New York: Simon & Schuster.

Carlson, K. J., Eisenstat, S. A., & Ziporyn, T. (2004). *The new Harvard guide to women's health*. Boston: Harvard University Press.

Gay, K. (2001). *Encyclopedia of women's health issues*. Portsmouth, NH: Greenwood.

Goldman, M. B., & Hatch, M. C. (Eds.). (2000). *Women and health*. San Diego, CA: Academic Press.

Loue, S., & Sajotovic, M. (Eds.). (2004). *Encyclopedia of women's health*. New York: Kluwer Academic.

Web Sites

Centers for Disease Control and Prevention, Office of Women's Health: http://www.cdc.gov/women.
Health Resources and Services Administration, Maternal and Child Health Bureau: http://mchb.hrsa.gov.
U.S. Department of Health and Human Services, Office on Women's Health, The National Women's Health Information Center: http://www.4women.gov.
World Health Organization, Women's Health: http://www.who.int/topics/womens_health/en.

WORLD HEALTH ORGANIZATION

The World Health Organization (WHO) is a specialized agency of the United Nations (UN). It was established on April 7, 1948, to promote international cooperation in improving health conditions. The WHO administrative office is headquartered in Geneva, Switzerland; however, WHO has six regional offices for Africa, the Americas, Southeast Asia, Europe, the Mediterranean, and the Western Pacific, located in major cities in each area.

The WHO mission is improving the health of all people of the world. The WHO definition of health is broad: As defined in the WHO constitution, "health is a state of complete physical, mental and social well-being and not merely the absence of disease or infirmity." A major aspect of this mission is to combat disease, especially infectious diseases, through the development and distribution of vaccines and by coordinating international efforts in monitoring outbreaks of diseases such as malaria and AIDS. However, WHO is also concerned with matters that affect health less directly, such as improving living conditions.

WHO work may be divided into three categories: (1) gathering and dissemination of health information through research services, (2) disease control through providing vaccination and medication, and (3) consultation and education through organizing conferences.

WHO has 192 member states: These include all UN member states, except Liechtenstein, and two non-UN members, Niue and the Cook Islands. These member states appoint delegations to the World Health Assembly, which is WHO's highest decision-making body. The World Health Assembly, which generally meets in May of each year, elects 32 members who are qualified in the field of health and are representatives from WHO's member states to be appointed to the Executive Board for 3-year terms. The main functions of the Board are to give effect to the decisions and policies of the Assembly, to advise it, and generally to facilitate its work.

The Assembly's main duty includes the supervision of the financial budgets, reviewing proposed projects, and appointing the Director General. WHO is financed based on annual contributions made by member governments on the basis of relative ability to pay and on the allocated resources that were assigned by the UN after 1951.

The day-to-day work of the WHO is carried out by its Secretariat, with regional offices throughout the world. These offices are staffed with health care workers who carry out the health projects designed for improving the human beings' health status in that specific region. In addition, WHO is represented by its Goodwill Ambassadors, who work independently and freely. These Ambassadors are usually celebrities, appointed in a nondiplomatic position to use their talent and fame in advocating for the health and well-being of human beings and in supporting WHO's goals and purposes.

WHO operates in 147 country and liaison offices in all its regions. The presence of a country office is motivated by a specific need and must be requested by that country. The country office is headed by a WHO Representative (WR), who is not a national of that country. The office consists of the WR and several health experts, both foreign and local. The main functions of WHO country offices include being the primary adviser of that country's government in matters of health and pharmaceutical policies, as well as coordinating a role for the action of other international and/or nongovernmental organizations when health is concerned and to provide leadership and coordination for emergency and disaster medical relief efforts.

—*Najood Ghazi Azar*

See also Disaster Epidemiology; Epidemiology in Developing Countries; Health, Definitions of; Vaccination

Web Sites

World Health Organization: http://www.who.org.

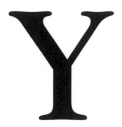

YELLOW FEVER

Yellow fever is a hemorrhagic fever that has a viral etiology. The virus is transmitted to humans by infected mosquitoes (*Aedes aegyptii*). It is called *yellow* fever due to the jaundice that affects some patients causing yellow eyes and yellow skin. The disease itself may be limited to mild symptoms or may cause severe illness or even death. Yellow fever occurs exclusively in Africa and South America. Annually, it is estimated to cause 200,000 cases, and the death toll is estimated to be around 30,000. It is a notifiable disease under the International Health Regulations of the World Health Organization (WHO), and member states are officially obliged to notify yellow fever cases to the WHO.

History

The first descriptions of a disease such as yellow fever can be found in historic texts as early as 400 years ago. It was especially common in American seaports. For instance, Philadelphia experienced an epidemic in 1793, which killed 10% of the city's population, and during which almost half of Philadelphia's residents fled the city. Yellow fever accounted for a significant number of casualties in the American army in the Spanish-American war of 1898: The impact was severe enough to warrant the setting up of the United States Army Yellow Fever Commission, also known as the Reed Commission, in 1900. Carlos Finlay, a Cuban physician, had proposed the mosquito-vector

theory in 1881. In collaboration with the Reed Commission and with the help of a few human volunteers, his theory was confirmed. By adopting mosquito control measures, yellow fever was controlled within 6 months in Havana.

At present, yellow fever is considered to be endemic in 33 African countries, 9 South American countries, and several Caribbean islands. Yellow fever has never been reported in Asia.

Transmission

Yellow fever affects mainly humans and monkeys. The virus spreads by *horizontal transmission* (from one person to another by mosquitoes) or by *vertical transmission* (transovarially in infected mosquitoes). There are three transmission cycles depending on whether the mosquitoes are domestic (urban yellow fever), wild (jungle or sylvatic yellow fever), or semidomestic (intermediate yellow fever). In South America, only the first two transmission cycles are found. Sylvatic yellow fever usually causes sporadic cases of yellow fever, mainly in young males who work in the forest. Intermediate yellow fever causes small-scale epidemics in African villages. Epidemics of urban yellow fever may occur when a person from an endemic area migrates to a nonendemic area (especially crowded urban areas) and introduces the virus in an unvaccinated population.

Clinical Manifestations

The virus (a *flavivirus*) enters the body through the bite of a female mosquito. This is followed by an incubation period of 3 to 6 days during which there are no signs or symptoms. Yellow fever has two phases. The acute phase is characterized by fever, chills, myalgia, headache, nausea, vomiting, anorexia, and general exhaustion. In the majority of the cases, these symptoms subside, and patients improve in 3 to 4 days. A few (about 15%), however, enter a toxic phase within 24 hr of the acute phase. This is characterized by reappearance of fever and deterioration of major organ systems of the body, mainly the liver and the kidneys signaled by jaundice, blood in stools, albuminuria, anuria, and so on. Half of the patients who enter the acute phase die within 10 to 14 days, while the others recover without significant residual organ damage. Yellow fever may be confused with many other diseases, especially in the initial stages, and it can be confirmed by serologic assays and other blood tests. As there is no specific drug for treating yellow fever, treatment is symptomatic.

Prevention

Since yellow fever is a zoonosis and cannot be eradicated, vaccination is the single most effective control measure in populations where it is endemic and for people traveling to endemic areas. Mosquito control can be used as an adjunct to vaccination. In case of low vaccination coverage, surveillance is very critical for early detection and rapid containment of outbreaks.

Yellow fever vaccine is a live viral vaccine that can be administered at 9 months of age, with a booster every 10 years. In countries where yellow fever is endemic, the WHO has recommended incorporation of yellow fever vaccine in routine childhood immunizations. It is contraindicated in cases of egg allergy, immune deficiency, pregnancy, and hypersensitivity to previous dose. Rare adverse reactions have included encephalitis in the very young, hepatic failure, and even death due to organ failure. The vaccine is not given before 6 months of age. In the past, intensive immunization campaigns have been successful in greatly decreasing the number of yellow fever cases.

—*Sangeeta Karandikar*

See also Epidemiology in Developing Countries; Insect-Borne Disease; Notifiable Disease; Public Health Surveillance; Reed, Walter

Further Readings

Atwater Kent Museum of Philadelphia. (2007). City history lesson 'Yellow Fever Epidemic of 1793.' Retrieved November 18, 2006, from http://www.philadelphia history.org/akm/lessons/yellowFever.

Chaves-Carballo, E. (2005). Carlos Finlay and yellow fever: Triumph over adversity. *Military Medicine,* *170*(10), 881–885.

Health Sciences Library at the University of Virginia. (2004). *Yellow fever and Reed Commission, 1898–1901.* Retrieved November 18, 2006, from http:// www.healthsystem.virginia.edu/internet/library/historical/ medical_history/yellow_fever.

Tomori, O. (2004). Yellow fever: The recurring plague. *Critical Reviews in Clinical Laboratory Sciences, 41*(4), 391–427.

World Health Organization. (2001). *Yellow fever fact sheet.* Retrieved November 18, 2006, from http://www.who.int/ mediacentre/factsheets/fs100/en.

YOUTH RISK BEHAVIOR SURVEILLANCE SYSTEM

The Youth Risk Behavior Surveillance System (YRBSS) is a project of the Centers for Disease Control and Prevention (CDC). Developed in 1990, the YRBSS consists of local, state, and national school-based surveys of youth to monitor the prevalence of and trends in health risk behaviors. Specific behaviors of interest include substance abuse, risky sexual practices, and unhealthy physical and dietary behaviors. These risk behaviors, often developed during childhood and adolescence, contribute to the leading causes of mortality and morbidity among youth and adults in the United States. The goals of YRBSS include documenting the prevalence and co-occurrence of health risk behaviors; monitoring trends in the prevalence of these behaviors; generating comparable national, state, and local data, as well as data on youth subpopulations; and tracking progress toward the objectives of Healthy People 2010 and other programs.

Surveys are conducted every 2 years and are representative of public and private high school students at the national level and public high school students at the local and state levels. Students are not tracked over time, and these data are publicly available. In addition to these biennial surveys, YRBSS also includes other national CDC surveys, including the

National College Health Risk Behavior and Alternative High School Youth Risk Behavior Surveys.

Methodology

National YRBSS surveys employ three-stage cluster sampling, while local and state surveys use two-stage cluster sampling. In the first stage of sampling in national surveys, primary sampling units (PSUs) are selected. PSUs are usually large-sized counties or groups of adjacent, smaller counties. During the second sampling stage, public and private schools are selected from the PSUs. Black and Hispanic students are oversampled at this stage to gain enough data to conduct analyses of these subgroups separately. Finally, classes are sampled in each grade of each selected high school. All students in selected classes are eligible for the survey. Local and state surveys use two stages of sampling: first, to select schools, and second, to sample classes within the selected schools.

The data are collected in a similar manner in the national, state, and local surveys. Parental permission is obtained in accordance with local standards for all YRBSS surveys. Students' participation in the self-administered surveys is anonymous and voluntary.

Between 1991 and 2003, student response rates ranged from 83% to 90%.

Limitations

There are several limitations of the YRBSS. Key limitations are all data are self-reported; the surveillance includes only in-school youth, who are less likely to engage in risky health behaviors; parental consent procedures are inconsistent; state-level data are not available for all 50 states; and the system is not able to evaluate specific interventions or programs.

—*Anu Manchikanti*

See also Behavioral Risk Factor Surveillance System; Child and Adolescent Health; Healthy People 2010

Further Readings

Centers for Disease Control and Prevention. (2004). Methodology of the youth risk behavioral survey system. *Morbidity and Mortality Weekly Report, 53*(RR-12), 1–16.
National Center for Chronic Disease Prevention and Health Promotion. (2006). YRBSS: Youth risk behavior surveillance system. Retrieved August 15, 2006, from http://www.cdc.gov/HealthyYouth/yrbs/index.htm.

Z

ZOONOTIC DISEASE

Infectious or communicable diseases of humans can be divided into those that are communicable only between humans and those that are communicable to humans by nonhuman vertebrate animals (those with backbones such as mammals, birds, reptiles, amphibians, and fish, referred to in this entry simply as "animals"). The latter diseases are called zoonoses or zoonotic diseases. Because of the large number of domestic and wild animals that can serve as a source of zoonotic diseases, and the numerous means of transmission including vectors, zoonotic diseases are often difficult to control. Public health veterinarians have a critical role in zoonotic disease surveillance, prevention, and control, but risk reduction increasingly requires application of multidisciplinary teams and a unified concept of medicine across human and animal species lines.

Zoonotic Disease Classification

All classes of disease agents cause zoonotic disease. These include bacteria (e.g., listeriosis), chlamydia (e.g., psittacosis), rickettsia (e.g., Rocky Mountain spotted fever), viruses (e.g., Hendra), parasites (e.g., leishmaniasis), and fungi (e.g., histoplasmosis).

Zoonoses can be subdivided into those transmitted from animals to humans (zooanthroponoses) or from humans to animals (anthropozoonoses, also called reverse zoonoses). *Mycobacterium tuberculosis* has been spread from humans to cattle and elephants, and methacillin-resistant *Staphylococcus aureus* (MRSA) has been transmitted from people to horses and then back to people. Diseases that are rarely transmitted between animals and humans are sometimes included, such as foot-and-mouth disease in cattle.

Zoonoses transmitted through direct contact are orthozoonoses (e.g., rabies). Cyclozoonoses (e.g., echinococcosis) require more than one vertebrate host for development. Metazoonoses are transmitted by an infected invertebrate vector (e.g., scrub typhus from mite bites). Zoonoses transmitted through physical contact with food, soil, or vegetation are saprozoonoses, sapronoses, or geonoses (e.g., fungal infections). Some diseases fit more than one category (e.g., tularemia from fly or tick bites, direct contact, or environmental exposure).

As noted by Enserink in *Science* in 2000, of 1,709 identified human disease agents, 832 (49%) are classified as zoonotic. Of the 156 "emerging" diseases, 114 (73%) are zoonotic. Thus, zoonotic diseases are disproportionately represented among those spreading into new areas.

Zoonotic disease agents account for most of the organisms in Categories A, B, and C of the U.S. government's Select Agent List of likely organisms for bioterrorism attacks. The diseases caused by Category A select agents include smallpox, anthrax, plague, tularemia, botulism, and viral hemorrhagic fevers.

Select agents in Categories B and C cause bacterial, chlamydial, and rickettsial diseases, including brucellosis, Q Fever, glanders, melioidosis, foodborne/waterborne disease, psittacosis, and typhus. Select viral agents include smallpox, Nipah, hanta, and the encephalitides viruses. Select agents that can lead to intoxications include *Staphylococcus* enterotoxin B, ricin, and *Clostridium perfringens* Epsilon toxin. All these select agents are considered zoonotic except for smallpox.

Populations at Increased Risk

Anyone who comes into contact with infected animals, vectors, or contaminated areas can become infected with zoonotic diseases; however, the risk of clinical signs and death is not uniformly distributed. The proportion who remain asymptomatic and the case fatality rate (proportion of ill persons who die) vary with certain risk factors.

Age is often associated with disease severity. Of those infected with *Escherichia coli* O157:H7 from contact with animals or their environment, children are more likely to develop potentially fatal hemolytic uremic syndrome (HUS). Younger, healthier people appear to be more susceptible to serious illness from the highly pathogenic avian influenza (HPAI) strain of Asian H5N1, compared with human influenza strains that differentially cause severe illness and death in older people. Similarly, hantavirus infection was first identified in physically fit young adults, and the very young and very old still seem to be relatively unaffected. Although the factors leading to these age differences are not understood, infection with both the Asian H5N1 HPAI virus and hantaviruses lead to pathologic changes caused by the body's own immune response to the viruses.

For some diseases, immunosuppression from disease or medication is a risk factor. Cryptosporidiosis is a common coinfection with acquired immunodeficiency syndrome (AIDS). Those without a functioning spleen have an increased risk of illness and death from *Capnocytophaga canimorsus* infection after dog bites. Those who take chloroquine for malaria prophylaxis concurrently with rabies pre-exposure immunizations are less likely to develop a sufficient immunologic response to survive a rabies exposure.

Other populations at risk include those who are cognitively impaired and cannot recognize or report bites from rabid bats. Pregnant women are at risk of fetal congenital malformations with lymphocytic choriomeningitis virus (LCMV) infection. Solid-organ transplant recipients have died from rabies and LCMV infections transmitted from the donors.

Zoonotic Disease Control

Zoonotic diseases are particularly difficult to control because of their animal reservoirs. Zoonoses are unlike diseases that can be eradicated with intensive human vaccination campaigns, such as smallpox and polio. It may be possible to eliminate some zoonotic disease variants from certain regions, as campaigns with oral rabies vaccines have attempted to do by distributing vaccine baits for vaccination of foxes, coyotes, and raccoons.

Global movement of animals has increased problems with zoonotic disease control. Inexpensive puppies of certain breeds are in great demand, and occasionally they are rabid when imported. Raccoon rabies was introduced to the central east coast of the United States by deliberate human movement of raccoons from the southeastern United States for hunting purposes, with subsequent spread to the entire east coast of the United States, as well as the midwestern United States and parts of Canada. Monkeypox virus infection of African rodents imported for the pet trade led to pet prairie dog and human cases and restrictions on the pet prairie dog trade. The spread of Asian H5N1 HPAI (avian flu) from Asia to Europe, the Middle East, and Africa appears to be a result of human movement of domestic birds as well as wild bird migration.

Zoonotic disease risk is increased when humans live in close proximity to domestic animals such as poultry and livestock. This allows efficient use of limited land resources and constant care and protection of the animals. But this practice increases the risk of humans becoming infected with disease agents such as HPAI.

Even in areas with greater separation between human homes and animal barns, zoonotic diseases still pose a risk because of human contact with animals. *Salmonella* infections (sometimes with multidrug resistant strains) have occurred from pets in homes, including reptiles and amphibians (turtles, iguanas, snakes), exotic pets (hedgehogs, sugar gliders), pocket pets (hamsters, mice, rats), pet birds (chicks, ducklings), dogs and cats, and from pet treats. Transmission can be directly from animal handling or by exposure to environmental contamination.

These transmission routes also apply to disease agents spread from livestock to people in public settings. Large *E. coli* O157:H7 outbreaks have been associated with dairy farms, children's day camps conducted in farm settings, social events in buildings previously used for animal exhibitions, fair petting zoos, and contaminated fair water systems. Critical control methods in homes and public settings include animal management to reduce disease burden, management of animal and human contacts, and education to reduce exposure particularly by handwashing.

Limiting contact between humans and wild animals is also critical to reducing risk. Most human rabies deaths in the United States are due to bites from bats, frequently in home settings. Although the human immunodeficiency virus (HIV) that causes AIDS is not zoonotic, it apparently evolved from similar monkey viruses through the practice of hunting and consuming bush meat (monkeys). Unprotected cleaning up of rodent feces is associated with hantavirus infection, and plague infection is associated with use of woodpiles and with outdoor recreational activities that bring people into contact with wild rodents and their fleas.

Contact between wild and domestic animals also increases the threat of zoonotic diseases for people. One example is Nipah virus, first identified in Indonesian pigs and pig farmers. Preliminary information about a possible association with fruit bats led to removal of fruit trees overhanging pig pens, which eliminated the pig and human cases in that area. This control method is reminiscent of John Snow's interruption of an 1854 London cholera outbreak after he identified a statistical association between use of a well pump and cases of cholera, even though cholera transmission was not fully understood.

Because zoonotic disease agents can be found in humans, animals, the environment, and vectors, management requires the collaboration of many types of health and disease control specialists. Disease control may include vector control programs for ticks (Lyme disease), fleas (plague), or mosquitoes (West Nile virus), and environmental cleanup or protection may be required to address disease agents that remain viable from days to years on surfaces (*Salmonella*), in soils (*Anthrax*), or in the water (*Leptospira*). In most state health agencies, public health veterinarians are available to assist in this critical disease control coordination.

—*Millicent Eidson*

See also Avian Flu; Bioterrorism; Influenza; Plague; Snow, John; Vector-Borne Disease

Further Readings

Beran, G. W., & Steele, J. H. (Eds.). (1994). *Handbook of zoonoses* (2nd ed.). Boca Raton, FL: CRC Press.
Enserink, M. (2000). Emerging diseases: Malaysian researchers trace Nipah virus outbreak to bats. *Science, 289,* 518–519.
Hugh-Jones, M. E., Hubbert, W. T., & Hagstad, H. V. (2000). *Zoonoses: Recognition, control, and prevention.* Ames: Iowa State University Press.
Krauss, H., Weber, A., Appel, M., Enders, B., Isenberg, H. D., Scheifer, H. G., et al. (Eds.). (2003). *Zoonoses: Infectious diseases transmissible from animals to humans.* Washington, DC: ASM Press.
Palmer, S. R., Soulsby, L., & Simpson, D. I. H. (Eds.). (1998). *Zoonoses: Biology, clinical practice, and public health control.* Oxford, UK: Oxford University Press.

Z Score

Z scores are also called standard units or standard scores. A *z* score standardizes values of a random variable from a normal (or presumed normal) distribution for comparison with known probabilities in a standard normal probability distribution table or *z* table. A *z* score is unitless and is simply a measure of the number of standard deviations a value is from the mean. The *z* score is especially useful to indicate where a particular data point is relative to the rest of the data. A positive *z* score indicates that the point is above the mean, while a negative *z* score indicates that the point is below the mean. The *z* score removes varying units (e.g., pounds or kilograms) and allows for easy determination of whether a particular result is unusual.

Most significance testing, hypothesis testing, and confidence intervals are based on an assumption that the data are drawn from an underlying normal distribution. However, the probabilities are dependent on the mean, μ, and standard deviation, σ, of the distribution. Since it is physically impossible to calculate the probabilities associated with infinitely many pairs of μ and σ, the *z* score allows a researcher to compare the sample data with the standard normal distribution. The standard normal distribution is a normal distribution with $\mu = 0$ and $\sigma = \sigma^2 = 1$, also denoted $N(0,1)$.

The *z* score finds the point *z* on the standard normal curve that corresponds to any point *x* on a nonstandard normal curve. To convert an *x* value from the original scale to a *z* score, center the distribution by subtracting the mean and then rescale by dividing by the standard deviation. The formula for this conversion is

$$z = \frac{\text{Data point} - \text{Mean}}{\text{Standard deviation}}.$$

In a population, the formula becomes $z = (x - \mu)/\sigma$. In a sample, the formula becomes $z = (x - \bar{x})/s$. This standardization ensures that the resulting distribution has a mean of 0 and standard deviation of 1. See Figure 1 for an illustration of how the *x* scales and *z* scores compare for a normal distribution with mean $\mu = 5$ and standard deviation $\sigma = 2$.

If the assumption of normality for the data is not grossly violated, then the *z* score will allow the researcher to compare the data with known probabilities and draw conclusions. If *x* did not have at least an approximately normal sampling distribution, then further use of the *z* score may result in erroneous conclusions. The central limit theorem does not apply since the researcher is interested in individual *x* values, not the mean of the *x* values.

Using the relationship between the *z* and *x* scales, a researcher can use a standard normal table or *z* table

to find the area under any part of any nonstandard normal curve. To calculate the area or probability of an *x* value occurring between two numbers *a* and *b* in the *x* scale, use

$$P(a < X < b) = p\left(\frac{a - \mu}{\sigma} < \frac{X - \mu}{\sigma} < \frac{b - \mu}{\sigma}\right)$$

$$= p\left(\frac{a - \mu}{\sigma} < z < \frac{b - \mu}{\sigma}\right).$$

In Figure 1 ($\mu = 5$, $\sigma = 2$), to find the probability of an *x* value between 3 and 10, use

$$P(3 < X < 10) = p\left(\frac{3 - 5}{2} < \frac{X - \mu}{\sigma} < \frac{10 - 5}{2}\right)$$

$$= p(-1 < z < 2.5)$$

$$= .3413 + .4938 = .8351.$$

A *z* score is sometimes confused with the *z* statistic, also denoted "*z*," which is used in the *z* test. The *z* statistic differs in that it measures the number of standard deviations a sample statistic (the mean, $\bar{x}$) is from some hypothesized value of a population parameter (a numerical value, μ_0). The differences between that formula and the *z* score formula are subtle,

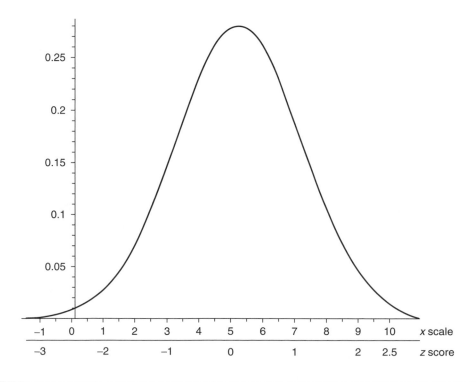

Figure 1   Comparison of *x* Scales and *z* Scores

including the change from the use of the standard deviation of *x*, σ, to the use of the standard error, $\sigma_{\bar{x}}$, which is also known as the standard deviation of the sampling distribution. The *z* statistic formula is

$$z = \frac{\bar{x} - \mu_0}{\sigma_{\bar{X}}} = \frac{\bar{x} - \mu_0}{\sigma/-\sqrt{n}}.$$

—*Stacie Ezelle Taylor*

See also Central Limit Theorem; Normal Distribution; Random Variable; Sampling Distribution

Further Readings

Munro, B. H. (2005). *Statistical methods for health care research* (5th ed.). Philadelphia: Lippincott Williams & Wilkins.

Petruccelli, J. D., Nandram, B., & Chen, M. (1999). *Applied statistics for engineers and scientists.* Upper Saddle River, NJ: Prentice Hall.

Index